Williams'
Basic Nutrition
&Diet Therapy

evolve

:•To access your Student Resources, visit:

http://evolve.elsevier.com/Williams/basic/

Evolve® Student Resources for **Nix:** *Williams' Basic Nutrition & Diet Therapy,* **Thirteenth edition,** offer the following features:

Student Resources (NOTE: Instructors also have access to student material.)

- **Case Studies**—Activities that help you gain further practice in problem solving and application of concepts.

- **Study Questions**—350 interactive self-assessment questions that provide instant feedback to ensure content mastery and help you prepare for the examination.

- **Infant and Child Growth Charts, United States, Centers for Disease Control and Prevention**—The most recent growth charts are now available electronically on Evolve in a format that makes it easier to print and to take with you.

- **Food Composition Table**—This detailed listing allows you to search the nutrient values of more than 3700 foods contained in the Nutritrac Nutrition Analysis Software CD-ROM located in the back of this textbook. It is separated and alphabetized into 18 different food categories.

- **ADA Nutrition Care Process**—This new standard for practice assures quality performance by providing steps to ensure consistent practices for more positive outcomes.

- **WebLinks**—Links to hundreds of Web sites carefully chosen to supplement the content of each chapter of the text.

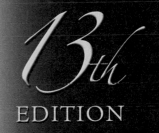

Williams'
Basic Nutrition
&Diet Therapy

Staci Nix, MS, RD, CD

Assistant Professor
Division of Nutrition
College of Health
University of Utah
Salt Lake City, UT

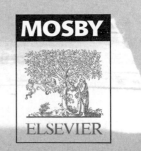

11830 Westline Industrial Drive
St. Louis, Missouri 63146

WILLIAMS' BASIC NUTRITION & DIET THERAPY   ISBN: 978-0-323-05199-6

NOTICE

Knowledge and best practice in this field are constantly changing. As new research and experience broaden our knowledge, changes in practice, treatment and drug therapy may become necessary or appropriate. Readers are advised to check the most current information provided (i) on procedures featured or (ii) by the manufacturer of each product to be administered, to verify the recommended dose or formula, the method and duration of administration, and contraindications. It is the responsibility of the practitioner, relying on their own experience and knowledge of the patient, to make diagnoses, to determine dosages and the best treatment for each individual patient, and to take all appropriate safety precautions. To the fullest extent of the law, neither the Publisher nor the Author assumes any liability for any injury and/or damage to persons or property arising out of or related to any use of the material contained in this book.

Library of Congress Cataloging-in-Publication Data

Nix, Staci.
    Williams' basic nutrition & diet therapy / Staci Nix. -- 13th ed.
        p. ; cm.
    Includes bibliographical references and index.
    ISBN 978-0-323-05199-6 (pbk. : alk. paper) 1. Diet therapy. 2. Nutrition. 3. Nursing. I. Williams, Sue Rodwell. Basic nutrition & diet therapy. II. Title. III. Title: Williams' basic nutrition and diet therapy. IV. Title: Basic nutrition & diet therapy.
    [DNLM: 1. Diet Therapy. 2. Food Habits. 3. Nutrition Physiology. 4. Nutritional Requirements. WB 400 N736w 2009]
    RM216.W6865 2009
    615.8′54--dc22

                                                                                2008024971

Acquisitions Editor: Yvonne Alexopoulos
Developmental Editor: Heather Bays
Publishing Services Manager: Jeff Patterson
Project Manager: Amy Rickles
Design Direction: Teresa McBryan
Cover Designer: Teresa McBryan

Printed in Canada

Last digit is the print number: 9 8 7 6 5 4 3 2 1

CONTRIBUTOR and REVIEWERS

CONTRIBUTOR

Sara E. Oldroyd, MS, RD
Assistant Professor and Extension Agent
Utah State University
Logan, Utah

REVIEWERS

Peter L. Beyer, MS, RD
Associate Professor
Dietetics and Nutrition
University of Kansas Medical Center
Kansas City, Kansas

Ardith R. Brunt, PhD, RD
Assistant Professor
Department of Health, Nutrition and Exercise Sciences
North Dakota State University
Fargo, North Dakota

Melanie Tracy Burns, PhD, RD
Associate Professor and DPD Coordinator
Family and Consumer Sciences
Eastern Illinois University
Charleston, Illinois

Lori M. Byrd, PhD, RN
Instructor
Christ Hospital School of Nursing
Essex County College
Newark, New Jersey;
Coordinator
LPN Program
Essex County College
Newark, New Jersey

Suzanne Carroll, RN, BSN
Instructor
LPN Program
Sandusky Career Center
Sandusky, Ohio

Pamela Charney, PhD, RD, CNSD
Consultant
Mercer Island, Washington

Suzanne M. Elbon, MS, PhD, MEd
Instructional Designer
U.S. Centers for Disease Control and Prevention
Coordinating Office of Global Health
Atlanta, Georgia;
Wellness Coordinator
Department of Foods and Nutrition
The University of Georgia
Athens, Georgia

Christine Filipowski, MS, RD, LDN
Clinical Dietitian
Rush University Medical Center
Chicago, Illinois

Pat Floro, RN
Instructor
Nancy J. Knight School of Nursing
Ohio Hi-Point Career Center
Bellefontaine, Ohio

Margie Lee Gallagher, MS, RD, PhD
Professor and Senior Scientist
College of Human Ecology
East Carolina University
Greensville, North Carolina

Susan Gollnick, MS, RD, BS, MS
Food Science and Nutrition Department
Cal Poly State University
San Luis Obispo, California

Janis E. Grimland, RN, BSN
Coordinator
Vocational Nursing Site
Hill College
Clifton, Texas

Janet Harbin, RN, MSN
Assistant Professor
Nursing
Roane State Community College
Oak Ridge, Tennessee

Dorothy G. Herron, PhD, APRN, BC, MS
Clinical Associate Professor
School of Nursing
University of North Carolina
Greensboro, North Carolina

Debra Hodge, BSN, MSN
Instructor
Clinical and Theory
Academy of Careers and Technology;
Adjunct Faculty
Mountain State University
Beckley, West Virginia

Sharon Hunt, RD, LD, BS
Associate Professor
Department of Family and Consumer Sciences
Fort Valley State University
Fort Valley, Georgia

Debra A. Indorato, RD, LDN
Owner
Approach Nutrition
Food Allergy Management
Norfolk, Virginia

Karla Kennedy-Hagen, PhD, RD, LDN
Assistant Professor
Dietetic Internship Coordinator
Eastern Illinois University
Charleston, Illinois

Betty Kenyon, RD, LMNT
Consultant Dietitian
Panhandle Community Services
Gering, Nebraska;
Adjunct Faculty
Western Nebraska Community College
Scottsbluff, Nebraska

Lauralee S. Krabill, RN, C, CNOR, MBA
Director
School of Practical Nursing
Sandusky Career Center
Sandusky, Ohio

Diane T. Kupensky, RN, MSN, CNS
Trauma Clinical Nurse Specialist
St. Elizabeth Health Center
Youngstown, Ohio

Ruth Leyse-Wallace, PhD, RD, MS, BS
Clinical Dietitian
Sharp Mesa Vista Hospital
San Diego, Califonia

Sheila M. Marquart, EdS, MSN, RN
Assistant Professor
School of Nursing
Middle Tennessee State University
Murfreesboro, Tennessee

Dennis McClure, MS, PhD
Instructor
Practical Nursing Program
University of the District of Columbia
Washington, D.C.

Alisa Montgomery, RN, MSN, CNE
Faculty
School of Nursing
Piedmont Community College
Roxboro, North Carolina

Juanita B. Nunley, RN, MSN
Associate Professor of Nursing
Division of Health Sciences
Rockingham Community College
Wentworth, North Carolina

Linda Kautz Osterkamp, RD, LMNT
Consultant Dietitian
Panhandle Community Services
Gering, Nebraska;
Adjunct Faculty
Western Nebraska Community College
Scottsbluff, Nebraska

Amy D. Ozier, PhD, RD
Assistant Professor and Facilitator
School of Family, Consumer, and Nutrition Sciences
Northern Illinois University
Dekalb, Illinois

Nancy Palmer, MSN, BSN
Professor
College of Nursing
Schoolcraft College
Livonia, Michigan

Jessie Pavlinac, MS, RD, CSR, LD
Clinical Nutrition Manager
Department of Food and Nutrition
Oregon Health and Science University
Portland, Oregon

Tracy Pekar, MSN, MBA, RN, CNE
Nursing Projects Manager
The Greene County Education Center
Westmoreland County Community College
Waynesburg, Pennsylvania

Beverly E. Peoples, RN, BS
Department Head of Health Services and Instructor
Practical Nursing
Louisiana Technical College, Northeast LA Campus
Winnsboro, Louisiana

Janet Peterson, RN, BSN
LPN Instructor
Columbiana County Career and Technical Center
Lisbon, Ohio;
Clinical Coordinator
ADN Program
Kent State University
East Liverpool, Ohio

Scott Peterson, MSN, BSN
Adjunct Faculty
Hill College
Hillsboro, Texas

Toni E. Pritchard, BSN, MSN
Department Head, Health Occupations
Louisiana Technical College, Lamar Salter Campus
Leesville, Louisiana

Rena Quinton, PhD
Assistant Professor
Texas A&M University
Kingsville, Texas

Ann Reisinger, RN, BSN
Practical Nursing Instructor
Pike-Lincoln Technical Center
Eolia, Missouri

Gretchen Schumacker, PhD, CRNP, NP-C
Assistant Professor
School of Nursing
Duquesne University
Pittsburgh, Pennsylvania

Erin Sawyer Spear, RN, MSN, NP-C
Moberly Area Community College
Moberly, Missouri

Ethel Stringham, RN, MSN
Assistant Professor
Bethel College
Mishawaka, Indiana

Lynne Sullivan, MSN, RN
Coordinator
Nursing Programs
Bristol-Plymouth Regional Technical School
Tauton, Massachusetts

Cyndy Sundstrom, RN, CRRN, MS
Coordinator
School of Practical Nursing
Fayette Institute of Tecnology
Oak Hills, Wisconsin

Sue G. Thacker, RNC, BSN, PhD
Professor
Nursing
Wytheville Community College
Wytheville, Virginia

Jule Traynor, MS, RN
Nursing Instructor
Lake Region State College
Devils Lake, North Dakota

Janet Willis, RN, BSN, MS
Senior Professor
Harrisburg Area Community College
Harrisburg, Pennsylvania

Beth Wolfgram, MS, RD, CD, CSCS
Nutrition and Fitness Consultant
Adjunct Faculty
Division of Nutrition
Sports Dietitian
Athletic Department
University of Utah
Salt Lake City, Utah

Meridan Zerner, MS, RD, LD
Dietitician
The Cooper Clinic and Cooper Fitness Center
Dallas, Texas

To my parents for their continuous support:
Ronnie and JoAnn Nix

PREFACE to the INSTRUCTOR

Our goal is to capture the excitement of nutrition knowledge and its application to human health in this thirteenth edition. The field of nutrition is a dynamic human endeavor that is continually expanding and evolving. Three main factors continue to change the modern face of nutrition. First, the science of nutrition continues to grow rapidly with exciting research. New knowledge in any science challenges some traditional ideas and lends to the development of new ones. Instead of primarily focusing on nutrition in the treatment of disease, we are expanding the search for disease prevention and general enhancement of life through nutrition. Thus was the spirit during the establishment of the current Dietary Reference Intakes. Second, the rapidly increasing multiethnic diversity of the United States population enriches our food patterns and presents a variety of health care opportunities and needs. Third, the public is more aware and concerned about health promotion and the role of nutrition, largely because of the media's increasing attention. Clients and patients are raising more questions and seeking intelligent answers. They want to be more involved in their own health care, and an integral part of that care is nutrition.

This new edition continues to reflect upon the evolving face of nutrition science. Its guiding principle is our own commitment, along with that of our publisher, to the integrity of the material. Our basic goal is to produce a new book for today's needs, with updated content, and to meet the expectations and changing needs of students, faculty, and practitioners of basic health care.

AUDIENCE

This text is primarily designed for students in licensed practical or vocational nursing (LPN/LVN) programs and associate degree programs (ADN/RN), as well as for diet technicians or aides. It is also appropriate for programs in various health-related professions.

CONCEPTUAL APPROACH

The general purpose of this text is to introduce basic principles of scientific nutrition and present their applications in person-centered care. As in previous editions, basic concepts are carefully explained when introduced.

In addition, our personal concerns are ever present, as follows: (1) that this introduction to the science and practice we love will continue to lead students and readers to enjoy learning about nutrition in the lives of people and stimulate further reading in areas of personal interest; (2) that caretakers will be alert to nutrition news and questions raised by their increasingly diverse clients and patients; and (3) that contact and communication with professionals in the field of nutrition will help build a strong team approach to clinical nutrition problems in all patient care.

ORGANIZATION

In keeping with the previous format, I have updated content areas to meet the needs of a rapidly developing science and society.

In **Part 1**, *Introduction to Basic Principles of Nutrition Science*, Chapter 1 focuses on the directions of health care and health promotion, risk reduction for disease prevention, and community health care delivery systems, with emphasis on team care and the active role of clients in educated self-care. A description and illustration accompany the MyPyramid guidelines. The **Dietary Reference Intakes (DRIs)** are incorporated throughout chapter discussions in Part 1 as well as throughout the rest of the text. Current research updates all the basic nutrient and energy chapters in the remainder of Part 1.

In **Part 2**, *Nutrition throughout the Life Cycle*, Chapters 10, 11, and 12 reflect current material on human growth and development needs in different parts of the life cycle. Current National Academy of Science guidelines for positive weight gain to meet the metabolic demands of pregnancy and lactation are reinforced. Positive growth support for infancy, childhood, and adolescence is emphasized. The expanding health maintenance needs of a growing adult population through the aging process focus on building a healthy lifestyle to reduce disease risks.

In **Part 3**, *Community Nutrition and Health Care*, a strong focus on community nutrition is coordinated with an emphasis on weight management and physical fitness as they pertain to health care benefits and risk reduction. The Nutrition Labeling and Education Act is discussed in terms of its current regulations and helpful label format as well as its effects on food marketing. Highlights of food-borne diseases reinforce concerns about food safety in a changing marketplace. Chapter 14 and Appendix H reinforce information on America's multiethnic cultural food patterns and various religious dietary practices. New information on the topics of obesity and genetics, along with the use of alternative weight loss methods, is included in Chapter 15. Chapter 16 discusses aspects of athletics to clarify the ongoing practice of glycogen loading for endurance events, the proliferation of sports drinks, and the dangerous illegal use of steroids by athletes.

In **Part 4**, *Clinical Nutrition*, chapters are updated to reflect current medical treatment and approaches to nutrition management. Special areas include developments in gastrointestinal disease, heart disease, diabetes mellitus, renal disease, surgery, cancer, and AIDS.

CONTENT AND FEATURES

- **Book format and design.** The chapter format and use of color continue to enhance the book's appeal. Basic chapter concepts and overview, illustrations, tables, boxes, definitions, headings, and subheadings make the content easier and more interesting to read.
- **Learning supplements**. Educational aids have been developed to assist both students and instructors in the teaching and learning process. Please see the *Ancillaries* section on the next page for more detailed information.
- **Illustrations.** Color illustrations, including artwork, graphs, charts, and photographs, help students and practitioners better understand the concepts and clinical practices presented.
- **Content threads.** This book shares a number of features—reading level; Key Concepts; Key Terms; Critical Thinking Questions; Chapter Challenge Questions; References; Further Reading and Resources; Glossary; and Cultural Considerations, For Further Focus, Drug-Nutrient Interactions, and Clinical Applications boxes—with other Elsevier books intended for students in demanding and fast-paced nursing curricula. These common threads help promote and hone the skills these students must master. (See the Content Threads page after this preface for more detailed information on these learning features.)

LEARNING AIDS

As indicated, this new edition is especially significant because of its use of many learning aids throughout the text.

- **Part openers.** To provide the "big picture" of the book's overall focus on nutrition and health, the four main sections are introduced as successive developing parts of that unifying theme.
- **Chapter openers.** To immediately draw students into the topic for study, each chapter opens with a short list of the basic concepts involved and a brief chapter overview leading into the topic to "set the stage."
- **Chapter headings.** Throughout each chapter, the major headings and subheadings in special type or color indicate the organization of the chapter material, providing easy reading and understanding of the key ideas. Main concepts and terms also are highlighted with color or bold type and italics.
- **Special boxes.** The inclusion of **For Further Focus, Cultural Considerations, Drug-Nutrient Interactions,** and **Clinical Applications** boxes leads students a step further on a given topic or presents a case study for analysis. These boxes enhance understanding of concepts through further exploration or application.
- **Case studies.** In clinical care chapters, case studies are provided in **Clinical Applications** boxes to focus students' attention on related patient care problems. Each case is accompanied by questions for case analysis. Students can use these examples for similar patient care needs in their own clinical assignments.
- **Diet therapy guides.** In clinical chapters, various diet therapy guides provide practical help in patient care and education.
- **Definitions of terms.** Key terms important to students' understanding and application of the material in patient care are presented in two ways. They are identified in the body of the text and are listed in a glossary at the back of the book for quick reference.
- **Summaries.** A brief summary at the end of each chapter reviews chapter highlights and helps students see how the chapter contributes to the book's "big picture." Students then can return to any part of the material for repeated study and clarification of details as needed.
- **Critical Thinking Questions.** To help students understand key parts of the chapter or apply it to patient care problems, critical thinking questions are posed after each chapter summary for review and analysis of the material presented.
- **Chapter Challenge Questions.** In addition, self-test questions in true-false, multiple choice, and matching formats are provided at the end of each chapter to allow students to test their basic knowledge of the chapter's contents. Answers are provided in the back of the book.
- **References.** Background references throughout the text provide resources used in each chapter for students who may want to probe a particular topic of interest.

- **Further Reading and Resources.** To encourage further reading of useful materials, expand students' knowledge of key concepts, and help students apply material in practical ways for patient care and education, a brief list of annotated resources—including books, journals, and Web sites—is provided at the end of each chapter.
- **Appendixes.** The numerous appendixes include information on the cholesterol, dietary fiber, sodium, and potassium content of food and on cultural and religious dietary patterns. The NEW **Choose Your Foods: Exchange Lists for Diabetes** is included, along with the revised **Eating Well with Canada's Food Guide**. These, and all the appendixes provided, serve as valuable reference tools and guides in learning and practice.

ANCILLARIES
For Instructors

- **Instructor's Manual:** This manual consists of chapter outlines; essay questions; and extensive print, audiovisual, software, and Web site resources that can be used for activities, projects, and further study.
- **Test Bank:** Includes approximately 700 questions in NCLEX style, multiple-choice format.
- **Image Collection:** With approximately 50 illustrations, these images can be used in a unique presentation or as visual aids.
- **PowerPoint Presentations:** PowerPoint slides to accompany each chapter guide classroom lectures.

For Students

- **Mosby's Nutritrac Nutrition Analysis CD-ROM:** A FREE nutrition analysis CD-ROM with a database of more than 3700 food items is included with every text. This software allows users to analyze nutrition and calculate food intake and energy expenditure for effective diet analysis.
- **Evolve Resources**
  - **Study Questions:** More than 350 self-assessment questions that provide students practice questions and immediate feedback to help them prepare for exams.
- **Infant and Child Growth Charts, United States, Centers for Disease Control and Prevention** and the **ADA Nutrition Care Process** are available as useful handouts to encourage use of these valuable resources inside and outside of the classroom.
- **Case Studies** engage students with the opportunity to apply the knowledge they have learned in real-life situations.
- **WebLinks** offer direct links to a wealth of Web sites on nutrition-related topics above and beyond information covered in the book.
- **Nutrition Resource Center Web site:** This informative Web site is available at *http://nutrition.elsevier.com* to provide the reader access to information about all Elsevier nutrition texts in one convenient location.

ACKNOWLEDGMENTS

Throughout this process, various staff members from Elsevier have kindly provided guidance and assistance, and I am grateful to all of them. I would like to especially acknowledge the professionalism, fortitude, and diligence of Yvonne Alexopoulos, Senior Editor; Heather Bays, Developmental Editor; Amy Whittier, Editorial Assistant; and Amy Rickles, Project Manager. Your vision for this text is the true power behind the print.

I would like to acknowledge the hard work and dedication of Elsevier's Nursing Marketing Department for supporting this book through its many editions. Their ability to bridge the gap between a product and the end point—students who will hopefully learn from and enjoy this text—is integral to the success of this project. In addition, I am grateful to the many reviewers who have critiqued this edition. Your involvement provides the strength and thoroughness that no author can accomplish alone.

Finally, I want to thank my family and friends who have compassionately dealt with me and "the book." Your abundant support sustains me.

Staci Nix

CONTENT THREADS

The thirteenth edition of *Williams' Basic Nutrition & Diet Therapy* shares a number of learning features with other Elsevier titles used in nursing programs. These user-friendly Content Threads are designed to streamline the learning process among the variety of books and content areas included in this fast-paced and demanding curriculum.

Shared elements included in *Williams' Basic Nutrition & Diet Therapy*, thirteenth edition, include the following:

- **Reading level:** The easy-to-read and user-friendly format, as well as the often personal writing style, engage the reader and help unfold the information simply and effectively.
- **Cover design:** Graphic similarities help readers to instantly recognize the book as containing content and features relevant to today's nursing curricula.
- Bulleted lists of **Key Concepts** on each chapter opening page help focus the student on the "big picture" content presented.
- **Key Terms** presented in color are readily apparent throughout the book. In addition, key terms boxes presented on the book pages in which the terms are discussed provide complete definitions to help with memory association.
- **Critical Thinking Questions** presented after each chapter's summary encourage the student to recall the information as well as analyze its implications and uses.
- **Chapter Challenge Questions** presented in true-false, multiple-choice, and matching formats help students test their comprehension of various content areas. Answers are provided in the back of the book.
- A complete list of **References** is accompanied by **Further Reading and Resources,** a section that includes a wealth of resources—books, journal articles, and Web sites—that supplement the information provided in the textbook.
- The **Glossary** is an alphabetical listing of the key terms presented throughout the textbook.
- Four types of boxes—**Cultural Considerations, For Further Focus, Clinical Applications, and Drug-Nutrient Interaction**—explore current hot topics in nutrition today and provide insight beyond the information presented in the chapter text.

PREFACE to the STUDENT

Williams' Basic Nutrition & Diet Therapy is a market leader in nutrition textbooks for support personnel in health care. It provides careful explanations of the basic principles of scientific nutrition and presents their applications in person-centered care in health and disease.

The author, Staci Nix, provides this important information in an easy-to-read, user-friendly format by including helpful learning tools throughout the text. Check out the following features to familiarize yourself with the book and help you get the most value out of this text:

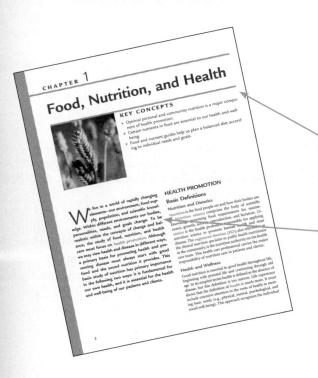

A short list of **Key Concepts** and a brief **chapter overview** begin each chapter to immediately draw you into the subject at hand.

Key terms boxes throughout the text identify and define key terms important to your understanding and application of the material.

health promotion active involvement in behaviors or programs that advance positive well-being.

nutrition the sum of the processes involved with the intake of nutrients as well as assimilating and using them to maintain body tissue and provide energy; a foundation for life and health.

nutrition science the body of science, developed through controlled research, that relates to the processes involved in nutrition—internationally, clinically, and in the community.

dietetics management of diet and the use of food; the science concerned with the nutrition planning and preparation of foods.

registered dietitian (RD) a professional dietitian, accredited with an academic degree of undergraduate or graduate study program, who has passed required registration examinations administered by the American Dietetic Association.

health a state of optimal physical, mental, and social well-being; relative freedom from disease or disability.

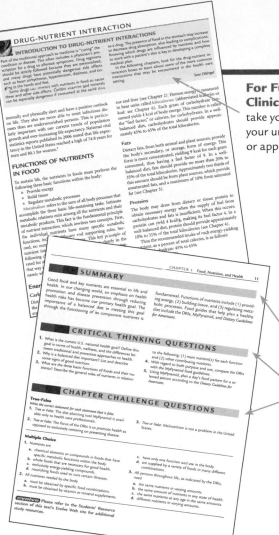

For Further Focus, Cultural Considerations, Clinical Applications, and **Drug-Nutrient Interaction** boxes take you one step further in the discussion of a given topic, enhancing your understanding of concepts through further exploration or application.

A brief **Summary** is included at the end of every chapter to review content highlights and help you see how particular chapters contribute to the book's overall focus.

Critical Thinking Questions and **Chapter Challenge Questions** are presented after each chapter summary for review and analysis and allow you to apply key concepts to patient care problems.

References and **Further Reading and Resources** complete the chapter with lists of relevant citations that provide a wealth of nutrition-related information above and beyond the book's content.

Your free copy of the latest version of the *Nutritrac Nutrition Analysis CD-ROM* is also included in the back of this text. *Nutritrac* provides the easiest way to analyze nutrition and calculate food intake and energy expenditure for effective diet analysis. Here is what you will find: an updated food database with more than 3700 foods, 18 food categories, and an updated *Detailed Energy Expenditure* section that includes more than 150 common/daily, sporting, recreational, and occupational activities.

Be sure to visit our two Web sites of interest.
1. An **Evolve** web site has been created specifically for this book at *http://evolve.elsevier.com/Williams/basic/*. (See the Evolve page at the beginning of this text for more information.) The following exciting features are available:
   - **Case Studies** are an integral tool to reinforce your understanding of key concepts and provide real-life examples.

- **Study Questions** give you a chance to practice for your exams and receive immediate feedback.
- **Infant and Child Growth Charts, United States, Centers for Disease Control and Prevention** and the **ADA Nutrition Care Process** are available as useful handouts to encourage use of these valuable resources inside and outside of the classroom.
- **WebLinks** offer direct links to a wealth of nutrition-related Web sites.
2. A **Nutrition Resource Center** Web site is available at *http://nutrition.elsevier.com* to provide you access to all the Elsevier nutrition texts in one convenient location.

We are pleased that you have included *Williams' Basic Nutrition & Diet Therapy* as a part of your nutrition education. Be sure to check out our Web site at *www.elsevier-health.com* for all your health science educational needs!

CONTENTS

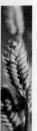

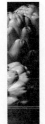

PART 2
Nutrition throughout the Life Cycle, 167

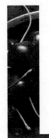

PART 3
Community Nutrition and Health Care, 231

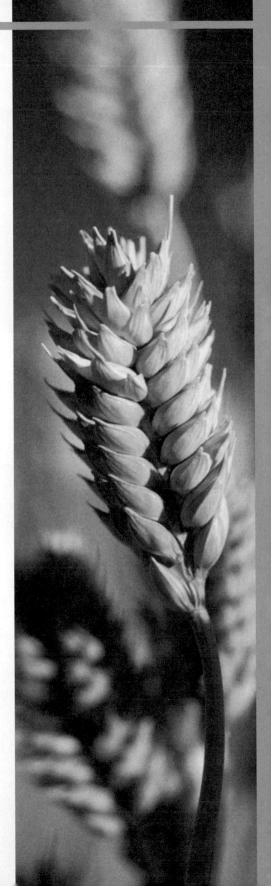

PART 1

Introduction to Basic Principles of Nutrition Science

Food, Nutrition, and Health

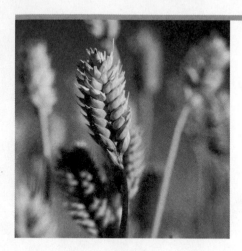

We live in a world of rapidly changing elements—our environment, food supply, population, and scientific knowledge. Within different environments our bodies, personalities, needs, and goals change. To be realistic within the concepts of change and balance, the study of food, nutrition, and health care must focus on health promotion. Although we may view health and disease in different ways, a primary basis for promoting health and preventing disease must always start with good food and the sound nutrition it provides. This basic study of nutrition has primary importance in the following two ways: it is fundamental for our own health, and it is essential for the health and well-being of our patients and clients.

HEALTH PROMOTION

Basic Definitions

Nutrition and Dietetics

Nutrition is the food people eat and how their bodies use it. Nutrition science comprises the body of scientific knowledge governing food requirements for maintenance, growth, activity, reproduction, and lactation. Dietetics is the health profession responsible for applying nutrition science to promote human health and treat disease. The registered dietitian (RD), also referred to as the *clinical nutrition specialist* or *public health nutritionist* in the community, is the nutrition authority on the health care team. This health care professional carries the major responsibility of nutrition care in patients and clients.

Health and Wellness

Good nutrition is essential to good health throughout life, beginning with prenatal life and continuing through old age. In its simplest terms health is defined as the absence of disease, but this definition is too narrow. Life experience shows that the definition of health is much more. It must include extensive attention to the roots of health in meeting basic needs (e.g., physical, mental, psychological, and social well-being). This approach recognizes the individual as a whole and relates health to both internal and external environments. The concept of *wellness* broadens this approach one step further. Wellness seeks the full development of potential for all persons, within whatever environment they may find themselves. It implies a balance between activities and goals: work vs. leisure, lifestyle choices vs. health risks, and personal needs vs. others' expectations. Wellness implies a positive dynamic state motivating a person to seek a higher level of functioning.

Wellness Movement and National Health Goals

The current wellness movement continues to be a fundamental response to the health care system's emphasis on illness and disease and the rising costs of medical care. Since the 1970s, holistic health and health promotion have focused on lifestyle and personal choice in helping persons and families develop plans for maintaining health and wellness. The U.S. national health goals continue to reflect this wellness philosophy. The most recent report in the *Healthy People* series published by the U.S. Department of Health and Human Services (USDHHS), *Healthy People 2010,* continues to focus on the nation's main objective of positive health promotion and disease prevention. This report outlines specific objectives for meeting the following broad public health goals[1]:

- Help individuals of all ages increase life expectancy *and* improve their quality of life.
- Eliminate health disparities among different segments of the population.

A major theme throughout the report is the encouragement of healthy choices in diet, weight control, and other risk factors for disease, especially in the report's specific nutrition objectives. Community health agencies continue to implement these goals and objectives in local, state, public, and private health programs, particularly in areas where malnutrition and poverty exist. Programs such as Supplemental Programs for Women, Infants and Children (WIC) and School Lunch Programs are well established throughout the United States. Each effort recognizes personal nutrition as an integral component of health and health care for all persons.

Traditional and Preventive Approaches to Health

The *preventive* approach to health involves identifying risk factors that increase a person's chances of developing a particular health problem. By knowing these factors, people can then choose behaviors that will prevent or minimize their risks for disease. On the other hand, the *traditional* approach to health only attempts change when symptoms of illness or disease already exist, at which point those who are ill seek a physician to diagnose, treat, and "cure" the condition (see the Drug-Nutrient Interaction box, "Introduction to Drug-Nutrient Interactions"). The traditional approach has little value for lifelong positive health. Major chronic problems (e.g., heart disease, cancer) may develop long before signs become apparent.

Importance of a Balanced Diet

Food and Health

Food is a necessity of life. However, many people are only concerned with food insofar as it relieves their hunger or satisfies their appetites, not with whether it supplies their bodies with all the components of good nutrition. The core practitioners of the health care team (i.e., physician, dietitian, and nurse) are all aware of the important part that food plays in maintaining good health and recovering from illness. Therefore assessing a patient's nutritional status and identifying nutrition needs are primary activities in the development of a health care plan.

Signs of Good Nutrition

A lifetime of good nutrition is evidenced by a well-developed body, the ideal weight for body composition (i.e., ratio of muscle mass to fat mass) and height, and good muscle development. In addition, a healthy person's skin is smooth and clear, the hair is glossy, and the eyes are clear and bright. Appetite, digestion, and elimination are normal. Well-nourished persons are more likely to be

---

health promotion active involvement in behaviors or programs that advance positive well-being.

nutrition the sum of the processes involved with the intake of nutrients as well as assimilating and using them to maintain body tissue and provide energy; a foundation for life and health.

nutrition science the body of science, developed through controlled research, that relates to the processes involved in nutrition—internationally, clinically, and in the community.

dietetics management of diet and the use of food; the science concerned with the nutrition planning and preparation of foods.

registered dietitian (RD) a professional dietitian, accredited with an academic degree of undergraduate or graduate study program, who has passed required registration examinations administered by the American Dietetic Association.

health a state of optimal physical, mental, and social well-being; relative freedom from disease or disability.

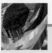

DRUG-NUTRIENT INTERACTION

INTRODUCTION TO DRUG-NUTRIENT INTERACTIONS

Part of the traditional approach to medicine is "curing" the condition or disease. This often includes a physician's prescription for a drug to alleviate symptoms. Drug regimens should be strictly followed because they are personalized, and many drugs have potentially dangerous side effects such as heart arrhythmias, hypertension, dizziness, and tingling in the hands and feet.

Some drugs can interact with nutrients in food to cause these and other side effects. Certain vitamins and minerals can be especially dangerous if consumed at the same time as a drug. The presence of food in the stomach may increase or decrease drug absorption, also leading to complications. Knowing which drugs are influenced by nutrients and how to work with a patient's diet is key to developing a complete medical plan.

In the following chapters, look for the drug-nutrient interaction boxes to learn about some of the more common interactions that may be encountered in the health care setting.

Sara Oldroyd

mentally and physically alert and have a positive outlook on life. They also are more able to resist infectious diseases than are undernourished persons. This is particularly important with our current trends of population growth and ever-increasing life expectancy. National vital statistics reports published in 2006 stated that life expectancy in the United States reached a high of 74.8 years for men and 80.1 for women.[2]

FUNCTIONS OF NUTRIENTS IN FOOD

To sustain life, the nutrients in foods must perform the following three basic functions within the body:

- Provide energy
- Build tissue
- Regulate metabolic processes

Metabolism refers to the sum of all body processes that accomplish the three basic life-sustaining tasks. Intimate metabolic relations exist among all the nutrients and their metabolic products. This fact is the fundamental principle of *nutrient interaction*, which involves two concepts. First, the individual nutrients have many specific metabolic functions, including primary and supporting roles. Second, no nutrient ever works alone. This key principle of nutrient interaction is demonstrated more clearly in the following chapters. Although the nutrients may be separated for study purposes, remember that they do not exist that way in the human body. They always interact as a dynamic whole to produce and maintain the body.

Energy Sources

Carbohydrates

Dietary carbohydrates (e.g., starches and sugars) provide the body's primary and preferred source of fuel for energy. They also maintain the body's backup store of quick energy as glycogen, or stored carbohydrate in muscle tissue and liver (see Chapter 2). Human energy is measured in heat units called kilocalories (abbreviated *kcalories* or *kcal;* see Chapter 6). Each gram of carbohydrate consumed yields 4 kcal of body energy. This number is called the "fuel factor," or calories, for carbohydrates. In a well-balanced diet, carbohydrates should provide approximately 45% to 65% of the total kilocalories.

Fats

Dietary fats, from both animal and plant sources, provide the body's secondary, or storage, form of energy. This form is more concentrated, yielding 9 kcal for each gram consumed, thus having a fuel factor of 9. In a well-balanced diet, fats should provide no more than 20% to 35% of the total kilocalories. Approximately two thirds of this amount should be from plant sources, which provide unsaturated fats, and a maximum of 10% from saturated fat (see Chapter 3).

Proteins

The body may draw from dietary or tissue protein to obtain necessary energy when the supply of fuel from carbohydrates and fats is insufficient. When this occurs, protein can yield 4 kcal/g, making its fuel factor 4. In a well-balanced diet, protein should provide approximately 10% to 35% of the total kilocalories (see Chapter 4).

Thus the recommended intake of each energy-yielding nutrient, as a percent of total calories, is as follows:

- Carbohydrate: 45% to 65%
- Fat: 20% to 35%
- Protein: 10% to 35%

Tissue Building

Proteins

The primary function of protein is tissue building. Dietary protein provides amino acids, which are the building blocks necessary for constructing and repairing body tissues (e.g., organs, muscle, cells, blood proteins). Tissue building is a constant process that ensures growth and maintenance of a strong body structure and vital substances for tissue functions.

Other Nutrients

Several other nutrients that contribute to building and maintaining tissues are described below.

Vitamins and Minerals. Vitamins and minerals are nutrients that help regulate many body processes. An example of the use of a vitamin in tissue building is that of vitamin C in developing collagen, the protein in fibrous tissues. Collagen helps build strong tissue such as cartilage, bone matrix, skin, and tendons. Two major minerals, calcium and phosphorus, participate in building and maintaining bone tissue. Another key mineral is iron, which contributes to building the oxygen carrier hemoglobin in red blood cells. Several other vitamins and minerals are discussed in greater detail in Chapters 7 and 8 with regard to their function, including tissue building.

Fatty Acids. Fatty acids, derived from fat metabolism, help build the central fat substance of cell membranes and promote the transport of fat-soluble nutrients throughout the body.

Regulation and Control

The multiple chemical processes in the body necessary for providing energy and building tissue are carefully regulated and controlled to maintain a constant dynamic balance among all body parts and processes.

Vitamins

Many vitamins function as coenzyme factors, which are components of cell enzymes, in governing chemical reactions during metabolism. For example, this is true for most of the B-complex vitamins.

Minerals

Many minerals also serve as coenzyme factors with enzymes in cell metabolism. For example, cobalt, which is a central constituent of vitamin B_{12} (cobalamin), functions with this vitamin in the synthesis of heme for hemoglobin formation.

Water and Fiber

Water and fiber also function as regulatory agents. In fact, water is the fundamental agent for life itself, providing the essential base for all metabolic processes. The adult body is approximately 50% to 60% water. Dietary fiber helps regulate the passage of food material through the

gastrointestinal tract and influences the absorption of various nutrients.

NUTRITIONAL STATES
Optimal Nutrition

Optimal nutrition means that a person receives and uses substances obtained from a *varied and balanced* diet of carbohydrates, fats, proteins, minerals, vitamins, and water in ideal amounts. The desired amounts of these nutrients should be balanced to cover variations in health and disease and provide reserve supplies without unnecessary excesses.

Malnutrition

Malnutrition refers to a condition caused by improper or insufficient diet. Both undernutrition and overnutrition are forms of malnutrition. Dietary surveys have shown that approximately one third of the U.S. population lives on suboptimal diets. That does not necessarily mean that all these Americans are undernourished. Some persons can maintain health on somewhat less than the optimal amounts of various nutrients in a state of borderline nutrition. However, on average someone receiving less than the desired amounts of nutrients has a greater risk for physical illness and compromised immunity than someone receiving the appropriate amounts.[3] Such nutritionally deficient people are limited in their physical work capacity, immune system function, and mental activity. They lack the nutritional reserves to meet any added

---

metabolism the sum of all chemical changes that take place in the body by which it maintains itself and produces energy for its functioning (products of the various reactions are called *metabolites*).

glycogen a polysaccharide, the main storage form of carbohydrate, largely stored in the liver and to a lesser extent in muscle tissue.

kilocalorie the general term *calorie* refers to a unit of heat measure and is used alone to designate the small calorie. The calorie used in nutrition science and the study of metabolism is the large calorie, or kilocalorie, to be more accurate and avoid the use of large numbers in calculations. A kilocalorie, or 1000 calories, is the measure of heat necessary to raise the temperature of 1000 g (1 L) of water 1° C.

amino acids nitrogen-bearing compounds that form the structural units of protein. After digestion amino acids are available for synthesis of specific tissue proteins.

physiologic or metabolic demands from injury or illness or to sustain fetal development during pregnancy or proper growth in childhood. This state may result from poor eating habits or a continuously stressful environment with little or no available food.

Undernutrition

Signs of more serious malnutrition appear when nutritional reserves are depleted and nutrient and energy intake is not sufficient to meet day-to-day needs or added metabolic stress. Many malnourished people live in conditions of poverty or illness. Such conditions influence the health of all involved, but especially that of the most vulnerable persons (pregnant women, infants, children, and elderly adults). In the United States, one of the wealthiest countries in the world, widespread hunger and malnutrition among the poor still exist, indicating that food security problems involve urban development issues, economic policy, and more general poverty issues (see the Cultural Considerations box, "Food Insecurity").

Malnutrition sometimes occurs in hospitals as well. For example, acute trauma or chronic illness, especially among older persons, places added stress on the body, and the daily nutrient and energy intake may be insufficient to meet their needs.

Overnutrition

Some persons may be in a state of overnutrition, which results from excess nutrient and energy intake over time. In a sense, overnutrition is another form of malnutrition, especially when excess caloric intake produces harmful body weight (i.e., morbid obesity; see Chapter 15). Harmful overnutrition can also occur in persons who consistently use excessive (e.g., "megadose") amounts of nutrient supplements, resulting in toxicities (see Chapter 7).

NUTRIENT AND FOOD GUIDES FOR HEALTH PROMOTION

Nutrient Standards

Most of the developed countries of the world have established standards for the major nutrients. These standards serve as a reference for intake levels of the essential nutrients to meet the known nutrition needs of most healthy population groups. Although these standards are similar in most countries, they may vary somewhat according to the philosophy of the scientists and practitioners on the purpose and use of such standards. In the United States, these standards have been updated and reorganized and are now called the Dietary Reference Intakes (DRIs).

U.S. Standards: Dietary Reference Intakes

Since 1941 the Recommended Dietary Allowances (RDAs), published by the National Academy of Sciences, has been the authoritative source setting standards for the minimum amounts of nutrients necessary to protect almost all persons against the risk for nutrient deficiency. The U.S. RDA standard was first published during World War II as a guide for planning and obtaining food sup-

CULTURAL CONSIDERATIONS

FOOD INSECURITY

Food insecurity is defined by the USDA as limited or uncertain availability of nutritious and adequate food. According to this definition, the Food Assistance and Nutrition Research Program of the USDA reported that 12.6 million households, or 11% of all U.S. households, qualified as having food insecurity in 2005. Furthermore, homes with children report double the rate of food insecurity of homes without children (15.6% vs. 8.5%, respectively).* Many studies document widespread hunger and malnutrition among the poor, especially in the growing number of homeless—including mothers with young children. Such problems can manifest into physical, psychological, and sociofamilial disturbances in all age groups, with a significant negative impact on health status (including mental health) and risk of chronic disease.† America's Second Harvest, the nation's largest organization of emergency food providers, estimated that 9 million children in the United States receive emergency food services each year.‡ Malnourished children are at an increased risk for stunted growth and episodes of infection and disease, which often have lasting effects on intellectual development. Hunger is a chronic issue (persisting 8 months or more per year) among most households reporting food insecurity. In 2005 the prevalence of food insecurity was substantially higher in households headed by single mothers and in African-American and Hispanic households.* A variety of federal and nonfederal programs are available to address hunger issues in all cultural and age groups. The American Dietetic Association has an extensive list of such programs in their position statement *Food Insecurity and Hunger in the United States.*†

*Nord M and others: *Household food security in the United States, 2005 (economic research report 29)*, Alexandria, VA, 2006, United States Department of Agriculture, Economic Research Services.
†Position statement of the American Dietetic Association: food insecurity and hunger in the United States, *J Am Diet Assoc* 106:446, 2006.
‡America's Second Harvest: *Hunger in America 2006,* Chicago, 2006, America's Second Harvest.

plies for national defense and providing average population standards as a goal for good nutrition. These standards are revised and expanded every 5 to 10 years to reflect increasing scientific knowledge and social concerns about nutrition and health.

Both public awareness and research attention have shifted to reflect an increasing emphasis on nutrient requirements for maintaining optimal health within the general population, as opposed to only preventing disease. This change of emphasis resulted in the DRIs project. The creation of the new DRIs involved distinguished U.S. and Canadian scientists, divided into six functional panels, who have examined hundreds of nutrition studies on the health benefits of nutrients and the hazards of taking too much of a nutrient (Box 1-1). The working group of nutrition scientists responsible for these standards forms the Food and Nutrition Board of the Institute of Medicine. The new DRI recommendations were published over several years in a series of six volumes.[4-9]

The DRIs include recommendations for each gender and age group as well as recommendations for pregnancy and lactation. For the first time, excessive amounts of nutrients are identified as tolerable upper intakes. The new DRIs incorporate and expand on the well-established RDAs. The DRIs encompass the following four interconnected categories of nutrient recommendations:

1. *Recommended Dietary Allowance (RDA)*. This is the daily intake of a nutrient that meets the needs of almost all (97.5%) healthy individuals of specific age and gender. Individuals should use the RDA as a guide to achieve adequate nutrient intake to decrease the risk of chronic disease. RDAs are only established when enough scientific evidence exists about a specific nutrient.
2. *Estimated Average Requirement (EAR)*. This is the intake level that meets the needs of half of the individuals in a specific group. This quantity is used as the basis for developing the RDA.

3. *Adequate Intake (AI)*. The AI is used as a guide when not enough scientific evidence is available to establish the RDA figure. Both the RDA and the AI may be used as goals for individual intake.
4. *Tolerable Upper Intake Level (UL)*. This indicator is not a recommended intake, but sets the maximal intake that is unlikely to pose adverse health risks in almost all healthy individuals. For most nutrients, the UL refers to the total daily intake from food, fortified food, and nutrient supplements.

Other Standards

Over the years Canadian and British standards have been similar to the U.S. standards. The current U.S. DRIs were developed with Canadian nutrition science associates and are similar to British standards. In less-developed countries, where factors such as the quality of available protein foods must be considered, individuals look to standards such as those set by the Food and Agriculture Organization and World Health Organization. Nonetheless, all these standards provide a guideline to help health care workers in a variety of population groups promote good health and prevent disease through sound nutrition.

Food Guides and Recommendations

To interpret and apply sound nutrient standards, health care workers need practical food guides to use in nutrition education and food planning with persons and families. Such tools include the U.S. Department of Agriculture (USDA) MyPyramid and the U.S. Dietary Guidelines.

My Pyramid

The MyPyramid food guidance system (Figure 1-1), released in early 2005 by the USDA, provides the public with a valuable nutrition education tool. The goal of this

---

BOX 1-1

DRI PANELS OF THE INSTITUTE OF MEDICINE OF THE NATIONAL ACADEMY OF SCIENCES

- Calcium, vitamin D, phosphorous, magnesium, and fluoride
- Folate and other B vitamins
- Antioxidants
- Macronutrients
- Trace elements
- Electrolytes and water

Dietary Reference Intakes (DRIs) nutrient recommendations for each gender and age group that can be used for assessing and planning diets for healthy populations.

Recommended Dietary Allowances (RDAs) recommended daily allowances of nutrients and energy intake for population groups according to age and sex, with defined weight and height.

MyPyramid a visual pattern of the current basic five food groups (bread/cereal, vegetable, fruit, milk/cheese, meat/dry beans/egg), arranged in a pyramid shape to indicate proportionate amounts of daily food choices.

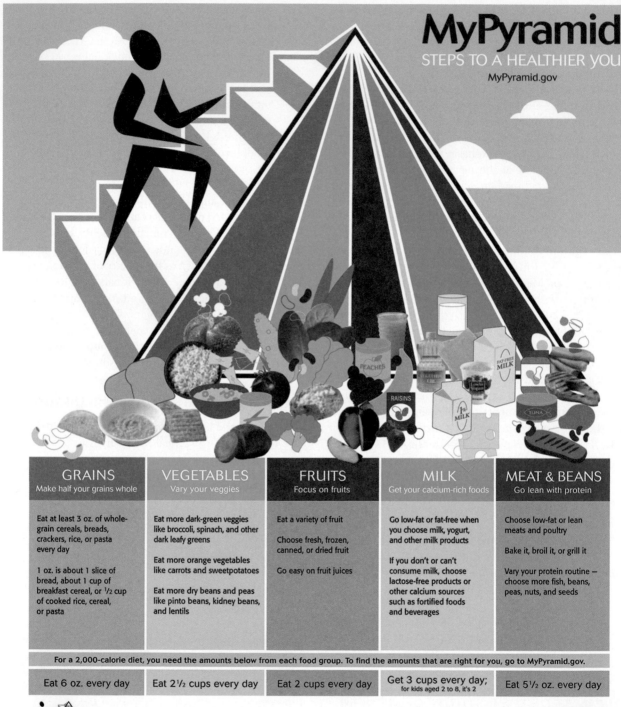

Figure 1-1 MyPyramid food guidance system mini-poster. (From U.S. Department of Agriculture, Center for Nutrition Policy and Promotion: *MyPyramid mini-poster, www.mypyramid.gov/downloads/MiniPoster.pdf.*)

Dietary Guidelines for Americans 2005

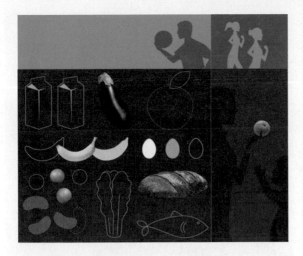

ADEQUATE NUTRIENTS WITHIN CALORIE NEEDS

- Consume a variety of nutrient-dense foods and beverages within and among the basic food groups while choosing foods that limit the intake of saturated and *trans* fats, cholesterol, added sugars, salt, and alcohol.
- Meet recommended intakes within energy needs by adopting a balanced eating pattern, such as the USDA Food Guide or the DASH Eating Plan.

WEIGHT MANAGEMENT

- To maintain body weight in a healthy range, balance calories from foods and beverages with calories expended.
- To prevent gradual weight gain over time, make small decreases in food and beverage calories and increase physical activity.

PHYSICAL ACTIVITY

- Engage in regular physical activity and reduce sedentary activities to promote health, psychological well-being, and a healthy body weight.
  - To reduce the risk of chronic disease in adulthood: Engage in at least 30 minutes of moderate-intensity physical activity, above usual activity, at work or home on most days of the week.
  - For most people, greater health benefits can be obtained by engaging in physical activity of more vigorous intensity or longer duration.
  - To help manage body weight and prevent gradual, unhealthy body weight gain in adulthood: Engage in approximately 60 minutes of moderate- to vigorous-intensity activity on most days of the week while not exceeding caloric intake requirements.
  - To sustain weight loss in adulthood: Participate in at least 60 to 90 minutes of daily moderate-intensity physical activity while not exceeding caloric intake requirements. Some people may need to consult with a healthcare provider before participating in this level of activity.
- Achieve physical fitness by including cardiovascular conditioning, stretching exercises for flexibility, and resistance exercises or calisthenics for muscle strength and endurance.

FOOD GROUPS TO ENCOURAGE

- Consume a sufficient amount of fruits and vegetables while staying within energy needs. Two cups of fruit and 2½ cups of vegetables per day are recommended for a reference 2,000-calorie intake, with higher or lower amounts depending on the calorie level.
- Choose a variety of fruits and vegetables each day. In particular, select from all five vegetable subgroups (dark green, orange, legumes, starchy vegetables, and other vegetables) several times a week.
- Consume 3 or more ounce-equivalents of whole-grain products per day, with the rest of the recommended grains coming from enriched or whole-grain products. In general, at least half the grains should come from whole grains.
- Consume 3 cups per day of fat-free or low-fat milk or equivalent milk products.

FATS

- Consume less than 10 percent of calories from saturated fatty acids and less than 300 mg/day of cholesterol, and keep *trans* fatty acid consumption as low as possible.
- Keep total fat intake between 20 to 35 percent of calories, with most fats coming from sources of polyunsaturated and mono-unsaturated fatty acids, such as fish, nuts, and vegetable oils.
- When selecting and preparing meat, poultry, dry beans, and milk or milk products, make choices that are lean, low-fat, or fat-free.
- Limit intake of fats and oils high in saturated and/or *trans* fatty acids, and choose products low in such fats and oils.

CARBOHYDRATES

- Choose fiber-rich fruits, vegetables, and whole grains often.
- Choose and prepare foods and beverages with little added sugars or caloric sweeteners, such as amounts suggested by the USDA Food Guide and the DASH Eating Plan.
- Reduce the incidence of dental caries by practicing good oral hygiene and consuming sugar- and starch-containing foods and beverages less frequently.

SODIUM AND POTASSIUM

- Consume less than 2,300 mg (approximately 1 tsp of salt) of sodium per day.
- Choose and prepare foods with little salt. At the same time, consume potassium-rich foods, such as fruits and vegetables.

ALCOHOLIC BEVERAGES

- Those who choose to drink alcoholic beverages should do so sensibly and in moderation—defined as the consumption of up to one drink per day for women and up to two drinks per day for men.
- Alcoholic beverages should not be consumed by some individuals, including those who cannot restrict their alcohol intake, women of childbearing age who may become pregnant, pregnant and lactating women, children and adolescents, individuals taking medications that can interact with alcohol, and those with specific medical conditions.
- Alcoholic beverages should be avoided by individuals engaging in activities that require attention, skill, or coordination, such as driving or operating machinery.

FOOD SAFETY

- To avoid microbial food-borne illness:
  - Clean hands, food contact surfaces, and fruits and vegetables. Meat and poultry should not be washed or rinsed.
  - Separate raw, cooked, and ready-to-eat foods while shopping, preparing, or storing foods.
  - Cook foods to a safe temperature to kill microorganisms.
  - Chill (refrigerate) perishable food promptly and defrost foods properly.
  - Avoid raw (unpasteurized) milk or any products made from unpasteurized milk, raw or partially cooked eggs or foods containing raw eggs, raw or undercooked meat and poultry, unpasteurized juices, and raw sprouts.

Figure 1-2 Summary of the nine focus areas included in the *Dietary Guidelines for Americans, 2005*. (Image from U.S. Department of Agriculture and Human Services: *Dietary Guidelines for Americans, 2005, www.health.gov/dietaryguidelines/dga2005/document*. Text reprinted from the U.S. Department of Health and Human Services, U.S. Department of Agriculture: *Dietary guidelines for Americans 2005*: *key recommendations,* Washington, DC, 2005, USDA.)

food guide is to promote physical activity, variety, proportionality, moderation, and gradual improvements.[10] Consumers are encouraged to personalize their own plans through the public Web site *(www.mypyramid.gov)* by entering their age, gender, weight, height, and activity level. The system will create a plan with individualized calorie levels and specific recommendations for serving amounts from each food group. The current recommendations reflect the DRIs and *Dietary Guidelines for Americans, 2005* (Figure 1-2). In addition, the MyPyramid site provides consumers with individualized Meal Tracking Worksheets and access to the MyPyramid Tracker, an online dietary and physical activity assessment tool.

Dietary Guidelines for Americans

The *Dietary Guidelines for Americans* were issued as a result of growing public concerns beginning in the 1960s and the subsequent Senate investigations studying hunger and nutrition in the United States. These guidelines are based on our developing alarm about chronic health problems in an aging population and changing food environment. They relate current scientific thinking to America's leading health problems. A new, updated statement is issued every 5 years. Recent review by expert committees has led to minimal changes over the past decade. The current set of guidelines, released in January 2005, also reflect the current DRIs. This issue encompasses a comprehensive evaluation of the scientific evidence between diet and health, based on findings in a current U.S. report jointly issued by the USDA and the Department of Health and Human Services.

The guidelines promote nine focus areas (see Figure 1-2), 23 general recommendations, and 18 specific population recommendations. The current guidelines continue to serve as a useful general guide for promoting dietary and lifestyle choices that reduce the risk for chronic disease. Although no guidelines can guarantee health or well-being, and people differ widely in their food needs and preferences, these general statements help people evaluate their food habits and move toward general improvements. Good food habits based on moderation and variety can help build sound, healthy bodies.

Other Recommendations

Other organizations, such as the American Cancer Society and American Heart Association, also have their own independent dietary guidelines. In most cases, the guidelines set by various national organizations are modeled after the U.S. Dietary Guidelines. This may seem a bit repetitive, but the difference is the emphasis on prevention of certain chronic diseases, such as heart disease and cancer.

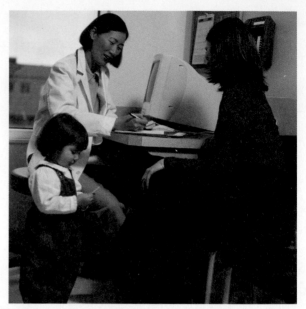

Figure 1-3 Nutrition education in the health care setting. (Copyright PhotoDisc.)

Individual Needs

Person-Centered Care

Regardless of the type of food guide or recommendations used, health care professionals must remember that food patterns vary with individual needs, tastes, habits, living situations, and energy demands. Persons who eat nutritionally balanced meals, spread fairly evenly throughout the day, usually can work more efficiently and sustain a more even energy supply.

Changing Food Environment

Our food environment has been rapidly changing in recent years. American food habits may have deteriorated in some ways, with a heightened reliance on fast, processed, prepackaged foods. Despite a plentiful food supply, surveys give evidence of malnutrition, even among hospitalized patients. Nurses and other health care professionals have an important responsibility to observe patients' food intake carefully (Figure 1-3). However, in general, Americans are recognizing the relation between food and health. Even fast food restaurants are beginning to respond to their customers' desires for lower-fat, health-conscious alternatives to the traditional fare. Other chain, family, and university restaurants are developing and testing similar patterns in new menu items. More than ever Americans are being selective about what they eat. Guided by the Food and Drug Administration nutrition labels, shoppers' choices indicate an increased awareness of nutritional values. Details of these marketing regulations are given in Chapter 14.

SUMMARY

Good food and key nutrients are essential to life and health. In our changing world, an emphasis on health promotion and disease prevention through reducing health risks has become our primary health goal. The importance of a balanced diet in meeting this goal through the functioning of its component nutrients is fundamental. Functions of nutrients include (1) providing energy, (2) building tissue, and (3) regulating metabolic processes. Food guides that help plan a healthy diet include the DRIs, MyPyramid, and *Dietary Guidelines for Americans*.

CRITICAL THINKING QUESTIONS

1. What is the current U.S. national health goal? Define this goal in terms of health, wellness, and the differences between traditional and preventive approaches to health.
2. Why is a balanced diet important? List and describe some signs of good nutrition.
3. What are the three basic functions of foods and their nutrients? Describe the general roles of nutrients in relation to the following: (1) main nutrient(s) for each function and (2) other contributing nutrients.
4. With regard to both purpose and use, compare the DRIs with the MyPyramid food guidelines.
5. Using MyPyramid, plan a day's food pattern for a selected person according to the *Dietary Guidelines for Americans*.

CHAPTER CHALLENGE QUESTIONS

True-False
Write the correct statement for each statement that is false.
1. *True or False:* The diet-planning tool MyPyramid is available only to health care professionals.
2. *True or False:* The focus of the DRIs is to promote health as opposed to exclusively centering on preventing disease.
3. *True or False:* Malnutrition is not a problem in the United States.

Multiple Choice
1. Nutrients are
   a. chemical elements or compounds in foods that have specific metabolic functions within the body.
   b. whole foods that are necessary for good health.
   c. exclusively energy-yielding compounds.
   d. nourishing foods used to cure certain illnesses.
2. All nutrients needed by the body
   a. must be obtained by specific food combinations.
   b. must be obtained by vitamin or mineral supplements.
   c. have only one function and use in the body.
   d. are supplied by a variety of foods in many different combinations.
3. All persons throughout life, as indicated by the DRIs, need
   a. the same nutrients in varying amounts.
   b. the same amount of nutrients in any state of health.
   c. the same nutrients at any age in the same amounts.
   d. different nutrients in varying amounts.

evolve Please refer to the Students' Resource section of this text's Evolve Web site for additional study resources.

REFERENCES

1. U.S. Department of Health and Human Services: *Healthy People 2010: understanding and improving health,* Washington, DC, 2000, U.S. Government Printing Office.
2. Hoyert DL and others: *Deaths: final data for* 2003. National vital statistics reports 54, Hyattsville, MD, 2006, National Center for Health Statistics.
3. Hughes S, Kelly P: Interactions of malnutrition and immune impairment, with specific reference to immunity against parasites, *Parasite Immunol* 28(11):577, 2006.
4. Food and Nutrition Board, Institute of Medicine: *Dietary reference intakes for calcium, phosphorous, magnesium, vitamin D, and fluoride,* Washington, DC, 1997, National Academies Press.
5. Food and Nutrition Board, Institute of Medicine: *Dietary reference intakes for thiamin, riboflavin, niacin, vitamin B_6, folate, vitamin B_{12}, pantothenic acid, biotin, and choline,* Washington, DC, 2000, National Academies Press.
6. Food and Nutrition Board, Institute of Medicine: *Dietary reference intakes for vitamin C, vitamin E, selenium, and carotenoids,* Washington, DC, 2000, National Academies Press.
7. Food and Nutrition Board, Institute of Medicine: *Dietary reference intakes for vitamin A, vitamin K, arsenic, boron, chromium, copper, iodine, iron, manganese, molybdenum, nickel, silicon, vanadium, and zinc,* Washington, DC, 2001, National Academies Press.
8. Food and Nutrition Board, Institute of Medicine: *Dietary reference intakes for energy, carbohydrate, fiber, fat, fatty acids, cholesterol, protein, and amino acids,* Washington, DC, 2002, National Academies Press.
9. Food and Nutrition Board, Institute of Medicine: *Dietary reference intakes for water, potassium, sodium, chloride, and sulfate,* Washington, DC, 2004, National Academies Press
10. Center for Nutrition Policy and Promotion, U.S. Department of Agriculture: *MyPyramid: steps to a healthier you,* http://mypyramid.gov, accessed June 2007.

FURTHER READING AND RESOURCES

The following organizations are key sources of up-to-date information and research about nutrition. Each site has a unique focus and may be helpful in keeping abreast on current topics.

USDA MyPyramid: *http://mypyramid.org*

Dietary Guidelines for Americans: *www.healthierus.gov/dietaryguidelines*

American Dietetic Association: *www.eatright.org*

American Society for Nutrition: *www.nutrition.org*

National Research Council (National Academies of Science): *www.nationalacademies.org/nrc*

Society for Nutrition Education: *www.sne.org*

American Cancer Society: *www.cancer.org*

American Heart Association: *www.americanheart.org*

Food and Agriculture Organization of the United Nations: *www.fao.org*

World Health Organization: *www.who.int*

Goldberg JP and others: The obesity crisis: don't blame it on the pyramid, *J Am Diet Assoc* 104(7):1141-1147, 2004.
> *The authors discuss the criticisms and praises of the Pyramid as a dietary guideline for Americans. A synopsis is provided for the history, concerns, and use of the Pyramid.*

Kretser AJ: The new Dietary Reference Intakes in food labeling: the food industry's perspective, *Am J Clin Nutr* 83(5):1231S-1234S, 2006.
> *Dietary Guidelines for Americans 2005, DRIs, and the MyPyramid food guidelines are collectively incorporated into food labels. The author looks at and discusses the industry's perspective in providing this information.*

CHAPTER 2

Carbohydrates

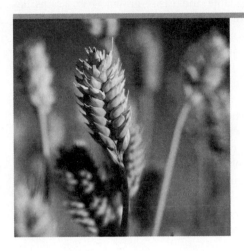

KEY CONCEPTS

- Carbohydrate foods provide practical energy sources because of their availability, relatively low cost, and storage capacity.
- Carbohydrate structures vary from simple to complex, providing both quick and extended energy for the body.
- Dietary fiber, an indigestible carbohydrate, serves separately as a regulatory agent within the gastrointestinal tract.

As discussed in Chapter 1, key nutrients in food sustain life and promote health. These results are possible because the human body's unique use of nutrients provides three essential elements for life: (1) energy to do its work, (2) building materials to maintain its form and functions, and (3) control agents to regulate these processes efficiently. These three basic life and health functions of nutrients are closely related; no nutrient ever works alone.

This chapter looks specifically at the body's primary fuel source—carbohydrates. Carbohydrates are plentiful in the food supply and are an important contribution to a well-balanced diet. Recent controversy surrounding the use, abuse, and misunderstanding of this critical macronutrient should be better interpreted after evaluating its functions within the body.

NATURE OF CARBOHYDRATES

Relation to Energy

Basic Fuel Source

Energy is necessary for life. It is the power an organism requires to do work. Any energy system must first have a basic fuel supply. In the earth's energy system, vast energy resources from the sun enable plants, through photosynthesis, to transform solar energy into carbohydrates, the stored fuel form of plants. Because the human body can rapidly break down these stores of quick and sustaining energy foods (sugars and starches), they provide the major source of energy in the form of calories.

Throughout this text the term *energy* is used interchangeably with the terms *calorie, kilocalorie,* and *kcal* (see definition of kilocalorie in Chapter 1). Our bodies need energy to survive. Both involuntary (heart pumping

---

photosynthesis process by which plants containing chlorophyll are able to manufacture carbohydrate by combining CO_2 and water. Sunlight is used as energy; chlorophyll is a catalyst.

$$6\ CO_2\ (gas) + 6\ H_2O\ (liquid) + Photons \rightarrow$$
$$C_6H_{12}O_6\ (aqueous) + 6\ O_2\ (gas)$$

and lungs breathing) and voluntary actions (walking and talking) require energy. That energy is derived from calories supplied by food.

Energy Production System

To produce energy from a basic fuel supply, a successful energy system must be able to do the following three things:

1. Change the basic fuel to a refined fuel that the machine is designed to use
2. Carry this refined fuel to the places that need it
3. Burn this refined fuel in the special equipment set up at these places

Far more efficient than any manmade machine, the body easily does these three things. It digests its basic fuel, carbohydrate, changing it to glucose. The body then absorbs and, through blood circulation, carries this refined fuel to cells that need glucose. Glucose is burned in the specific and intricate equipment in these cells, and energy is released through the process of cell metabolism. Because the human body can rapidly break down the starches and

sugars that are eaten to yield energy, carbohydrates are called quick energy foods.

Dietary Importance

Practical reasons also exist for the large quantities of carbohydrates in diets all over the world. First, carbohydrates are widely available and easily grown (e.g., grains, legumes, vegetables, and fruits). In some countries carbohydrate foods make up almost the entire diet. Second, carbohydrates are relatively low in cost when compared with many other food items. Third, carbohydrates may be easily stored. They can be kept in dry storage for relatively long periods without spoilage. Modern processing and packaging extend the shelf life of carbohydrate products for years.

The USDA regularly surveys individual food intake. These reports usually indicate that approximately half of the total kilocalories in the American diet come from carbohydrates, with children consuming somewhat more than adults.[1] Daily intake of grain products by Americans accounts for roughly 39% of total carbohydrate kilocalo-

---

TABLE 2-1

SUMMARY OF CARBOHYDRATE CLASSES

CHEMICAL CLASS NAME	CLASS MEMBERS	SOURCES
Monosaccharides (single sugars, simple carbohydrates)	Glucose (dextrose) Fructose Galactose	Corn syrup (commonly used in processed foods) Fruits, honey Lactose (milk)
Disaccharides (double sugars, simple carbohydrates)	Sucrose Lactose Maltose	Table sugar (sugar cane, sugar beets) Molasses Milk Starch digestion, intermediate Sweetener in food products Starch digestion, final
Polysaccharides (multiple sugars, complex carbohydrates)	Starch Glycogen	Grains and grain products (cereal, bread, crackers, baked goods) Rice, corn, bulgur Legumes Potatoes and other vegetables Storage form of carbohydrate in animal tissue (not a dietary source)

Illustrations from Mahan LK, Escott-Stump S: *Krause's food, nutrition, & diet therapy,* ed 11, Philadelphia, 2004, Saunders.

ries. An equal proportion of kilocalories comes from added sugars and sweeteners, with the remainder of the carbohydrate kilocalories coming from dairy, fruit, and vegetable products.[2]

Classes of Carbohydrates

The term *carbohydrate* comes from its chemical nature. A carbohydrate is composed of carbon (C), hydrogen (H), and oxygen (O). Its abbreviated name, CHO, which is the combination of the chemical symbols of its three components, often is used in medical charts or various notations. The term saccharide is used as a carbohydrate class name and comes from the Latin word *saccharum*, meaning sugar. Thus a saccharide unit is a single sugar unit. Carbohydrates are classified according to the number of sugar, or saccharide, units making up their structure: *mono*saccharides have one sugar unit; *di*saccharides have two sugar units; and *poly*saccharides have many sugar units. Monosaccharides and disaccharides are small, simple structures of only one- and two-sugar units, so they are called simple carbohydrates. However, polysaccharides are large, complex compounds of many saccharide units in long chains; thus they are called complex carbohydrates. For example, starch, the most significant polysaccharide in human nutrition, is composed of many coiled and branching chains in a treelike structure. Each of the multiple branching chains is composed of 24 to 30 sugar units of glucose, which gradually split off in digestion to supply a steady source of energy over time. Table 2-1 summarizes these classes of carbohydrates.

Monosaccharides

The three single sugars in nutrition are glucose, fructose, and galactose. Monosaccharides, the building blocks for all carbohydrates, require no further digestion. They are quickly absorbed from the intestine into the blood stream and carried to the liver. In the liver, they are stored as glycogen for a constant backup energy supply or used for immediate energy needs.

Glucose. The basic single sugar in body metabolism is glucose, which is the form of sugar circulating in the blood and is the primary fuel for cells. It usually is not found as such in the diet, except in corn syrup used alone or in processed food items. The body supply mainly comes from the digestion of starch. Glucose is a moderately sweet sugar. Glucose also is called *dextrose* to denote the structure of the molecule (six carbons).

Fructose. Fructose is mainly found in fruits, from which it gets its name, or in honey. Although honey is sometimes thought of as a sugar substitute, it is a sugar itself; therefore it cannot be considered a substitute. The

amount of fructose in fruits depends on the degree of ripeness. As a fruit ripens, some of its stored starch turns to sugar. Fructose is the sweetest of the simple sugars.

High-fructose corn syrups, manufactured by changing the glucose in cornstarch to fructose, are increasingly being used in processed food products, canned and frozen fruits, and soft drinks. It is an inexpensive sweetener and a major source of increased sugar intake in the United States. Per capita consumption of high-fructose corn syrup has increased from 0.12 tsp daily in 1970 to 12.44 tsp daily in 2004 (Figure 2-1).[3]

Galactose. Galactose usually is not found as a free monosaccharide in the diet; it mainly comes from the digestion of milk sugar, or lactose.

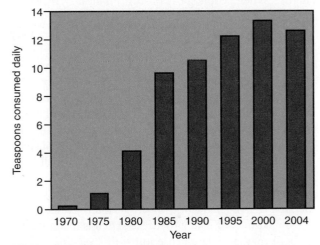

Figure 2-1 High-fructose corn sweetener consumption per capita from 1970 to 2004. (From USDA/Economic Research Service: *High fructose corn sweetener [HFCS]: per capita consumption adjusted for loss, www.ers.usda.gov/Data/FoodConsumption/FoodGuideIndex.htm,* accessed July 2006.)

saccharide chemical name for sugar molecules. May occur as single molecules in monosaccharides (glucose, fructose, galactose), two molecules in disaccharides (sucrose, lactose, maltose), or multiple molecules in polysaccharides (starch, dietary fiber, glycogen).

simple carbohydrates sugars with a simple structure of one or two single-sugar (saccharide) units. A monosaccharide is composed of one sugar unit; a disaccharide is composed of two sugar units.

complex carbohydrates large, complex molecules of carbohydrates composed of many sugar units (polysaccharides). Complex forms of dietary carbohydrates are starch, which is digestible and provides a major energy source, and dietary fiber, which is indigestible (human beings lack the necessary enzymes) and thus provides important bulk in the diet.

Disaccharides

Disaccharides are simple double sugars composed of two single-sugar units linked together. The three disaccharides important in nutrition are sucrose, lactose, and maltose.

Sucrose = Glucose + Fructose
Lactose = Glucose + Galactose
Maltose = Glucose + Glucose

Sucrose. Sucrose is common table sugar. Its two single-sugar units are glucose and fructose. Sucrose is used in the form of granulated, powdered, or brown sugar and is made from sugar cane or sugar beets. Molasses, a by-product of sugar production, also is a form of sucrose. When people speak of sugar in the diet, they usually mean sucrose.

Lactose. The sugar in milk, formed in mammary glands, is lactose. Its two single-sugar units are glucose and galactose. Lactose is the only common sugar not found in plants. It is less soluble and less sweet than sucrose. Lactose remains in the intestine longer than other sugars and encourages the growth of certain useful bacteria. Cow's milk contains 4.8% lactose, and human milk contains 7% lactose. Because lactose aids in the absorption of calcium and phosphorus, the presence of all three nutrients in milk is a fortunate circumstance.

Maltose. Maltose usually is not found as such in the diet. It is derived in the body from the intermediate digestive breakdown of starch. Because starch is made up entirely of many single-glucose units, the two single-sugar units that compose maltose are both glucose. Synthetically derived maltose is used as a sweetener in various processed foods.

Polysaccharides

Polysaccharides are complex carbohydrates composed of many single-sugar units. The important polysaccharides in nutrition include starch, glycogen, and dietary fiber.

Starch. Starches are by far the most significant polysaccharides in the diet. They are found in grains, legumes and other vegetables, and some fruits in minute amounts. Starches are more complex in structure than simple sugars. Thus they break down more slowly and supply energy over a longer period. For starch to be used more promptly by the body, the outer membrane can be broken down by grinding or cooking. Cooking starch improves its flavor and also softens and ruptures the starch cells, making digestion easier. Starch mixtures thicken when cooked because the portion that encases the starch granules has a gel-like quality, thickening the starch mixture in the same way that pectin causes jelly to set.

Starch is the most important dietary carbohydrate worldwide. The DRIs (see Chapter 1) recommend that 45% to 65% of total kilocalories consumed come from carbohydrates, with a greater portion of that intake coming from complex carbohydrates.[4] In countries where starch is the staple food, it makes up an even higher portion of the diet. The major food sources of starch (Figure 2-2) include grains in the form of cereal, pasta, crackers, bread, and other baked goods; legumes in the form of beans and peas; potatoes, rice, corn, and bulgur; and other vegetables, especially of the root variety.

The term *whole grain* is used for food products such as flours, breads, or cereals produced from unrefined grain, which is grain that still retains its outer bran layers and inner germ and endosperm (Figure 2-3) and their nutrients (dietary fiber, minerals, and vitamins). *Enriched grains* are refined grain products to which key nutrients—usually minerals (e.g., iron) and vitamins (e.g., A, C, D, thiamin, riboflavin, and niacin)—have been added back. Ready-to-eat breakfast cereals usually contain additional nutrients such as vitamins D, E, B_6, and folic acid as well as the minerals phosphorus, magnesium, and zinc. These cereals, which are a favorite breakfast item for children, have become a major source of vitamin and mineral intake.

Glycogen. Glycogen, found in animal muscle tissue, is similar in structure to starch. Glycogen, sometimes called *animal starch,* is not a significant source of carbohydrate in the diet. Rather, it is a carbohydrate formed within the body's tissues and is crucial to the body's metabolism and energy balance. Glycogen is found in the liver and muscles, where it is constantly recycled (broken down to form glucose for immediate energy needs and synthesized for storage in the liver and muscles). These small stores of glycogen help sustain normal blood glucose during short-term fasting periods (e.g., sleep) and provide immediate fuel for muscle action. These reserves also protect cells from depressed metabolic function and injury. The process of blood glucose regulation, with regard to glycogen breakdown, is discussed in greater detail in Chapter 20.

Dietary Fiber. Several types of dietary fiber are polysaccharides. Because human beings lack the necessary enzymes to digest dietary fiber, these substances do not have a direct energy value like other carbohydrates. However, their inability to be digested makes these materials important dietary assets. Increasing attention has focused on the relation of fiber to health promotion and disease prevention, especially to gastrointestinal (GI) problems, cardiovascular disease, and the management of diabetes.[5-7]

As a means of simplification, dietary fiber usually is divided into two groups on the basis of solubility. Cellu-

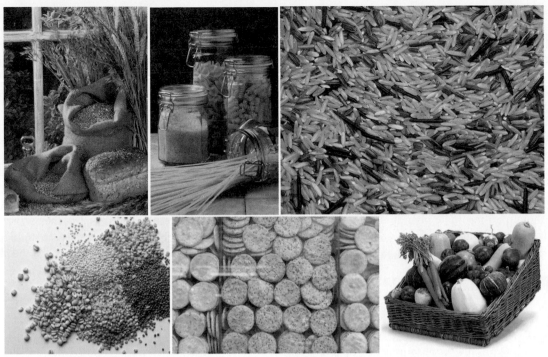

Figure 2-2 Complex carbohydrate foods. (Copyright JupiterImages Corporation.)

lose, lignin, and most hemicelluloses are not soluble in water. The rest of the dietary fibers (e.g., most pectins and other polysaccharides, such as gums and mucilages), however, are water soluble. These two classes of dietary fiber are summarized in Box 2-1. The looser physical structure and greater water-holding capacity of gums, mucilages, pectins, and algal polysaccharides (e.g., those

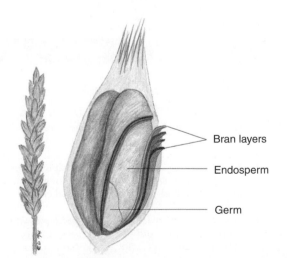

Figure 2-3 Kernel of wheat showing bran layers, endosperm, and germ. (Courtesy Eileen Draper.)

Bran layers

Endosperm

Germ

BOX 2-1

SUMMARY OF SOLUBLE AND INSOLUBLE FIBERS

Insoluble
Cellulose
Most hemicelluloses
Lignin

Soluble
Gums
Mucilages
Algal polysaccharides
Most pectins

derived from seaweed) partly account for their greater water solubility. Recommendations for specific types of fiber to consume often are based on the water solubility distinction. Soluble fiber is noted for its ability to bind bile acids and thus lower blood cholesterol levels. Insoluble fiber, on the other hand, is recommended for relief from constipation. The types of dietary fiber important in human nutrition are described below.

Cellulose. Cellulose is the chief part of the framework of plants. It remains undigested in the GI tract and provides important bulk to the diet. This bulk helps move the food mass along, stimulates normal muscle action in the intestine, and forms feces for elimination of waste products. The main sources of cellulose are the stems and leaves of vegetables and the coverings of seeds and grains. Within the same area of the plant, phosphorus is stored in the form of phytic acid—a compound undigested in humans because of the lack of a necessary enzyme (phytase). Phytic acid is a strong chelator of important minerals (see the Drug-Nutrient Interaction box, "Phytic Acid and Mineral Absorption").

Lignin. Lignin, the only noncarbohydrate type of dietary fiber, is a large compound that forms the woody part of certain plants. It binds the cellulose fibers in plants, giving added strength and stiffness to plant cell walls. Although an insoluble fiber, it also combines with bile acids and cholesterol in the human intestine, preventing their absorption.

Noncellulose Polysaccharides. Hemicellulose, pectins, gums and mucilages, and algal substances are noncellulose polysaccharides. They absorb water and swell to a larger bulk, thus slowing the emptying of the food mass from the stomach, binding bile acids (including cholesterol)[8] in the intestine, and preventing spastic colon pressure by providing bulk for normal muscle action. Noncellulose polysaccharides also provide fermentation material on which colon bacteria can work.

Table 2-2 provides a summary of these dietary fiber classes along with the sources and functions of each.

In general, the food groups that provide needed dietary fiber include whole grains, legumes, vegetables, and fruits in their many food forms with as much of their skin remaining as possible. Whole grains provide a special natural "package" of both the complex carbohydrate starch and the fiber in its

DRUG-NUTRIENT INTERACTION

PHYTIC ACID AND MINERAL ABSORPTION

Some compounds naturally found in food bind minerals, making them unavailable for absorption. Phytic acid is one such compound found in legumes, wheat bran, and seeds. Iron also is naturally found in these foods, but because of the phytic acid interference as little as 2% of the available iron is absorbed.

This can especially be a problem in the developing world.* A diet that consists of high-fiber foods containing phytic acid and a low intake of iron-rich foods such as meat and poultry may exacerbate iron deficiency.

In the developed world, including the United States, iron deficiency is rarely seen from this cause. However, iron deficiency is still common in pregnant and premenopausal women. If the anemia is severe enough, a physician may prescribe an iron supplement. Intake of foods containing

high amounts of phytic acid with the supplement would inhibit iron absorption just as it would if the iron were part of the food.

Phytic acid binds to other minerals that have a similar charge as iron, namely calcium, magnesium, and zinc. Calcium supplements are often prescribed for those who may be losing bone mass, such as postmenopausal women, or those who do not get enough calcium in the diet, such as teens and the elderly. Food sources of phytic acid eaten with calcium supplements may inhibit absorption. When recommending patients take an iron or calcium supplement, also advise them to take the supplement with non-phytate-containing foods.

Sara Oldroyd

*Coutinho GG and others: Iron deficiency anemia in children: a challenge for public health and for society, *Sao Paulo Med J* 123(2):88, 2005.

TABLE 2-2

SUMMARY OF DIETARY FIBER CLASSES

DIETARY FIBER CLASS	SOURCE	FUNCTION
Cellulose	Main cell wall constituent of plants (stalks and leaves of vegetables, outer covering of seeds)	Holds water; reduces elevated colonic intraluminal pressure
Noncellulose polysaccharides		Slow gastric emptying; provide fermentable material for colonic bacteria with production of gas and volatile fatty acids; bind bile acids and cholesterol
Gums and mucilages	Secretions of plants and seeds	
Algal polysaccharides	Algae, seaweeds	
Pectin substances	Intercellular plant material (fruit)	
Hemicellulose	Cell wall plant material (bran and whole grains)	Hold water and increase stool bulk; reduce elevated colonic pressure; bind bile acids
Lignin	Woody part of plants (broccoli stems and fruits with edible seeds, such as strawberries and flaxseeds)	Antioxidant; binds bile acids, cholesterol, and metals

CLINICAL APPLICATIONS

CASE STUDY: IDENTIFYING CARBOHYDRATES AND FIBER

A patient comes to you for dietary analysis. He is trying to eat a diet consistent with the dietary guidelines of 45% to 65% carbohydrate and 38 g of dietary fiber per day. Based on his 1-day diet, answer the questions that follow regarding his dietary analysis.

Breakfast:
- 2 cups Cheerios
- 1.25 cups skim milk
- 1 medium banana
- 16 oz coffee with 1 Tbsp sugar and 2 Tbsp whole milk creamer

Lunch:
- Turkey sandwich (2 slices whole-wheat bread, 3 oz lean turkey, 1 oz cheddar cheese, 1 slice tomato, 2 lettuce leaves, 2 tsp yellow mustard, and ½ Tbsp mayonnaise)
- 1 oz pretzels
- 1½ cups mixed green salad with 2 Tbsp crushed pecans and 2 Tbsp fat-free Italian dressing
- 20 oz water

Snack:
- 1 medium apple
- 1 package peanut butter crackers (6 crackers)

Dinner:
- 4 oz grilled chicken breast
- ½ cup green beans
- ¾ cup mashed potatoes made with skim milk and butter
- ½ cup roasted red peppers
- 1 whole wheat roll
- 16 oz sweet tea

Questions for Analysis
1. Identify all foods containing carbohydrates.
2. Using the dietary analysis CD-ROM included in this book, or MyPyramid Tracker (*http://.mypyramid.gov*), analyze this 1-day diet to determine:
   a. How many total grams of carbohydrate he consumed
   b. How many grams of sugar he consumed
   c. How many grams of soluble, insoluble, and total fiber he consumed
   d. The percentage of total calories from carbohydrates
3. Did he meet the dietary guidelines for percent of calories from carbohydrates and grams of fiber on this day?
4. What additional recommendations would you make for improvement?

coating. In addition, whole grains contain an abundance of vitamins and minerals (see the Clinical Applications box, "Case Study: Identifying Carbohydrates and Fiber").

Many health organizations have recommended increasing the intake of complex carbohydrates in general and dietary fiber in particular.[4,9] The Food and Nutrition Board has always indicated that a desirable fiber intake should not be exclusively achieved by adding concentrated fiber supplements to the diet but by eating a higher fiber diet of whole grains, fruits, vegetables, and legumes, which also provide vitamins and minerals. The recommended daily intake of fiber for men and women aged 50 years and younger is 38 and 25 g/day, respectively. The DRIs are reduced to 30 and 21 g/day for men and women older than 50 years.[4] This intake requires consistent use of whole grains, legumes, vegetables, fruits, seeds, and nuts. Unfortunately, Americans, on average, do not meet the recommended servings of grains, vegetables, and fruit on a daily basis. The most recent National Health and Nutrition Examination Survey revealed that based on appropriate calorie levels, only 34% of individuals meet the recommended servings of grains and vegetables and a mere 24% consume the recommended fruit servings per day.[10] A table of the dietary fiber content of some commonly used foods is provided in Table 2-3 and Appendix B (see the For Further Focus box, "Fiber: What's All the Fuss About?").

As with many things in nutrition, too much of a good thing also can be problematic. Sudden increases in fiber intake can result in gas, bloating, and constipation. Fiber intake should be gradually increased, along with water intake, to an appropriate amount for the individual. In addition, excessive amounts of dietary fiber can trap small amounts of minerals and prevent their absorption in the GI tract. This function of fiber is beneficial when trapping or binding bile acids, but it may compromise nutritional status if fiber intake greatly exceeds the recommendations to the point of reducing mineral absorption.

Other Sweeteners

Sugar alcohols and alternative sweeteners often are used as a sugar replacement. Sweeteners, such as sugar alco-

chelator a ligand that binds to a metal to form a metal complex.

sugar alcohols nutritive sweeteners that provide 2 to 3 kcal/g; examples include sorbitol, mannitol, and xylitol. Produced in food industry laboratories for use as sweeteners in candies, chewing gum, beverages, and other foods; excess consumption may result in diarrhea.

TABLE 2-3

DIETARY FIBER AND CALORIC VALUE FOR SELECTED FOODS

FOOD	SERVING SIZE	DIETARY FIBER (g)	KILOCALORIES
Breads and Cereals			
All Bran	⅓ cup	13	75
Complete Oat Bran	¾ cup	4	105
Complete Wheat Bran	¾ cup	5	92
Cracklin' Oat Bran	¾ cup	6.4	225
Fiber One	½ cup	14.4	60
Oatmeal	1 cup	4	138
Popcorn, air popped	1 cup	1.2	30
Raisin Bran	½ cup	3.5	94
100% Bran	⅓ cup	8.3	83
Shredded Wheat n' Bran	⅔ cup	4	98
Whole-wheat bread	1 slice	2	69
Fruit			
Apple, raw with skin	1 medium (2¾ inches in diameter)	3.7	81
Apricot	1 medium	0.7	17
Banana	1 medium (7-8 inches long)	2.8	108
Blueberries	½ cup	2	40
Cherries	½ cup	0.8	26
Dates, dried	1	0.6	23
Grapefruit	½ cup pieces	1.25	38
Orange	1 medium (2½ inches in diameter)	3.1	61
Peach	1 medium (2½ inches in diameter)	2	42
Prunes, dried	1	0.6	20
Raisins, seedless	½ cup (not packed)	3	217
Strawberries	½ cup sliced	1.9	25
Legumes			
Black beans	½ cup	7.5	113
Garbanzo beans	½ cup	6.2	134
Kidney beans	½ cup	5.6	112
Lima beans	½ cup	6.5	108
Vegetables			
Asparagus, cooked	½ cup	1.4	21
Black-eyed peas	½ cup	4.1	80
Broccoli, cooked	½ cup	2.3	22
Carrots, raw strips	½ cup	1.8	26
Cauliflower, cooked	½ cup	1.7	14
Corn	½ cup	2.2	88
Green beans (snap beans), cooked	½ cup	2	22
Green peas	½ cup	4.4	67
Potato, baked, with skin	1 medium (2¼-3¼ inches in diameter)	3.8	160
Sweet potato, baked in skin	1 medium (2 × 5 inches)	3.4	117
Tomato, raw, chopped	½ cup	1	19

Data from the USDA, Agricultural Research Service, Nutrient Data Laboratory: *USDA nutrient database for standard reference, release 20,* www.ars. usda.gov/ba/bhnrc/ndl.

FOR FURTHER FOCUS

FIBER: WHAT'S ALL THE FUSS ABOUT?

The National Institutes of Health and World Health Organization, along with most all other health-related agencies in the world, have been promoting the intake of fiber for years. The benefits have been defined in several clinical trials relating to a variety of chronic illnesses.[5-8] However, the average fiber intake in American diets remains at less than half the recommendation. Scientists are confident that consuming adequate amounts of fiber confer the following health benefits:

- Lowers blood cholesterol levels
- Promotes normal bowel function and movements and prevents constipation
- Increases satiety, which aids in obesity prevention
- Protects against colon cancer

- Slows glucose absorption, thereby reducing blood glucose spikes and reducing insulin secretion
- Prevents and helps manage diverticulosis

Health professionals can assist the public in evaluating their fiber intake by educating and encouraging the use of food labels. Food labels list the total dietary fiber found in each serving of food. Manufacturers also voluntarily list the specific type of fiber (soluble and/or insoluble). Increases in dietary fiber intake should be made gradually and with extra attention to fluid intake. A sudden boost in dietary fiber can lead to uncomfortable bloating, gas, and cramping. This can be avoided by making small changes over time with an appropriate fluid intake of 8 glasses of water per day.

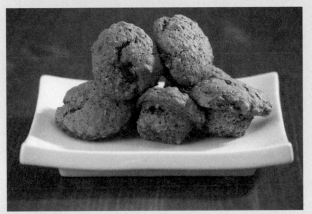

(Copyright JupiterImages Corporation.)

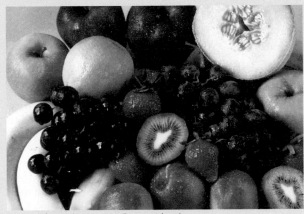

(Copyright JupiterImages Corporation.)

hols, that contribute to total calorie intake are considered nutritive sweeteners. Nonnutritive sweeteners, or alternative sweeteners, are sugar substitutes that do not have any caloric value.

Nutritive Sweeteners. The sugar alcohols (sorbitol, mannitol, and xylitol) are the alcohol forms of sucrose, mannose, and xylose. Sugar alcohols provide 2 to 3 kcal/g, similar to other carbohydrates providing 4 kcal/g. The most well known probably is sorbitol, which has been widely used as a sucrose substitute in various foods, candies, chewing gum, and beverages. Sugar alcohols share absorption with glucose in the small intestine. However, they are absorbed more slowly and do not increase the blood sugar as rapidly as glucose. Therefore sugar alcohols often are used in products intended for individuals who cannot tolerate a high blood sugar level, such as those with diabetes. The downside of using excessive amounts of sugar alcohols in food products is that the slowed digestion may result in diarrhea. The advantage of using a sugar al-

cohol to replace sugar is lowered risk of dental caries because oral bacteria cannot use the alcohol for fuel.

Nonnutritive Sweeteners. Nonnutritive sweeteners are specifically manufactured to be used as alternative, or artificial, sweeteners in food products. Because nonnutritive sweeteners do not supply any kilocalories, they provide the sweet taste without contributing to total energy intake. People typically associate these sweeteners with diet foods. Alternative sweeteners most commonly used in the United States are aspartame, saccharin, and sucralose. Nonnutritive sweeteners are much sweeter than sucrose, or table sugar. Therefore extremely small quanti-

---

sorbitol a sugar alcohol formed in mammals from glucose and converted to fructose. Named for its initial discovery in nature, it is found in ripe berries of the tree Sorbus aucuparia and also occurs in small quantities in various other berries, cherries, plums, and pears.

TABLE 2-4

SWEETNESS OF SUGARS AND ARTIFICIAL SWEETENERS

SUBSTANCE	SWEETNESS VALUE
Sugar or Sugar Product	
Levulose, fructose	173
Invert sugar	130
Sucrose	100
Glucose	74
Sorbitol	60
Mannitol	50
Galactose	32
Maltose	32
Lactose	16
Artificial Sweeteners	
Cyclamate (banned in United States)	30
Aspartame (Nutra-Sweet and Equal)*	180
Acesulfame-K (Sunette and Sweet One)	200
Saccharin (Sweet 'N Low and Sugar Twin)	300
Sucralose (Splenda)	600
Alitame (approval pending)	2000

Reprinted from Mahan LK, Escott-Stump S: *Krause's food & nutrition therapy,* ed 12, Philadelphia, 2008, Saunders.
*Nutritive (has calories).

ties can be used to produce the same sweet taste. Table 2-4 provides a summary of artificial sweeteners and their relative sweetness value compared with table sugar.

FUNCTIONS OF CARBOHYDRATES

Primary Energy Function

Basic Fuel Supply

The main function of carbohydrates is to provide fuel for the body. Carbohydrates burn in the body at the rate of 4 kcal/g; thus, the fuel factor for carbohydrates is 4. Carbohydrates furnish readily available energy needed for physical activities as well as the work of the body cells. Fat also is a fuel, but the body only needs a small amount of dietary fat, mainly to supply the essential fatty acids (see Chapter 3).

Reserve Fuel Supply

The total amount of carbohydrate in the body, including both stored glycogen and blood sugar, is relatively small. Without refueling, the total amount of available glucose only provides enough energy for approximately a half-day of moderate activity. Therefore to maintain a normal blood glucose level and prevent a breakdown of fat and protein in tissue, individuals must eat carbohydrate foods regularly to meet energy demands.

Special Tissue Functions

Carbohydrates also serve special functions in many body tissues and organs.

Liver

Glycogen reserves in the liver and muscle tissue provide a constant exchange with the body's overall energy balance system. These reserves, especially in the liver, protect cells from depressed metabolic function and resulting injury.

Protein and Fat

Carbohydrates help regulate both protein and fat metabolism. If dietary carbohydrate is sufficient to meet general body energy needs, protein does not have to be broken down to supply energy. This *protein-sparing action* of carbohydrate protects protein, allowing it to be used for its major role in tissue growth and maintenance. Likewise, with sufficient carbohydrate for energy, fat is not needed to supply large amounts of energy. Such a rapid breakdown of fat would produce excess materials called *ketones,* a product of incomplete fat oxidation in the cells. Ketones are strong acids. The condition of acidosis, or *ketosis,* upsets the normal acid-base balance of the body and can become serious. This protective action of carbohydrate is called its *antiketogenic* effect.

Heart

The constant action of the heart muscle sustains life. Although fatty acids are the preferred fuel for the heart muscle, glycogen is a vital emergency fuel. In a damaged heart, low glycogen stores or inadequate carbohydrate intake may cause symptoms of cardiac disorder and angina.

Central Nervous System

Constant carbohydrate intake and reserves are necessary for proper functioning of the central nervous system (CNS). The master center of the CNS, the brain, has no stored supply of glucose; therefore it is especially dependent on a minute-to-minute supply of glucose from the blood. Sustained and profound shock from low blood sugar may cause brain damage and can result in coma and/or death.

FOOD SOURCES OF CARBOHYDRATES

Starches

Starches are the central type of food for a balanced diet. In unrefined forms, they also provide important sources of fiber and other nutrients. Table 2-5 outlines the carbohydrate content of commonly consumed foods.

TABLE 2-5

CARBOHYDRATE CONTENT OF FOODS (GRAMS PER SERVING)

FOOD SOURCE	SERVING SIZE	GRAMS OF CARBOHYDRATE	TOTAL KILOCALORIES
Concentrated Sweets			
Sugar:			
Granulated	1 tsp	4.2	16
Powdered	1 tsp	2.49	10
Brown	1 tsp, packed	4.48	17
Maple	1 tsp	2.73	11
Honey	1 Tbsp	17.3	64
Syrup:			
High-fructose corn	1 Tbsp	14.44	53
Maple	1 Tbsp	13.42	52
Jam and Preserves	1 Tbsp	13.77	56
Carbonated beverage, cola (containing caffeine)	12 oz	35.18	136
Candy:			
Starburst fruit chews	1 package (2.07 oz)	49.85	234
Gummy bears	10 pieces	21.76	87
Skittles	1 package (2 oz)	51.66	231
Baked goods:			
Doughnut, glazed	1 medium (3-inch diameter)	22.86	192
Butter cookie	1 medium (1 oz)	19.53	132
Brownie	1 square (1 oz)	18.12	115
Fruit			
Apple, with skin	1 medium (2¾-inch diameter)	19.06	72
Banana	1 medium (7.5 inches long)	26.95	105
Cherries, sweet, raw	15 cherries	16.33	64
Orange	1 medium (2½-inch diameter)	15.39	62
Pineapple	1 slice (3½-inch diameter × ¾-inch thick)	10.6	40
Strawberries	10 medium (1¼-inch diameter)	9.22	38
Dried fruit, mixed (prune, apricot, pear)	1 package (5.5 oz)	93.85	356
Vegetables			
Beans, kidney, cooked	½ cup	19.34	109
Carrots, raw	½ cup chopped, raw	6.13	26
Corn, sweet, yellow, cooked	½ cup, drained	20.59	89
Lettuce, green leaf, raw	1 cup shredded	1	5
Potato, with skin, baked	1 medium (2¼-3¼-inch diameter)	36.59	161
Squash, summer	½ cup cooked slices	3.88	18
Tomatoes, red, raw	½ medium (2⅗-inch diameter)	2.4	11
Dairy Products			
Milk:			
Skim	1 cup	12.15	88
2%	1 cup	13.5	138
Whole	1 cup	11.03	146
Cheese:			
Cheddar	½ cup, shredded	0.72	228
Cottage, 2% milk fat	½ cup	4.1	102

Data from the USDA, Agricultural Research Service, Nutrient Data Laboratory: *USDA nutrient database for standard reference, release 20, www.ars. usda.gov/ba/bhnrc/ndl.*

Continued

TABLE 2-5

CARBOHYDRATE CONTENT OF FOODS (GRAMS PER SERVING)—cont'd

FOOD SOURCE	SERVING SIZE	GRAMS OF CARBOHYDRATE	TOTAL KILOCALORIES
Grain Products			
Bread:			
White	1 slice	12.6	66
Rye	1 slice	15.46	83
Wheat	1 slice	11.8	65
Cereal (dry):			
Corn flakes	1 cup	24.28	101
Wheat, shredded, presweetened	1 cup	43.58	183
Rice, puffed	1 cup	12.57	56
Cereal (cooked):			
Oatmeal, cooked with water	1 cup	25.27	147
Wheat, cooked with water	1 cup	32.96	160
Grits, corn, cooked with water	1 cup	31.15	143
Crackers, saltines	5	10.72	65
Pasta, cooked	1 cup	39.07	176
Rice:			
White	½ cup, cooked	26.59	121
Brown	½ cup, cooked	22.92	109

Data from the USDA, Agricultural Research Service, Nutrient Data Laboratory: *USDA nutrient database for standard reference, release 20, www.ars. usda.gov/ba/bhnrc/ndl.*

Sugars

Sugar per se is not the villain in the story of health. The problem lies in the large quantities of sugar that many people consume, often to the exclusion of other important foods. The average American consumes approximately 10 Tbsp of added sugar per day.[11] As with most things, moderation is the key (see the For Further Focus box, "The Carb Confusion Continues").

DIGESTION OF CARBOHYDRATES

Mouth

The digestion of carbohydrate foods, starches, and sugars begins in the mouth and progresses through the successive parts of the GI tract, accomplished by two types of actions: (1) mechanical or muscle functions that break the food mass into smaller particles and (2) chemical processes in which specific enzymes break down the food nutrients into still smaller usable metabolic products. The chewing of food, a process called *mastication,* breaks food into fine particles and mixes it with saliva. During this process, the salivary enzyme *salivary amylase* (also referred to as *ptyalin*) is secreted by the *parotid* glands, which lie under each ear at the back of the jaw. Salivary amylase acts on starch to begin its breakdown into dextrins (i.e., intermediate starch breakdown products) and disaccharides (primarily maltose). Carbohydrates eaten in the form of monosaccharides travel to the stomach and small intestines for absorption without further digestion.

Stomach

Wavelike contractions of the muscle fibers of the stomach continue the mechanical digestive process. This action, called *peristalsis,* further mixes food particles with gastric secretions to facilitate chemical digestion. The gastric secretions contain no specific enzyme for the breakdown of carbohydrates. Hydrochloric acid in the stomach stops the action of salivary amylase in the food mass. Before the food completely mixes with the acidic stomach secretions, however, up to 20% to 30% of the starch may have been changed to maltose. Muscle action continues to mix the food mass and move it to the lower part of the stomach. Here the food mass is a thick creamy *chyme,* ready for its controlled emptying through the *pyloric valve* into the *duodenum,* the first portion of the small intestine.

FOR FURTHER FOCUS

THE CARB CONFUSION CONTINUES

Glycemic Index

The glycemic index, developed by researchers at the University of Toronto in 1987, initially was thought to be an ideal tool for controlling blood glucose levels, specifically for individuals with diabetes. The use of this tool, however, has been less than promising and quite controversial in recent years.

The glycemic index ranks foods according to how fast blood glucose levels rise after consuming a specific amount (50 g) when compared with a reference food such as white bread or pure glucose. The higher glycemic index rankings are associated with higher peaks in blood sugar within 2 hours of eating the food and vice versa for low glycemic index rankings.

The claim that consuming only foods low on the glycemic index will control appetite, manage blood glucose, and promote weight loss currently is not supported by research. The primary reason why this tool is unsupported is because of its high variability. The glycemic index of a food can very significantly in the following ways:

- Between person to person
- From one time of day to another
- When a food is eaten alone versus with other foods
- Depending on the ripeness, its variety, cooking method used, degree of processing, and site of origin
- With the quantity of food eaten

Additionally, the glycemic index of a food does not indicate the nutritious quality of the food. For example, soft drinks, candies, sugars, and high-fat foods such as hot dogs all qualify as low glycemic index foods.

In light of such controversy, the American Dietetic Association continues to recommend that people with diabetes monitor total grams of carbohydrates and use the concept of the glycemic index to fine tune their food choices.

Net Carbs

Food manufacturers invented a new category of carbohydrates called "net carbs" as a marketing ploy to capitalize on the low-carb diet craze. The Food and Drug Administration regulates all information provided in the Nutrition Facts label, including total carbohydrates, dietary fiber, and sugars, and does not acknowledge or approve of the net carb category.

The concept was derived from the controversial use of the glycemic index. Because dietary fiber and sugar alcohols have a lower impact on blood glucose levels after eating than do other high glycemic index foods, these sources of carbohydrates have simply been subtracted from existence as far as net carbs are concerned. For example, a food may have 30 g of total carbohydrates, 18 g of sugar alcohols, and 3 g of fiber, thus leaving 9 net carbs, also referred to as impact carbs or active carbs.

Problems with this mode of thinking include the following:

- Sugar alcohols do have calories and can raise blood sugar.
- Excessive use of sugar alcohols in foods has not been studied, but this type of labeling encourages manufacturers to increase the use of products such as sorbitol to lower their net carb claim.
- Excess sugar alcohols can cause diarrhea.
- The idea of zero net carbs does not explain the fact that the food still has calories.

Bottom line, the FDA maintains that regarding weight management, no substitute exists for the formula of "calories in must equal calories out." Total calories count more than the quantity, or lack thereof, of high glycemic index carbohydrates, low glycemic index carbohydrates, or net carbohydrates.

Small Intestine

Peristalsis continues to aid digestion in the small intestine by mixing and moving the chyme along the length of the tube. Chemical digestion of carbohydrate is completed in the small intestine by specific enzymes from both the pancreas and intestine.

Pancreatic Secretions

Secretions from the *pancreas* enter the duodenum through the common bile duct. These secretions contain the starch enzyme *pancreatic amylase* for continued breakdown of starch to disaccharides and monosaccharides.

enzymes proteins produced in cells that digest or change nutrients in specific chemical reactions without being changed themselves in the process. Their action is therefore that of a catalyst. Digestive enzymes in GI secretions act on food substances to break them down into simpler compounds. An enzyme usually is named according to the substance (substrate) on which it acts, with the common word ending of -ase; for example, sucrase is the specific enzyme for sucrose, which it breaks down into glucose and fructose.

Intestinal Secretions

Enzymes from the brush border (microvilli) of the intestinal tract contain three disaccharidases: *sucrase, lactase,* and *maltase.* These specific enzymes act on their respective disaccharides to render the monosaccharides—glucose, galactose, and fructose—ready for absorption directly into the portal blood circulation.

Lactose intolerance, the inability to break lactose down into its monosaccharide units (glucose and galactose), results from a lack of the enzyme lactase. Symptoms include bloating, gas, abdominal pain, and diarrhea. Lactose intolerance affects approximately 75% of adults worldwide, with a much higher prevalence in some countries and ethnic groups (see the Cultural Considerations box, "Ethnicity and Lactose Intolerance").

A summary of the major aspects of carbohydrate digestion through the successive parts of the GI tract is shown in Figure 2-4. The overall processes of absorption and metabolism of all energy-yielding nutrients together (carbohydrate, fat, and protein) are discussed in Chapter 5.

RECOMMENDATIONS FOR DIETARY CARBOHYDRATE

Dietary Reference Intakes

In the nutrient standards, energy needs are listed as total kilocalories, which includes caloric intake from fat and protein as well as carbohydrate. According to the most recent DRIs, 45% to 65% of an adult's total caloric intake should come from carbohydrate foods.[4] This translates to 225 to 325 g of carbohydrates for a 2000-kcal/day diet. The recommended fiber intake can be achieved by choosing carbohydrate foods consisting of whole-grain cereals, legumes, vegetables, and fruits, which also provide minerals and vitamins. In addition, the DRIs recommend limiting added sugar to no more than 25% of total calories consumed. See the Clinical Applications box, "What Is Your Dietary Reference Intake for Carbohydrates?" to calculate specific carbohydrate recommendations.

CULTURAL CONSIDERATIONS

ETHNICITY AND LACTOSE INTOLERANCE

Lactose intolerance or malabsorption results when the enzyme necessary for lactose digestion is absent or deficient from the brush border cells of the small intestine, a condition known as hypolactasia. If the disaccharide lactose cannot be hydrolyzed to its respective monosaccharides (glucose and galactose), the unabsorbed sugar attracts excess fluid into the gut. Lactose then entering into the large intestine can be partially metabolized by normal bacteria found in the colon, thus producing large amounts of gas.

In the United States, several ethnic groups have significantly higher rates of lactose intolerance than do Americans from northern European decent. Approximately 80% of African Americans, 80% to 100% of American Indians, and 90% to 100% of Asian Americans endure some level of lactose intolerance compared with 2% to 15% of persons from northern European decent.* Other ethnic groups commonly experiencing discomfort caused by the lack of lactase are Hispanics (50% to 80% intolerant) and Jews (60% to 80% intolerant). The Swiss, Swedish, and northern and central Europeans have significantly less trouble with lactose digestion; less than 20% of their populations report any discomfort.

Individuals with lactose intolerance can usually tolerate some low-lactose milk products such as cheese. Lactose intolerance is not an allergy. Most affected individuals can handle varying levels of lactose in their diet. The amount tolerated varies and should be explored by gradually introducing small amounts of lactose-containing foods into the diet while keeping note of any side effects. In general, the equivalent of 8 oz of milk can be tolerated before symptoms arise in most people. The strong genetic link to lactose intolerance indicates little chance is likely for a drastic change in response to dietary lactose over a lifetime. However, many individuals do experience slight changes. Most people become more intolerant with age, whereas others are able to gradually accept more.

*National Digestive Diseases Clearinghouse, National Institute of Diabetes and Digestive and Kidney Diseases, National Institutes of Health: *Lactose intolerance, www.niddk.nih.gov/health/digest/pubs/lactose/lactose.htm,* accessed June 2007.

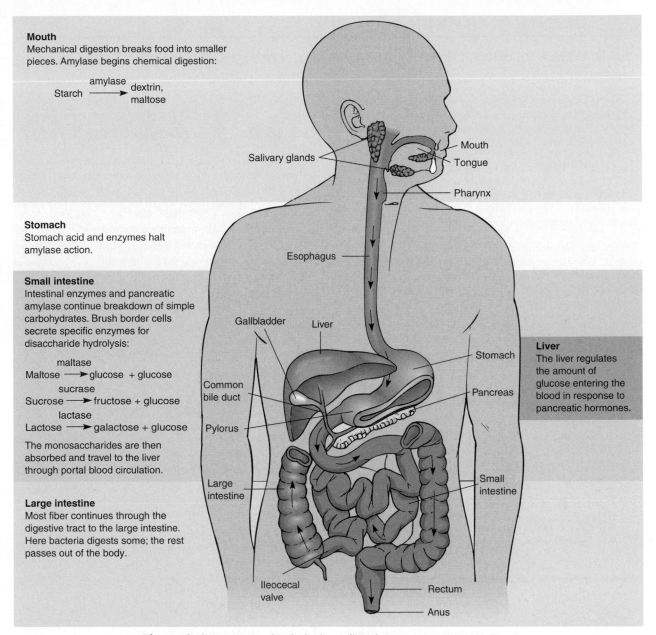

Mouth
Mechanical digestion breaks food into smaller pieces. Amylase begins chemical digestion:

$$\text{Starch} \xrightarrow{\text{amylase}} \text{dextrin, maltose}$$

Stomach
Stomach acid and enzymes halt amylase action.

Small intestine
Intestinal enzymes and pancreatic amylase continue breakdown of simple carbohydrates. Brush border cells secrete specific enzymes for disaccharide hydrolysis:

$$\text{Maltose} \xrightarrow{\text{maltase}} \text{glucose} + \text{glucose}$$
$$\text{Sucrose} \xrightarrow{\text{sucrase}} \text{fructose} + \text{glucose}$$
$$\text{Lactose} \xrightarrow{\text{lactase}} \text{galactose} + \text{glucose}$$

The monosaccharides are then absorbed and travel to the liver through portal blood circulation.

Large intestine
Most fiber continues through the digestive tract to the large intestine. Here bacteria digests some; the rest passes out of the body.

Liver
The liver regulates the amount of glucose entering the blood in response to pancreatic hormones.

Salivary glands
Mouth
Tongue
Pharynx
Esophagus
Gallbladder
Liver
Stomach
Common bile duct
Pancreas
Pylorus
Large intestine
Small intestine
Ileocecal valve
Rectum
Anus

Figure 2-4 Summary of carbohydrate digestion. (Courtesy Rolin Graphics.)

Dietary Guidelines for Americans

The *Dietary Guidelines for Americans* are general guidelines to promote health; therefore they do not outline specifics in terms of calorie consumption or where those kilocalories should come from. Instead, the *Guidelines* advise individuals to do the following[9]:

- Choose fiber-rich fruits, vegetables, and whole grains often.
- Choose and prepare foods and beverages with little added sugars or caloric sweeteners, such as the amounts suggested by the USDA Food Guide and

brush border cells located on the microvilli within the lining of the intestinal tract. The microvilli are tiny hair-like projections that protrude from the mucosal cells that help increase surface area for the digestion and absorption of nutrients.

portal an entrance or gateway; for example, the portal blood circulation designates the entry of blood vessels from the intestines into the liver, carrying nutrients for major liver metabolism, then draining into the body's main systemic circulation to deliver metabolic products to body cells.

CLINICAL APPLICATIONS

WHAT IS YOUR DIETARY REFERENCE INTAKE FOR CARBOHYDRATES?

Based on the current DRIs, calculate the amount of calories and grams of carbohydrates you are recommended to consume on a daily basis. This requires you to know how many total calories you consume on a daily basis.

Step 1: Keep track of everything you eat for 1 day. You can use the CD-ROM included with this book to calculate your daily food intake. This is your *total energy intake.* (Chapter 6 discusses the evaluation of total energy intake relative to weight.)

Step 2: Total energy intake = _____ kcal.

Step 3: Multiply your total energy intake by 45% (0.45) and 65% (0.65) to get the recommended number of *kilocalories from carbohydrates*. The DRIs recommend consuming a minimum intake of 130 g of nutrient-dense carbohydrates per day.

$$\text{\_\_\_ total kcal} \times 0.45 = \text{\_\_\_ kcal}$$
$$\text{\_\_\_ total kcal} \times 0.65 = \text{\_\_\_ kcal}$$

Example:

$$2200 \text{ total kcal} \times 0.45 = 990 \text{ kcal}$$
$$2200 \text{ total kcal} \times 0.65 = 1430 \text{ kcal}$$

Recommended range of total kilocalories from CHO = 990−1430 kcal/day

How many *grams of CHO* do you need based on these recommendations?

Step 4: Divide your recommended range of kilocalories from CHO by 4. Each gram of CHO has 4 kcal.

$$\text{\_\_\_ kcal/day from CHO/4} = \text{\_\_\_ g of CHO/day}$$

Example:

$$990 - 1430 \text{ kcal/day from CHO/4} =$$
$$247.5 - 357.5 \text{ g of CHO/day}$$

Recommended range of total grams of CHO for this example = 247.5−357.5 g of CHO/day

What is the maximum amount of total kilocalorie consumption that can come from *added sugars,* according to the DRIs? Added sugars are added to food and beverages during production. The majority of added sugars in American diets come from candy, soft drinks, fruit drinks, pastries, and other sweets. The DRIs recommend limiting added sugar intake to no more than 25% of total kilocalories consumed.

Step 5: Multiply your total energy intake by 25% (0.25) to get the maximum number of *kilocalories from added sugars*.

$$\text{\_\_\_ total kcal} \times 0.25 = \text{\_\_\_ kcal}$$

Example:

$$2200 \text{ total kcal} \times 0.25 = 550 \text{ kcal}$$

Maximum amount of total kilocalories from added sugar = 550 kcal/day

Step 6: Determine how many grams of added sugar by dividing the maximum kcal/day of added sugar by 4.

$$\text{\_\_\_ kcal/day from added sugar/4} = \text{\_\_\_ g of added sugar/day}$$

Example:

$$550 \text{ kcal/day from added sugar/4} = 137.5 \text{ g of added sugar/day}$$

Therefore the 137.5 g of added sugar is the recommended *limit* per day.

http://MyPyramid.gov is a helpful resource to assess your diet quality with the MyPyramid Tracker.

---

the Dietary Approaches to Stop Hypertension Eating Plan.

■ Reduce the incidence of dental caries by practicing good oral hygiene and consuming sugar- and starch-containing foods and beverages less frequently.

MyPyramid

The MyPyramid food guidance system provides recommendations specific to age, gender, height, weight, and physical activity when reported on the MyPyramid Plan (see Figure 1-1). Once this basic information is entered, the system will produce a plan with recommendations for each of the food groups. Other helpful information

found on the Web site *(www.mypyramid.gov)* includes the following [12]:

■ Tips for consuming more whole grains, fruits, and vegetables
■ Serving size information
■ Health benefits and nutrients associated with each food group
■ Sample menus

In addition, the MyPyramid Tracker is an assessment tool that allows the user to enter his or her own menu for evaluation of diet quality. This is a great resource for feedback on dietary sources of carbohydrate, including fiber, whole grain, fruits, vegetables, and added sugar consumption.

SUMMARY

The primary source of energy for most of the world's population comes from carbohydrate foods. These foods are from widely distributed plant sources such as grains, legumes, vegetables, and fruits. For the most part, these food products store easily and are relatively low in cost.

Two basic types of carbohydrates supply energy: simple and complex. Simple carbohydrates are single- and double-sugar units (monosaccharides and disaccharides). Because simple carbohydrates are easy to digest and absorb, they provide quick energy. Complex carbohydrates, or polysaccharides, are composed of many sugar units. They break down more slowly and thus provide sustained energy over a longer period.

Dietary fiber in most of its forms is a complex carbohydrate that is not digestible by humans. It mainly oc-curs as the structural parts of plants and provides important bulk in the diet, affects nutrient absorption, and benefits health.

Carbohydrate digestion starts briefly in the mouth with the initial action of salivary amylase to begin breaking down starch into smaller units. No enzyme for starch breakdown is present in the stomach, but muscle action continues to mix the food mass and move it to the small intestine, where pancreatic amylase continues the chemical digestion. Final starch and disaccharide digestion occurs in the small intestine with the action of specific enzymes (sucrase, lactase, and maltase) to produce single-sugar units of glucose, fructose, and galactose, which are then directly absorbed into the portal blood circulation to the liver.

CRITICAL THINKING QUESTIONS

1. Why are carbohydrates the predominant type of food in the world's diets? Give some basic examples of these carbohydrate foods.
2. How would you describe each of the main classes of carbohydrates in terms of general nature, functions, and main food sources to an individual who comes to you for advice on a no- or low-carbohydrate diet?
3. Compare starches and sugars as a basic fuel. Why are complex carbohydrates a significant part of a healthy diet? What is the recommendation about the use of sugars in such a diet? Why?
4. Describe the types and functions of dietary fiber. What are the main food sources? How would you recommend increasing dietary fiber consumption, and how much per day would you recommend for an adult?
5. What is glycogen? Why is it a vital tissue carbohydrate?

CHAPTER CHALLENGE QUESTIONS

True-False

Write the correct statement for each statement that is false.
1. *True or False:* Carbohydrates are composed of carbon, hydrogen, oxygen, and nitrogen.
2. *True or False:* Starch is the main source of carbohydrate in the diet.
3. *True or False:* Lactose is a very sweet, simple monosaccharide found in a number of foods.
4. *True or False:* Glucose is the form of sugar circulating in the blood.
5. *True or False:* Glycogen is an important long-term storage form of energy because large amounts are stored in the liver and muscles.
6. *True or False:* Modern food processing and refinement have reduced dietary fiber.

Multiple Choice

1. Which of the following carbohydrate foods provides energy the *quickest*?
   a. Slice of bread
   b. Oat bran muffin
   c. Milk
   d. Orange juice
2. A quickly available but limited form of energy is stored in the liver by conversion of glucose to

a. glycerol.
b. glycogen.
c. protein.
d. fat.

3. The current DRIs recommend _____ of a person's total daily caloric intake to come from carbohydrate sources.

  a. 5% to 15%
  b. 20% to 35%
  c. 35% to 50%
  d. 45% to 65%

4. Which of the following is not a monosaccharide?

  a. Lactose
  b. Glucose

c. Galactose
d. Fructose

5. The disaccharide sucrose is hydrolyzed to the monosaccharides glucose and

  a. galactose.
  b. glucose.
  c. fructose.
  d. starch.

6. Which type of fiber would be specifically beneficial for someone with elevated blood cholesterol levels?

  a. Soluble
  b. Insoluble

evolve Please refer to the Students' Resource section of this text's Evolve Web site for additional study resources.

References

1. United States Department of Agriculture, Center for Nutrition Policy and Promotion: *U.S. food supply: nutrients and other food components, per capita per day, 1909 to 2004,* www.ers.usda.gov/Data/FoodConsumption/NutrientAvailIndex.htm, accessed June 2007.
2. United States Department of Agriculture, Center for Nutrition Policy and Promotion: *U.S. food supply: nutrients contributed from major food groups, 1970 and 2000,* www.ers.usda.gov/Data/FoodConsumption/NutrientAvailIndex.htm, accessed June 2007.
3. USDA, Economic Research Service: *High fructose corn sweetener (HFCS): per capita consumption adjusted for loss,* www.ers.usda.gov/Data/FoodConsumption/FoodGuideIndex.htm, accessed June 2007.
4. Food and Nutrition Board, Institute of Medicine: *Dietary reference intakes for energy, carbohydrate, fiber, fat, fatty acids, cholesterol, protein, and amino acids,* Washington, DC, 2002, National Academies Press.
5. Hadley SK, Gaarder SM: Treatment of irritable bowel syndrome, *Am Fam Physician* 72(12):2501, 2005.
6. Olendzki B and others: Nutritional assessment and counseling for prevention and treatment of cardiovascular disease, *Am Fam Physician* 73(2):257, 2006.
7. Kelley DE: Sugars and starch in the nutritional management of diabetes mellitus, *Am J Clin Nutr* 78:858S, 2003.
8. Behall KM and others: Diets containing barley significantly reduce lipids in mildly hypercholesterolemic men and women, *Am J Clin Nutr* 80:1185, 2004.
9. U.S. Department of Health and Human Services: *Dietary guidelines for Americans, 2005,* Washington, DC, 2005, U.S. Government Printing Office.
10. Cook AJ, Friday JE. *Pyramid servings intakes in the United States 1999-2002, 1 day.* Agricultural Research Service, Community Nutrition Research Group, CNRG Table set 3.0, www.ba.ars.usda.gov/cnrg/services/ts_3-0.pdf, accessed June 2007.
11. USDA, Economic Research Service: *Average daily per capita servings from the U.S. food supply, adjusted for spoilage and other waste,* www.ers.usda.gov/Data/FoodConsumption/FoodGuideIndex.htm, accessed June 2007.
12. Center for Nutrition Policy and Promotion, U.S. Department of Agriculture: *MyPyramid plan,* http://mypyramid.gov, accessed June 2007.

FURTHER READING AND RESOURCES

The following organizations are valuable resources of nutrition and health-related information.

U.S. Department of Health and Human Services: *www.dhhs.gov*

Centers for Disease Control and Prevention: *www.cdc.gov*

Whole Grains Council: *www.wholegrainscouncil.org*

International Food Information Council Foundation: *www.ific.org*

Continuum Health Partners, Dietary Fiber: *www.slrhc.org/healthinfo/dietaryfiber/fibercontentchart.html*

Saris WH: Sugars, energy metabolism, and body weight control, *Am J Clin Nutr* 78(4):850S, 2003.
  Are Americans eating more calories? Where are the majority of the calories coming from? This author reviews a considerable amount of research to summarize the trends in energy intake and the results on weight control.

Last AR, Wilson SA: Low-carbohydrate diets, *Am Fam Physician* 73(11):1942, 2006.
  Carbohydrates are the topic of much debate in weight loss programs. This article gives an overview of various low-carbohydrate diets, their effectiveness, safety, relationship with the glycemic index, and key recommendations for practice.

CHAPTER 3

Fats

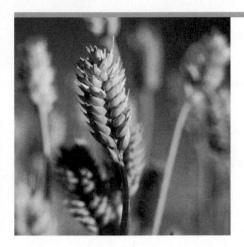

KEY CONCEPTS

- Dietary fat supplies essential body tissue needs, both as an energy fuel and structural material.
- Foods from animal and plant sources supply distinct forms of fat that affect health in different ways.
- Excess dietary fat, especially from animal food sources, is a negative risk factor in overall health.

Americans are beginning to show dietary modifications in the types of fat they are choosing in response to health concerns regarding the risk of chronic disease from excess dietary fat, especially saturated fat.

This chapter examines the various aspects of fat: an essential nutrient, concentrated storage fuel, and savory food component. In addition, the types of fat and health implications when dietary fat or body fat goes unchecked are explored.

THE NATURE OF FATS

Dietary Importance

Fats are a storage form of concentrated fuel for the human energy system. As such, they supplement carbohydrates, the primary fuel, as an available energy source. In food, fats may be in the form of either solid fat or liquid oil. Fats are not soluble in water and have a greasy texture.

Structure and Classes of Fats

The overall name for the chemical group of fats and fat-related compounds is lipids, which comes from the Greek word *lipos,* meaning fat. The word *lipid* appears in combination words used for fat-related health problems. For example, the condition of an elevated level of blood fats is called *hyperlipidemia.*

All lipids are composed of the same basic chemical elements as carbohydrates: carbon, hydrogen, and oxygen. The majority of dietary fats are glycerides because they are composed of *glycerol* with *fatty acids* attached. Most natural fats, whether in animal or plant sources,

---

lipids the chemical group name for organic substances of a fatty nature. The lipids include fats, oils, waxes, and other fat-related compounds such as cholesterol.

glycerides chemical group name for fats; formed from the glycerol base with one, two, or three fatty acids attached to make monoglycerides, diglycerides, and triglycerides, respectively. Glycerides are the principal constituents of adipose tissue and are found in animal and vegetable fats and oils.

have three fatty acids attached to their glycerol base, providing the chemical name of triglyceride (Figure 3-1).

Fatty Acids

The main building blocks of triglycerides are fatty acids. Fatty acids can be classified by their length as short-, medium-, or long-chain fatty acids. The chains contain carbon atoms with a methyl group ($-CH_3$) on one end and an acid carboxyl group ($-COOH$) on the other end. Short-chain fatty acids have two to four carbons, whereas medium and long chains have 6 to 10 and more than 12 carbons, respectively. Fatty acids have two significant characteristics, one of which relates to the concept of saturation and the other to essentiality.

Saturated, Unsaturated, and *Trans*-Fatty Acids

Saturated Fatty Acid. When a substance is described as saturated, it contains all the material it is capable of holding (Figure 3-2). For example, a sponge is saturated with water when it holds all the water it can hold. Similarly, fatty acids are saturated or unsaturated according to whether each carbon is filled with hydrogen. Thus a saturated fatty acid has a structure filled with all the hydrogen bonds it can hold and, as a result, is heavier, denser, and more solid (e.g., meat fats). If most of the fatty acids in a fat are saturated, that fat is said to be a *saturated fat.* Most saturated fats are of animal origin. Figure 3-3 shows a variety of foods with saturated fat, including meat, dairy, and eggs.

Unsaturated Fatty Acid. A fatty acid that is not completely filled with all the hydrogen it can hold is unsaturated, and as a result is less heavy and less dense (e.g., a liquid oil). If most of the fatty acids in a given fat are unsaturated, that fat is said to be an *unsaturated fat.* If the component fatty acids have *one* unfilled spot, the fat is called a *mono*unsaturated fat. For example, olives and olive oil, peanuts and peanut oil, canola oil (rapeseed), almonds, pecans, and avocados supply monounsaturated fats. If the component fatty acids have two or more unfilled spots, the fat is called a *poly*unsaturated fat. Examples of such fats, in order of their degree of unsaturation, are the vegetable oils: safflower, corn, cottonseed, and soybean. Fats from plant and fish sources usually are unsaturated (Figure 3-4). However, notable exceptions are the tropical oils, which are saturated. Although world production of saturated tropical oils (e.g., palm, palm kernel, and coconut) has increased rapidly since the 1970s, use of these oils in the United States has not followed suit.

Essential Fatty Acid. The term *essential* or *nonessential* is applied to a nutrient according to its relative necessity in the diet. A nutrient is essential if either of the following is true: (1) its absence will create a specific deficiency disease or (2) the body cannot manufacture it in sufficient amounts and must obtain it from the diet. A diet with 10% or less of its total kilocalories from fat cannot supply adequate amounts of essential fatty acids. The only fatty acids known to be essential for complete human nutrition are the polyunsaturated fatty acids linoleic (omega-6), and alpha-linolenic (omega-3). Both essential fatty acids serve important functions related to tissue strength, cholesterol metabolism, muscle tone, blood clotting, and heart action. Essential fatty acids must come from the foods we eat. The body is capable of producing saturated fatty acids, monounsaturated fatty acids, and cholesterol. Therefore no set recommendations of daily intake exist for these.

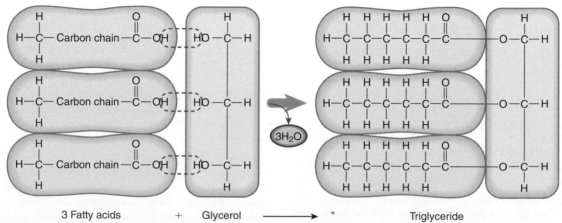

3 Fatty acids   +   Glycerol   ⟶   Triglyceride

Figure 3-1 Triglyceride containing three fatty acids bound to a glycerol molecule.

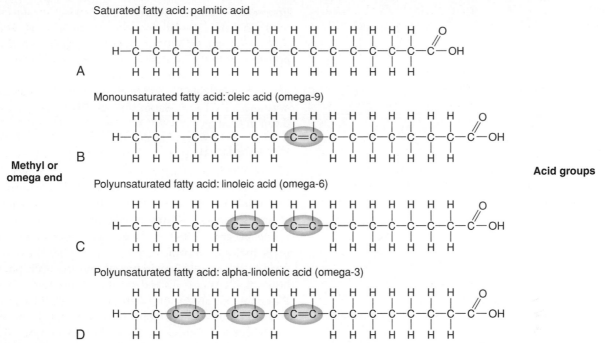

Figure 3-2 Types of fatty acids. **A,** Saturated palmitic acid. **B,** Monounsaturated oleic acid (omega-9). **C,** Polyunsaturated linoleic acid (omega-6). **D,** Polyunsaturated alpha-linolenic acid (omega-3). (Modified from Grodner M and others: *Foundations and Clinical Applications of Nutrition*, ed 4, St Louis, 2007, Mosby.)

***Trans*-Fatty Acid.** Naturally occurring fatty acid molecules have a bend in the chain of atoms at the point of the double bond in the chain. This form is called *cis* (meaning same side) because all atoms are on the same side of the bond. When vegetable oils are partially hydrogenated to produce a more solid, self-stable fat, the normal bend is changed so that the chains of atoms are on opposite sides of the central bond. This form is called *trans* (meaning opposite side), and the process is termed hydrogenation. The illustration on page 34 shows the two structures in a molecule of oleic acid, which is a common monounsaturated fatty acid with a chain of 18 carbon atoms.

Commercially hydrogenated fats in margarine, snack items, fast food, and many other food products are high in the *trans* form. Increased use of these products has stirred debate about accumulating *trans*-fatty acids in the body.

Lipoproteins

Lipoproteins, the major vehicles for lipid transport in the blood stream, are combinations of triglycerides, protein *(apoprotein)*, and other fat-related substances (e.g., cholesterol, fat-soluble vitamins). Because fat is insoluble in water and blood is mainly water, fat cannot freely travel in the blood stream; it needs a water-soluble carrier. The body solves this problem by wrapping small particles of

triglycerides chemical name for fats in the body or in food; compound of three fatty acids attached to a glycerol base.

fatty acids the major structural components of fats.

saturated state of being filled; state of fatty acid components of fats being filled in all their available carbon bonds with hydrogen, making the fat harder and more solid. Such solid food fats are generally from animal sources.

linoleic acid (omega-6) essential fatty acid consisting of 18 carbons and two double bonds; found in vegetable oils.

alpha-linolenic acid (omega-3) essential fatty acid with 18 carbon atoms and three double bonds; found in soybean, canola, and flaxseed oil.

lipoproteins chemical complexes of fat and protein that serve as the major carriers of lipids in the plasma. They vary in density according to the size of the fat load being carried; the lower the density, the higher the fat load. The combination package with water-soluble protein makes possible the transport of non-water-soluble fatty substances in the water-based blood circulation.

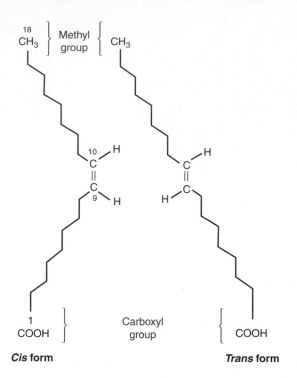

Cis form   Trans form

fat in a covering of protein, which is hydrophilic ("water loving"). The blood then carries these packages of fat to and from the cells to supply needed nutrients. A lipoprotein's relative load of fat and protein determines its density. The higher the protein load, the higher the lipoprotein's density. The higher the fat load, the lower the lipoprotein's density (Figure 3-5). *Low-density lipoproteins* (LDLs) carry fat and cholesterol to cells. *High-density lipoproteins* (HDLs) carry free cholesterol from body tissues to the liver for breakdown and excretion. All lipoproteins are closely associated with lipid disorders and the underlying blood vessel disease in heart attacks, *atherosclerosis*. These relationships are discussed in greater detail in Chapter 19.

Phospholipids

Phospholipids are triglyceride derivatives in which the third fatty acid has been replaced with a phosphate group. The result is a molecule that is partially hydrophobic ("water fearing") and partially hydrophilic (because of the phosphate group). This combination is called an **amphophilic** molecule, in which the hydrophilic heads face outward to the aqueous environment and the hydrophobic heads bind fats and oils and face each other (Figure 3-6). Phospholipids are major constituents in cell membranes and allow transport of fats through the blood stream.

Lecithin. Lecithin, produced by the liver, is a key building block for cell membranes. It is a combination of **glycolipids**, triglycerides, and phospholipids. The amphophilic quality in lecithin makes it ideal for transporting fats and cholesterol.

Eicosanoids. Eicosanoids are signaling hormones exerting control over multiple functions in the body, such as the inflammatory response and immunity, and are messengers for the CNS. Eicosanoids are divided into

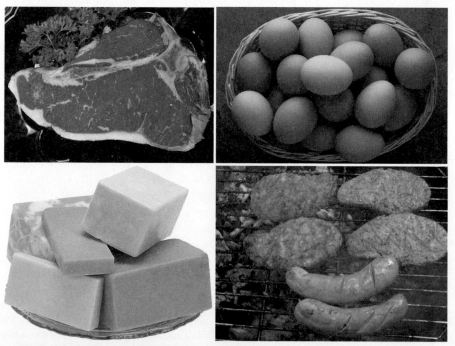

Figure 3-3 Dietary sources of saturated fats. (Copyright JupiterImages Corporation.)

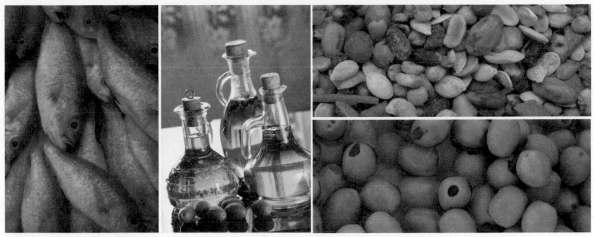

Figure 3-4 Dietary sources of monounsaturated and polyunsaturated fats. (Copyright JupiterImages Corporation.)

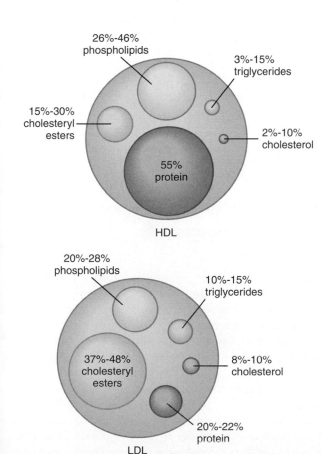

HDL

26%-46% phospholipids

3%-15% triglycerides

15%-30% cholesteryl esters

2%-10% cholesterol

55% protein

LDL

20%-28% phospholipids

10%-15% triglycerides

37%-48% cholesteryl esters

8%-10% cholesterol

20%-22% protein

Figure 3-5 Composition of HDL and LDL lipoproteins.

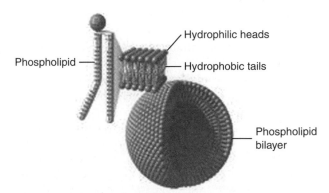

Phospholipid

Hydrophilic heads

Hydrophobic tails

Phospholipid bilayer

Figure 3-6 Phospholipid bilayer. (Reprinted from NASA Astrobiology Institute, Washington, DC, *http://nai.nasa.gov,* accessed July 6, 2007.)

four classes: (1) prostaglandins, (2) prostacyclins, (3) thromboxanes, and (4) leukotrienes. Eicosanoids are derived from omega-3 or omega-6 essential fatty acids.

Sterols

Sterols are a subgroup of steroids and are amphipathic in nature. Sterols made by plants are called phytosterols and sterols produced by animals are zoosterols. Sterols play a

amphophilic molecule containing both hydrophilic and hydrophobic groups.

glycolipids a lipid with a carbohydrate attached.

variety of important roles, such as membrane fluidity and cellular signaling. Cholesterol is the most important zoosterol.

Cholesterol. Cholesterol is vital to membranes and plays other important roles in human metabolism. It occurs naturally in animal foods and is not present in plant products. The main food sources of cholesterol are egg yolks and organ meats, such as liver and kidney, as well as other meats (see Appendix A). To ensure that it always has the relatively small amount of cholesterol necessary for sustaining life, the human body synthesizes the *endogenous* cholesterol in many body tissues, particularly in the liver, as well as small amounts in the adrenal cortex, skin, intestines, testes, and ovaries. Consequently, no biologic requirement for dietary cholesterol exists, and no DRI has been set for cholesterol consumption. The *Dietary Guidelines for Americans* recommend consuming a diet low in cholesterol. Epidemiologic studies have found links between cholesterol intake and increased risk for coronary heart disease.[1]

FUNCTIONS OF FAT

Fat in Foods

Energy

In addition to carbohydrates, fats serve as a fuel for energy production. Fat is also an important storage form of body fuel. Excess carbohydrate and protein intake are converted into stored fat. Fat is a much more concentrated form of fuel, yielding 9 kcal/g when burned by the body compared with carbohydrate's yield of 4 kcal/g.

Essential Nutrients

Dietary triglycerides supply the body with essential fatty acids. As long as an adequate amount of essential fatty acids are consumed, the body is capable of endogenously producing other fats and cholesterol as needed. Food fats also carry fat-soluble vitamins (see Chapter 7) and aid in their absorption.

Flavor and Satisfaction

Some fat in the diet adds flavor to foods and contributes to a feeling of *satiety,* or satisfaction after a meal. These effects are partly caused by the slower rate of digestion of fats compared with that of carbohydrates. This satiety also results from the fuller texture and body that fat gives to food mixtures and the slower emptying time of the stomach that it necessitates. The absence of this satiation and hunger delay experienced by some people on low-fat diets may contribute to dissatisfaction and problems with

necessary changes in food habits to establish a lowered fat and cholesterol intake.

Fat Substitutes

Several fat substitutes, compounds that are not absorbed and thus contribute little or no kilocalories, are being marketed or tested to provide improved flavor and physical texture to low-fat foods and help reduce total dietary fat. Fat substitutes currently on the market are considered safe by the Food and Drug Administration (FDA); however, the safety of long-term use is not well established. Two examples of these fat substitutes are Simplesse (CP Kelco, Atlanta, Ga.), which is made by reshaping the protein of milk whey or egg whites, and Olestra (Procter & Gamble, Cincinnati, Ohio), which is an indigestible form of sucrose.

Fat in the Body

Adipose Tissue

Fat stored in various parts of the body is called adipose tissue, from the Latin word *adiposus,* meaning fatty. A weblike padding of this tissue supports and protects vital organs, and a layer of fat directly under the skin is important in regulating body temperature. Additionally, a special fat covering protects nerve fibers and helps relay nerve impulses.

Cell Membrane Structure

Fat forms the fatty center of cell membranes, making the semipermeable lipid bilayer. Proteins are embedded within this layer and allow transport of various nutrient material in and out of cells.

FOOD SOURCES OF FAT

Variety of Sources

Animal Fats

The predominant supply of saturated fats comes from animal sources, the most concentrated of which include meat fats (e.g., bacon and sausage), dairy fats and products (e.g., cream, ice cream, butter, and cheese), and egg yolk. Because these are animal sources, they also contain considerable amounts of cholesterol. The exceptions are coconut and palm oils, which also contain saturated fatty acids. The American diet traditionally has featured meats and other foods of animal origin. The USDA reports that animal products in particular (e.g., meat, poultry, fish, eggs, and dairy products) contribute 36.8% of the total fat to U.S. diets, half of the saturated fat, and all the cholesterol.[2]

CULTURAL CONSIDERATIONS

ETHNIC DIFFERENCES IN LIPID METABOLISM

Dietary patterns and habits form at an early age as a result of both family influence and environmental factors. The dietary fat intake in some individuals is much lower than others simply because of how the individuals were raised. However, since the unveiling of the human genome, we are learning that biologic differences also exist that may affect dietary patterns and determine the way in which our bodies handle the nutrients we eat. The prevalence for obesity has long been known to differ among ethnic and racial populations, but the exact cause remains ambiguous.

Women often are the subjects for study in obesity research. A significant difference in ethnicity exists in the incidence of adult women older than 20 years who are overweight in the United States: 76.8% of African-American women, 69.3% of Hispanic women, and 58.2% of Caucasian women.* Evidence is accumulating that suggests bio-

logic differences in lipid metabolism among ethnic groups may be the cause. Bower and colleagues found that African-American women have an increased capacity to synthesize fat from glucose in adipose tissue compared with Caucasian women.† Thus they are more efficient at converting excess kilocalories into stored fat, contributing to the higher rate of obesity among African-American women.

These types of differences continue to unfold with ongoing studies of the human genome. Differences such as these also will guide individuals in their dietary choices regarding how their bodies will respond to specific nutrients. The path from fat in our food to fat on our bodies continues to provide many locations for inspection and evaluation. The science of lipid digestion, metabolism, and utilization will remain a hot topic for debate and research for years to come.

* U.S. Department of Health and Human Services, Centers for Disease Control and Prevention, National Center for Health Statistics: *Heath, United States, 2005, www.cdc.gov/nchs/data/hus/hus05.pdf#073,* accessed July 2007.
†Bower JF and others: Ethnic differences in *in vitro* glyceride synthesis in subcutaneous and omental adipose tissue, *Am J Physiol Endocrinol Metab* 283(5):E988, 2002.

In light of the saturated fat and cholesterol source that animal products supply to the diet, all types of animal protein are not created equal. A recent study found that regardless of the protein source, when consuming lean beef, lean fish, and poultry without skin, in a well-balanced diet that also includes a high polyunsaturated to saturated fat ratio and ample fiber, similar benefits are found in blood cholesterol levels.[3] In other words, even though animal products can have a hefty supply of cholesterol and saturated fat, lean portions do not have the same hypercholesterolemic effects as their full-fat counterparts when consumed with diets high in fiber. However, even greater cholesterol-lowering effects can be achieved from a diet low in *trans*-fatty acids and regular moderate use of polyunsaturated oils in the place of saturated fat.[4]

Some animal fats contain small amounts of unsaturated fats. Specifically, fish oils are a good source of the polyunsaturated essential fatty acids.

Plant Fats

Plant foods supply mostly monounsaturated and polyunsaturated fats. Food sources for unsaturated fats include vegetable oils (e.g., safflower, corn, cottonseed, soybeans, peanuts, and olives; see Figure 3-4) but, as indicated, coconut and palm oils are exceptions. These oils are saturated fats used mainly in commercially processed food items.

Food Label Information

The FDA food-labeling regulations regarding the nutrition panel content provide the following mandatory and voluntary (italicized below) information relating to dietary fat in food products[5]:

- Calories from fat
- *Calories from saturated fat*
- Total fat
- Saturated fat
- *Trans* fat
- *Polyunsaturated fat*
- *Monounsaturated fat*
- Cholesterol

The nature and amount of dietary fat and cholesterol are special health concerns related to some cancers, coronary heart disease, diabetes, and obesity (see the Cultural Considerations box, "Ethnic Differences in Lipid Metabolism"). The FDA has approved a series of *health claims*

---

cholesterol a fat-related compound, a sterol, synthesized only in animal tissues; a normal constituent of bile and a principal constituent of gallstones. In the body, cholesterol is mainly synthesized in the liver. In the diet, it is found primarily in animal food sources.

adipose fat present in cells of adipose (fatty) tissue.

that link one or more dietary components to the reduced risk of a specific disease.[6] Approved health claims include the following:

- *Fat and cancer:* A diet low in total fat may reduce the risk of some cancers.
- *Saturated fat and cholesterol and coronary heart disease:* Diets low in saturated fat and cholesterol may reduce the risk of coronary heart disease.

The following are claims pending approval:

- *Omega-3 fatty acid and coronary heart disease:* Consumption of eicosapentaenoic acid (EPA) and docosahexanoic (DHA) omega-3 fatty acids may reduce the risk of coronary heart disease.
- *Monounsaturated fatty acids and coronary heart disease:* Replacing saturated fat with monounsaturated olive oil may reduce the risk of coronary heart disease.

See *A Food Labeling Guide* published by the FDA's Center for Food Safety and Applied Nutrition at *http://vm.cfsan.fda.gov/~dms/flg-6c.html* for more information on FDA-approved health claims. This Web site provides a table with approved claims, food requirements, and model claim statements. Food labels and health claims are discussed further in Chapter 13.

Characteristics of Food Fat Sources

For practical purposes, food fats can be classified as *visible* or *invisible* fats to help individuals become aware of all food sources of fat.

Visible Fat

The obvious fats are easy to see and include butter, margarine, separate cream, salad oils and dressings, lard, shortening, fat meat (e.g., bacon, sausage, salt pork), and the visible fat of any meat. Visible fats are easier to control in the diet than those that are less apparent.

Invisible Fat

Some dietary fats are less visible, so individuals who want to control dietary fat also must be aware of these food sources. Invisible fats include cheese, the cream portion of homogenized milk, egg yolk, nuts, seeds, olives, avocados, and lean meat. Even when all the visible fat has been removed from meat (e.g., the skin on poultry and the obvious fat on the lean portions), approximately 6% of the total fat surrounding the muscle fibers remains.

Table 3-1 provides a list of commonly eaten foods and their fat contents.

DIGESTION OF FATS
Mouth

As with other macronutrients (carbohydrates and proteins), fats are broken down into their basic building blocks, fatty acids, through the process of digestion (Figure 3-7). When foods are eaten, some initial fat breakdown may begin in the mouth by action of *lingual lipase,* which is secreted by Ebner's glands at the back of the tongue. Of note, lingual lipase is only important for digestion during infancy. For adults, the primary digestive action occurring in the mouth is mechanical. Foods are broken up into smaller particles through chewing and moistened for passage into the stomach.

TABLE 3-1

FAT IN FOOD SERVINGS

FOOD	SERVING SIZE	FAT CONTENT
Butter or margarine	1 Tbsp	11 g
Salad dressing	1 Tbsp	7 g
Mayonnaise	1 Tbsp	11 g
Cream cheese	1 Tbsp	10 g
Carrots	½ cup	Trace
Broccoli	½ cup	Trace
Potato, baked	1	Trace
French fries	1 cup	8 g
Apple	1	Trace
Orange	1	Trace
Banana	1	Trace
Fruit juice	1 cup	Trace
Rice or pasta	½ cup	Trace
Bagel	1	Trace
Muffin	1 medium	6 g
Danish pastry	1 medium	13 g
Skim milk	1 cup	Trace
Low-fat milk	1 cup	5 g
Whole milk	1 cup	8 g
American cheese	2 oz	18 g
Cheddar cheese	1½ oz	14 g
Frozen yogurt	½ cup	2 g
Ice cream	⅓ cup	7 g
Lean beef	3 oz	6 g
Poultry	3 oz	6 g
Fish	3 oz	6 g
Ground beef	3 oz	16 g
Bologna (2 slices)	1 oz	16 g
Egg	1	5 g
Nuts (⅓ cup)	1 oz	22 g

From Grodner M and others: *Foundations and clinical applications of nutrition*, ed 4, St Louis, 2007, Mosby.

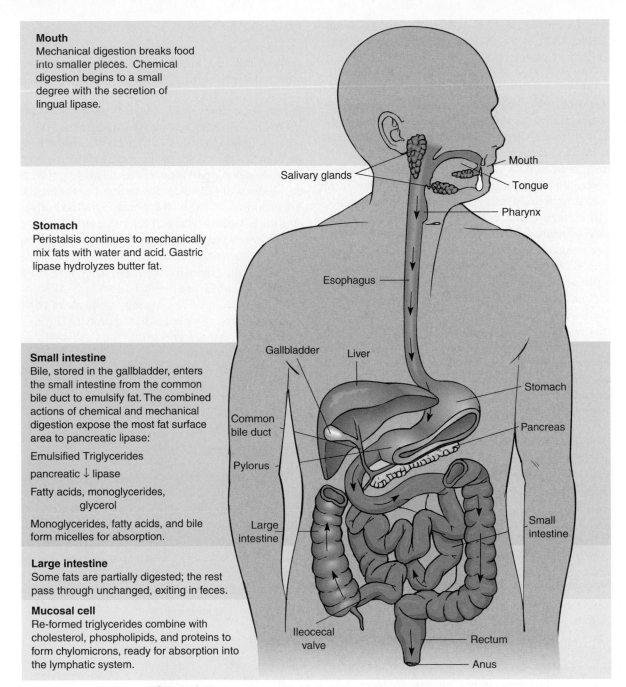

Mouth
Mechanical digestion breaks food into smaller pieces. Chemical digestion begins to a small degree with the secretion of lingual lipase.

Stomach
Peristalsis continues to mechanically mix fats with water and acid. Gastric lipase hydrolyzes butter fat.

Small intestine
Bile, stored in the gallbladder, enters the small intestine from the common bile duct to emulsify fat. The combined actions of chemical and mechanical digestion expose the most fat surface area to pancreatic lipase:

Emulsified Triglycerides

pancreatic ↓ lipase

Fatty acids, monoglycerides, glycerol

Monoglycerides, fatty acids, and bile form micelles for absorption.

Large intestine
Some fats are partially digested; the rest pass through unchanged, exiting in feces.

Mucosal cell
Re-formed triglycerides combine with cholesterol, phospholipids, and proteins to form chylomicrons, ready for absorption into the lymphatic system.

Salivary glands — Mouth — Tongue — Pharynx — Esophagus — Gallbladder — Liver — Stomach — Common bile duct — Pancreas — Pylorus — Large intestine — Small intestine — Ileocecal valve — Rectum — Anus

Figure 3-7 Summary of lipid digestion. (Courtesy Rolin Graphics.)

Stomach

Little, if any, chemical fat digestion occurs in the stomach. General muscle action continues to mix the fat with the stomach contents. No significant amount of fat enzymes is present in the gastric secretions except *gastric lipase* (tributyrinase), which acts on emulsified butterfat. As the main gastric enzymes act on other specific nutrients in the food mix, fat is separated out and prepared for its major, enzyme-specific breakdown in the small intestine.

Small Intestine

Fat digestion primarily occurs in the small intestine where the major enzymes necessary for the chemical changes are present. These digestive agents come from three major sources: an emulsification agent from the gallbladder and two specific enzymes from the pancreas and the small intestine itself.

Bile from the Gallbladder

The fat coming into the duodenum, the first section of the small intestine, stimulates the secretion of *cholecystokinin,* a hormone released from glands in the intestinal walls. In turn, cholecystokinin causes the gallbladder to contract, relax its opening muscle, and subsequently secrete bile into the intestine by way of the common duct. The bile is first produced in large, dilute amounts in the liver, which then sends it to the gallbladder for concentration and storage so that it is ready for use with fat digestion as needed. Bile is not an enzyme that acts in the chemical digestive process, but functions as an emulsifier. This preparation process accomplishes two important tasks: (1) it breaks the fat into small particles, greatly enlarging the total surface area available for action of the enzyme, and (2) it lowers the surface tension of the finely dispersed and suspended fat particles, allowing the enzymes to penetrate more easily. This process is similar to the emulsification action of detergents. The bile also provides an alkaline medium necessary for the action of the fat enzyme *pancreatic lipase.*

Enzymes from the Pancreas

Pancreatic juice flowing into the small intestine contains an enzyme for triglycerides and another for cholesterol. First, *pancreatic lipase,* a powerful fat enzyme, breaks off one fatty acid at a time from the glycerol base of fats (triglycerides). One fatty acid plus a diglyceride, then another fatty acid plus a monoglyceride, are produced in turn. Each succeeding step of this breakdown occurs with increasing difficulty. In fact, separation of the final fatty acid from the remaining monoglyceride is such a slow process that less than one third of the total fat present reaches complete breakdown. The final products of fat digestion to be absorbed are fatty acids, monoglycerides, and glycerol. Some remaining fat may pass into the large intestine for fecal elimination. The enzyme *cholesterol esterase* acts on cholesterol esters (not free cholesterol) to form a combination of free cholesterol and fatty acids in preparation for absorption into the lymph vessels and finally into the blood stream (see Chapter 5).

Enzyme from the Small Intestine

The small intestine secretes an enzyme in the intestinal juice called *lecithinase,* which acts on lecithin, another lipid compound, breaking it down for absorption. Figure 3-7 summarizes fat digestion in the successive parts of the GI tract.

Absorption

Fat absorption into the GI cells and blood stream is more involved than the absorption of either carbohydrates or protein because triglycerides are not soluble in water and cannot enter the blood stream, which is mostly water. Within the small intestines, bile salts surround the monoglycerides and fatty acids to form micelles. The non-water-soluble fat particles (fatty acids, monoacylglycerols) are found in the middle of the packaged micelle, whereas the water-soluble part faces outward. This structure allows the products of lipid digestion to travel to the brush border membrane. Once there, fats are absorbed separately into the intestinal cells, and bile is absorbed and transported by the portal vein to the liver for reprocessing—a process called enterohepatic circulation. Once inside the intestinal cell, monoglycerides and fatty acids re-form triglycerides, which are then packaged into a lipoprotein called chylomicron. Chylomicrons are made of triglycerides, cholesterol, phospholipids, and proteins (Figure 3-8). Again, this structure forms within the enterocyte (intestinal cell) and allows the products of fat digestion to enter the circulation. Chylomicrons first enter the lymphatic circulatory system and then eventually the blood stream.

Digestibility and Market Availability of Food Fats

The digestibility of fats varies somewhat according to the food source and cooking method. Butter digests more completely than meat fat. Fried foods, especially those saturated with fat in the frying process, are digested more slowly than baked or broiled foods. When fried foods are cooked at too high of a temperature, they are more difficult to digest because substances in the fat break down into irritating materials. Fried foods should be consumed

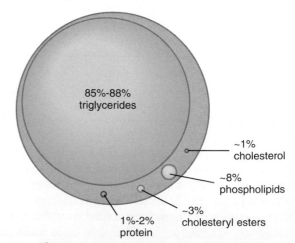

Figure 3-8 Composition of a chylomicron.

CLINICAL APPLICATIONS

HOW MUCH FAT ARE YOU EATING?

Keep an accurate record of everything you eat and drink for 1 day. Be sure to include all fat or other nutrient seasonings used with your foods (salad dressing, sugar, mayonnaise, etc.). If you want a more representative picture, use the nutrient analysis program that came with this text or another program to which you have access and keep a 3- to 7-day record.

Step 1: Calculate the total kilocalories and grams of each of the energy-yielding nutrients (carbohydrates, fat, and protein) in everything you eat. Multiply the total grams of each energy nutrient by its respective fuel value:

$$\text{Fat } \underline{\hspace{1cm}} \text{ g} \times 9 = \underline{\hspace{1cm}} \text{ kcal}$$
$$\text{Protein } \underline{\hspace{1cm}} \text{ g} \times 4 = \underline{\hspace{1cm}} \text{ kcal}$$
$$\text{Carbohydrate } \underline{\hspace{1cm}} \text{ g} \times 4 = \underline{\hspace{1cm}} \text{ kcal}$$

Step 2: Calculate the percentage of each energy nutrient in your total diet:

$$(\text{Fat kcal/Total kcal}) \times 100 = \% \text{ fat kcal in diet}$$

Step 3: Compare your diet with the fat in a typical American diet (30% to 45% fat) and with the U.S. dietary goal (20% to 35% fat).

---

sparingly, and the temperature of the fat should be carefully controlled during frying. Although lower fat food products are now generally more available in food markets, many high-fat products still compete for the customer's attention. In any case, fat is an essential part of a healthy, well-balanced diet. Our overall health goal is to reduce the amount of *excessive* fat used in the diet.

RECOMMENDATIONS FOR DIETARY FAT

Dietary Fat and Health

American Diet

Fats in the diet supply flavor to food, providing a sense of satisfaction and an enhancement to eating pleasure. The American diet has traditionally been high in fat. USDA nutrient intake records show 31% of the total kilocalories came from fat in 1909, with an increase to 41% in 2004. However, Americans have succeeded in reducing the amount of fat coming from decidedly unhealthy saturated fat, from 43% of total fat to 31% over the same timeframe.[7] Still, the average amount of total fat and saturated fat consumed per person in the United States, for all individuals ages 2 years and older, exceeds the recommendations based on the DRIs. Total kilocalories coming from fat should not exceed 20% to 35%, with a maximum of 10% of total kilocalories from saturated and *trans* fats combined.[1] Many individuals with health problems are encouraged to adjust to lower amounts of fat, with goals such as 15% to 25% of the total kilocalories and no more than 7% of total kilocalories from saturated and *trans* fats combined. This amount could easily provide an adequate amount of the essential fatty acids, linolenic and linoleic acid, to meet the physiologic needs of the body.

Health Problems

If fat is vital to human health, what is the concern about fat in the diet? Research continues to validate results indicating that health problems from fat relate to too much dietary fat, specifically saturated fat.

Amount of Fat. Too many kilocalories in the diet, regardless of the source (fat, carbohydrates, or protein), will exceed the requirement of immediate energy needs. The excess is stored as body fat. Increased body fat and weight have been associated with risk factors for health problems such as diabetes, hypertension, and heart disease. How much fat is in your own daily diet? See the Clinical Applications box, "How Much Fat Are You Eating?"

---

bile a fluid secreted by the liver and transported to the gallbladder for concentration and storage; it is released into the duodenum with the entry of fat to facilitate enzymatic fat digestion by acting as an emulsifying agent.

emulsifier an agent that breaks down large fat globules into smaller, uniformly distributed particles; the action is chiefly accomplished in the intestine by bile acids, which lower the surface tension of the fat particles, breaking the fat into many smaller droplets and thus greatly increasing the surface area of fat and facilitating contact with the fat-digesting enzymes.

micelles packages of free fatty acids, monoglycerides, and bile salts. The non-water-soluble fat particles are found in the middle of the package, whereas the water-soluble part faces outward and allows for the absorption of fat into the intestinal mucosal cell.

chylomicron lipoprotein formed in the intestinal cell composed of triglycerides, cholesterol, phospholipids, and protein. Allows for absorption of fat into the lymphatic circulatory system before entering the blood circulation.

Type of Fat. An excess of cholesterol and saturated fat in the diet, which comes from animal food sources, has been identified as a specific risk factor for atherosclerosis, the underlying blood vessel disease that contributes to heart attacks and strokes (see Chapter 19). A decrease in dietary saturated fats (e.g., using polyunsaturated and monounsaturated fats instead) has been shown to produce favorable lipid profiles in many individuals.[4,8] When substituted for saturated fat in the diet, monounsaturated fats reduce LDL cholesterol and also may increase HDL levels.

Essential Fatty Acid Deficiency. Fat-free diets may lead to essential fatty acid deficiency with clinical manifestations. Because essential fatty acids play an important role in maintaining the integrity of biologic membranes, one indication of essential fatty acid deficiency is dermatitis. Omega-3 fatty acids especially are required for normal function of the brain, CNS, and cell membranes. Low levels of omega-3 and omega-6 fatty acids are linked to hair loss, low blood platelets, impaired vision, altered mental states, learning problems, and growth retardation in children.

Trans-Fatty Acids. Some observed effects from diets high in *trans*-fatty acids include elevation of total cholesterol, LDL cholesterol, and risk of cardiovascular disease, alterations in the cell membrane, and increased production of atherosclerotic inflammatory cytokines. In response to these growing health concerns, the FDA now requires that all food products identify the amount of *trans* fats on the Nutrition Facts Label, making identification of these products much easier. This has motivated the food industry to develop alternative fats and oils to avoid the use of *trans* fats and improve the fatty acid composition in relation to cardiovascular health risk.[9]

Health Promotion

The ongoing movement in American health care is toward health promotion and disease prevention through reduction of risk factors related to chronic disease. Heart disease continues to be a leading cause of death in developed countries, and much attention is given to reducing the various risk factors leading to this disease. Excess dietary fat, particularly saturated fat and cholesterol, contributes to these risk factors, which include obesity, diabetes, elevated blood fats, and elevated blood pressure. Such risk factors have previously been thought of as only affecting adults but are becoming increasingly apparent in obese children and adolescents.[10-12] Healthier eating habits are especially important for children in high-risk families (e.g., families with identified lipid disorders and heart disease at young ages) who should develop modera-

tion in fat use, as well as other aspects of a healthy lifestyle, at an early age.

Additional lifestyle risk factors include smoking, increased stress, and lack of exercise, especially in middle-aged and older individuals. Thus a middle-aged or older adult who eats a high-fat diet, is overweight, and has high blood cholesterol and blood pressure should reduce both weight and amount of dietary fat, especially animal fat. Today increasing emphasis—especially for persons 40 years of age and older—is placed on the importance of keeping the body's total daily energy use in balance with the total daily caloric intake.

In addition, changes are gradually being made in the fast-food industry to reduce the traditional high-fat content of menu items. For example, most of the fast-food chains are shifting to leaner meat for hamburgers and more variety in food choices (e.g., grilled chicken and fish sandwiches; breakfast items such as fruit, waffles, pancakes, and hot and cold cereals; baked potatoes; chili; and fresh and packaged salads and fruit) and using vegetable oil for frying. Many fast-food restaurants are experimenting and surveying customers about the use of fat substitutes.

Low-fat diets, fad diets, and other issues about weight loss are discussed in more detail in Chapter 15.

Dietary Reference Intakes

Healthy diet guidelines stress the benefits of a diet low in fat, saturated fat, *trans*-fatty acids, and cholesterol. All guidelines recommend that the fat content of the diet not exceed 20% to 35% of the total kilocalories, that less than 10% of the kilocalories should come from saturated fats, and that dietary cholesterol be limited to 300 mg/day (see Chapter 1). No DRI or UL is set for *trans*-fatty acids. The National Academy of Sciences recommends limiting trans fat intake to as low as possible while maintaining a nutritionally adequate diet.[1] As mentioned, fat is an essential part of the diet; therefore diets completely devoid of fat are equally unhealthy and can result in essential fatty acid deficiency.

The DRIs for linoleic acid, found in polyunsaturated vegetable oils, are set at 17 g/day for men and 12 g/day for women. Linolenic acid is primarily found in fish, soybeans, and flaxseed oil and is necessary in much lesser quantities than linoleic acid. The recommendations for linolenic acid intake are 1.6 and 1.1 g/day for men and women, respectively.[1] American diets have an omega-6/omega-3 fatty acid ratio of approximately 8:1 to 12:1. However, consuming more omega-3 fatty acids (from vegetables and fish) would help achieve a preferred omega-6/omega-3 ratio of between 2:1 to 3:1.

Dietary Guidelines for Americans

In line with the current national health goal of health promotion through disease prevention by reducing identified risks of chronic disease, the *Dietary Guidelines for Americans, 2005* recommend general control of fat in the diet, especially saturated fat and cholesterol. The following guidelines address dietary fat intake[13]:

- Consume a variety of nutrient-dense foods and beverages within and among the basic food groups while choosing foods that limit the intake of saturated and *trans* fats, cholesterol, added sugars, salt, and alcohol.
- Consume less than 10% of calories from saturated fatty acids and less than 300 mg/day of cholesterol, and keep *trans*-fatty acid consumption as low as possible.
- Keep total fat intake between 20% to 35% of calories, with most fats coming from sources of polyunsaturated and monounsaturated fatty acids, such as fish, nuts, and vegetable oils.
- When selecting and preparing meat, poultry, dry beans, and milk or milk products, make choices that are lean, low fat, or fat free.
- Limit intake of fats and oils high in saturated and/or *trans*-fatty acids, and choose products low in such fats and oils.

MyPyramid

The MyPyramid food guidance system provides recommendations on designing a diet relative to the DRI and *Dietary Guidelines* recommendations for fat intake within a well-balanced diet. Once an individual plan is determined on the basis of age, gender, and physical activity level, other helpful tips and resources are available through the free Web site, such as how to choose lean meats, where to find essential fatty acids, how to avoid saturated fat intake, tips for eating out, and sample menus.[14]

SUMMARY

Fat is an essential body nutrient, serving important body needs as a backup storage fuel, secondary to carbohydrate, for energy. Fat also supplies important tissue needs as a structural material for cell membranes, protective padding for vital organs, insulation to maintain body temperature, and covering for nerve fibers.

Food fats have different forms and body uses. Saturated fats primarily come from animal food sources and carry health risks for the body. Plant food sources are the richest source for unsaturated fats and help reduce health risks. Cholesterol is a sterol synthesized only by animals. When consumed in excessive amounts,

cholesterol also contributes to health risks for developing cardiovascular disease. Americans generally consume more fat than they need or is healthy. Reducing total fats and saturated fat and maintaining a low-cholesterol diet are recommended for health promotion and disease prevention.

When various foods containing triglycerides and cholesterol are eaten, specific digestive agents, including bile and pancreatic lipase, prepare and break down the fats (triglycerides). Fatty acids and monoglycerides are incorporated into chylomicrons and absorbed by the lymphatic system into the blood stream.

CRITICAL THINKING QUESTIONS

1. Compare fat and carbohydrate as a fuel source in the body's energy system. Name several other important functions of fat in human nutrition and health.

2. Differentiate the components of *lipids, triglycerides, fatty acids, cholesterol,* and *lipoproteins*.

3. Compare the structure of a saturated fat, monounsaturated fat, polyunsaturated fat, and a *trans* fat. Give food sources for each.

4. Why is a controlled amount of dietary fat recommended for health promotion? How much fat should a healthy diet contain?

CHAPTER CHALLENGE QUESTIONS

True-False
Write the correct statement for each statement that is false.

1. *True or False:* Fat has the same energy value as carbohydrate.

2. *True or False:* Fat is composed of the same basic chemical elements as carbohydrate.

3. *True or False:* Corn oil is a saturated fat.

4. *True or False:* Polyunsaturated fats predominantly come from animal food sources.

5. *True or False:* Lipoproteins, produced mainly in the liver, carry fat in the blood.

Multiple Choice

1. The fuel form of fat found in food sources is
   a. triglyceride.
   b. fatty acid.
   c. glycerol.
   d. lipoprotein.

2. Which of the following statements about the saturation of fats is correct?
   a. The degree of saturation does not depend on the amount of hydrogen in the fatty acids that make up the fat.
   b. Unsaturated fats come from animal food sources.
   c. The more saturated the fat, the softer it tends to be.
   d. Fats composed of fatty acids with two or more "unfilled" spaces in their structure are called *polyunsaturated.*

3. If an individual implemented a low saturated fat diet to lower the risk for heart disease, which of the following foods would more frequently be consumed?
   a. Whole milk
   b. Olive oil and vinegar salad dressing
   c. Butter
   d. Cheddar cheese

4. Once absorbed into the enterocyte, monoglycerides and fatty acids re-form triglycerides, which are then packaged into a lipoprotein called_____ for absorption into the lymphatic structure.
   a. LDL cholesterol
   b. HDL cholesterol
   c. micelles
   d. chylomicrons

evolve Please refer to the Students' Resource section of this text's Evolve Web site for additional study resources.

REFERENCES

1. Food and Nutrition Board, Institute of Medicine: *Dietary reference intakes for energy, carbohydrate, fiber, fat, fatty acids, cholesterol, protein, and amino acids,* Washington, DC, 2002, National Academies Press.
2. United States Department of Agriculture/Center for Nutrition Policy and Promotion: *U.S. food supply: nutrients contributed from major food groups, 1970 and 2000,* www.ers.usda.gov/Data/FoodConsumption/NutrientAvailIndex.htm, accessed June 2007.
3. Beauchesne-Rondeau E and others: Plasma lipids and lipoproteins in hypercholesterolemic men fed a lipid-lowering diet containing lean beef, lean fish, or poultry, *Am J Clin Nutr* 77:587, 2003.
4. Binkoski AE and others: Balance of unsaturated fatty acids is important to a cholesterol-lowering diet: comparison of mid-oleic sunflower oil and olive oil on cardiovascular disease risk factors, *J Am Diet Assoc* 105(7):1080, 2005.
5. U.S. Food and Drug Administration, Center for Food Safety and Applied Nutrition: *Examples of revised nutrition facts panel listing* trans *fat,* Washington, DC, www.cfsan.fda.gov/~dms/labtr.html, accessed June 2007.
6. U.S. Food and Drug Administration, Center for Food Safety and Applied Nutrition: *Food labeling and nutrition,* www.cfsan.fda.gov/label.html, accessed June 2007.
7. United States Department of Agriculture/Center for Nutrition Policy and Promotion: *U.S. food supply: nutrients and other food components, per capita per day, 1909 to 2004,* www.ers.usda.gov/Data/FoodConsumption/NutrientAvailIndex.htm, accessed June 2007.
8. Montoya MT and others: Fatty acid saturation of the diet and plasma lipid concentrations, lipoprotein particle concentrations, and cholesterol efflux capacity, *Am J Clin Nutr* 75(3):484, 2002.
9. Flickinger BD, Huth PJ: Dietary fats and oil: technologies for improving cardiovascular health, *Curr Atheroscler Rep* 6(6):468, 2004.
10. Meyer AA and others: Impaired flow-mediated vasodilation, carotid artery intima-media thickening, and elevated endothelial plasma markers in obese children: the impact of cardiovascular risk factors, *Pediatrics* 117(5):1560, 2006.
11. Zhu W and others: Arterial intima-media thickening and endothelial dysfunction in obese Chinese children, *Eur J Pediatr* 164(6):337, 2005.
12. Woo KS and others: Overweight in children is associated with arterial endothelial dysfunction and intima-media thickening, *Int J Obes Relat Metab Disord* 28(7):852, 2004.

13. U.S. Department of Health and Human Services, U.S. Department of Agriculture: *Dietary guidelines for Americans 2005: executive summary,* Washington, DC, 2005, USDA.
14. Center for Nutrition Policy and Promotion, U.S. Department of Agriculture: *MyPyramid Plan,* Washington, DC, *http://mypyramid.gov,* accessed June 2007.

FURTHER READING AND RESOURCES

USDA Nutrient Data Laboratory: *www.nal.usda.gov/fnic/foodcomp/search*
A useful Web site to find the nutrient content, including trans fats, of the foods you most enjoy.

Mayo Clinic: *www.mayoclinic.com*
A site search for "dietary fat" results in several informative articles.

Lipids in Health and Disease: *www.lipidworld.com*
An online journal of peer-reviewed articles on all aspects of lipids that are open access and free to the public.

The following articles focus on the negative effects of excess fat in the diet, specifically saturated fat, and the long term consequences.

Haag M, Dippenaar NG: Dietary fats, fatty acids and insulin resistance: short review of a multifaceted connection, *Med Sci Monit* 11(12):RA359, 2005.

Baer DJ and others: Dietary fatty acids affect plasma markers of inflammation in healthy men fed controlled diets: a randomized crossover study, *Am J Clin Nutr* 79(6):969, 2004.

Hu FB: Plant-based foods and prevention of cardiovascular disease: an overview, *Am J Clin Nutr* 78(3):544S, 2003.
The authors discuss the benefits of a diet based mostly on plant foods, with an emphasis on monounsaturated and polyunsaturated fats as opposed to animal-derived saturated fats. Health care professionals should explore a variety of methods for encouraging positive dietary change in patients.

CHAPTER 4

Proteins

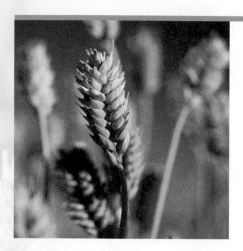

KEY CONCEPTS

- Food proteins provide the amino acids necessary for building and maintaining body tissue.
- Protein balance, both within the body and in the diet, is essential to life and health.
- The quality of a protein food and its ability to meet the body's needs are determined by the composition of amino acids.

Many different proteins in the body make human life possible. Each of these thousands of specific body proteins has a unique structure designed to perform an assigned task. Amino acids are the building blocks of all protein. People obtain amino acids from the variety of food proteins. This chapter looks at the specific nature of proteins, both in food and in human bodies, and explains why protein balance is essential to life and health and how that balance is maintained.

THE NATURE OF PROTEINS

Amino Acids: Basic Building Material

Role as Building Units

All protein, whether in our bodies or in the food we eat, is composed of building units known as amino acids. Amino acids are joined in unique chain sequences to form specific proteins. Each amino acid is joined by a peptide bond (Figure 4-1). Two amino acids joined together are called a *dipeptide*. *Polypeptides* are chains of up to 100 amino acids. Hundreds of amino acids are linked together to form a single protein. When foods rich in protein are eaten, the protein is broken down into amino acids in the digestive process. The specific types of protein found in different foods are unique. For example, casein is the protein found in milk and cheese, albumin is in egg whites, and gluten is in wheat products. Amino acids are then reassembled in the body in a specific order to form a variety of proteins needed by the body. To maintain its solvency, each protein chain adopts a folded form, which can fold and unfold according to metabolic need. Because proteins are relatively large, complex molecules, they often are subject to mutations, or malformations in structure. For example, protein-folding mistakes are involved in Alzheimer's disease, which robs many older adults of their mental capacity.

Dietary Importance

Amino acids are named for their chemical nature. The word *amino* refers to compounds containing nitrogen. Like carbohydrates and fats, proteins have a basic structure of carbon, hydrogen, and oxygen. However, unlike carbohydrates and fats, protein is approximately 16% nitrogen. As such, protein is the primary source of nitrogen in the diet. In addition, some proteins contain small but valuable amounts of the minerals sulfur, phosphorus, iron, and iodine.

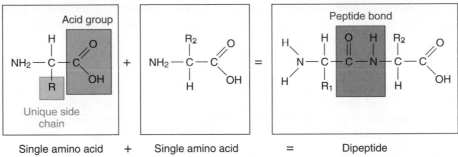

Figure 4-1 Amino acid structure. (Modified from Mahan LK, Escott-Stump S: *Krause's food & nutrition therapy,* ed 12, Philadelphia, 2008, Saunders.)

Classes of Amino Acids

Twenty common amino acids have been identified, all of which are vital to life and health. These amino acids are classified as indispensable, dispensable, or conditionally indispensable *in the diet* according to whether the body can make them (Box 4-1).[1] These classifications were formerly known as essential, nonessential, or conditionally essential, respectively.

Indispensable Amino Acids

Nine amino acids are classified as indispensable because the body cannot manufacture them in sufficient quantity or at all (see Box 4-1). Thus as the word *indispensable* implies, these amino acids are necessary in the diet and cannot be left out. Under normal circumstances, the remaining 11 amino acids are synthesized by the body to meet continuous metabolic demands throughout the life cycle.

Dispensable Amino Acids

The word *dispensable* can be misleading; all amino acids have essential tissue-building and metabolic functions in the body. However, the term refers to five amino acids that the body can synthesize from other amino acids provided the necessary building blocks and enzymes are present (see Box 4-1). These amino acids are needed by the body for healthy life but are dispensable (not necessary) in the diet.

Conditionally Indispensable Amino Acids

The remaining six amino acids are classified as *conditionally indispensable* (see Box 4-1). Under certain physiologic conditions these amino acids, which are normally synthesized in the body like the dispensable amino acids, must be consumed in the diet. Arginine, cysteine, glutamine, glycine, proline, and tyrosine are indispensable when endogenous sources cannot meet the metabolic demands. For example, the human body can make cysteine from the

essential amino acid methionine. However, when the diet is deficient in methionine, cysteine must be consumed in the diet, therefore making it an indispensable amino acid during that time. Severe physiologic stress, illness, and

BOX 4-1

INDISPENSABLE, DISPENSABLE, AND CONDITIONALLY INDISPENSABLE AMINO ACIDS

INDISPENSABLE	DISPENSABLE	CONDITIONALLY INDISPENSABLE
Histidine	Alanine	Arginine
Isoleucine	Aspartic acid	Cysteine
Leucine	Asparagine	Glutamine
Lysine	Glutamic acid	Glycine
Methionine	Serine	Proline
Phenylalanine		Tyrosine
Threonine		
Tryptophan		
Valine		

amino acids nitrogen-bearing compounds that form the structural units of protein. When digested, the various food proteins yield their constituent amino acids, which are then available for use by the cells to synthesize specific tissue proteins.

indispensable amino acids nine amino acids that must be obtained from the diet because the body does not make adequate amounts to support body needs.

dispensable amino acids five amino acids that the body can synthesize from other amino acids supplied through the diet and thus do not have to be consumed on a daily basis.

conditionally indispensable amino acids six amino acids that normally are considered dispensable amino acids because the body can make them. However, under certain circumstances such as illness, the body cannot make them in high enough quantities and they become indispensable in the diet.

genetic disorders also may render an amino acid conditionally indispensable. Phenylketonuria (PKU) is a genetic disorder in which the affected individual lacks the enzyme needed to convert phenylalanine to tyrosine. Because conversion of phenylalanine cannot take place, amounts in the blood may rise to toxic levels. A specific PKU diet must be followed and certain foods avoided (see the Drug-Nutrient Interaction box, "Aspartame and PKU"). With this condition, tyrosine must be supplied in the diet and is conditionally indispensable.

Balance

The term *balance* refers to the relative intake and output of substances in the body to maintain equilibrium necessary for health in various circumstances throughout life. This concept of balance can be applied to life-sustaining protein and the nitrogen it supplies.

Protein Balance

The body's tissue proteins are constantly being broken down into amino acids, a process called *catabolism,* and then resynthesized into tissue proteins as needed, a process called *anabolism.* To maintain nitrogen balance, the part of the amino acid that contains nitrogen may be removed by *deamination,* then converted to ammonia (NH_3), and excreted as urea in the urine. The remaining nonnitrogen residue can be used to make carbohydrate or fat or reattached to make another amino acid if necessary. The rate of this protein and nitrogen turnover varies in different tissues according to the degree of metabolic activity.

Tissue turnover is a continuous process of reshaping, rebuilding, and adjusting as necessary to maintain overall protein balance within the body. The body also maintains a balance between tissue protein and plasma protein, which are then further balanced with dietary protein intake. With this finely balanced system, a pool of amino acids from both tissue protein and dietary protein is always available to meet construction needs (Figure 4-2).

Nitrogen Balance

The body's nitrogen balance indicates how well its tissues are being maintained. The intake and use of dietary protein is measured by the amount of nitrogen intake in food protein and the amount of nitrogen excreted in the urine. For example, 1 g of urinary nitrogen results from the digestion and metabolism of 6.25 g of protein. Thus if 1 g of nitrogen is excreted in the urine for every 6.25 g of protein consumed, the body is said to be in nitrogen balance. This balance is the normal pattern in adult health, but at different times of life or in states of malnutrition or illness, the balance may shift to be either positive or negative.

Positive Nitrogen Balance. A positive nitrogen balance exists when the body takes in more nitrogen than it excretes, thus storing more nitrogen (by building tissue) than it is losing (by breaking down tissue). This situation occurs normally during periods of rapid growth such as during infancy, childhood, adolescence, pregnancy, and lactation. A positive nitrogen balance also occurs in individuals who have been ill or malnourished and are being "built back up" with increased nourishment. In such cases protein is stored to meet increased needs for tissue building and associated metabolic activity.

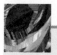

DRUG-NUTRIENT INTERACTION BOX

ASPARTAME AND PKU

Aspartame is a nonnutritive sweetener (it does not provide any nutrients or calories) composed of two amino acids: aspartic acid and phenylalanine. It is made synthetically and its structure more closely resembles a protein than a carbohydrate. However, by adding a methanol group, a sweet taste results. It is used in foods and beverages as a high-potency sweetener, called such because it is approximately 200 times sweeter than table sugar, or sucrose. Therefore much less is needed to sweeten a food to the same degree.*

As previously mentioned, PKU is a disease in which an individual lacks the enzyme phenylalanine hydroxylase. Without this enzyme, phenylalanine cannot be made into a usable form and accumulates in the blood. High levels in the blood cause toxicity to brain tissue, resulting in mental degradation and possibly death. Those with PKU should eliminate or avoid foods containing aspartame because of its phenylalanine content.

Foods containing phenylalanine, and therefore aspartame, indicate so on their packages. Also look on packaging for aspartame's trade names *NutraSweet* and *Equal.* Following is a list of common foods containing aspartame:

- Diet sodas
- Yogurt
- Chewing gum
- Frozen desserts
- Gelatins
- Puddings
- Sugar-free candies

Sara Oldroyd

*FDA: *Artificial sweeteners: no calories . . . sweet!* www.fda.gov/fdac/features/2006/406_sweeteners.html, accessed June 2007.

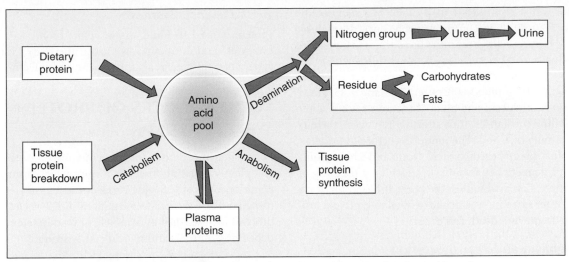

Figure 4-2 Balance between protein compartments and amino acid pool.

Negative Nitrogen Balance. A negative nitrogen balance occurs when the body takes in less nitrogen than it excretes. This means that the body has an inadequate protein intake and is losing nitrogen by breaking down more tissue than it is building up. This situation arises in states of malnutrition and illness. For example, this nitrogen imbalance is seen in individuals when protein deficiency—even when kilocalories from carbohydrate and fat are adequate—causes the classic protein deficiency disease *kwashiorkor*. Failure to maintain nitrogen balance may not become apparent for some time but eventually causes loss of muscle tissue, impairment of body organs and functions, and increased susceptibility to infection. In children, negative nitrogen balance for an extended period causes growth retardation.

FUNCTIONS OF PROTEIN
Primary Tissue Building

Protein is the fundamental structural material of every cell in the body. In fact, the largest dry weight portion of the body is protein. Body protein, such as the lean mass of muscles, accounts for approximately three fourths of the dry matter in most tissues, excluding bone and adipose fat. Protein makes up the bulk of the muscles, internal organs, brain, nerves, skin, hair, and nails and also is a vital part of regulatory substances such as enzymes, hormones, and blood plasma. All these tissues must be constantly repaired and replaced. The primary functions of protein are to repair worn-out, wasted, or damaged tissue and build new tissue. Thus protein meets growth needs and maintains tissue health during adult years. In fact, protein is central to the biochemical machinery that makes cells work.

Additional Body Functions

In addition to its basic tissue-building function, protein has other body functions relating to energy, water balance, metabolism, and the body's defense system. Box 4-2 lists the primary functions of protein.

Energy System

As described in previous chapters, carbohydrates are the primary fuel source for the body's energy system, assisted by fat as a stored fuel. In times of need, protein may furnish additional fuel to sustain body heat and energy, but this is a less-efficient, backup source for use only when the supply of carbohydrate and fat is insufficient. The available fuel factor of protein is 4 kcal/g.

Water and pH Balance

Fluids within the body are divided into three compartments: intravascular, intracellular, and interstitial (see Chapter 9). The body compartments are separated with cell membranes that are not freely permeable to protein.

BOX 4-2

FUNCTIONS OF PROTEIN

Structural tissue building
Source of energy (4 kcal/g)
Water balance through osmotic pressure
Digestion and metabolism through enzymatic action
Cell signaling (insulin) and transport (hemoglobin and transferring)
Immunity (antibodies)

Because water is attracted to protein, plasma proteins such as albumin help control water balance throughout the body by exerting osmotic pressure. This pressure maintains normal circulation of tissue fluids within the appropriate compartments.

Normal pH of blood is between 7.35 and 7.45. However, constantly occurring bodily functions release acidic and alkaline substances, thus affecting the overall acidity and alkalinity of blood. The unique structure of proteins, a combination of a carboxyl acid group and a base group, allows proteins to act as buffering agents by releasing or taking up excess acid within the body. If blood reaches a pH in either extreme (too acidic or alkaline), plasma proteins denature and death can occur.

Metabolism and Transportation

Protein aids metabolic functions through enzymes, transport agents, and hormones. Digestive and cell enzymes are proteins that control metabolic processes. Enzymes necessary for the digestion of carbohydrates (amylase), fats (lipase), and proteins (proteases) are all proteins in nature. Proteins also act as the vehicle in which nutrients are carried throughout the body. Lipoproteins are necessary to transport fats in the water-soluble blood supply. Other examples are hemoglobin, the vital oxygen carrier in the red blood cells, and transferrin, the iron transport protein in the blood. Hormones, such as insulin and glucagon, also are proteins that play a major function in the metabolism of glucose (see Chapter 20).

Body Defense System

Protein is used to build special white blood cells (lymphocytes) and antibodies as part of the body's immune system to help defend against disease and infection.

FOOD SOURCES OF PROTEIN
Types of Food Proteins

Fortunately most foods contain a mixture of proteins that complement one another. In a mixed diet, animal and plant foods provide a wide variety of many nutrients and proteins. Thus the key to a balanced diet is *variety*. Food proteins are classified as complete or incomplete proteins depending on their amino acid composition.

Complete Proteins

Protein foods that contain all nine indispensable amino acids in sufficient quantity and ratio to meet the body's needs are called *complete proteins* (Figure 4-3). These proteins are primarily of animal origin (e.g., egg, milk, cheese, meat, poultry, and fish). However, soybeans and soy products are the exception. Soy products are the only plant sources of complete proteins. Another exception is gelatin. Although gelatin is a protein food of animal origin, it is a relatively insignificant protein because it lacks three essential amino acids (tryptophan, valine, and isoleucine) and has only small amounts of leucine.

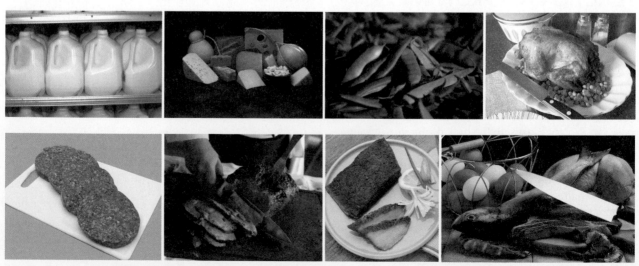

Figure 4-3 Sources of complete proteins. (Copyright JupiterImages Corporation.)

Incomplete Proteins

Protein foods that are deficient in one or more of the nine indispensable amino acids are called *incomplete proteins*. These proteins generally are of plant origin (e.g., grains, legumes, nuts, seeds) but are found in foods that make valuable contributions to the total dietary protein.

Vegetarian Diets

Complementary Protein

Current knowledge of protein metabolism and the pooling of amino acid reserves (see Figure 4-2) indicates that a mixture of plant proteins can provide adequate amounts of amino acids when the basic use of various grains is expanded to include soy protein and other dried legume proteins (i.e., beans and peas). Because most plant proteins are incomplete, lacking one or more indispensable (or essential) amino acids, vegetarians can match plant foods so that the amino acids missing in one food are supplied in another. This is the art of combining plant protein foods so that they complement one another and supply all nine indispensable amino acids.

A normal eating pattern through the day, together with the body's reserve supply of protein, usually ensures a complementary amino acid balance. The underlying requirement for vegetarians, as for all people, is to eat a sufficient amount of varied foods to meet normal nutrient and energy needs (see the Cultural Considerations box, "Indispensable Amino Acids and Their Complementary Food Proteins").

Types of Vegetarian Diets

Vegetarian diets differ according to the beliefs or needs of individuals following these food patterns. Approximately 2.8% of the U.S. population, or roughly 5.7 million people, followed a vegetarian diet in 2003.[2] A variety of reasons lead people to choose a vegetarian diet, including environmental or animal cruelty concerns, health incentives, religious adherence (e.g., Buddhism, Hinduism, Seventh-Day Adventists), and aversion to consuming animal products. On the other hand, a diet void of animal products is not always a choice. In some areas in the world, vegetarianism is simply a result of the lack of resources and availability of animal products.

In general, vegetarians can be described as one of the following four basic types:

1. *Lacto-ovo-vegetarians:* Vegetarians who follow a food pattern that allows dairy products and eggs (Figure 4-4). Their mixed diet of plant and animal food sources, excluding only meat and fish, poses no nutritional concerns.
2. *Lacto-vegetarians:* These vegetarians accept only dairy products from animal sources to comple-

CULTURAL CONSIDERATIONS

INDISPENSABLE AMINO ACIDS AND THEIR COMPLEMENTARY FOOD PROTEINS

More than 5.7 million Americans currently follow a vegetarian diet. This trend in dietary pattern has gained significant followers in the past decade, especially female adolescents and young adults. A large percentage of the worldwide population follows various forms of vegetarian diets for religious, traditional, or economic reasons. Seventh-Day Adventists follow a lacto-ovo-vegetarian diet, whereas individuals of the Hindu and Buddhist faith generally are lacto-vegetarian. The Mediterranean diet has such a strong emphasis on grains, pastas, vegetables, and cheese that little other animal products (beef, chicken, and fish) are consumed. In other areas of the world, the economic burden of animal products does not allow the consumption of such foods. Any form of a vegetarian diet can be healthy; however, a good understanding of how to achieve complete protein balance is necessary.

All nine indispensable, or essential, amino acids must be supplied by the diet. Protein from both animal and plant sources is believed to meet protein requirements. One concern related to a vegetarian diet is getting a balanced amount of the indispensable amino acids to complement each other and make complete food combinations.

In making complementary food combinations to balance the needed amino acids, families of foods (e.g., grains, legumes, and dairy) must be mixed. For example, grains are low in threonine and high in methionine, whereas legumes are the opposite—low in methionine and high in threonine. Therefore grains and legumes help balance one another in the accumulation of all indispensable amino acids. The addition of milk products and eggs enhances the amino acid adequacy for lacto-ovo-vegetarians. Following are sample food combination dishes to illustrate complementary protein combinations:

- *Grains and peas, beans, or lentils:* brown rice and beans, whole-grain bread with pea or lentil soup, wheat or corn tortilla with beans, peanut butter on whole wheat bread, Indian dishes of rice and dal (a legume), Chinese dishes of tofu and rice
- *Legumes and seeds:* falafel, soybeans and pumpkin or sesame seeds, Middle Eastern hummus (garbanzo beans and sesame seeds) or tahini
- *Grains and dairy:* whole-wheat pasta and cheese, yogurt and a multigrain muffin, cereal and milk, cheese sandwich with whole-grain bread

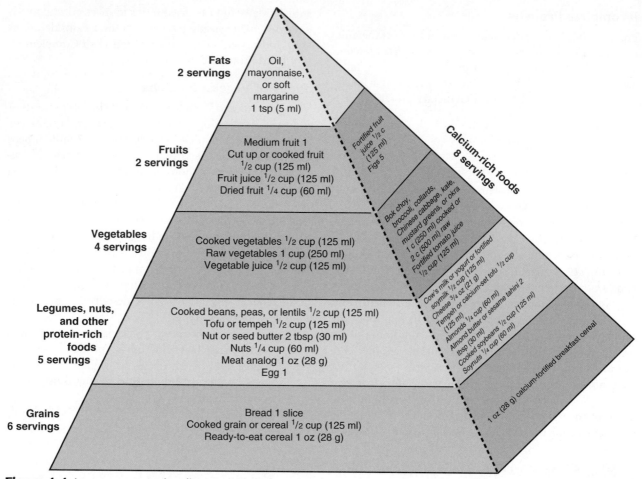

Figure 4-4 Lacto-ovo-vegetarian diet pyramid. (Reprinted from Messina V and others: A new food guide for North American vegetarians, *J Am Diet Assoc* 103(6):771-775, 2003.)

ment their basic diet of plant foods. The use of milk and milk products (e.g., cheese) with a varied mixed diet of whole or enriched grains, legumes, nuts, seeds, fruits, and vegetables in sufficient quantities to meet energy needs provides a balanced diet.

3. *Ovo-vegetarians:* The only animal foods included in the ovo-vegetarian diet are eggs. Because eggs are an excellent source of complete proteins, individuals following this diet do not have to be overly concerned with complementary proteins on a daily basis.

4. *Vegans:* Vegans follow a strict vegetarian diet and consume no animal foods. Their food pattern consists entirely of plant foods (e.g., whole or enriched grains, legumes, nuts, seeds, fruits, and vegetables). The use of soybeans, soy milk, soybean curd (tofu), and processed soy protein products

enhances the nutritional value of the diet, and these products are well tolerated and accepted. Careful planning and sufficient food intake ensure adequate nutrition.

The most recent position paper from the American Dietetic Association and Dietitians of Canada states that a vegetarian diet, including vegan, can meet the current recommendations for all essential nutrients, including protein.[3] The experts also indicate that the former mindful combination of complementary plant proteins within every given meal is unnecessary. Achieving a balance throughout the day is more important. In addition, vegetarian diets are appropriate throughout all stages of life, including pregnancy, infancy, childhood, adolescence, and older age as well as for competitive athletes. *The Dietary Guidelines for Americans, 2005* state that "vegetarians of all types can achieve recommended nutrient intakes through careful selection of foods."[4]

Health Benefits and Risk

Some of the most notable benefits of vegetarianism include the following[3]:

- Lower levels of dietary saturated fat and cholesterol from animal products
- Higher levels of carbohydrates, fiber, magnesium, boron, folate, carotenoids, phytochemicals, and antioxidants such as vitamins C and E
- Lower body mass index and prevalence of obesity
- Lower rates of death from cardiovascular disease, including ischemic heart disease, high blood cholesterol, and hypertension
- Lower risk of type 2 diabetes and some forms of cancer (e.g., prostate and colon)
- Lowered risk of renal disease from high glomerular filtration rates
- Lowered risk of dementia

After extensive review of the effects of vegetarian diets in various medical conditions, researchers have concluded that "dietary intervention with a vegetarian diet seems to be a cheap, physiologic, and safe approach for the prevention and possible management of modern lifestyle diseases."[5] The preventive mechanism at work in the vegetarian diet is the rich supply of monounsaturated and polyunsaturated fatty acids, fiber, complex carbohydrates, and antioxidants and a restriction in saturated fat. To reap the benefits of a vegetarian diet, a well-balanced diet from a variety of foods is necessary.[6]

Key nutrients of concern for practicing vegetarians are protein, iron, zinc, calcium, vitamin D, vitamin B_{12}, vitamin A, and omega-3 fatty acids (alpha-linolenic acid).[7] Reasons for concern and effective ways to overcome these barriers are outlined in Table 4-1.

TABLE 4-1

NUTRIENT CONSIDERATIONS FOR VEGETARIANS

NUTRIENT	PROBLEM	SOLUTION
Protein	Plant protein quality varies; lower digestibility than animal protein	Consume a variety of plant foods throughout the day
Iron	Plant foods contain nonheme iron, which is less bioavailable than heme iron found in animal foods and is sensitive to inhibitors such as phytate, calcium, teas, coffee, and fiber	Iron intake recommendations are 1.8 times higher than for nonvegetarians. Consume high-iron plant foods with dietary sources of vitamin C, an enhancer of iron absorption
Zinc	Plant foods high in phytates bind zinc	Regularly consuming foods such as soaked and sprouted beans, grains, and seeds will increase the bioavailability of dietary zinc
Calcium	Oxalates reduce calcium absorption (found in spinach, beet greens, and Swiss chard)	Regularly consume plant foods high in calcium and low in oxalates such as Chinese cabbage, broccoli, Napa cabbage, collards, kale, okra, and turnip greens, in addition to calcium fortified foods
Vitamin D	Other than endogenously produced vitamin D from sunlight exposure, the primary source of this vitamin is fortified cow's milk	Sun exposure to the face, hands, and forearms for 5-15 min/day during the summer provides enough sunlight for light-skinned people to produce adequate vitamin D. Dark-skinned people need more time. Otherwise, choose foods or dietary supplements fortified with vitamin D, such as soymilk, rice milk, or breakfast cereal
Vitamin B_{12}	No plant food contains active vitamin B_{12}	Choose foods fortified with B_{12} such as soy milk, breakfast cereal, nutritional yeast, or dietary supplements
Vitamin A (beta-carotene)	Preformed vitamin A is only found in animal foods	Beta-carotene from plant foods can be converted to vitamin A; consume 3 servings/day of yellow or orange vegetables, leafy green vegetables, or fruits rich in beta-carotene
Omega-3 fatty acid (alpha-linolenic)	Few plant foods are good sources of alpha-linolenic acid	Include good sources of alpha-linolenic acid in the diet with foods such as flaxseed, flaxseed oil, canola oil, walnuts, walnut oil, soybeans, and soybean oil on a regular basis

Modified from Mangels AR and others: Position of the American Dietetic Association and Dietitians of Canada: vegetarian diets, *J Am Diet Assoc* 103(6):748, 2003.

DIGESTION OF PROTEINS
Mouth

After protein is eaten, it must be changed into the necessary, ready-to-use building units, amino acids. This work is done through the successive parts of the GI tract by the mechanical and chemical processes of digestion. The mechanical breaking down of protein foods occurs by chewing in the mouth. The food particles are mixed with saliva and passed on to the stomach as a semisolid mass.

Stomach

Because proteins are such large, complex structures, a series of enzymes is necessary to break them down and produce individual amino acids, the primary form for absorption. Unlike enzymes needed for carbohydrate and fat digestion, all enzymes involved in protein digestion (proteases) are stored as inactive proenzymes called zymogens. Zymogens are then activated upon need. Enzymes needed for protein digestion cannot be stored in an active form or the cells and organs (made of structural proteins) that produce and store them would be digested as well.

Chemical digestion of protein begins in the stomach. In fact, the stomach's chief digestive function overall is the first stage in the enzymatic breakdown of protein. The following three agents in the gastric secretions help with this task.

Hydrochloric Acid

Hydrochloric acid provides the acid medium necessary to convert pepsinogen to active pepsin, the gastric enzyme specific to proteins. Hydrochloric acid also begins the unfolding and denaturing of the complex protein chains. This unfolding makes the individual amino acids more available for enzymatic action.

Pepsin

Pepsin is first produced as an inactive proenzyme, *pepsinogen,* by a single layer of chief cells in the stomach wall. The hydrochloric acid within gastric juices then changes pepsinogen to the active enzyme pepsin. Pepsin begins splitting the links between the protein's amino acids, which changes the large protein into smaller short chains called *polypeptides.* If the protein were held in the stomach longer, pepsin could continue this breakdown until only the individual amino acids of the protein remained. However, with normal gastric emptying time, pepsin only completes the first stage of breakdown.

Rennin

The gastric enzyme rennin is only present in infancy and childhood and is especially important in the infant's digestion of milk. Rennin and calcium act on the casein of milk to produce a curd. By coagulating milk into a more solid curd, rennin prevents the food from passing too rapidly from the infant's stomach to the small intestine.

Small Intestine

Protein digestion begins in the acidic medium of the stomach and is completed in the alkaline medium of the small intestine. Enzymes from secretions of both the pancreas and intestine take part.

Pancreatic Secretions

The following three enzymes produced by the pancreas continue breaking down proteins into simpler and simpler substances:

1. Trypsin, secreted first as inactive trypsinogen, is activated by the enzyme enterokinase. Enterokinase is secreted from the intestinal cells on contact with food entering the duodenum, the first section of the small intestine. The active trypsin then works on proteins and large polypeptide fragments carried from the stomach. This enzymatic action produces small polypeptides and dipeptides.
2. Chymotrypsin, secreted first as the inactive chymotrypsinogen, is activated by the trypsin already present. The active enzyme then continues the same protein-splitting action of trypsin.
3. Carboxypeptidase attacks the acid (carboxyl) end of the peptide chains, producing small peptides and some free amino acids. Carboxypeptidase also is first released as the inactive proenzyme procarboxypeptidase and is activated by trypsin.

Intestinal Secretions

Glands in the intestinal wall produce the following two protein-splitting enzymes to complete the breakdown and free the remaining amino acids:

1. Aminopeptidase attacks the nitrogen-containing (amino) end of the peptide chain and releases amino acids one at a time, producing peptides and free amino acids.
2. Dipeptidase, the final enzyme in the protein-splitting system, completes the large task by breaking the remaining dipeptides into two free amino acids.

This finely coordinated system of protein-splitting enzymes breaks down the large, complex proteins into progressively smaller peptide chains and frees each individual amino acid, a tremendous overall task. The free amino acids are now ready to be absorbed directly into the portal blood circulation for use in building body tissues. This remarkable system of protein digestion is summarized in Figure 4-5.

RECOMMENDATIONS FOR DIETARY PROTEIN

Influential Factors of Protein Needs

The following three factors influence the requirement for protein: (1) tissue growth, (2) quality of the dietary protein, and (3) additional needs resulting from illness or disease.

Tissue Growth

During rapid growth periods of the human life cycle, more protein per unit of body weight is necessary to build new tissue and maintain present tissue. Human growth is most rapid during fetal growth, infant growth during the first year of life, and adolescent growth. Young childhood is a sustained time of continued growth but at a somewhat slower rate. For adults, protein requirements level off to meet tissue-maintenance needs, but individual needs may vary.

Dietary Protein Quality

The nature of protein and pattern of amino acids significantly influence its dietary quality. Sufficient kilocalories or energy intake—especially from nonprotein foods—also is necessary to conserve protein for tissue building. Finally, the digestion and absorption of the protein consumed are affected by the comparative complexity of its structure as well as its preparation and cooking. The comparative quality of protein foods has been determined by the following:

1. *Chemical score (CS):* derived from the amino acid pattern of the food. A high-quality protein food, such as an egg (with a value of 100) is compared with other foods according to their amino acid ratios.
2. *Biological value (BV):* based on nitrogen balance.
3. *Net protein utilization (NPU):* based on the biologic value and the degree of the food protein's digestibility.
4. *Protein efficiency ratio (PER):* based on the weight gain of a growing test animal in relation to its protein intake.

Table 4-2 compares various protein food scores on the basis of these measures of protein quality. As seen in the table, egg and milk proteins lead all the lists. The quality

and digestibility of most plant proteins are significantly less than animal proteins; therefore the dietary protein needs of vegans who rely solely on plant foods for protein may be higher than those for nonvegetarians.[3] In other words, because the protein provided by whole-wheat products is only approximately half as bioavailable as protein from eggs, twice as much protein from whole-wheat products would have to be eaten to get the same amount of useable protein.

proenzyme an inactive precursor (forerunner substance from which another substance is made) converted to the active enzyme by the action of an *acid,* another enzyme, or other means.

zymogen an inactive enzyme precursor.

pepsin the main gastric enzyme specific for proteins. Pepsin begins breaking large protein molecules into shorter chain polypeptides; gastric hydrochloric acid is necessary to activate.

rennin milk-curdling enzyme of the gastric juice of human infants and young animals such as calves. Should not be confused with renin, which is an important enzyme produced by the kidney that plays a vital role in producing angiotensin, a potent vasoconstrictor and stimulant for release of the hormone aldosterone from the adjacent adrenal glands.

trypsin a protein-splitting enzyme secreted as the inactive proenzyme *trypsinogen* in the pancreas that is activated and acts in the small intestine to reduce proteins to shorter chain polypeptides and dipeptides.

enterokinase an enzyme produced and secreted in the duodenum in response to food entering the small intestine; activates trypsinogen to its active form, trypsin.

chymotrypsin a protein-splitting enzyme secreted as the inactive proenzyme *chymotrypsinogen* in the pancreas that is activated and acts in the small intestine to continue breaking down proteins into shorter chain polypeptides and dipeptides.

carboxypeptidase specific protein-splitting enzyme secreted as the inactive proenzyme procarboxypeptidase in the pancreas that is activated by trypsin in the small intestine to break off the acid (*carboxyl*) end of the peptide chain, producing smaller chained peptides and free amino acids.

aminopeptidase specific protein-splitting enzyme secreted by small glands in the walls of the small intestine that breaks off the nitrogen-containing amino ($-NH2$) end of the peptide chain, producing smaller chained peptides and free amino acids.

dipeptidase specific final enzyme in the protein-splitting system that produces the last two free amino acids.

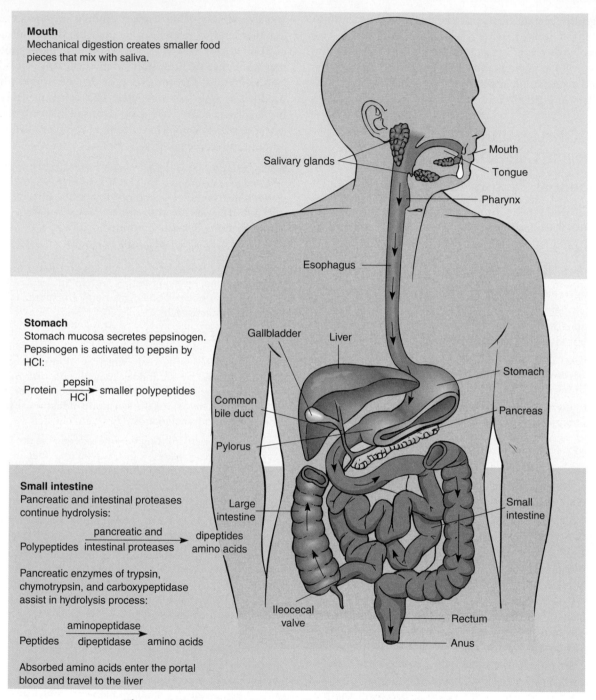

Mouth
Mechanical digestion creates smaller food pieces that mix with saliva.

Stomach
Stomach mucosa secretes pepsinogen. Pepsinogen is activated to pepsin by HCl:

$$\text{Protein} \xrightarrow[\text{HCl}]{\text{pepsin}} \text{smaller polypeptides}$$

Small intestine
Pancreatic and intestinal proteases continue hydrolysis:

$$\text{Polypeptides} \xrightarrow{\text{pancreatic and intestinal proteases}} \begin{array}{l}\text{dipeptides}\\\text{amino acids}\end{array}$$

Pancreatic enzymes of trypsin, chymotrypsin, and carboxypeptidase assist in hydrolysis process:

$$\text{Peptides} \xrightarrow[\text{dipeptidase}]{\text{aminopeptidase}} \text{amino acids}$$

Absorbed amino acids enter the portal blood and travel to the liver

Labels: Salivary glands, Mouth, Tongue, Pharynx, Esophagus, Gallbladder, Liver, Stomach, Common bile duct, Pancreas, Pylorus, Large intestine, Small intestine, Ileocecal valve, Rectum, Anus

Figure 4-5 Summary of protein digestion. (Courtesy Rolin Graphics.)

Regardless of dietary preferences for protein foods, a sound diet is the best way for a healthy person to obtain quality protein. Amino acid and whole-protein dietary supplements are not advantageous over whole foods. The body cannot store large quantities of protein and therefore must break it down and excrete the nitrogen waste product.

Illness or Disease

An illness or disease, especially when accompanied by fever and increased tissue breakdown (catabolism), increases the body's need for protein and kilocalories for rebuilding tissue and meeting the demands of an increased metabolic rate. Traumatic injury requires extensive tissue rebuilding. After surgery, extra protein is needed for wound healing

TABLE 4-2

COMPARATIVE PROTEIN QUALITY OF SELECTED FOODS

FOOD	CHEMICAL SCORE*	BV	NPU	PER
Egg	100	100	94	3.92
Cow's milk	95	93	82	3.09
Fish	71	76	—	3.55
Beef	69	74	67	2.30
Unpolished rice	67	86	59	—
Peanuts	65	55	55	1.65
Oats	57	65	—	2.19
Polished rice	57	64	57	2.18
Whole wheat	53	65	49	1.53
Corn	49	72	36	—
Soybeans	47	73	61	2.32
Sesame seeds	42	62	53	1.77
Peas	37	64	55	1.57

BV, Biologic value; *NPU*, net protein utilization; *PER*, protein efficiency ratio.
*Amino acid.
Modified from Guthrie H: *Introductory nutrition*, ed 6, New York, 1986, McGraw-Hill; and Food and Nutrition Board, Institute of Medicine: *Recommended dietary allowances*, ed 10, Washington, DC, 1989, National Academies Press.

and restoring losses. Extensive tissue destruction, such as occurs with burns, requires a large protein increase for the healing and grafting processes.

Dietary Deficiency or Excess

As with any nutrient, moderation and balance are the keys to health. Too much or too little dietary protein can be problematic in overall body function.

Protein-Energy Malnutrition

Protein-energy malnutrition (PEM) can occur in a variety of situations. The most severe cases are found in less-industrialized countries where all foods are in short supply, not just protein-rich foods. Children are at the highest risk for developing PEM because of their elevated needs during rapid growth and development. However, PEM can affect anyone at any age. Persons with poor nutrient intake, such as the elderly or those with eating disorders, may have PEM as well. PEM rarely exists without overall energy deficiency. However, individuals with high protein needs during infection or disease, such as acquired immunodeficiency syndrome, cancer, and liver failure, sometimes have PEM despite seemingly adequate total energy intake. As previously mentioned, protein has many critical functions in the body. Thus a dietary deficiency has multiple consequences directly related to these functions. Without the amino acid building blocks, the body cannot synthesize needed struc-

tural (muscle) or functional (enzymes, antibodies, hormones, etc.) proteins.

Two severe forms of PEM are kwashiorkor and marasmus. Characteristics of the two forms of PEM are quite different, as described below. Kwashiorkor is thought to result from an acute deficiency of protein, whereas marasmus results from a more chronic deficiency. The end result with either form is stunted growth, a weakened immune system, and poor development.

Kwashiorkor. Kwashiorkor is more common in children between the ages of 18 to 24 months who have been breastfed all their lives and then are rapidly weaned, often because of the arrival of a younger sibling. These children are switched from nutritionally balanced breast milk to a dilute diet of mostly carbohydrates and little protein. The term kwashiorkor is a Ghanaian word that refers to the disease that takes over the first child when the second child is born. The children may receive adequate total kilocalories but lack enough kilocalories from protein sources. Characteristics of kwashiorkor include edema in the feet and legs and a bloated abdomen, both from lack of protein in the blood to maintain fluid balance and transport fat from the liver (Figure 4-6).

Marasmus. Individuals with marasmus have an emaciated appearance with little or no body fat. This is a chronic form of energy and protein deficiency—basic starvation. Stunted growth and development are even

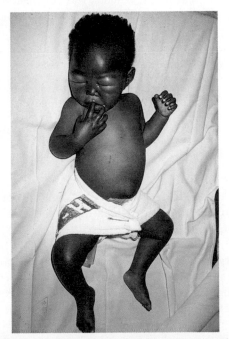

Figure 4-6 Kwashiorkor. The infant shows generalized edema, seen in the form of puffiness of the face, arms, and legs. (Reprinted from Kumar V and others: *Robbins basic pathology*, ed 8, Philadelphia, 2007, Saunders.)

FOR FURTHER FOCUS

THE HIGH-PROTEIN DIET

The per capita consumption of protein by Americans continues to rise, along with total caloric intake. In the United States the per capita daily consumption of kilocalories and grams of protein rose from 3200 kcal and 86 g protein in 1935 to 3900 kcal and 113 g protein in 2004.* Not coincidentally, significant weight gains and the health risks associated with obesity (heart disease, diabetes, hypertension, some forms of cancer, etc.) have been noted. As a result, 24% of men and 38% of women are actively trying to lose weight.†

Many health care professionals are concerned about the rising rate of obesity in this country as well as the methods by which people are trying to combat it. In a survey of more than 32,000 people, only 34% reported using the recommended strategy of eating fewer calories and exercising more to lose weight.† Some of the more popular diets are the high-protein, low-carbohydrate diets, although the safety of such diets has yet to be clearly determined. Long-term studies are beginning to emerge that will hopefully shed light on this controversial practice in weight loss.

High-protein diets generally are higher in total fat, saturated fat, and cholesterol. Initial weight loss associated with a high-protein, high-fat diet is caused by the induction of metabolic ketosis and fluid loss from a lack of carbohydrates. Ketosis eventually suppresses the appetite, ultimately leading to reduced caloric intake and weight loss. The debate concerns the side effects of the diet.

In the past, excessive protein intake was thought to present many health risks, including increased blood cholesterol, increased uric acid levels, increased triglycerides, and calcium loss from bones. However, recent studies have addressed and overturned some initial worries. One such study found that high-protein diets followed for 10 days significantly increased dietary absorption of calcium that parallels the observed loss in urine. Thus the calcium loss is not detrimental to bone loss (as was previously thought) in the short term.‡ How high-protein intake affects calcium deposits in bone long term is still not clear. Another study comparing the Zone diet (high protein), Atkins diet (high fat), and a control diet of high-carbohydrates in insulin-resistant obese women found that the Zone diet was the most appropriate for short-term weight loss without increasing the risk of cardiovascular disease.§ However, the subjects were only followed for 6 months; thus long-term effects cannot be determined. At least one long-term study (1 year) has reported greater loss of abdominal adipose tissue in a high-protein, low-fat group when compared with a medium-protein, low-fat group.||

Regardless of these findings, the American Heart Association has not changed its view regarding high-protein diets. In a statement for health care professionals from the Nutrition Committee of the Council on Nutrition, Physical Activity, and Metabolism of the American Heart Association researchers concluded that "high-protein diets are not recommended because they restrict healthful foods that provide essential nutrients and do not provide the variety of foods needed to adequately meet nutritional needs."¶

*United States Department of Agriculture, Center for Nutrition Policy and Promotion: *U.S. food supply: Nutrients contributed from major food groups, 1970 and 2000,* www.ers.usda.gov/Data/FoodConsumption/NutrientAvailIndex.htm, accessed August 2006.
†Kruger J and others: Attempting to lose weight: specific practices among U.S. adults, *Am J Prev Med* 26(5):402, 2004.
‡Kerstetter J and others: The impact of dietary protein on calcium absorption and kinetic measures of bone turnover in women, *J Clin Endocrinol Metab* 90:26, 2005.
§McAuley KA and others: Comparison of high-fat and high-protein diets with a high-carbohydrate diet in insulin-resistant obese women, *Diabetologia* 48:8, 2005.
||Due A and others: Effects of normal-fat diets, either medium or high in protein, on body weight in overweight subjects: a randomized 1-year trial, *Int J Obes Relat Metab Disord* 28(20):1283, 2004.
¶Sachiko T and others: Dietary protein and weight reduction, *Circulation* 104(15):1869, 2001.

more severe with this form of PEM. Marasmus can affect individuals of all ages with inadequate food sources.

Excess Dietary Intake

Contrary to popular belief, the ingestion of too much dietary protein can occur (see the Further Focus box, "The High-Protein Diet"). The body has a finite need for protein. In other words, once a person has met the dietary protein needs, additional protein is deaminated (the nitrogen is removed) and stored as fat or used as energy. Eating excess protein does not build muscle. Only exercis-

ing with enough protein to support growth can do that. The following problems can occur with diets heavily laden with protein:

1. They are often high in saturated fats, a known risk for cardiovascular disease.
2. If a person fills up on protein foods, little room is left for fruits, vegetables, and other whole grains packed with essential vitamins, minerals, and fiber.
3. The kidneys have the extra burden of getting rid of excess nitrogen.

Although most protein and amino acid supplements are not harmful, they are unnecessary in a balanced diet.

Dietary Guides

Dietary Reference Intakes

The RDAs continue to be the principal dietary guide for protein consumption and are part of the DRI standards. Similar to carbohydrate and fat recommendations, the National Academy of Sciences has set the DRIs for proteins as a percentage of the total kilocalorie consumption. Children and adults should get 10% to 35% of their total caloric intake from protein. The RDA standards relate to the age, sex, and weight of the average person and are based on analysis of available nitrogen balance studies. Protein RDAs are highest at birth and slowly decline into adulthood. The RDA for both men and women is set at 0.8 g of high-quality protein per kilogram of desirable body weight per day (0.8 g/kg per day) (see the Clinical Applications box, "Calculating Dietary Reference Intake for Protein").[1] Needs are higher for infants, pregnant and breastfeeding women, and possibly vegans.

Of note, the RDAs are set to meet the nutritional requirements of most healthy people. Severe physical stress, such as illness, disease, and surgery, can increase a person's need for protein. The USDA recently reported that 97% of men older than 19 years consumed dietary protein from whole foods sources alone that meet their needs based on the DRI. Approximately 93% of women older than 19 years meet their needs through usual dietary patterns.[8]

Dietary Guidelines for Americans

No known benefits exists from the consumption of a diet with a high animal protein content, which also carries added fat. However, some potential health risks do exist. These risks relate to certain cancers, coronary heart disease associated with increased animal fat, kidney stones, and chronic renal failure (see Chapter 21) associated with the excess protein intake. Therefore the *Dietary Guidelines for Americans* recommend that individuals choose foods from each of the five food groups according to the MyPyramid food guide system, consuming moderate amounts of foods from the meat and bean group (two to three servings per day).

Americans generally eat more protein than necessary, especially in the form of meat, which carries considerable animal fat. Cutting down consumption of meat to leaner, more moderate portions would also bring the health benefits of reducing the intake of saturated animal fat. Table 4-3 provides a comparison of protein food portions.

MyPyramid

As with the other macronutrient recommendations from the MyPyramid site, Americans are encouraged to consume a variety of foods to meet all nutrient needs. The site includes tips for choosing lean sources of meat, poultry, fish, or protein alternatives such as beans, nuts, and seeds. An individualized plan can be obtained by entering a person's age, sex, height, weight, and physical activity level. Sample menus for nonvegetarians and eating tips for vegetarian lifestyles are also available.

CLINICAL APPLICATIONS

CALCULATING DIETARY REFERENCE INTAKE FOR PROTEIN

To calculate the protein needs of an individual consuming 2200 kcal/day based on the DRI recommendation of 10% to 35% of total kilocalories, perform the following calculations:

(1) 2200 kcal × 0.10 = 220 kcal/day *and*
(2) 2200 kcal × 0.35 = 770 kcal/day,
thus giving a range of 220-770 kcal/day from protein
(3) 220 kcal/4 kcal/g = 55 *and*
(4) 770 kcal/4 kcal/g = 192.5 g of protein per day,
thus providing a range of 55-192.5 g of protein per day

To calculate the protein needs of a woman who is 5 feet, four inches tall with an ideal body weight (see Chapter 15) of 120 lb, based on the RDA of 0.8 g protein/kg body weight per day, perform the following calculations:

(1) Convert weight in pounds to weight in kg (2.2 lb = 1 kg) as follows: 120 lb/2.2 lb/kg = 54.5 kg
(2) 54.5 kg × 0.8 g/kg = 43.6 g protein per day
Therefore a woman measuring 5 feet, four inches tall consuming 2200 kcal/day with a minimum of 10% of calories coming from high-quality protein will exceed her RDA for protein (43.6 g per day).

TABLE 4-3

FOODS HIGH IN PROTEIN

FOOD	APPROXIMATE AMOUNT	PROTEIN (g)
Veal, leg, meat only, braised	3 oz cooked	31.2
Beef, top round, trimmed of fat	3 oz cooked	30.7
Chicken, breast, meat only, roasted	½ breast (3 oz)	26.7
Tuna, fresh, bluefin, cooked with dry heat	3 oz cooked	25.4
Turkey, meat only, roasted	3 oz cooked	24.9
Goose, meat only, roasted	3 oz cooked	24.6
Pork, sirloin, boneless, roasted	3 oz cooked	24.5
Halibut, fresh, cooked with dry heat	3 oz cooked	22.7
Liver, chicken, pan fried	3 oz cooked	21.9
Lamb, shoulder, trimmed to ¼-inch fat, broiled	3 oz cooked	21.7
Tuna, canned in water, drained	3 oz cooked	21.7
Beef, ground, 70% lean, 30% fat, pan browned	3 oz cooked	21.7
Haddock, cooked with dry heat	3 oz cooked	20.6
Duck, meat only, roasted	3 oz cooked	20
Scallops, steamed	3 oz cooked	19.7
Salmon, Atlantic, cooked with dry heat	3 oz cooked	18.8
Soy burger	3 oz cooked	16.1
Oysters, cooked with moist heat	3 oz cooked	16.1
Tofu, fried	3 oz	14.6
Ham, sliced, 11% fat	3 oz cooked	14.1
Cottage cheese, 2% milkfat	3 oz	11.7
Soy milk	1 cup	11
Milk, 1% fat	1 cup	9.7
Peanut butter, smooth	2 Tbsp	8
Lentils, boiled	3 oz cooked	7.7
Kidney beans, boiled	3 oz cooked	7.4
Cheddar cheese	1 oz	7
Egg, whole, scrambled	1 large	6.8
Yogurt, plain, skim milk	3 oz	4.9

Data from the USDA, Agricultural Research Service, Nutrient Data Laboratory: *USDA nutrient database for standard reference, release 20*, www.ars.usda.gov/ba/bhnrc/ndl.

SUMMARY

Proteins provide the human body with its primary tissue-building units, amino acids. Of the 20 common amino acids, nine are indispensable in the diet because the body cannot manufacture them as it can the remaining 11. Foods that supply all the indispensable amino acids are called complete proteins. These foods are mostly of animal origin (e.g., egg, milk, cheese, and meat). Plant protein foods (e.g., grains, legumes, nuts, seeds, and vegetables) are considered incomplete proteins because they lack one or more of the indispensable amino acids. The exception is soy protein, which is of plant origin and provides complete proteins. Strict vegan diets use only plant proteins, but other vegetarian diets may include dairy, egg, and sometimes fish.

Constant turnover of tissue protein occurs between tissue building (anabolism) and tissue breakdown (catabolism). Adequate dietary protein and a reserve pool of amino acids help maintain this overall protein balance. Nitrogen balance is a measure of overall protein balance. A mixed diet of a variety of foods, together with sufficient nonprotein kilocalories from the primary fuel foods, supplies a balance of protein and other nutrients. Only strict vegetarians (vegans) risk protein imbalance and other nutritional deficiencies in iron, zinc, calcium, and vitamin B_{12}.

After protein foods are eaten, a powerful digestive team of six protein-splitting enzymes frees individual unique amino acids for their vital tissue-building tasks.

Protein requirements are mainly influenced by growth needs and the nature of the diet in terms of protein quality and energy intake. Clinical influences on protein needs include fever, disease, surgery, and other trauma to body tissues.

CRITICAL THINKING QUESTIONS

1. What is the difference between indispensable and dispensable amino acids? Why is this difference important?
2. Compare complete and incomplete protein foods. Give examples of each.

3. Describe the different types of vegetarian diets. Compare each in terms of protein quality and risk for nutrient deficiencies. What recommendations would you offer someone following a vegan diet?
4. Describe the factors that influence protein requirements.

CHAPTER CHALLENGE QUESTIONS

True-False

Write the correct statement for each statement that is false.

1. *True or False:* Complete proteins of high biologic value are found in whole grains, dried beans and peas, and nuts.

2. *True or False:* The primary function of dietary protein is to supply the necessary amino acids to build and repair body tissue.

3. *True or False:* Protein provides a main source of body heat and muscle energy.

4. *True or False:* The average American diet contains a relatively small amount of protein.

5. *True or False:* Because they are smaller, infants and young children need less protein per unit of body weight than do adults.

6. *True or False:* Healthy adults are in a state of nitrogen balance.

7. *True or False:* Positive nitrogen balance exists during periods of rapid growth (e.g., in infancy and adolescence).

8. *True or False:* When negative nitrogen balance exists, an individual is less able to resist infection and general health deteriorates.

9. *True or False:* Egg protein has a higher biologic value than meat protein.

Multiple Choice

1. Nine of the 20 amino acids are indispensable, meaning that
   a. the body cannot make them and must obtain them from the diet.
   b. they are indispensable in body processes and the rest are not.
   c. the body makes them because they are the life-essential ones.
   d. after making them, the body uses them for growth.

2. A complete protein food of high biologic value contains
   a. all 20 of the amino acids in sufficient amounts to meet human requirements.
   b. the nine indispensable amino acids in any proportion because the body can always fill in the necessary differences.
   c. all the 20 amino acids from which the body can make additional amounts of the nine indispensable ones as necessary.
   d. all nine of the indispensable amino acids in correct proportion to meet human requirements.

3. A state of negative nitrogen balance may occur during periods of
   a. pregnancy.
   b. adolescence.
   c. injury or surgery.
   d. infancy.

evolve Please refer to the Students' Resource section of this text's Evolve Web site for additional study resources.

REFERENCES

1. Food and Nutrition Board, Institute of Medicine: *Dietary reference intakes for energy, carbohydrate, fiber, fat, fatty acids, cholesterol, protein, and amino acids,* Washington, DC, 2002, National Academies Press
2. The Vegetarian Resource Group: *How many vegetarians are there?* www.vrg.org/journal/vj2003issue3/vj2003issue3poll.htm, accessed June 2007.
3. Mangels AR and others: Position of the American Dietetic Association and Dietitians of Canada: vegetarian diets, *J Am Diet Assoc* 103(6):748, 2003.
4. U.S. Department of Health and Human Services, U.S. Department of Agriculture: *Dietary guidelines for Americans, 2005,* Washington, DC, 2005, USDA.
5. Segasothy M, Phillips PA: Vegetarian diet: panacea for modern lifestyle diseases? *J Med* 92:531, 1999.
6. Leitzmann C: Vegetarian diets: what are the advantages? *Forum Nutr* 57:147, 2005.
7. Key TJ and others: Health effects of vegetarian and vegan diets, *Proc Nutr Soc* 65(1):35, 2006.
8. Moshfegh A and others: *What we eat in America, NHANES 2001-2002: Usual nutrient intakes from food compared to dietary reference intakes,* Washington, DC, 2005, U.S. Department of Agriculture, Agricultural Research Service.

FURTHER READING AND RESOURCES

The following organizations provide a good source of information about vegetarian diets.

Food and Nutrition Information Center: *www.nal.usda.gov/fnic/etext/000058.html*

Vegetarian Union of North America: *www.ivu.org/vuna*

North American Vegetarian Society: *www.navs-online.org*

The Vegetarian Resource Group: *www.vrg.org*

Vegetarian Nutrition Dietetic Practice Group: *www.vegetariannutrition.net*

Medline Plus (key search word "vegetarianism"): *www.nlm.nih.gov/medlineplus/vegetarianism.html*

Messina V and others: A new food guide for North American vegetarians, *J Am Diet Assoc* 103(6):771, 2003.
  The authors design and explain a new Food Guide Pyramid appropriate for vegetarians. This article reviews the nutrient needs from each food group and the best sources for achieving nutritional balance. A great resource for vegetarians.

The following articles explore the scientific evidence to support the advantages of vegetarianism while explaining that poor meal planning in any type of diet can negate the benefits.

Key TJ and others: Health effects of vegetarian and vegan diets, *Proc Nutr Soc* 65(1):35, 2006.

Leitzmann C: Vegetarian diets: what are the advantages? *Forum Nutr* 57:147, 2005.

CHAPTER 5

Digestion, Absorption, and Metabolism

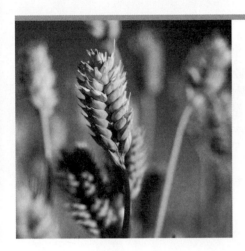

KEY CONCEPTS

- Through a balanced system of mechanical and chemical digestion, food is broken down into smaller substances and the nutrients are released for biologic use.
- Special organ structures and functions conduct these tasks through the successive parts of the overall system.

As described in previous chapters, nutrients the body requires do not come ready to use, but rather packaged as foods in a variety of forms. Therefore whole food must be broken down into smaller substances to meet the body's needs. Digestion of the macronutrients (carbohydrates, fat, and protein) has been discussed in preceding chapters.

This chapter views the overall process of food digestion and nutrient absorption as one continuous whole with a series of successive events. In addition, metabolism and the unique body structures and functions that make this process possible—as well as life—are reviewed.

DIGESTION

Basic Principles

Principle of Change

Body cells cannot use food as it is eaten. Food must be changed into simpler substances for absorption and then into even simpler substances that cells can use to sustain life. Preparing food for the body's use involves many steps including digestion, absorption, transport, and metabolism.

---

digestion process in which food is broken down in the GI tract, releasing many nutrients in forms the body can use.

absorption process in which nutrients are taken into the cells lining the GI tract.

transport movement of nutrients through the circulatory system from one area of the body to another.

metabolism the sum of the vast number of chemical changes in the cell, the functional unit of life, which finally produces the essential materials necessary for energy, tissue building, and metabolic controls.

Principle of Wholeness

The parts of this overall process of change do not exist separately. The different parts of the GI tract and their accessory organs are shown in Figure 5-1. Food components travel through this system until they ultimately are delivered to the cells or excreted as waste.

Mechanical and Chemical Changes

For nutrients to be delivered to cells, food must go through a series of mechanical and chemical changes. Together, these two actions encompass the overall process of digestion.

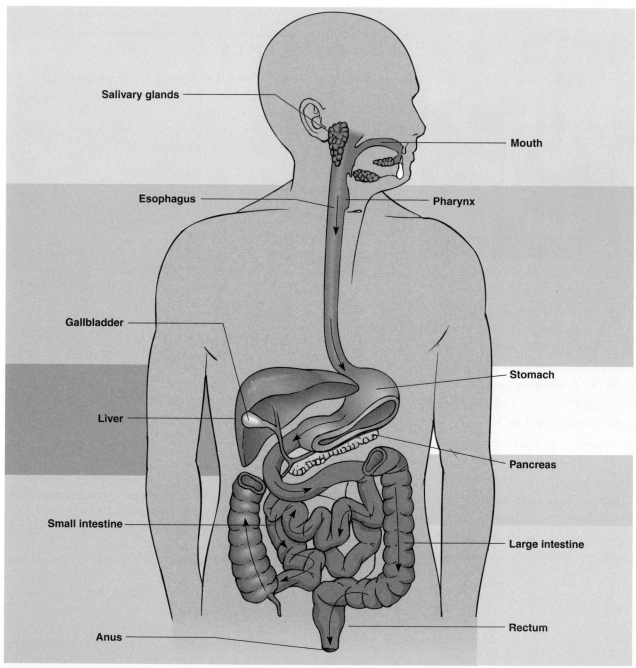

Figure 5-1 The GI system. Through the successive parts of the system, multiple activities of digestion liberate food nutrients for use. (Courtesy Rolin Graphics.)

The specific mechanical and chemical actions that occur during digestion of carbohydrates, proteins, and fats have previously been discussed. This chapter touches on those actions as a whole and as an interdependent process.

Mechanical Digestion: Gastrointestinal Motility

Beginning in the mouth, muscles and nerves in the walls of the GI tract coordinate their actions to provide the necessary motility for digestion to proceed. *Motility* is the ability to move spontaneously. This automatic response to the presence of food enables the system to break up the food mass and move it along the digestive pathway. Muscles and nerves work together to produce smooth-running motility.

Muscles. Layers of smooth muscle in the GI wall interact to provide two general types of movement: (1) *muscle tone,* or tonic contraction, which ensures continuous passage of the food mass and valve control along the way; and (2) *periodic muscle contraction and relaxation,* which are rhythmical waves that mix the food mass and move it forward. These alternating muscular contractions and relaxations that force the contents forward are known as *peristalsis,* a term from two Greek words: *peri,* meaning around, and *stalsis,* meaning contraction.

Nerves. Specific nerves regulate muscle action along the GI tract. A complex network of nerves in the GI wall extends from the esophagus to the anus. This network is called the *intramural nerve plexus.* These nerves do three things: (1) control muscle tone in the wall, (2) regulate the rate and intensity of the alternating muscle contractions, and (3) coordinate all the various movements. When all is well, these finely tuned movements flow together like those of a great symphony, without conscience awareness. But when all is not well, the discord is felt as pain. Such problems and diseases with the GI tract are discussed in Chapter 18.

Chemical Digestion: Gastrointestinal Secretions

A number of secretions work together to make chemical digestion possible. Five types of substances generally are involved.

Hydrochloric Acid and Buffer Ions. Hydrochloric acid and buffer ions are needed to produce the correct pH (degree of acidity or alkalinity) necessary for enzyme activity.

Enzymes. Digestive enzymes are proteins, specific in kind and quantity for breaking down nutrients.

Mucus. Secretions of mucus lubricate and protect the mucosal tissues lining the GI tract as well as help mix the food mass.

Water and Electrolytes. The products of digestion are carried and circulated through the GI tract and into the tissues by water and electrolytes.

Bile. Made in the liver and stored in the gallbladder, bile divides fat into smaller pieces to expose more surface area for the actions of fat enzymes.

Secretory cells in the intestinal tract and nearby accessory organs (i.e., pancreas and liver) produce each of the preceding substances for specific jobs in chemical digestion. The secretory action of these cells or glands is stimulated by (1) the presence of food, (2) nerve impulse, or (3) hormones specific for certain nutrients.

Digestion in the Mouth and Esophagus

Mechanical Digestion

In the mouth, the process of *mastication* (i.e., biting and chewing) begins to break down food into smaller particles. The teeth and oral structures are particularly suited for this work. After the food is chewed, the mixed mass of food particles is swallowed and passes down the esophagus largely by peristaltic waves controlled by nerve reflexes. Muscles at the base of the tongue facilitate the swallowing process. Then, if the body is in the upright position, gravity aids the movement of food down the esophagus. At the entrance to the stomach, the gastroesophageal sphincter muscle relaxes, much like a one-way valve, to allow the food to enter, then constricts again to retain the food within the stomach cavity. If the sphincter is not working properly, it may allow acid-mixed food to seep back into the esophagus. The result is a discomforting feeling of heartburn.

Heartburn has nothing to do with the heart but has been called this because sensations are perceived as originating in the region of the heart. A hiatal hernia is another common cause of heartburn. This occurs when part of the stomach protrudes upward into the chest cavity (thorax).

Chemical Digestion

The salivary glands secrete material containing salivary amylase, also called *ptyalin. Amylase* is the general name for any starch-splitting enzyme. Small glands at the back of the tongue (Ebner's glands) secrete a *lingual lipase. Lipase* is the general name for any fat-splitting enzyme, but in this case food does not remain in the mouth long

salivary amylase a starch-splitting enzyme in the mouth, commonly called ptyalin (from the Greek word *ptyalon,* meaning spittle), that is secreted by the salivary glands.

enough for much chemical action to occur. During infancy, lingual lipase is a more relevant enzyme for milk fat. The salivary glands also secrete a mucous material that lubricates and binds food particles to facilitate the swallowing of each food *bolus,* or lump of food material. Mucous glands also line the esophagus, and their secretions help move the food mass toward the stomach.

Digestion in the Stomach

Mechanical Digestion

Under sphincter muscle control from the esophagus, which joins the stomach at the cardiac notch, the food enters the *fundus,* the upper portion of the stomach, in individual bolus lumps. Within the stomach, muscles gradually knead, store, mix, and propel the food mass forward in slow, controlled movements. By the time the food mass reaches the *antrum,* the lower portion of the stomach, it is now a semiliquid, acid-food mix called chyme. A constricting sphincter muscle at the end of the stomach, the *pyloric valve,* controls the flow at this point. This valve slowly releases acidic chyme so that it can be quickly buffered by the alkaline intestinal secretions and not irritate the mucosal lining of the *duodenum,* which is the first section of the small intestine. The caloric density of a meal, which mainly results from its fat component, not just its volume or particular composition, influences the rate of stomach emptying at the pyloric valve. The major parts of the stomach are shown in Figure 5-2.

Chemical Digestion

The gastric secretions contain three types of materials that aid chemical digestion in the stomach.

Acid. Parietal cells within the lining of the stomach secrete hydrochloric acid to create the necessary degree of acidity for gastric enzymes to work. Hydrochloric acid also works on denaturing proteins in the stomach.

Mucus. Mucous secretions protect the stomach lining from the erosive effect of the hydrochloric acid. Secretions also bind and mix the food mass and help move it along.

Enzymes. The inactive enzyme *pepsinogen* is secreted by stomach cells and is activated by hydrochloric acid to become the protein-splitting enzyme pepsin. Other cells produce small amounts of a specific gastric lipase called *tributyrinase,* which works on tributyrin (butterfat), but this is a relatively minor activity in the stomach.

Various sensations, emotions, and foods stimulate nerve impulses that trigger these secretions. The concept that the stomach is said to "mirror the person within" is not without merit. For example, anger and hostility increase secretions. Fear and depression decrease secretions and inhibit blood flow and motility. Additional hormonal stimulus occurs when food enters the stomach.

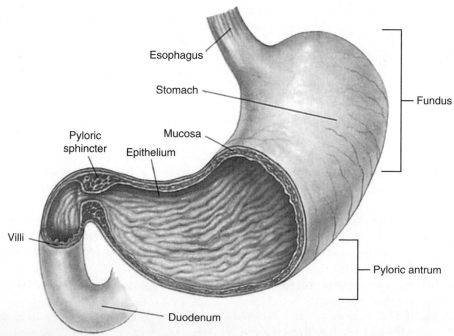

Figure 5-2 Stomach. (Reprinted from Raven PH, Johnson GB: *Biology,* ed 3, New York, 1992, McGraw-Hill.)

Digestion in the Small Intestine

Up to this point, digestion of food has largely been mechanical, delivering a semifluid mixture of fine food particles and watery secretions to the small intestine. Chemical digestion has been minimal. Thus the major task of digestion, and the absorption that follows, occurs in the small intestine. The structural parts, synchronized movements, and array of specific enzymes of the small intestine are highly developed for the final task of mechanical and chemical digestion.

Mechanical Digestion

Under the control of nerve impulses, walls stretch from the food mass or hormonal stimuli, and the intestinal muscles produce several types of movement that aid digestion, as follows:

- *Peristaltic waves* slowly push the food mass forward, sometimes with long, sweeping waves over the entire length of the intestine.
- *Pendular movements* from small, local muscles sweep back and forth, stirring the chyme at the mucosal surface.
- *Segmentation rings* from the alternating contraction and relaxation of circular muscles progressively chop the food mass into successive soft lumps and mix them with secretions.
- *Longitudinal rotation,* by long muscles running the length of the intestine, rolls the slowly moving food mass in a spiral motion, mixing it and exposing new surfaces for absorption.
- *Surface villi motions* stir and mix the chyme at the intestinal wall, exposing additional nutrients for absorption.

Chemical Digestion

The small intestines, together with the GI accessory organs (pancreas, liver, and gallbladder), supply many secretory materials to meet the major burden of chemical digestion. The pancreas and intestines secrete enzymes specific for the digestion of carbohydrates, proteins, and fat.

Pancreatic Enzymes

1. *Carbohydrate:* Pancreatic amylase converts starch to the disaccharides maltose and sucrose.
2. *Protein:* Trypsin and chymotrypsin split large protein molecules into smaller and smaller peptide fragments and finally into single amino acids. Carboxypeptidase removes end amino acids from peptide chains.
3. *Fat:* Pancreatic lipase converts fat to glycerides and fatty acids.

Intestinal Enzymes

1. *Carbohydrate:* Disaccharidases (maltase, lactase, and sucrase) convert their respective disaccharides (maltose, lactose, sucrose) to monosaccharides (glucose, galactose, and fructose). A large percent of the world's population does not produce enough lactase to digest lactose (milk sugar). As a result, these individuals cannot tolerate milk and milk products well unless they are in a predigested form (e.g., yogurt, buttermilk, aged cheese, or lactase-treated milk).[1] Lactose-affected individuals also can take commercially available oral lactase capsules to help with digestion.
2. *Protein:* The intestinal enzyme enterokinase activates trypsinogen (from the pancreas) to become the protein-splitting enzyme trypsin. Amino peptidase removes end amino acids from polypeptides. Dipeptidase splits dipeptides into their two remaining amino acids.
3. *Fat:* Intestinal lipase splits fat into glycerides and fatty acids.

Mucus. Large quantities of mucus, secreted by intestinal glands, protect the mucosal lining from irritation and erosion caused by the highly acidic gastric contents entering the duodenum.

Bile. Bile is an emulsifying agent and an important aid to fat digestion and absorption. It is produced by the liver and stored in the adjacent gallbladder, ready for use when fat enters the intestine.

---

chyme semifluid food mass in the GI tract present after gastric digestion.

pepsin the main gastric enzyme specific for proteins. Pepsin begins breaking large protein molecules into shorter chain polypeptides; gastric hydrochloric acid is necessary for activation.

pancreatic amylase a major starch-splitting enzyme secreted by the pancreas that acts in the small intestine.

trypsin a protein-splitting enzyme formed in the small intestine. The inactive precursor trypsinogen is activated by enterokinase.

chymotrypsin one of the protein-splitting and milk-curdling pancreatic enzymes activated in the small intestine from the precursor chymotrypsinogen; breaks specific amino acid peptide links of protein.

carboxypeptidase a protein enzyme that splits off the chemical group carboxyl ($-COOH$) at the end of peptide chains.

pancreatic lipase a major fat-splitting enzyme produced by the pancreas and secreted into the small intestine to digest fat.

Hormones. The hormone *secretin,* produced by the mucosal glands in the first part of the intestine, controls the acidity and secretion of enzymes from the pancreas. The resulting alkaline environment in the small intestine, with a pH >8, is necessary for the activity of the pancreatic enzymes. The hormone *cholecystokinin,* secreted by intestinal mucosal glands when fat is present, triggers the release of bile from the gallbladder to emulsify fat.

The arrangement of accessory organs to the duodenum, the first section of the small intestine, is shown in Figure 5-3. These organs make up the biliary system and have vital roles in digestion and metabolism. The liver is sometimes called the "metabolic capital" of the body because it has numerous functions in the metabolism of all converging nutrients (Box 5-1). The liver's many metabolic functions are reviewed in greater detail in Chapter 18.

The various nerve and hormone controls of digestion are illustrated in Figure 5-4. Although small individual summaries of digestion are given in each of the major nutrient chapters, a general summary of the entire digestive processes is shown in Figure 5-5 so that the overall process can be viewed as it is—one continuous, integrated *whole.*

ABSORPTION AND TRANSPORT

When digestion is complete, food has been changed into simple end products ready for cell use. Carbohydrate foods are reduced to the *simple sugars* glucose, fructose, and galactose. Fats are transformed into *fatty acids* and *glycerides.* Protein foods are changed to single *amino acids.* Vitamins and minerals are also liberated. With a water base for solution and transport in addition to the necessary electrolytes, the whole fluid food-derived mass is now prepared for absorption. For many nutrients, especially certain vitamins and minerals, the point of absorption becomes the vital gatekeeper that determines how much of a given nutrient is kept for body use. Although the GI tract is quite efficient, 100% of all the nutrients consumed are not absorbed because of varying degrees of *bioavailability.* A nutrient's bioavailability depends on (1) the amount of nutrient present in the GI tract, (2) competition between nutrients for common absorptive sites, and (3) the form in which the nutrient is present. This degree of bioavailability is a factor in setting dietary intake standards for all macronutrients and micronutrients.[2-7]

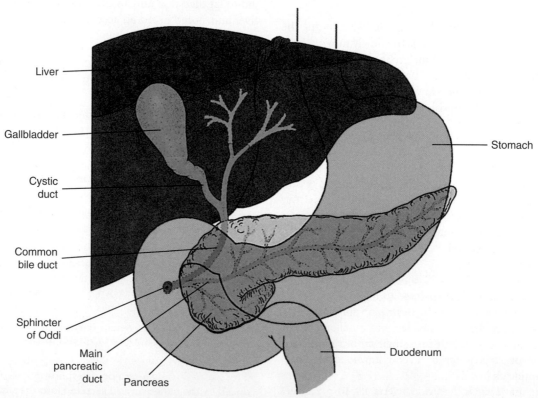

Figure 5-3 Organs of the biliary system and the pancreatic ducts.

BOX 5-1

FUNCTIONS OF THE LIVER

Major Functions
Bile production (for fat digestion)
Synthesis of proteins and blood clotting factors
Metabolism of hormones and medications
Regulation of blood glucose levels
Urea production (to remove waste products of normal metabolism)

Specific Metabolic Functions of the Energy-Yielding Nutrients
Lipolysis: breaking down lipids to fatty acids and glycerol
Lipogenesis: building up of lipids from fatty acids and glycerol
Glycolysis: breaking down glucose to pyruvate to enter the Krebs cycle
Gluconeogenesis: converting noncarbohydrate substances into glucose
Glycogenolysis: breaking down glycogen to individual glucose units
Glycogenesis: combining units of glucose to store as glycogen
Protein degradation: breaking down proteins to single amino acids
Protein synthesis: building complete proteins from individual amino acids

Absorption in the Small Intestine

Special Absorbing Structures

Three important structures of the intestinal wall surface are particularly adapted to ensure maximal absorption of essential nutrients in the digestive process (Figure 5-6), as follows:

- *Mucosal folds:* Like the hills and valleys of a mountain range, the surface of the small intestine piles into many folds. Mucosal folds can easily be seen when such tissue is examined.
- *Villi:* Closer examination under a regular light microscope reveals small, fingerlike projections, the villi, covering the piled-up folds of mucosal lining. These little villi further increase the area of exposed surface. Each villus has an ample supply of blood vessels to receive protein and carbohydrate materials as well as a special lymph vessel to receive fat materials. This lymph vessel is called a *lacteal* because the fatty chyme is creamy at this point and looks like milk.
- *Microvilli:* Even closer examination with an electron microscope reveals a covering of smaller projections on the surface of each tiny villus. The covering of microvilli on each villus is called a *brush border* because it looks like bristles on a brush.

These three unique structures of the inner intestinal wall—folds, villi, and microvilli—combine to make the inner surface some 600 times greater than the area of the outer surface of the intestine. The length of the small intestine is approximately 660 cm (22 feet). This remarkable organ is well adapted to deliver nutrients into circulation to the body's cells. If its entire surface were spread out on a flat plane, the total surface area is estimated to be as large as half a basketball court. Far from being the lowly gut, the small intestine is one of the most highly developed, exquisitely fashioned, specialized tissues in the human body.

Absorption Processes

A number of absorbing processes complete the task of moving vital nutrients across the inner intestinal wall and into body circulation. These processes include diffusion, energy-driven active transport, and pinocytosis (Figure 5-7), as follows:

- *Simple diffusion* is the force by which particles move outward in all directions from an area of greater concentration to an area of lesser concentration. Small materials that do not need the help of a specific protein channel to move across the mucosal cell wall use this method.
- *Facilitated diffusion* is similar to simple diffusion but uses a protein channel for carrier-assisted movement of larger items across the mucosal cell membrane.
- *Active transport* is the force by which particles move against their concentration gradient. Active transport mechanisms usually require some sort of carrier partner to help ferry the particles across the membrane. For example, glucose enters absorbing cells through an active transport mechanism involving sodium (Na^+) as a ferrying partner.
- *Pinocytosis* is the penetration of larger materials by attaching to the thicker cell membrane and being engulfed by the cell (see Chapter 9).

mucosal folds large visible folds of the mucous lining of the small intestine that increase the absorbing surface area.

villi small protrusions from the surface of a membrane; fingerlike projections covering mucosal surfaces of the small intestine that further increases the absorbing surface area; visible through a regular microscope.

microvilli extremely small, hairlike projections covering all villi on the surface of the small intestine that greatly extend the total absorbing surface area; visible through an electron microscope.

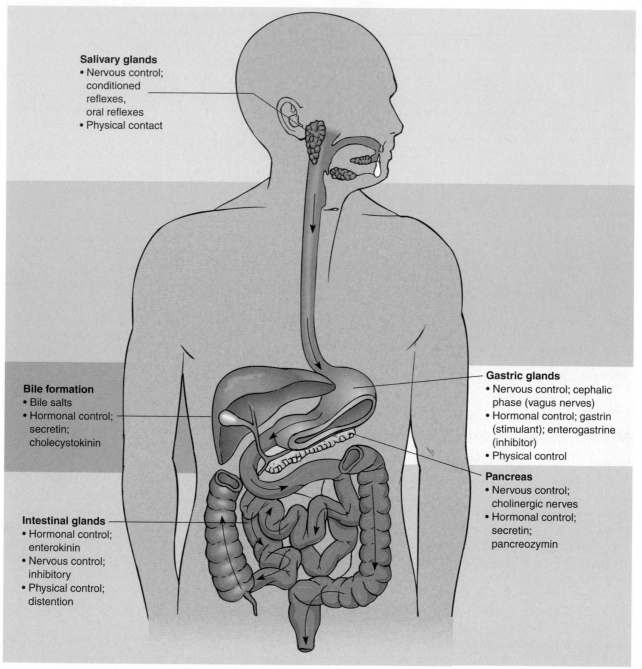

Salivary glands
• Nervous control;
  conditioned
  reflexes,
  oral reflexes
• Physical contact

Bile formation
• Bile salts
• Hormonal control;
  secretin;
  cholecystokinin

Intestinal glands
• Hormonal control;
  enterokinin
• Nervous control;
  inhibitory
• Physical control;
  distention

Gastric glands
• Nervous control; cephalic
  phase (vagus nerves)
• Hormonal control; gastrin
  (stimulant); enterogastrine
  (inhibitor)
• Physical control

Pancreas
• Nervous control;
  cholinergic nerves
• Hormonal control;
  secretin;
  pancreozymin

Figure 5-4 Summary of the factors influencing secretions of the GI tract. (Courtesy Rolin Graphics.)

Absorption in the Large Intestine

Water

The main absorptive task remaining for the large intestine is to take up needed body water. Most water in the chyme entering the large intestine is absorbed in the first half of the colon. Only a small amount (approximately 100 mL) remains to form and eliminate the feces.

Dietary Fiber

Food fiber is not digested because human beings lack the specific enzymes required. Dietary fiber, however, contributes important bulk to the food mass throughout the process of digestion and helps form the feces. The formation and passage of intestinal gas is a normal process but is embarrassing to some individuals (see the Clinical Ap-

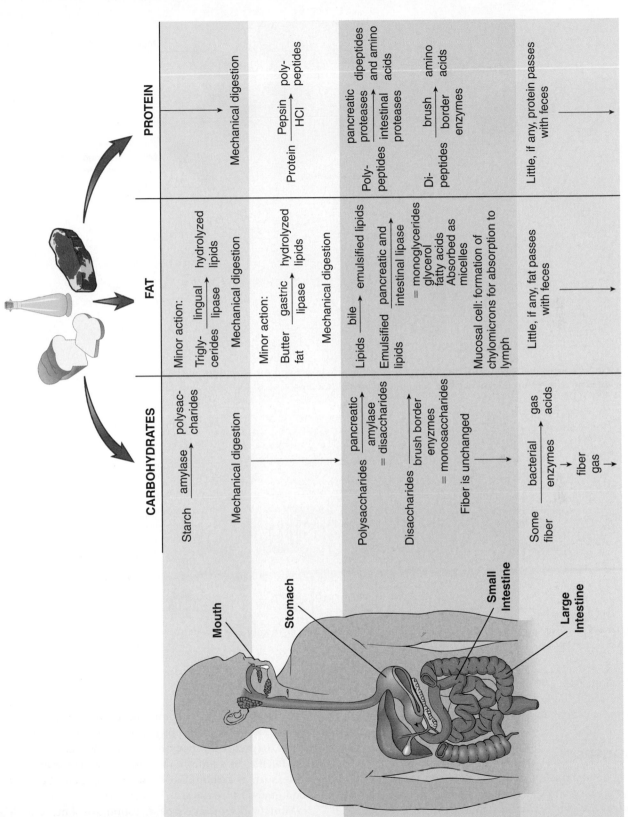

Figure 5-5 Summary of digestive processes. (Courtesy Rolin Graphics.)

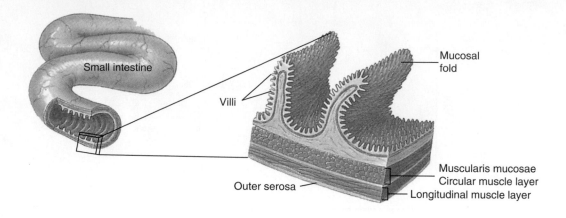

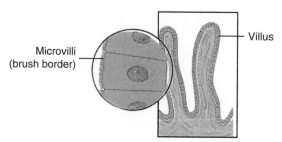

Figure 5-6 Intestinal wall. Note the arrangement of muscle layers and the structures of the mucosa that increase the surface area for absorption: mucosal folds, villi, and microvilli. (Courtesy Medical and Scientific Illustration.)

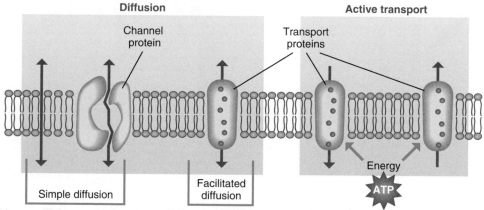

Figure 5-7 Diagram illustrating transport pathways through the cell membrane. (Reprinted from Mahan LK, Escott-Stump S: *Krause's food & nutrition therapy*, ed 12, Philadelphia, 2008, Saunders.)

plications box, "The Sometimes Embarrassing Effects of Digestion"). Table 5-1 summarizes major features of intestinal nutrient absorption.

Transport

After being broken down from food and absorbed, nutrients must be transported to various cells throughout the body. This transportation requires the work of both the vascular and lymphatic systems (Figure 5-8).

Vascular System

The vascular system is composed of veins and arteries and is responsible for supplying the entire body with nutrients, oxygen, and many other vital substances necessary for life. In addition, the vascular system transports waste, such as carbon dioxide and nitrogen, to the lungs and kidneys for removal.

Most of the products of digestion are water-soluble nutrients, which therefore can be absorbed into the vas-

THE SOMETIMES EMBARRASSING EFFECTS OF DIGESTION

After eating a meal or certain foods, some people complain of the discomfort or embarrassment of gas. Gas is a normal by-product of digestion, but when it becomes painful or apparent to others it may become a physical and social problem.

The GI tract normally holds approximately 3 oz of gas that move along with the food mass and are silently absorbed into the blood stream. Sometimes extra gas collects in the stomach or intestine, creating an embarrassing, although usually harmless, situation.

Stomach Gas

Gas in the stomach results from trapped air bubbles and occurs when a person eats too fast, drinks through a straw, or otherwise takes in extra air while eating. Burping relieves this gas, but the following tips may help to avoid uncomfortable situations:

- Avoid carbonated beverages
- Do not gulp
- Chew with your mouth closed
- Do not drink from a can or through a straw
- Do not eat when you are nervous

Intestinal Gas

The passing of gas from the intestine can be a social embarrassment. This gas forms in the colon, where bacteria attack undigested items, causing them to decompose and produce gas. Carbohydrates release hydrogen, carbon dioxide, and—in some people with certain types of bacteria in the gut—methane. All three products are odorless (although noisy) gases. Protein produces hydrogen sulfide and such volatile compounds as indole and skatole, which add a distinctive aroma to the expelled air. The following suggestions may help to control the problem:

- Cut down on simple carbohydrates (e.g., sugars). Especially observe milk's effect because lactose intolerance may be the culprit. Substitute cultured forms such as yogurt or milk treated with a lactase product such as Lactaid (McNeil Nutritionals, Fort Washington, Pa.).
- Use a prior leaching process before cooking dry beans to remove indigestible saccharides such as raffinose and stachyose. Although human beings cannot digest these substances, they provide a feast for bacteria in the intestines. This simple procedure eliminates a major portion of these gas-forming saccharides. First, put washed, dry beans into a large pot, add 4 cups of water for each pound (approximately 2 cups) of beans, and boil beans uncovered for 2 minutes. Remove pot from heat, cover, and let stand for 1 hour. Finally, drain and rinse the beans, add 8 cups fresh water, bring to a boil, reduce heat, and simmer in covered pot for 1 to 2 hours or until beans are tender. Season as desired.
- Eliminate known food offenders. These vary among individuals, but some of the most common offenders are beans (if not prepared for cooking as described above), onions, cabbage, and high-fiber wheat products.

Once relief is achieved, slowly add more complex carbohydrates and high-fiber foods back to the diet. Once small amounts are tolerated, try moderate increases. If no relief occurs, medical help may be needed to rule out or treat an overactive GI tract.

TABLE 5-1

INTESTINAL ABSORPTION OF SOME MAJOR NUTRIENTS

NUTRIENT	FORM	MEANS OF ABSORPTION	CONTROL AGENT OR REQUIRED COFACTOR	ROUTE
Carbohydrate	Monosaccharides (glucose or galactose)	Competitive Selective Active transport by sodium pump	— — Sodium	Blood
	Fructose	Facilitated diffusion	Protein carrier	Blood
Protein	Amino acids	Selective	—	Blood
	Some dipeptides	Facilitated diffusion	Pyridoxine (pyridoxal phosphate)	Blood
	Whole protein (rare)	Pinocytosis	Protein carrier	Blood
Fat	Fatty acids Glycerides (mono-, di-)	Fatty acid/bile complex (micelles)	Bile	Lymph
	Few triglycerides (neutral fat)	Pinocytosis	—	Lymph
Vitamins	B_{12}	Facilitated diffusion	Intrinsic factor	Blood
	A, D, E, K	Bile complex	Bile	Blood
	K from bacterial synthesis			From large intestine to blood
Minerals	Sodium	Active transport by sodium pump	—	Blood
	Calcium	Active transport	Vitamin D	Blood
	Iron	Active transport	Ferritin mechanism	Blood (as transferrin)
Water	Water	Osmosis	—	Blood, lymph, interstitial fluid

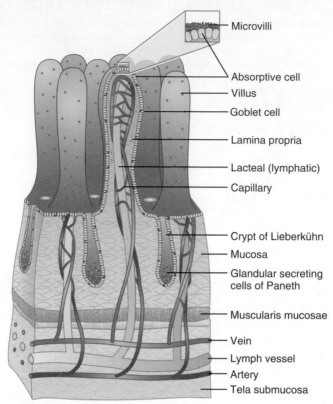

Figure 5-8 Diagram of villi of the human intestine showing the structure and blood and lymph vessels. (Reprinted from Mahan LK, Escott-Stump S: *Krause's food & nutrition therapy,* ed 12, Philadelphia, 2008, Saunders.)

cular system, or blood circulatory system, directly from the intestinal cells. The nutrients travel first to the liver for immediate cell enzyme work in energy production before being dispersed to other cells throughout the body. The portion of circulation from the intestines to the liver is called *portal circulation.*

Lymphatic System

Because fatty materials are not water soluble, another route must be provided. These fat molecules pass into the lymph vessels in the villi (e.g., the lacteals), flow into the larger lymph vessels of the body, and eventually enter the blood stream.

METABOLISM

Finally, the individual macronutrients in food (carbohydrates, protein, and fat) have been broken down through digestion into the basic building blocks (monosaccharides, amino acids, and fatty acids) and absorbed into the blood stream. Now these nutrients can be converted into needed energy or stored in the body for later use.

Energy for Fuel

Metabolism is the sum of chemical reactions occurring within a living cell to maintain life. The mitochondrion of the cell is the work center in which all metabolic reactions take place. The two types of metabolism are catabolism and anabolism. Catabolism is the breaking down of large substances into smaller units. The process of breaking down large carbohydrate and protein chains into their smaller building blocks, monosaccharides and amino acids, is a catabolic reaction. Anabolism is the opposite; it is the process by which cells build large substances from smaller particles, such as building a complex protein from single amino acids within the body.

The Krebs cycle, also known as the *citric acid cycle* or TCA cycle, is the hub of energy formation from food particles occurring in the mitochondria of the cell. The combined processes of metabolism ensure that the body has much needed energy in the form of adenosine triphosphate (ATP). The rate of ATP production fluctuates. It speeds up or slows down depending on energy needs at a given time. Energy needs are minimal during sleep but increase dra-

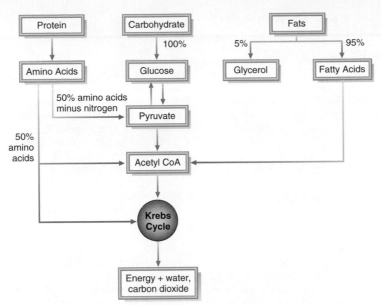

Figure 5-9 Metabolic pathways. (Reprinted from Peckenpaugh NJ: *Nutrition essentials and diet therapy,* ed 10, Philadelphia, 2007, Saunders.)

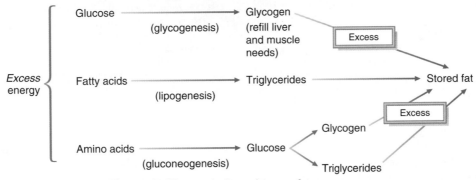

Figure 5-10 Metabolic pathways of excess energy.

matically during strenuous physical activity. Energy supply and demand are discussed further in Chapter 6. Figure 5-9 illustrates a brief breakdown of the macronutrients and how they enter the final step in energy production.

Because carbohydrates have 4 kcal/g and fat has 9 kcal/g, the metabolism of glucose yields less energy than the metabolism of fat, gram for gram. However, the body prefers to use glucose as its primary source of energy. Protein can be used as a source of energy as well, but this is a relatively inefficient method of creating energy and results in extra nitrogen waste. The body only breaks down protein for energy when glucose and fatty acids are in short supply.

Energy for Storage

If the amount of food consumed yields more energy than is needed, the remaining energy is stored for later use in the body (Figure 5-10). The human body is a highly efficient organism. Energy, or kilocalories, in excess of needs is not wasted. Excess glucose can easily be stored as glycogen in the liver and muscles for quick energy at a later time. The anabolic process of converting extra glucose into glycogen is called glycogenesis. Although alcohol is not considered a nutrient, it does provide 7 kcal/g. Therefore alcohol intake adds to the overall supply of energy (see the For Further Focus box "What About Alcohol?").

Once the glycogen reserves are full, additional excess energy (from carbohydrates, fat, or protein) are stored as fat in adipose tissue. Lipogenesis is the building up of triglycerides for storage in the adipose tissue of the body.

---

catabolism metabolic process of breaking down large substances to yield smaller building blocks.

anabolism metabolic process of building large substances from smaller parts; the opposite of catabolism.

glycogenesis formation of stored glycogen from glucose.

FOR FURTHER FOCUS

WHAT ABOUT ALCOHOL?

Does Alcohol Provide Energy?

Yes. Alcohol contributes to the overall energy intake in the form of calories. Alcohol yields 7 kcal/g consumed, which is more than both carbohydrates and protein, which yield 4 kcal/g each.

Is Alcohol a Nutrient?

No. Unlike carbohydrates, fats, proteins, vitamins, minerals, and water, alcohol performs no essential function in the body. Alcohol is not stored in the body and can be toxic in large amounts.

How Is Alcohol Digested?

The majority (85% to 95%) of alcohol is absorbed without any chemical digestion. Alcohol is one of the few substances that can be absorbed directly into circulation from the stomach. Small amounts of alcohol can enter the blood circulation from the mouth and esophagus. What is not absorbed in the stomach is absorbed in the small intestine and sent directly to the liver for metabolism.

How Is Alcohol Metabolized?

Alcohol metabolism takes precedence over the metabolism of any other nutrient in the body because it is technically a toxin. The primary by-product of alcohol metabolism is acetaldehyde, the culprit for destruction of healthy tissue associated with alcoholism. After detoxification, the liver uses remaining by-products to produce fatty acids. Fatty acids are converted into triglycerides and stored in the liver. A single drinking binge can result in an accumulation of fat in the liver. Repeated episodes over time can lead to fatty liver disease, the first stage of alcoholic liver disease.

Alcohol metabolism is a priority for the liver. Blood alcohol concentrations peak at approximately 30 to 45 minutes after one drink (defined as 12 oz of beer, 5 oz of wine, or 1.5 oz of 80-proof distilled spirits). The liver can only work so fast to metabolize and rid the body of alcohol, regardless of how much has been consumed, after which alcohol and its metabolites begin to accumulate in the blood.

Several factors influence an individual's ability to metabolize alcohol, such as gender, food intake, body weight, sex hormones, and medications.

More Information

To find out more about alcohol (dangers, benefits, associated diseases, etc.), refer to the following Web sites:

- National Clearinghouse for Alcohol and Drug Information: *http://ncadi.samhsa.gov*
- National Institute on Alcohol Abuse and Alcoholism: *www.niaaa.nih.gov*
- Alcoholics Anonymous: *www.aa.org*
- The National Council on Alcoholism and Drug Dependence: *www.ncadd.org*

Contrary to popular belief, excess protein intake is not stored as muscle. The body does use amino acids to build needed functional and structural proteins, and the liver stores some free amino acids to meet rapid needs of the body. However, protein intake above and beyond the body's requirements is broken down further so that the nitrogen unit is removed and the remaining carbon chain can be converted to glucose, if needed, or to fat for storage. The conversion of amino acids to glucose is referred to as gluconeogenesis. Figure 5-10 demonstrates the pathways of excess energy from carbohydrates, fats, or protein.

Both glycogen and stored fat are available for use when energy demands require it. Energy balance and the factors that influence it are discussed in Chapter 6.

GENETIC DISEASE AND FOOD INTOLERANCE

The Genetic Defect

Certain food intolerances stem from underlying genetic disease. In each genetic disease, the specific cell enzyme (all enzymes are proteins) controlling the cell's metabolism of a specific nutrient is missing, thus blocking the normal handling of the nutrient at that point. Three examples of genetic defects are phenylketonuria (PKU), galactosemia, and lactose intolerance.

Phenylketonuria

PKU is an autosomal recessive genetic disorder that results when phenylalanine hydroxylase, the enzyme responsible for breaking down the essential amino acid phenylalanine to tyrosine (another amino acid), is not produced by the body. If left untreated, this condition causes profound mental retardation and CNS damage, with irritability, hyperactivity, convulsive seizures, and bizarre behavior. PKU affects approximately 1 in every 10,000 infants born in the United States. Today mandatory newborn screening programs in all areas of the United States can identify affected infants so treatment can start immediately. With treatment, these children can grow normally and have healthy lives. The treatment is a low-phenylalanine diet of special formulas and low-protein food products for life. Intensive family counseling by the metabolic team at each care center is also needed.

Galactosemia

This genetic disease affects carbohydrate metabolism. The missing enzyme, GALT (galactose-1-phosphate uridyl-transferase), is one that converts galactose to glucose. Because galactose comes from the breakdown of lactose (milk sugar), all sources of lactose in an infant's diet must be eliminated. When not treated, this condition causes brain and liver damage. Newborn screening programs also identify affected infants so treatment can begin immediately to avoid such damage and enable the child to grow normally. Treatment is a galactose-free diet, with special formulas for infants and lactose-free food guides. Similar to PKU, galactosemia also is an autosomal recessive disorder and the treatment diet must be followed for life.

Lactose Intolerance

A deficiency of any one of the disaccharidases (e.g., lactase, sucrase, or maltase) in the small intestine may produce a wide range of GI problems and abdominal pain because the specific sugar involved cannot be digested. Lactose intolerance is the most common. In this condition, there is insufficient lactase to break down the milk sugar lactose; thus lactose accumulates in the intestine, causing abdominal cramping and diarrhea. Milk and all products containing lactose are carefully avoided. Milk treated with a commercial lactase product or soy milk products are safe substitutes.

lipogenesis formation of fat.

adipose tissue storage site for excess fat.

gluconeogenesis formation of glucose from noncarbohydrate substances such as amino acids.

SUMMARY

Necessary nutrients as they occur in food are not usable by the human body but must be changed, released, regrouped, and rerouted into forms body cells can use. The closely related activities of digestion, absorption, and transport ensure that key food nutrients are delivered to the cells so that the multiple metabolic tasks that sustain life can be completed.

Mechanical digestion consists of spontaneous muscular activity responsible for the following: (1) initial mechanical breakdown by mastication and (2) movement of the food mass along the GI tract by motions such as peristalsis. Chemical digestion involves enzymatic action that breaks food down into smaller and smaller components and releases its nutrients for absorption.

Absorption involves the passage of nutrients from the intestines into the mucosal lining of the intestinal wall. It mainly occurs in the small intestine by highly efficient intestinal wall structures that, together with a number of effective absorbing mechanisms, increase the absorbent surface area. Nutrients absorbed are then transported throughout the body by blood circulation.

Finally, the nutrients we eat are converted into energy through the cycles of metabolism. *Metabolism* is the sum of the body processes that change food energy from the three energy nutrients (mainly carbohydrate, some fat, and protein as backup) into various forms of energy. Throughout this cycling of body energy, metabolism is balanced by two types of metabolic actions: (1) *anabolism,* which builds tissue and stores energy, and (2) *catabolism,* which breaks down tissue and releases energy.

Genetic diseases of metabolism result from missing enzymes that control the metabolism of specific nutrients. Special diets in each case limit or eliminate the particular nutrient involved.

CRITICAL THINKING QUESTIONS

1. Describe the types of muscle movement involved in mechanical digestion. What does the word *motility* mean?
2. Identify digestive enzymes and any related substances secreted by the following: salivary and mucosal glands, pancreas, and liver. What activities do they perform on carbohydrates, proteins, and fats? What stimulates the release of these enzymes? What inhibits their activity?
3. Describe four mechanisms of nutrient absorption from the small intestine. Describe the routes taken by the breakdown products of carbohydrates, proteins, and fats after absorption. Why must an alternate route to the blood stream be provided for fat?
4. What functions does the large intestine perform?

CHAPTER CHALLENGE QUESTIONS

True-False

Write the correct statement for each statement that is false.

1. *True or False:* The digestive products of a large meal are difficult to absorb because the overall area of the absorbent surface of the intestines is relatively small.
2. *True or False:* Before they can work, some enzymes must be activated by hydrochloric acid or other enzymes.

3. *True or False:* Bile is an enzyme specifically used for the chemical breakdown of fat.

4. *True or False:* The GI circulation provides a constant supply of water and electrolytes to carry digestive secretions and substances being produced.

5. *True or False:* Secretions from the GI accessory organs, the gallbladder and the pancreas, mix with gastric secretions in the stomach to aid digestion.

6. *True or False:* One enzyme may work on both carbohydrate and fat breakdown.

7. *True or False:* Bile is released from the gallbladder in response to a hormonal stimulus.

Multiple Choice

1. During digestion, the major muscle action that moves the food mass forward in regular rhythmic waves is called

   a. valve contraction.
   b. segmentation ring motion.
   c. muscle tone.
   d. peristalsis.

2. Mucus is an important GI secretion because it

   a. causes chemical changes in substances to prepare for enzyme action.
   b. helps create the proper degree of acidity for enzymes to act.
   c. lubricates and protects the GI lining.
   d. helps emulsify fats for enzyme action.

3. Pepsin is

   a. produced in the small intestine to act on protein.
   b. a gastric enzyme that acts on protein.
   c. produced in the pancreas to act on fat.
   d. produced in the small intestine to act on fat.

4. Bile is an important secretion that is

   a. produced by the gallbladder.
   b. stored in the liver.
   c. an aid to protein digestion.
   d. a fat-emulsifying agent.

5. The route of fat absorption is

   a. the lymphatic system by way of the villi lacteals.
   b. directly into the portal blood circulation.
   c. with the aid of bile directly into the villi blood capillaries.
   d. with the aid of protein directly into the portal blood circulation.

---

evolve Please refer to the Students' Resource section of this text's Evolve Web site for additional study resources.

REFERENCES

1. National Institute of Diabetes and Digestive and Kidney Diseases, National Institutes of Health: *Lactose intolerance,* www.niddk.nih.gov/health/digest/pubs/lactose/lactose.htm, accessed June 2007.
2. Food and Nutrition Board, Institute of Medicine: *Dietary reference intakes for calcium, phosphorous, magnesium, vitamin D, and fluoride,* Washington, DC, 1997, National Academies Press.
3. Food and Nutrition Board, Institute of Medicine: *Dietary reference intakes for thiamin, riboflavin, niacin, vitamin B_6, folate, vitamin B_{12}, pantothenic acid, biotin, and choline,* Washington, DC, 2000, National Academies Press.
4. Food and Nutrition Board, Institute of Medicine: *Dietary reference intakes for vitamin C, vitamin E, selenium, and carotenoids,* Washington, DC, 2000, National Academies Press.
5. Food and Nutrition Board, Institute of Medicine: *Dietary reference intakes for vitamin A, vitamin K, arsenic, boron, chromium, copper, iodine, iron, manganese, molybdenum, nickel, silicon, vanadium, and zinc,* Washington, DC, 2001, National Academies Press
6. Food and Nutrition Board, Institute of Medicine: *Dietary reference intakes for energy, carbohydrate, fiber, fat, fatty acids, cholesterol, protein, and amino acids,* Washington, DC, 2002, National Academies Press.
7. Food and Nutrition Board, Institute of Medicine: *Dietary reference intakes for water, potassium, sodium, chloride, and sulfate,* Washington, DC, 2004, National Academies Press.

FURTHER READING AND RESOURCES

The following organizations provide up-to-date research and reliable information regarding matters of the GI tract and metabolism.

The American College of Gastroenterology: *www.acg.gi.org*

American Gastroenterological Association: *www.gastro.org*

The American Journal of Gastroenterology: *www.amjgastro.com*

Metabolism: *www.metabolism.com*

Nutrition & Metabolism: *www.nutritionandmetabolism.com*

MacDonald A and others: Protein substitute dosage in PKU: how much do young patients need? *Arch Dis Child* 91(7):588, 2006.

Bosch AM and others: Living with classical galactosemia: health-related quality of life consequences, *Pediatrics* 113(5):e423, 2004.

CHAPTER 6

Energy Balance

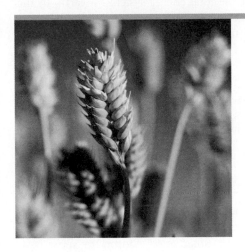

KEY CONCEPTS

- Food energy is changed into body energy to do work.
- The body uses most of its energy supply for basal metabolic needs.
- A balance between intake of food energy and output of body work maintains life and health.
- States of being underweight and overweight reflect degrees of energy imbalance.

Efficient human bodies constantly convert energy from food into the energy used for work and rest. Fuel is used and stored as necessary according to intake and output demands.

This chapter looks at the big picture of energy balance among all the energy nutrients and shows how energy intake is measured, cycled, and used to meet all the body's energy needs.

HUMAN ENERGY SYSTEM

Basic Energy Needs

The body needs constant energy to do work necessary for maintenance of life and health. Both voluntary and involuntary actions are involved.

Voluntary Work and Exercise

Voluntary work includes all actions related to a person's usual activities as well as any additional physical exercise. Although this visible, conscious action seems to require most of the energy output, this usually is not true.

Involuntary Body Work

The greatest energy output is the result of involuntary work, which includes all activities in the body not consciously performed. These activities include such vital processes as circulation, respiration, digestion, and absorption (referred to as the thermic effect of food) as well as many other internal activities that maintain life. Involuntary body functions require energy in various forms, such as *chemical* energy (in many metabolic products), *electrical* energy (in brain and nerve activities), *mechanical* energy (in muscle contraction), and *thermal* (heat) energy to keep the body warm.

---

thermic effect of food an increase in energy expenditure caused by the activities of digestion, absorption, and storage of ingested food. A meal consisting of a usual mixture of carbohydrates, protein, and fat increases the energy expenditure equivalent to approximately 10% of the food's energy content. For example, a 300-kcal piece of pizza would elicit an increase in energy expenditure of 30 kcal.

Sources of Fuel

Energy needed for voluntary and involuntary body work requires fuel, provided in the form of ATP. As previously explained, the only three energy-yielding nutrients are carbohydrate, fat, and protein. Carbohydrates are the body's primary fuel, with fat assisting as a storage fuel. Protein is used for energy only when other fuel sources are not available. The body must have an adequate supply of fuel to balance energy demands for healthy weight maintenance.

Measurement of Energy

Unit of Measure: Kilocalorie

In common usage, the word calorie refers to the amount of energy in food or expended in physical actions. However, in human nutrition the term kilocalorie (1000 calories) is used to designate the large calorie unit used in nutrition science to avoid dealing with such large numbers. A kilocalorie, abbreviated as *kcalorie* or *kcal,* is the amount of heat necessary to raise 1 kg of water 1° C. Sometimes the international unit of measure for energy, the *joule (J),* is used. The conversion factor for changing kilocalories (kcal) to kilojoules (kJ) is 4.184; therefore 1 kcal equals 4.184 kJ.

Food Energy: Fuel Factors

As discussed, the energy-yielding nutrients have basic fuel factors. Ethanol, or beverage alcohol from fermented grains and fruits, also supplies fuel. These factors reflect their relative fuel densities: carbohydrate, 4 kcal/g; fat, 9 kcal/g; protein, 4 kcal/g; and alcohol, 7 kcal/g.

Caloric and Nutrient Density

The term *density* refers to the degree of concentrated material in a given substance. More material in a smaller amount of substance increases the density. Thus the concept of *caloric density* refers to a higher concentration of energy (kilocalories) in a smaller amount of food. Therefore, of the three energy nutrients, fat or foods high in fat have the highest caloric density. Similarly, foods may be evaluated in terms of their relative *nutrient density.* High nutrient density refers to a relatively high concentration of all nutrients, including vitamins and minerals, in smaller amounts of a given food. A number of food guides do not base their listed food scores on the concentration of nutrients in given foods, but on the overall nutrient density in those foods as a general indicator of a food's contribution to health goals.

ENERGY BALANCE

Energy, like matter, is not created or destroyed. When energy is referred to as being produced, it really means that it is transformed (i.e., changed in form and cycled throughout a system). Consider the human energy system as part of the total energy system on earth. In this sense, two energy systems support human life: one within the body and the much larger one surrounding us, as follows:

1. *External energy cycle:* In the environment, the ultimate source of energy is the sun and its vast nuclear reactions. Using water and carbon dioxide as raw materials, plants transform the sun's radiation into stored chemical energy (mainly carbohydrate with some fat and protein). The food chain continues as animals, including human beings, eat plants and the flesh of other animals.
2. *Internal energy cycle:* When people eat plant and animal foods, the stored energy changes into body fuels—glucose and fatty acids—and cycles them into various other energy forms to serve body needs. These forms include the involuntary actions mentioned above: chemical, electrical, mechanical, and thermal energy. As this internal energy cycle continues, water is excreted, carbon dioxide is exhaled, and heat is radiated, returning these end products to the external environment. The overall energy cycle continually repeats, sustaining life.

Energy Intake

The total overall energy balance within the body depends on the energy intake in relation to the energy output. The main source of energy for all body work is food, backed up by stored energy in body tissues.

Sources of Food Energy

The three energy-yielding nutrients in food keep human bodies supplied with fuel. Personal energy intake can easily be estimated by recording a day's actual food consumption and calculating its energy value. Nutritrac, the nutrition analysis CD-ROM that accompanies this text, is an excellent tool to evaluate energy intake as well as several other components of an individual's diet (e.g., vitamins, minerals, fat, carbohydrates, sugar, protein).

Sources of Stored Energy

When food is not available, such as during sleep, longer periods of fasting, or the extreme stress of starvation, the body draws from its stored energy.

Glycogen. A 12- to 48-hour reserve of glycogen exists in liver and muscles and is quickly depleted if not replenished by daily food intake. For example, glycogen stores maintain normal blood glucose levels for body functions during sleep hours. The first meal, breakfast (so-named because it "breaks the fast"), has a significant function for energy intake.

Adipose Tissue. Although fat storage is larger than glycogen, the supply varies from person to person. As an additional energy resource, stored fat provides more kilocalories per gram than any other fuel source.

Muscle Mass. Energy in the form of protein exists in muscle mass, but this lean muscle mass must be maintained for health. Only during longer periods of fasting or starvation does the body turn to this tissue for energy.

Energy Output

The necessary activities to sustain life, such as normal body functions, regulation of body temperature, and the processes of tissue growth and repair, use energy from food and body reserves. The total chemical changes that occur during all these activities are called *metabolism*. This exchange of energy in overall balance usually is expressed in kilocalories. The following three demands for energy determine the body's total energy requirements: (1) resting energy expenditure, (2) physical activity, and (3) the thermic effect of food.

Resting Energy Expenditure and Basal Energy Expenditure

The term resting energy expenditure (REE), or *resting metabolic rate (RMR)*, refers to the sum of all internal working activities of the body at rest and is expressed in kilocalories per day. For instance, if an individual's REE were 1500 kcal, that would be the amount of energy that individual would need to consume over a 24-hour period to maintain his or her current weight while at complete rest. In general use, the terms REE, RMR, and basal energy expenditure (BEE) are used interchangeably, describing a vast amount of physiologic work. However, a technical difference exists between BEE and REE. BEE must be measured when an individual is at *complete* digestive, physical, mental, thermal, and emotional rest. Because maintaining the stringent conditions representing a true BEE often is difficult, the measurement is most often expressed as REE. REE is slightly higher than a true BEE measurement.[1]

Most of the body's total energy expenditure is spent maintaining necessary bodily functions in the form of BEE. The majority of that energy is used by small but highly active tissues (e.g., liver, brain, heart, kidney, and GI tract), which amount to less than 5% of the total body weight.[2] However, these tissues account for 60% to 75% of basal metabolic needs. Although *resting* muscle and adipose fat are far larger in mass, they contribute much less to the body's metabolic rate.

Measuring Basal Metabolic Rate or Resting Metabolic Rate. A measure of basal metabolic rate (BMR) or RMR is sometimes made in clinical practice (e.g., on metabolic wards or research laboratories) using *indirect calorimetry* (Figure 6-1). This method indirectly measures the amount of energy a person uses while at rest. A portable metabolic cart allows the person to breathe into an attached mouthpiece or ventilated hood system while lying in bed, and the normal exchange of oxygen and carbon dioxide is measured. From the rate of oxygen utilization, the metabolic rate can be calculated with a high degree of accuracy.

The MedGem and BodyGem (Microlife USA, Inc., Dunedin, Fla.) are alternative methods for determining RMR with much faster and more portable devices (Figure 6-2). Both devices are handheld and come with disposable mouthpieces and nose clips. The individual being tested holds the device while breathing exclusively into the mouthpiece. The MedGem and BodyGem measure oxygen consumption to determine an individual's RMR by using a modified Weir equation with a constant respiratory quotient of 0.85 ($RMR = 6.931 \times VO_2$).

---

calorie a measure of heat. The energy necessary to do work is measured as the amount of heat produced by the body's work. The energy value of a food is expressed as the number of kilocalories a specified portion of the food will yield when oxidized in the body.

kilocalorie the calorie used in nutrition science and the study of metabolism (1000 calories) to be more accurate and avoid the use of very large numbers in calculations. The general term *calorie* often is used as a general term in common language for the kilocalorie.

resting energy expenditure (REE) the amount of energy needed by the body for maintenance of life at rest over a 24-hour period; often used interchangeably with basal energy expenditure but is slightly higher.

basal energy expenditure (BEE) the amount of energy (in kcal) needed by the body for maintenance of life when a person is at complete digestive, physical, mental, thermal, and emotional rest (10 to 12 hours after eating, 12 to 18 hours after physical activity, and measured immediately on waking).

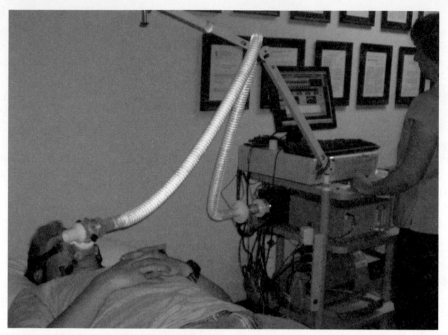

Figure 6-1 Measuring RMR.

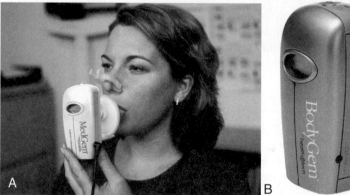
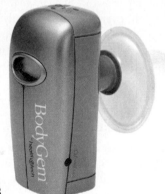

Figure 6-2 MedGem (A) and BodyGem (B) devices used to determine RMR. (Courtesy Microlife, Inc., Dunedin, Fla.)

Predicting Basal Metabolic Rate or Resting Metabolic Rate. A general formula for calculating basal energy needs is to multiply 0.9 or 1 kcal/kg body weight by the number of hours in a day. Thus the daily basal metabolic needs (in kilocalories) are calculated as follows. Example for a 154-lb man:

1 kcal × kg body weight × 24 hours
(1) Convert pounds to kilograms: 154/2.2 = 70 kg
(2) 1 kcal × 70 kg × 24 hr = 1680 kcal/24 hr

Example for a 121-lb woman:

0.9 kcal × kg body weight × 24 hours
(1) Convert pounds to kilograms: 121/2.2 = 55 kg
(2) 0.9 kcal × 55 kg × 24 hr = 1188 kcal/24 hr

The classic Harris-Benedict equations, Mifflin-St. Jeor equations, and equations used for the 2002 DRI values provide an alternate method of estimating the BMR or RMR for adults that is more specific to the individual (Box 6-1). Of these equations, recent studies found the Mifflin-St. Jeor equation to give the most reliable RMR measures.[3]

In addition, *thyroid function tests* may be used as an indicator of BMR because the thyroid hormone regulates metabolism. Thyroid function tests measure the activity of the thyroid, serum thyroxin levels and serum protein-bound iodine (PBI) and radioactive iodine uptake. Iodine's basic function is in the synthesis of thyroxine. Such tests are not associated with a kilocalorie amount in terms of total energy needs. They can be used, however, as

BOX 6-1

EQUATIONS FOR ESTIMATING RESTING ENERGY NEEDS

Mifflin-St. Jeor   *multiply before addition*

Men:

TEE (kcal/day) = (Weight [kg] × 10 + Height [cm] × 6.25 − Age × 5 − 5) × PA

Women:

TEE (kcal/day) = (Weight [kg] × 10 + Height [cm] × 6.25 − Age × 5 − 161) × PA

PA coefficient:
1.200 = Sedentary (little or no exercise)
1.375 = Lightly active (light exercise/sports 1-3 day/wk)
1.550 = Moderately active (moderate exercise/sports 3-5 day/wk)
1.725 = Very active (hard exercise/sports 6-7 day/wk)
1.900 = Extra active (very hard exercise/sports and physical job)

Harris Benedict

Men:

TEE (kcal/day) = 66.5 + (13.75 × Weight (kg)) + (5 × Height (cm)) − (6.78 × Age) × PA

Women:

TEE (kcal/day) = 655 + (9.56 × Weight (kg)) + (1.85 × Height (cm)) − (4.68 × Age) × PA

PA coefficient:
1.2 = Sedentary (little or no exercise, desk job)
1.375 = Lightly active (light exercise/sports 1-3 day/wk)
1.55 = Moderately active (moderate exercise/sports 3-5 day/wk)
1.725 = Heavy exercise (hard exercise/sports 6-7 day/wk)

2002 DRI Energy Calculation

EER = TEE + Energy deposition

Children 0-36 Months:
0-3 months: (89 × Weight [kg] − 100) + 175 kcal
4-6 months: (89 × Weight [kg] − 100) + 56 kcal
7-12 months: (89 × Weight [kg] − 100) + 22 kcal
13-36 months: (89 × Weight [kg] − 100) + 20 kcal

Boys 3-8 Years:
EER = 88.5 − (61.9 × Age [yr]) + PA × (26.7 × Weight [kg] + 903 × Height [m]) + 20 kcal

PA coefficient:
1.00 if PAL is estimated to be ≥1.0 but <1.4 (sedentary)
1.13 if PAL is estimated to be ≥1.4 but <1.6 (low active)
1.26 if PAL is estimated to be ≥1.6 but <1.9 (active)
1.42 if PAL is estimated to be ≥1.9 but <2.5 (very active)

Girls 3-8 Years:
EER = 135.3 − (30.8 × Age [yr]) + PA × (10.0 × Weight [kg] + 934 × Height [m]) + 20 kcal

PA coefficient:
1.00 if PAL is estimated to be ≥1.0 but <1.4 (sedentary)
1.16 if PAL is estimated to be ≥1.4 but <1.6 (low active)
1.31 if PAL is estimated to be ≥1.6 but <1.9 (active)
1.56 if PAL is estimated to be ≥1.9 but <2.5 (very active)

Boys 9-18 Years:
EER = 88.5 − (61.9 × Age [yr]) + PA × (26.7 × Weight [kg] + 903 × Height [m]) + 25 kcal

PA coefficient:
1.00 if PAL is estimated to be ≥1.0 but <1.4 (sedentary)
1.13 if PAL is estimated to be ≥1.4 but <1.6 (low active)
1.26 if PAL is estimated to be ≥1.6 but <1.9 (active)
1.42 if PAL is estimated to be ≥1.9 but <2.5 (very active)

Girls 9-18 Years:
EER = 135.3 − (30.8 × Age [yr]) + PA × (10.0 × Weight [kg] + 934 × Height [m]) + 25 kcal

PA coefficient:
1.00 if PAL is estimated to be ≥1.0 but <1.4 (sedentary)
1.16 if PAL is estimated to be ≥1.4 but <1.6 (low active)
1.31 if PAL is estimated to be ≥1.6 but <1.9 (active)
1.56 if PAL is estimated to be ≥1.9 but <2.5 (very active)

Men Ages 19 Years and Older:
EER = 662 − (9.53 × Age [yr]) + PA × (15.91 × Weight [kg] + 539.6 × Height [m])

PA coefficient:
1.00 if PAL is estimated to be ≥1.0 but <1.4 (sedentary)
1.11 if PAL is estimated to be ≥1.4 but <1.6 (low active)
1.25 if PAL is estimated to be ≥1.6 but <1.9 (active)
1.48 if PAL is estimated to be ≥1.9 but <2.5 (very active)

Women Ages 19 Years and Older:
EER = 354 − (6.91 × age [y]) + PA × (9.36 × Wt [kg] + 726 × Ht [m])

PA coefficient:
1.00 if PAL is estimated to be ≥1.0 but <1.4 (sedentary)
1.12 if PAL is estimated to be ≥1.4 but <1.6 (low active)
1.27 if PAL is estimated to be ≥1.6 but <1.9 (active)
1.45 if PAL is estimated to be ≥1.9 but <2.5 (very active)

TEE, Total energy expenditure; *PA,* physical activity; *EER,* estimated energy requirement.

a gauge of normal metabolic function. Abnormal results require the care of a physician.

Factors Influencing Basal Metabolic Rate. Several factors influence BMR and should be kept in mind when related test results are interpreted. The major factors affecting BMR relate to lean body mass, growth periods, body temperature, and hormonal status, as follows:

- *Lean body mass*: One of the greatest factors affecting metabolism is the percent of lean body mass. This is caused by the greater metabolic activity in lean tissues (muscles and organs) compared with fat and bones. The metabolic rate is higher in lean bodies, thus requiring more energy.[4] It is lower in fat bodies, thus requiring less energy. Other factors, such as surface area and sex, only influence the metabolic rate as they relate to the lean body mass.[2] Even though lean body mass is lost with advanced age,[5] lowered metabolic rate in the elderly is not exclusively caused by changes in body composition.[6]

- *Growth periods*: During growth periods the growth hormone stimulates cell metabolism and raises BMR 15% to 20%. BMR slowly rises during the first few years of life, levels off somewhat, rises again just before and during puberty, and then gradually declines into old age. BMR rises significantly during pregnancy, which is a rapid growth period requiring an additional 300 kcal/day on average—a value that is highly variable between women and also is correlated to weight gain and prepregnancy body composition.[7,8] During the following period of lactation, the breastfeeding mother's BMR further increases to cover the added metabolic process of producing milk.[9]

- *Body temperature*: Fever increases BMR approximately 7% for each 1° F (0.83° C) rise in temperature. Diseases involving increased cell activity (e.g., cancer and cardiac failure) and respiratory problems (e.g., emphysema) usually increase the BMR. In the abnormal states of starvation and malnutrition, the BMR is lowered because of the sacrifice of lean muscle mass for energy. In cold weather, especially in freezing temperatures, the BMR rises somewhat to generate more body heat to maintain normal body temperature.

- *Hormonal status*: Energy expenditure also is influenced by hormonal secretions. As previously mentioned, the thyroid function test is a means of measuring metabolism. Individuals with an underactive thyroid gland develop hypothyroidism, resulting in a decreased metabolic rate. Conversely, hyperthyroidism occurs when the thyroid gland is overactive (see the Cultural Considerations box,

"Hypermetabolism and Hypometabolism: What Are They, and Who Is at Risk?"). The fight-or-flight reflexes increase metabolic rate because of the hormone epinephrine. Other hormones, such as growth hormone, insulin, and cortisol, also increase metabolism and may fluctuate daily.

Physical Activity

Exercise involved in work or recreation (Figure 6-3) accounts for wide individual variations in energy output (see Chapter 16). Regular physical activity, balanced with adequate energy intake, is especially important to help offset the risks for heart disease and diabetes.[10,11] Physical activity has beneficial effects on both the body and mind throughout the adult years. Table 6-1 gives some representative kilocalorie expenditures of different types of work and recreation. Mental work or study does not require additional kilocalories; emotional states do not increase kcalorie needs but may require energy intake to compensate for muscle tension, restlessness, and agitated movements.

Energy expenditure used for physical activity goes above and beyond RMR. Keeping track of all energy used explicitly for physical activity to calculate total energy needs is somewhat difficult. Instead, the energy used for physical activity can be estimated as a factor of RMR by categorizing physical activity level (PAL) according to standard values (1.2 to 2.4, depending on lifestyle). This factor is then multiplied by the RMR. For example, an individual who works at a desk job and has little or no leisure activity would have a PAL of 1.4 to 1.5. To get a range of total energy expenditure, multiply the person's RMR by 1.4 to 1.5 (see the Clinical Applications box, "Evaluate Your Daily Energy Requirements," for PAL factors).

Thermic Effect of Food

After eating, food stimulates metabolism and requires extra energy for digestion, absorption, and transportation of nutrients to the cells. This overall stimulating effect is called the *thermic effect of food*. Approximately 5% to 10% of the body's total energy needs for metabolism relates to the handling of food.

Total Energy Requirement

RMR, physical activities, and the thermic effect of food make up a person's overall total energy requirements (Figure 6-4). To maintain daily energy balance, food energy intake must match body energy output. An energy imbalance, when energy intake exceeds energy output, can lead to weight gain (Table 6-2). Treatment should include a decrease in food kilocalories and an increase in

CULTURAL CONSIDERATIONS

HYPERMETABOLISM AND HYPOMETABOLISM: WHAT ARE THEY, AND WHO IS AT RISK?

Hypermetabolism and hypometabolism are conditions in which the metabolic rate is either significantly higher (hyper) or lower (hypo) than normal. Because the thyroid gland is responsible for producing the hormone thyroxine, which controls the metabolic rate, such conditions usually result from malformations or malfunctions of the thyroid gland. Clinically, hypermetabolism and hypometabolism are referred to as hyperthyroidism and hypothyroidism, respectively.

An individual with hyperthyroidism has a significantly higher metabolic rate, and energy needs, than normal. Such increases in energy needs are not explained by lean tissue, age, or gender. This individual has an overactive thyroid gland, producing too much thyroxine. As a result, the normal energy intake recommendations do not meet his or her needs. For example, a woman aged 25 years, height 5 feet, 5 inches, and weight 125 lb normally needs approximately 2200 kcal/day to maintain her weight at a moderate level of activity. However, the same woman with hyperthyroidism may need 1.5 to 2.5 times as many kilocalories per day to maintain her current weight.

Hypothyroidism is the opposite of hyperthyroidism. Individuals with hypothyroidism do not produce enough thyroxine and therefore require less energy than normal to maintain their current body weight. The DRIs for energy intake for a hypothyroid individual are too high and thus result in weight gain. However, effective medications are available for hypothyroidism. Typically both hyperthyroidism and hypothyroidism are discovered in young adulthood.

Congenital hypothyroidism (CH), occurring in 1 of every 3000 to 4000 live births, is a type of hypothyroidism present at birth and can result in mental retardation if not treated. Studies have found that the risk of CH is linked with birth weight, gender, and ethnicity. Both male and female infants weighing less than 4.5 lb or greater than 10 lb have a significantly higher risk of developing CH, and females of any weight have twice the prevalence of males. In a study conducted in California, African-American infants had the lowest rate of CH, whereas most ethnic groups (including Hispanics, Chinese, Filipinos, Vietnamese, Middle Easterners, Asian Indians, and Hawaiians) had an increased prevalence when compared with Caucasian infants.* A follow-up study published in 2004 confirmed these findings while also pointing out that Latino/Hispanic females had a significantly higher prevalence of CH.†

Another risk factor for developing abnormal thyroid function, and thus abnormal metabolism, is iodine intake. The mineral iodine is an important part of the hormone thyroxine, and one of the symptoms of iodine deficiency is abnormal thyroid function and metabolism. The incidence of hyperthyroidism and hypothyroidism has been linked to iodine intake.‡ Both high and low intakes of iodine are associated with thyroid disease.

Close monitoring of basal metabolism and total energy expenditure is an important aspect of the treatment of thyroid disease. Medications and energy intake are then modified to control weight and prevent complications.

*Waller DK and others: Risk factors for congenital hypothyroidism: an investigation of infant's birth weight, ethnicity, and gender in California, 1990-1998, *Teratology* 62:36, 2000.
†Schoen EJ and others: The key role of newborn thyroid scintigraphy with isotopic iodide (123I) in defining and managing congenital hypothyroidism, *Pediatrics* 114(6):e683, 2004.
‡Pedersen IB and others: Large differences in incidences of overt hyper and hypothyroidism associated with a small difference in iodine intake: a prospective comparative register-based population study, *J Clin Endo Metab* 87(10):4462, 2002.
Additional resource: Polak M and others: Congenital hyperthyroidism: the fetus as a patient, *Horm Res* 65(5):235, 2006.

physical activity. Extreme weight loss (e.g., anorexia nervosa or starvation) results when food energy intake does not meet body energy requirements for extended periods. Treatment should include a gradual increase in food kilocalories along with moderate activity and rest (see Chapter 15).

The Clinical Applications box "Evaluate Your Daily Energy Requirements" provides a step-by-step example for evaluating a person's energy needs. You also may wish to record your food and activities for a day and calculate your energy intake (kilocalories) and output (kilocalorie expenditure in activities). Total your day's activity and compare it with the general type of similar activities given in Table 6-1. Estimate the total time you spent on a given

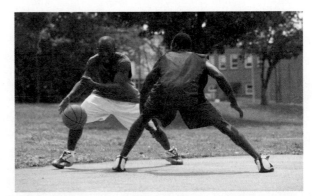

Figure 6-3 Energy output in exercise. (Copyright Photo-Disc.)

TABLE 6-1

convert Kgs to lbs.

ENERGY EXPENDITURE PER POUND PER HOUR DURING VARIOUS ACTIVITIES

ACTIVITY	Kcal/lb/hr*
Aerobics, moderate	2.95
Bicycling	
Light: 10-11.9 mph	2.72
Moderate: 12-13.9 mph	3.63
Fast: 14-15.9 mph	4.54
Mountain biking	3.85
Daily Activities	
Cleaning	1.36
Cooking	0.91
Driving a car	0.91
Eating, sitting	0.68
Gardening, general	1.81
Office work	0.82
Reading, writing while sitting	0.70
Sleeping	0.41
Shoveling snow	2.72
Running	
5 mph (12 min/mile)	3.63
7 mph (8.5 min/mile)	5.22
9 mph (6.5 min/mile)	6.80
10 mph (6 min/mile)	7.26
Sports	
Boxing, in ring	5.44
Field hockey	3.63
Golf	2.04
Rollerblading	4.42
Soccer	3.85
Skiing, downhill, moderate	2.72
Skiing, cross country, moderate	3.63
Swimming, moderate	3.14
Tennis, doubles	2.27
Tennis, singles	3.63
Ultimate Frisbee	3.63
Volleyball	1.81
Walking	
Moderate: ~3 mph (20 min/mile), level	1.50
Moderate: ~3 mph (20 min/mile), uphill	2.73
Brisk: ~3.5 mph (17.14 min/mile), level	1.72
Fast: ~ 4.5 mph (13.33 min/mile), level	2.86
Weight Training	
Light or moderate	1.36
Heavy or vigorous	2.72

Energy expenditure depends on the physical fitness of the individual and continuity of exercise.

Modified from Nieman DC: *Exercise testing and prescription: a health-related approach,* ed 5, New York, 2003, McGraw-Hill.

*Multiply activity factor by weight in pounds by fraction of hour performing activity. *Example:* A 150-lb person plays soccer for 45 minutes, as follows: 3.18 (Factor) × 150 (lb) × 0.75 (hr) = 357.75 calories burned.

activity by adding the minutes you spent at any time on that activity and then converting those minutes to hours (or decimal fractions of hours) for the day. For example, if you spent 10 minutes at one point and 5 minutes at another point doing the same thing, then your day's total for that activity is 15 minutes, or 0.25 hr. Multiply this total time for a given type of activity by the average kilocalories per hour for that activity (see Table 6-1) and add them up for the day's total kilocalories. Use the following

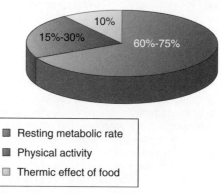

Figure 6-4 Contributions of RMR, physical activity, and the thermic effect of food to total energy expenditure.

TABLE 6-2

ENERGY BALANCE: 32-YEAR-OLD, 120 LB, 5 FEET, 4 INCH WOMAN

ENERGY INTAKE	ENERGY OUTPUT	
Breakfast: 450 kcal	RMR: 1240.5 kcal (includes the thermic effect of food)	Mifflin-St. Jeor equation
Midmorning snack: 175 kcal	Physical activity: additional 899.4 kcal	Very active (RMR × 1.725)
Lunch: 500 kcal		
Afternoon snack: 250 kcal		
Dinner: 600 kcal		
Evening snack: 200 kcal		
Total intake: 2175 kcal	**Total output: 2140 kcal**	**Positive energy balance with an extra 35 kcal/day**

Although not much, an extra 35 kcal/day could lead to weight gain. Approximately 3500 kcal are in 1 lb of fat mass. Therefore, if maintained, this woman could gain 1 lb of fat in 100 days despite her very active lifestyle. By decreasing her energy intake by 35 kcal/day or further increasing her energy expenditure by 35 kcal/day, she would then be in energy balance and weight stable.

CLINICAL APPLICATIONS

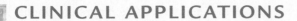

EVALUATE YOUR DAILY ENERGY REQUIREMENTS

Your estimated energy requirement (in kilocalories) per day is the sum of your body's three uses of energy, as follows:

1. RMR
2. Thermic effect of food
3. Physical activity

Estimated Energy Requirement (EER) as calculated by the 2002 DRIs

Men ages 19 years and older = 662 − (9.53 × age [yr]) + Physical activity (PA) × (15.91 × Weight [kg] + 539.6 × Height [m])
Women ages 19 years and older = 354 − (6.91 × Age [yr]) + PA × (9.36 × Weight [kg] + 726 × Height [m])

Physical Activity

Estimate your general average level of physical activity (PA). PA level is the ratio of the total energy expenditure to the BEE.

Lifestyle	PA Factor for Men	PA Factor for Women
Sedentary: Mostly resting with little or no planned strenuous activity and only performing those tasks required for independent living	1.0	1.0
Low Active: In addition to activities of a sedentary lifestyle, the added equivalent of a 1.5- to 3-mile walk at a speed of 3-4 mph for the average-weight person*	1.11	1.12
Active: In addition to the activities identified with a sedentary lifestyle, an average of 60 minutes of daily moderate-intensity physical activity (e.g., walking at 3 to 4 mph for 3 to 6 miles/day) or shorter periods of more vigorous exertion (e.g., jogging for 30 minutes at 5.5 mph)	1.25	1.27
Very Active: In addition to activities of a sedentary lifestyle, an activity level equivalent to walking at 3 to 4 mph for 12 to 22 miles/day (approximately 5-7 hours per day) or shorter periods of more vigorous exertion (e.g., running 7 mph for approximately 2.5 hours/day)	1.48	1.45

*Man weighing 70 kg and 1.77 m tall and a woman weighing 57 kg at 1.63 m tall based on the reference body weights for adults.

Example 1

A 32-year-old woman who weighs 130 lb (59 kg), is 5 feet, 4 inches tall, and who has started and maintains a regular physical exercise program. She is currently consuming approximately 2600 kcal/day:

Conversions: 1 pound = 2.2 kg, 39.37 in = 1 m. Thus 130/2.2 = 59 kg and 5 feet 4 inches = 64/39.37 = 1.626 m.

EER = 354 − (6.91 × 32) + 1.27 [PA] × (9.36 × 59 + 726 × 1.626)
EER = 354 − 221.12 + 1.27 × (552.24 + 1180.5)
EER = 2334 kcal/day

Result: This woman will gain weight. Her energy output is approximately 266 kcal/day less than her food intake. Because 1 lb of body weight equals approximately 3500 kcal, she will gain approximately 1 lb every 13 days with the preceding eating and exercise routine.

Example 2

A 41-year-old man who weighs 180 lb (82 kg), is 6 feet tall and eats an average of 3300 kcal/day while maintaining a very active lifestyle:

EER = 662 − (9.53 × 41) + 1.48 [PA] × (15.91 × 82 + 539.6 × 1.829 [m])
EER = 662 − 390.73 + 1.48 × (1304.62 + 986.93)
EER = 3663 kcal/day

Result: This man will tend to lose weight on his current exercise and meal plan because he is consuming approximately 163 kcal less than he is expending. Approximately how many pounds will he lose per month?

Handwritten notes:

1.2 bed bound
1.4 - 1.5 sedentary
1.6 - 1.7 light
1.8 - 1.9 moderate
2.0 - 2.4 heavy

basic steps to estimate your energy expenditure for a day's activities:

1. Total minutes of an activity/60 = Hours of that activity
2. Total time (hr) × kcal/hr = Total kcal/day for that activity
3. Total kcal/day of all activities = Total kcal energy expenditure for day from activities

RECOMMENDATIONS FOR DIETARY ENERGY INTAKE

General Life Cycle

Growth Periods

During periods of rapid growth, extra energy per unit of body weight is necessary to build new tissue. In childhood, the most rapid growth occurs during infancy and adolescence, with continuous but slower growth in between (Table 6-3). The rapid growth of the fetus, placenta, and other maternal tissues makes increased energy intake during pregnancy and lactation highly important.

Adulthood

With full adult growth achieved energy needs level off, meeting requirements for tissue maintenance and usual physical activities.

As the aging process continues the gradual decline in BMR and physical activity decreases the total energy requirement (Table 6-4). Therefore food choices should reflect a decline in caloric density and place greater emphasis on increased nutrient density.

Dietary Reference Intakes

To determine recommendations for energy intake, the Food and Nutrition Board of the Institute of Medicine considered the average energy intake of individuals who were healthy, free living, and maintaining a healthy body weight as determined by body mass index (BMI) measurements.[1] Table 6-5 gives the average total energy expenditure throughout life for those individuals. Note the average height, weight, BMI, and PAL within each age and gender group. Because a balance of energy intake and energy expenditure helps maintain a healthy weight, the DRIs for energy intake are equal to the total energy expenditure in kilocalories.

Dietary Guidelines for Americans

The *Dietary Guidelines* for healthy Americans address energy needs by the following recommendations[12]:

- To maintain body weight in a healthy range, balance calories from foods and beverages with calories expended.
- To prevent gradual weight gain over time, make small decreases in food and beverage calories and increase physical activity.
- Meet recommended intakes within energy needs by adopting a balanced eating pattern, such as the USDA Food Guide or the Dietary Approaches to Stop Hypertension eating plan.

TABLE 6-3

APPROXIMATE CALORIC ALLOWANCES FROM BIRTH TO 18 YEARS

AGE (yr)	Kcal/lb
Infants	
0-0.5	33.4
0.6-1.0	35.6
Children	
1-2	36.2
Boys	
3-8	32
9-13	26.3
14-18	24
Girls	
3-8	29.7
9-13	23.8
14-18	19.3

Modified from Food and Nutrition Board, Institute of Medicine: *Dietary reference intakes for energy, carbohydrate, fiber, fat, fatty acids, cholesterol, protein, and amino acids,* Washington, DC, 2005, National Academies Press.

TABLE 6-4

GRADUAL REDUCTION OF KILOCALORIE NEEDS DURING ADULTHOOD

AGE (yr)	KILOCALORIE REDUCTION (%) FOR MAINTENANCE OF IDEAL WEIGHT*
30-40	3
40-50	3
50-60	7.5
60-70	7.5
70-80	10

*Added percent decreases for each decade past the age of 25 years.

TABLE 6-5

MEDIAN HEIGHT, WEIGHT, AND RECOMMENDED ENERGY INTAKE

AGE (yr)	MEAN WEIGHT (kg [lb])	MEAN HEIGHT (m [in])	MEAN BMI (kg/m²)	BEE (kcal/day)	MEAN PAL	MEAN TEE (kcal/day)
Infants						
0-0.5	6.9 (15)	0.64 (25)	16.86	—	—	501
0.6-1.0	9 (20)	0.72 (28)	17.20	—	—	713
Children						
1-2	11 (24)	0.82 (32)	16.19	—	—	869
Males						
3-8	20.4 (45)	1.15 (45)	15.42	1035	1.39	1441
9-13	35.8 (79)	1.44 (57)	17.20	1320	1.56	2079
14-18	58.8 (130)	1.70 (67)	20.37	1729	1.80	3116
19-30	71 (156)	1.80 (71)	22.02	1769	1.74	3081
31-50	71.4 (157)	1.78 (70)	22.55	1675	1.81	3021
51-70	70 (154)	1.74 (69)	22.95	1524	1.63	2469
71+	68.9 (152)	1.74 (69)	22.78	1480	1.52	2238
Females						
3-8	22.9 (50)	1.20 (47)	15.63	1004	1.48	1487
9-13	36.4 (80)	1.44 (57)	17.38	1186	1.60	1907
14-18	54.1 (119)	1.63 (64)	20.42	1361	1.69	2302
19-30	59.3 (131)	1.66 (65)	21.42	1361	1.80	2436
31-50	58.6 (129)	1.64 (65)	21.64	1322	1.83	2404
51-70	59.1 (130)	1.63 (63)	22.18	1226	1.70	2066
71+	54.8 (121)	1.58 (62)	21.75	1183	1.33	1564
Pregnant						
First trimester						+0
Second to third trimester						+300/day
Lactating						
First 12 months						+500/day

TEE, Total energy expenditure.
Modified from Food and Nutrition Board, Institute of Medicine: *Dietary reference intakes for energy, carbohydrate, fiber, fat, fatty acids, cholesterol, protein, and amino acids,* Washington, DC, 2005, National Academies Press.

MyPyramid

The *http://mypyramid.gov* Web site can outline an individualized calorie level and corresponding serving sizes from each of the food groups to meet nutrient and energy density needs on the basis of age, gender, weight, height, and activity level. The site also gives a variety of helpful information for maintaining balance between food intake and energy output through physical activity.

SUMMARY

Energy is the force or power to do work. In the human energy system, food provides energy. Energy is measured in kilocalories (1000 calories). Energy from food is cycled through the body's internal energy system in balance with the external environment's energy system, powered by the sun.

Metabolism is the sum of the body processes involved in converting food into various forms of energy. These forms of energy include chemical, electrical, me-chanical, and thermal energy. When food is not available, the body draws on its stored energy: glycogen, fat, and muscle protein.

Total body energy requirements are based on the following: (1) basal metabolism needs, which make up the largest portion of energy needs; (2) energy for physical activities; and (3) the thermal effect of food (digesting food and absorbing and transporting nutrients). Energy requirements vary throughout life.

CRITICAL THINKING QUESTIONS

1. What are the fuel factors of the three energy nutrients? What is the fuel factor for alcohol? What do these figures mean? What is the primary energy nutrient? Why? Give examples of foods providing these nutrients.

2. Define RMR. What body tissues contribute most to resting metabolic needs? Why? What factors influence basal energy requirements, and how?

3. What factors influence nonbasal energy needs? Identify each as either voluntary or involuntary.

CHAPTER CHALLENGE QUESTIONS

True-False
Write the correct statement for each statement that is false.

1. *True or False:* Vitamins are energy-yielding nutrients in foods.

2. *True or False:* RMR takes into account energy used for physical activity.

3. *True or False:* The thyroid hormone, thyroxine, controls the rate of body metabolism.

4. *True or False:* Because children are smaller, their energy requirements are less per kilogram (or pound) of body weight than those of adults.

5. *True or False:* The thermic effect of food refers to the energy necessary for the digestion of food.

6. *True or False:* Different persons doing the same amount of physical activity require the same amount of energy in kilocalories.

Multiple Choice

1. In human nutrition, the kilocalorie is used to
   a. provide vitamins and water.
   b. measure energy input and output.
   c. control energy reactions.
   d. measure electrical energy.

2. In the following family of four, who has the highest energy needs per unit of body weight?
   a. 32-year-old mother
   b. 35-year-old father
   c. 2-month-old son
   d. 70-year-old grandmother

3. An overactive thyroid causes
   a. decreased energy need.
   b. no effect on energy need.
   c. increased energy need.
   d. decreased protein need.

4. Which of the following persons is using the most energy?
   a. Teenager playing basketball
   b. Woman walking uphill
   c. Student studying for final examinations
   d. Man driving a car

5. Which of these foods has the highest energy value per unit of weight?
   a. Bread
   b. Meat
   c. Potato
   d. Butter

6. A slice of bread contains 2 g protein, 1 g fat, and 15 g carbohydrate in the form of starch. What is its kilocalorie value?
   a. 17 kcal
   b. 68 kcal
   c. 77 kcal
   d. 92 kcal

evolve Please refer to the Students' Resource section of this text's Evolve Web site for additional study resources.

REFERENCES

1. Food and Nutrition Board, Institute of Medicine: *Dietary reference intakes for energy, carbohydrate, fiber, fat, fatty acids, cholesterol, protein, and amino acids,* Washington, DC, 2002, National Academies Press.

2. Wang Z and others: Resting energy expenditure-fat-free mass relationship: new insights provided by body composition modeling, *Am J Physiol Endocrinol Metab* 279(3):E539, 2000.

3. Frankenfield D and others: Comparison of predictive equations for resting metabolic rate in healthy nonobese and obese adults: a systematic review, *J Am Diet Assoc* 105(5):775, 2005.

4. Luke A and others: Positive association between resting energy expenditure and weight gain in lean adult population, *Am J Clin Nutr* 83(5):1076, 2006.

5. Roberts SB, Dallal GE: Energy requirements and aging, *Public Health Nutr* 8(7A):1028, 2005.

6. Krems C and others: Lower resting metabolic rate in the elderly may not entirely due to changes in body composition, *Eur J Clin Nutr* 59(2):255, 2005.

7. Lof M and others: Changes in basal metabolic rate during pregnancy in relation to changes in body weight and composition, cardiac output, insulin-like growth factor I, and thyroid hormones and in relation to fetal growth, *Am J Clin Nutr* 81(3):678, 2005.

8. Butte NF and others: Energy requirements during pregnancy based on total energy expenditure and energy deposition, *Am J Clin Nutr* 79(6), 2004.

9. Butte NF, King JC: Energy requirements during pregnancy and lactation, *Public Health Nutr* 8(7A):1010, 2005.

10. Vatten LJ and others: Combined effect of blood pressure and physical activity on cardiovascular mortality, *J Hypertens* 24(10):1939, 2006.

11. Hamman RF and others: Effect of weight loss with lifestyle intervention on risk of diabetes, *Diabetes Care* 29(9):2102, 2006.

12. U.S. Department of Health and Human Services: *Dietary guidelines for Americans 2005*, Washington, DC, 2005, U.S. Government Printing Office.

FURTHER READING AND RESOURCES

The following Web sites provide methods for predicting total energy needs and evaluating energy expenditure.

Children's energy needs calculator: *www.kidsnutrition.org/consumer/nyc/vol1_03/energy_calculator.htm*

Adult energy needs and BMI calculator: *www.bcm.edu/cnrc/caloriesneed.htm*

Mayo Clinic: "Metabolism and weight loss: how you burn calories": *www.mayoclinic.com/health/metabolism/WT00006*

Frenkenfield D and others: Comparison of predictive equations for resting metabolic rate in healthy nonobese and obese adults: a systematic review, *J Am Diet Assoc* 105(5):775, 2005.
    This review article evaluates the four most common prediction equations for RMR for accuracy and usefulness.

CHAPTER 7

Vitamins

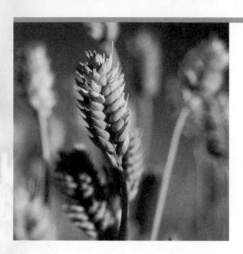

KEY CONCEPTS

- Vitamins are noncaloric essential nutrients necessary for many metabolic tasks.
- Certain health problems are related to inadequate or excessive vitamin intake.
- Vitamins occur in a wide variety of foods packaged with the energy- and tissue-building macronutrients (carbohydrate, fat, and protein). The body uses vitamins to make coenzymes required for some enzymes to function.
- The need for particular vitamin supplements depends on a person's vitamin status.

More than any other group of nutrients, vitamins have captured public interest and concern. This chapter answers some of the questions about vitamins: What do they do? How much of each vitamin does the human body need? What foods do they come from? Because of the attention vitamins receive in the media, we can assume people want real answers to these questions rather than unfounded claims. The scientific study of nutrition, on which the DRI guidelines are based, continues to expand the body of nutrition knowledge.

This chapter looks at the vitamins as a group and as individual nutrients. It explores general and specific vitamin needs as well as reasonable and realistic supplement use.

DIETARY REFERENCE INTAKES

The study of vitamins and minerals and their many functions in human nutrition is a subject of intense scientific investigation. As discussed in Chapter 1, the DRIs are recommendations for nutrient intake by healthy population groups. The continuing development of DRIs, under the direction of the National Academy of Sciences, takes place over several years and involves numerous scientists from the United States and Canada. They include recommendations for each gender and age group and incorporate and expand the well-known RDAs.

Within the DRIs are the following four interconnected categories of recommendations, defined in Chapter 1:

1. *RDA,* the daily intake that meets the needs of almost all healthy individuals in a specified group
2. *EAR,* the basis for developing the RDA, is the intake that meets the needs of half of the individuals in the reference population

3. *AI*, a guideline used when not enough scientific data are available to establish an RDA
4. *UL*, a new guideline that sets the maximum nutrient intake that is unlikely to pose a risk of toxicity in healthy individuals

This chapter's discussion of vitamins and the following chapters that discuss minerals, fluids, and electrolytes refer to the various DRI recommendations (especially the RDAs) whenever possible.

THE NATURE OF VITAMINS

Discovery

Early Observations

Vitamins were largely discovered while searching for cures for classic diseases suspected to be associated with dietary deficiencies. As early as 1753 a British naval surgeon, Dr. James Lind, observed that many sailors became ill and died on long voyages when they had to live on rations without fresh foods. When Lind provided the sailors fresh lemons and limes (which were easily stored) on a later voyage, no one became ill. Dr. Lind had discovered that scurvy, the curse of sailors, was caused by a dietary deficiency and was prevented by adding lemons or limes to the diet. Because British sailors carried limes on these long voyages, they got the nickname "limeys."

Early Animal Experiments

In 1906, Dr. Frederich Hopkins of Cambridge University performed an experiment in which he fed a group of rats a synthetic mixture of protein, fat, carbohydrate, mineral salts, and water. All the rats became ill and died. In another experiment he added milk to the purified ration, and all the rats grew normally. This important discovery, that accessory factors are present in *natural* foods that are essential to life, provided the necessary foundation for the individual vitamin discoveries that followed.

Era of Vitamin Discovery

Most of the vitamins known today were discovered during the first half of the 1900s. The nature of these vital molecules became more evident over time. A form of the name *vitamin* was first used in 1911 when Casimir Funk, a Polish chemist working at the Lister Institute in London, discovered a nitrogen-containing substance (in organic chemistry known as an *amine*) that he speculated might be a common characteristic of all vital agents. He coined the word *vitamine* from "vital amine." The final *e* was dropped later when other vital substances turned out not to be amines, and the name *vitamin* was retained to designate compounds of this class of essential substances.

At first scientists assigned letters of the alphabet to each vitamin in the order they were discovered; however, as more vitamins were discovered, this practice was abandoned in favor of more specific names based on a vitamin's chemical structure or body function.

Definition

As each vitamin was discovered during the first half of the 1900s, the following two characteristics clearly emerged that define a vitamin:

1. It must be a vital, organic substance that is not a carbohydrate, fat, or protein and must be necessary in only extremely *small* amounts to perform its specific metabolic function or prevent its associated deficiency disease.
2. It cannot be manufactured by the body in sufficient quantities to sustain life, so it must be supplied by the diet.

Because the body only needs them in small amounts, vitamins are designated micronutrients. The total volume of vitamins a healthy person normally requires each day would barely fill a teaspoon. Thus the units of measure for vitamins (e.g., milligrams or micrograms) are exceedingly small and difficult to visualize (see the For Further Focus box, "Small Measures for Small Needs"). Nonetheless, all vitamins are essential to life.

Functions of Vitamins

Although each vitamin has its specific metabolic task, general functions of vitamins are (1) components of coenzymes, (2) antioxidants, (3) hormones that affect gene expression, (4) a component of cell membranes, and/or (5) a component of the light-sensitive rhodopsin molecule in the eyes (vitamin A).

Metabolism: Enzymes and Coenzymes

Coenzymes derived from vitamins are an integral part of some enzymes, without which these enzymes cannot catalyze their metabolic reactions. For example, several of the B vitamins (thiamin, niacin, and riboflavin) are part of coenzymes. These coenzymes are, in turn, integral parts of enzymes that metabolize glucose, fatty acids, and amino acids

---

scurvy a hemorrhagic disease caused by a lack of vitamin C characterized by diffuse tissue bleeding, painful limbs and joints, thickened bones, and skin discoloration from bleeding; bones fracture easily, wounds do not heal, gums are swollen and bleed, and teeth loosen.

FOR FURTHER FOCUS

SMALL MEASURES FOR SMALL NEEDS

By definition, vitamins are essential nutrients necessary in small amounts for human health. But just how small those amounts are is sometimes hard to imagine. Vitamins are measured in metric system terms such as milligram and microgram, but how much is that? Perhaps comparing these amounts with commonly used household measures may be helpful.

Early in the age of scientific development, scientists realized that they needed a common language of measures that could be understood by all nations to exchange rapidly developing scientific knowledge. Thus the metric system was born. Like American money, it is a simple decimal system, here applied to weights and measures. This system was developed in the mid-1800s by French scientists and named Le Système International d'Unités, which is abbreviated as SI units. Use of these more precise units is now widespread, especially because it is mandatory for all purposes in most countries besides the United States. The U.S. Congress passed the official Metric Conversion Act in 1975, but this country has been slower to apply it to common use than have other countries (see Appendix G). The use of this system in scientific work, however, is worldwide.

Compare the two metric measures used for vitamins in the United States. Following are the RDAs with common measures to see how small our need really is:

- One *milligram* (mg) equals one-thousandth of a gram (28 g = 1 oz; 1 g = approximately ¼ tsp). RDAs are measured in milligrams for vitamins E, C, thiamin, riboflavin, niacin, B_6, pantothenic acid, and choline.
- A *microgram* (mcg or μg) equals one-millionth of a gram. RDAs are measured in micrograms for vitamins A (REs), D, K, folate, B_{12}, and biotin.

Small wonder that the total amount of vitamins we need in a day would scarcely fill a teaspoon; but that small amount makes the big difference between life and death.

to extract energy. Enzymes act as *catalysts*. Catalysts increase the rate at which their specific chemical reactions proceed but are not themselves consumed in the reactions.

Tissue Structure and Protection

Some vitamins are involved in tissue or bone building. For example, vitamin C is involved in the synthesis of collagen, a structural protein in skin, ligaments, and bones. In fact, the word *collagen* comes from a Greek word meaning glue. Collagen is gluelike in its capacity to add tensile strength to body structures. Vitamins also act as antioxidants to protect cell structures and prevent free radical damage.

Prevention of Deficiency Diseases

When a vitamin deficiency becomes severe, the nutritional deficiency disease associated with the specific function of that vitamin becomes apparent. For example, the classic vitamin deficiency disease *scurvy* is caused by insufficient dietary vitamin C. Scurvy is a hemorrhagic disease characterized by bleeding in joints and other tissues and by the breakdown of fragile capillaries under normal blood pressure—all symptoms related to vitamin C's role in producing the collagen in strong capillary walls. Internal membranes disintegrate and death occurs, as previously mentioned in British sailors of earlier centuries. The name *ascorbic acid* comes from the Latin word *scorbutus,* meaning scurvy, and the combining form, *a,* means without, so the term *ascorbic* means without scurvy. In developed countries today, we do not see frank scurvy often, but we do see vitamin C deficiency in combination with other forms and degrees of malnutrition among low-income and poverty-stricken population groups.

Vitamin Metabolism

The way in which our bodies digest, absorb, and transport vitamins depends on the vitamin's solubility. Vitamins traditionally are classified as either *fat soluble* or *water soluble.* The fat-soluble vitamins are A, D, E, and K. The water-soluble vitamins are C and all the B vitamins.

Fat-Soluble Vitamins

Intestinal cells absorb fat-soluble vitamins with fat and incorporate both the fat and fat-soluble vitamins into chylomicrons. From the intestinal cells, chylomicrons enter the lymphatic circulation and then the blood. The absorption of fat-soluble vitamins is enhanced by dietary fat. For instance, the vitamin A in a glass of vitamin A–fortified milk is better absorbed from whole or 2% milk than from skim milk because skim milk contains no fat.

Unlike water-soluble vitamins, fat-soluble vitamins can be stored in the liver and in adipose tissue for long periods. The body uses this reserve in times of inadequate intake. Fat-soluble vitamin accumulation in the liver and in adipose tissue is the reason excess intake can result in toxicity over time.

Water-Soluble Vitamins

Intestinal cells easily absorb water-soluble vitamins. From these cells they move directly into the portal blood circulation. Because blood is mostly water, transport of water-soluble vitamins does not require the assistance of carrier proteins.

With the exception of vitamins B_{12} and B_6 the body does not store water-soluble vitamins to any significant extent. Therefore the body does not have a reserve supply and requires foods rich in water-soluble vitamins daily. The potential toxicity of each vitamin is determined by the body's capacity to store it and the capacity of the liver and kidneys to clear it.

SECTION | FAT-SOLUBLE VITAMINS

VITAMIN A (RETINOL)

Functions

Vitamin A performs the following functions in the body.

Vision

The chemical name retinol was given to vitamin A because of its major function in the retina of the eye. The aldehyde form, retinal, is part of a light-sensitive pigment in retinal cells named *rhodopsin,* commonly known as *visual purple.* Rhodopsin enables the eye to adjust to different amounts of available light. A mild vitamin A deficiency may cause night blindness, slow adaptation to darkness, or glare blindness. Vitamin A–related compounds—the carotenoids, lutein and zeaxanthin—are specifically associated with the prevention of age-related macular degeneration.

Tissue Strength and Immunity

The other retinoids, retinoic acid and retinol, help maintain healthy *epithelial* tissue, the protective tissue covering body surfaces (e.g., the skin and the inner mucous membranes in the nose, throat, eyes, GI tract, and genitourinary tract). These tissues are the primary barrier to infection. Vitamin A also is important as an antioxidant and in the production of immune cells responsible for fighting bacterial, parasitic, and viral attacks.

Growth

Retinoic acid and retinol are involved in skeletal growth and soft tissue growth through their roles in protein synthesis and cell membrane stabilization. The constant need to replace old cells in the bone matrix, the GI tract, and so forth requires adequate vitamin A intake.

Requirements

Vitamin A requirements are based on its two basic forms in foods—preformed A or provitamin A (discussed below)—and its storage in the body. The established RDA for adults is 700 mcg retinol equivalents (RE) for women and 900 mcg RE for men.

Food Forms and Units of Measure

Vitamin A occurs in two forms, as follows:

1. *Preformed vitamin A* or *retinol* is the active vitamin A found in foods derived from animals.
2. Provitamin A, or beta-carotene, is a pigment in yellow, orange, and deep green fruits or vegetables that the human body can convert to retinol. Carotenoids are a family of compounds similar in structure, of which beta-carotene and lutein are the most common in foods (Box 7-1).

In the typical American diet, a significant amount of vitamin A is in the provitamin A form, beta-carotene. To account for all food forms, individual carotenoids and preformed vitamin A are measured and the amounts are converted to REs. For the body to make 1 mcg of retinol, 12 mcg of dietary beta-carotene, 2 mcg of supplemental

---

retinol the chemical name of vitamin A; derived from its visual function relating to the retina of the eye, which is the back inner lining of the eyeball that catches the lens light refractions to form images interpreted by the optic nerve and brain and makes the necessary light-dark adaptations.

carotenoids organic pigments found in plants. Known to have functions such as scavenging free radicals, reducing the risk of certain types of cancer, and helping prevent age-related eye diseases. More than 600 carotenoids have been identified, with beta-carotene being the most well known.

carotene a group name for three red and yellow pigments (alpha-, beta-, and gamma-carotene) found in dark green and yellow vegetables and fruits. Beta-carotene is most important to human nutrition because the body can convert it to vitamin A, thus making it a primary source of the vitamin.

BOX 7-1

CAROTENOIDS

Carotenes: orange pigments
- α-Carotene
- β-Carotene
- γ-Carotene
- δ-Carotene
- Lycopene
- Neurosporene
- Phytofluene
- Phytoene

Xanthophylls: yellow pigments
- Astaxanthin
- Canthaxanthin
- Cryptoxanthin
- Lutein
- Zeaxanthin

beta-carotene, and 24 mcg of the two carotenoids, alpha-carotene or beta-cryptoxanthin, are necessary. An older measure sometimes used to quantify vitamin A is International Units (IU). One IU of vitamin A equals 0.3 mcg retinol, or 0.6 mcg beta-carotene.

Body Storage

The liver can store large amounts of retinol. In healthy individuals the liver stores more than 50% of ingested retinol and contains approximately 90% of the body's total store. Thus when people take large supplements of retinol in addition to dietary sources, they can ingest a toxic quantity.

Deficiency Disease

Adequate vitamin A intake prevents two eye conditions: (1) *xerosis,* or itching, burning, and red, inflamed eyelids; and (2) *xerophthalmia,* or blindness caused by severe deficiency. Dietary vitamin A deficiency is the leading cause of blindness in children worldwide.

Deficiency symptoms are directly related to vitamin A's functions. Therefore a lack of dietary vitamin A results in epithelial and immune system disorders.

Toxicity Symptoms

The condition created by excessive vitamin A intake is called *hypervitaminosis A.* Symptoms include joint pain, thickening of long bones, loss of hair, and jaundice. Excessive vitamin A intake may cause liver injury with (1) *portal hypertension,* which is elevated blood pressure in the portal vein; and (2) *ascites,* or fluid accumulation in the abdominal cavity. Because of the potential for toxicity,

the UL of retinol for adults has been set at 3000 mcg/day. Although vitamin A deficiency is more common worldwide than toxicity, people in the United States may consume excess vitamin A in fortified foods and dietary supplements.[1] Toxicity symptoms usually result from overconsumption of preformed vitamin A, not carotenoids. Absorption of dietary carotenoids is dose dependent at high intake levels. However, prolonged excessive intake of foods high in beta-carotene will cause a harmless orange skin tint that disappears when excessive intakes are discontinued. Beta-carotene supplements, on the other hand, can reach concentrations in the body that promote oxidative damage, cell division, and destruction of other forms of vitamin A.

Food Sources

Fish liver oils, liver, egg yolk, butter, and cream are sources of preformed, natural vitamin A. Preformed vitamin A only occurs naturally in milk fat. Low-fat and nonfat milks and margarine are good sources of vitamin A because they are fortified. Some good sources of beta-carotene are dark-green, leafy vegetables such as Swiss chard, turnip greens, kale, and spinach and dark-orange vegetables and fruits such as carrots, sweet potatoes or yams, pumpkin, mango, and apricots. Table 7-1 provides some comparative food sources of vitamin A.

Beta-carotene and preformed vitamin A require emulsification by bile salts to be absorbed by the intestine. Inside intestinal cells both forms are incorporated into chylomicrons with fat, and the chylomicrons traverse the lymphatic system to the blood stream.

Stability

Retinol is unstable when exposed to heat and oxygen. Cooking vegetables in uncovered pots inactivates much of their vitamin A. Quicker cooking with little water helps preserve vitamin A. If fats are rancid or vegetables are wilted, most of the vitamin A is inactive.

VITAMIN D (CHOLECALCIFEROL)

Vitamin D is not truly a vitamin because the human body makes it with the help of the sun's ultraviolet rays. It was mistakenly classified as a vitamin in 1922 by its discoverers because they cured rickets with fish oil, a natural source of vitamin D. Today we know that the compound made by the sun's ultraviolet rays in our skin is a prohormone named cholecalciferol, often shortened to *calciferol.* The precursor of calciferol in the skin is *7-dehydrocholesterol,* which is made by the liver. Calciferol made in

TABLE 7-1

FOOD SOURCES OF VITAMIN A

ITEM	QUANTITY	AMOUNT (mcg RE)
Vegetables		
Beet greens, boiled	½ cup	276
Chinese cabbage	½ cup	790
Carrots, raw	½ cup (1 medium)	538
Collards, boiled	½ cup	386
Dandelion greens, boiled	½ cup	260
Kale, raw	½ cup	258
Mustard greens, boiled	½ cup	221
Pumpkin, boiled	½ cup	306
Spinach, boiled	½ cup	472
Sweet potato, baked, in skin	1 medium (114 g)	1096
Winter squash	½ cup	268
Fruits		
Cantaloupe	1 cup, diced	264
Meat, Poultry, Fish, Dry Beans, Eggs, Nuts		
Beef liver, pan fried	3 oz	6582
Chicken liver, pan fried	3 oz	3652
Milk, Dairy Products		
Milk, low fat 2%, fortified	8 oz	134
Milk, skim, fortified	8 oz	149
Ricotta cheese, whole milk	½ cup	149

Data from the USDA, Agricultural Research Service, Nutrient Data Laboratory: *USDA nutrient database for standard reference, release 20, www.ars.usda.gov/ba/bhnrc/ndl.*

the skin and vitamin D from dietary sources must be activated in two successive hydroxylation steps, the first occurring in the liver and the second occurring in the kidneys. The activated, functional form of vitamin D is calcitriol (1,25-dihydroxycalciferol, 1,25-dihydroxycholecalciferol, or 1,25-dihydroxy vitamin D_3) (Figure 7-1).

Functions

Absorption of Calcium and Phosphorus and Bone Mineralization

Calcitriol acts physiologically with two other hormones, parathyroid hormone and the thyroid hormone calcitonin to control calcium and phosphorus metabolism. Calcitriol stimulates (1) intestinal cell absorption of calcium and phosphorus, (2) kidney reabsorption of calcium and phosphorus, and (3) osteoclastic removal of calcium and phosphorus from trabecular bone—all

mechanisms that increase blood calcium and phosphorus concentrations (see Figure 7-1).

Osteoporosis Treatment

Because calcitriol regulates the rate of calcium and phosphorus resorption from bone, it has been clinically used to treat osteoporosis, a loss of bone density that leads to brittle bones and spontaneous fractures.

Requirements

A number of factors influence vitamin D requirements and excessive intake is possible, especially by young infants. Establishing requirements for vitamin D is difficult because (1) it is made in the skin by the sun's ultraviolet rays from *7-dehydrocholesterol*, and (2) the number of food sources are limited. Vitamin D requirement varies with individual exposure to sunlight, which is affected by season, the latitude where a person resides, and even a person's skin color.

In general, people who are regularly exposed to sunlight (face and hands for 10 to 20 minutes per day) have no dietary requirement for vitamin D. However, in the northern hemisphere, particularly above 40 degrees latitude, less sunlight is present in fall and winter, between the autumnal equinox and vernal equinox (September 23 to March 21), than in spring and summer, between the vernal and autumnal equinoxes (March 21 to September 23). This particularly affects the vitamin D_3 requirement of people with darker skin because darker skin produces even less vitamin D_3 in low-intensity sunlight than does lighter skin.

The DRI committee has not established an RDA for vitamin D. Instead, it proposed AI levels of 5 mcg/day (200 IU) for both women and men from birth to age 50 years. Dietary recommendations triple for individuals older than 70 years because of their skin's decreased ability to synthesize vitamin D.

prohormone a precursor substance that the body converts to a hormone. For example, a cholesterol compound in the skin is first irradiated by sunlight and then converted through successive enzyme actions in the liver and kidney into the vitamin D hormone, which then regulates calcium absorption and bone development.

cholecalciferol the chemical name for vitamin D in its inactive dietary form; often shortened to calciferol.

calcitriol the activated hormone form of vitamin D.

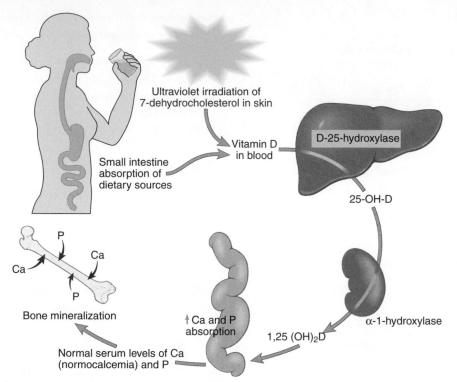

Figure 7-1 Vitamin D activation from skin synthesis and dietary sources. Normal vitamin D metabolism maintains blood calcium levels. (Reprinted from Kumar V and others: *Robbins basic pathology*, ed 8, Philadelphia, 2007, Saunders.)

Deficiency Disease

A calcitriol deficiency causes rickets, a condition in growing children characterized by malformation of bones (Figure 7-2). Children with rickets have soft long bones that bend under the child's weight. In addition to skeletal malformations, inadequate vitamin D intake prevents children from attaining their peak bone mass, contributing to the development of osteoporosis or osteomalacia as adults. Although the fortification of milk with vitamin D has reduced the prevalence of deficiency, an estimated 36% of healthy young adults still have inadequate vitamin D stores.[2]

Toxicity Symptoms

Excessive intake of vitamin D, especially in infants, can be toxic. Symptoms of toxicity, or *hypervitaminosis D,* include calcification of soft tissues, such as kidneys and lungs, and fragile bones. Prolonged elevated intake of cholecalciferol (more than 50 mcg/day [2000 IU], or 10 times the AI) produces elevated blood calcium concentration in infants and calcium deposits in the kidney nephrons in both infants and adults, interfering with overall kidney function. For example, when fortified milk

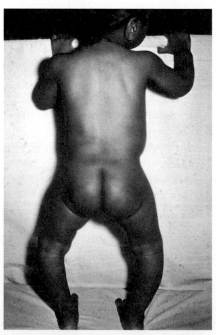

Figure 7-2 Child with rickets; note the bowlegs. (Reprinted from Kumar V and others: *Robbins basic pathology*, ed 8, Philadelphia, 2007, Saunders.)

TABLE 7-2

FOOD SOURCES OF VITAMIN D

ITEM	QUANTITY	AMOUNT (IU)
Bread, Cereal, Rice, Pasta		
All Bran, Kellogg's cereal	½ cup	50
Total Whole Grain, General Mill's cereal	1 cup	53
Meat, Poultry, Fish, Dry Beans, Eggs, Nuts		
Herring or trout, cooked	3 oz	177
Salmon, Atlantic, cooked	3 oz	255
Salmon, canned (includes Chinook, Coho, pink, Sockeye)	3 oz	689
Sardines, Pacific, canned	3 oz	408
Tuna, canned, Albacore or Ahi	3 oz	119
Tuna, bluefin, cooked	3 oz	782
Milk, Dairy Products		
Milk, vitamin D fortified	1 cup (8 fl oz)	100
Soy or rice milk, fortified with vitamin D	1 cup (8 fl oz)	80
Fats, Oils, Sugar		
Fish oil, cod liver	1 Tbsp	1360

Data from the USDA, Agricultural Research Service, Nutrient Data Laboratory: *USDA nutrient database for standard reference, release 20, www.ars.usda.gov/ba/bhnrc/ndl.*, and British Columbia Ministry of Health: *Food sources of calcium and vitamin D, www.bchealthguide.org/healthfiles/hfile68e.stm#hf004,* accessed August 2007.

and fortified cereal are used in addition to vitamin supplements, infants may consume excessive cholecalciferol. An infant (from birth to 1 year) only needs 5 mcg (200 IU) of cholecalciferol daily.[3] The UL for vitamin D in persons older than 1 year is 50 mcg/day. Vitamin D intoxication cannot occur from cutaneous production of vitamin D. For most people vitamin D intake from food and dietary supplements is not likely to exceed the UL. However, individuals consuming diets high in fatty fish, and fortified milk, in addition to dietary supplements containing vitamin D, may be at risk of toxicity.

Food Sources

Yeast and fatty fish are the only good natural sources of vitamin D. Therefore a large portion of daily vitamin D intake comes from fortified foods (Table 7-2). Because it is a common food and also contains calcium and phosphorus, milk is the most practical food to fortify with vitamin D. The standard commercial practice is to add 10 mcg/qt (400 IU). Butter substitutes, such as margarines, also are fortified with vitamin D. Children consuming vitamin D–deficient diets (e.g., a rigid macrobiotic pattern with no milk products) are especially vulnerable to stunted bone development and rickets.

Stability

Vitamin D is stable to heat, aging, and storage.

VITAMIN E (TOCOPHEROL)

Early vitamin studies identified a substance necessary for animal reproduction. This substance was named **tocopherol,** from two Greek words: *tophos,* meaning childbirth, and *phero,* meaning to bring, with the *-ol* ending to indicate its alcohol functional group. Tocopherol became known as the antisterility vitamin, but it was soon demonstrated to have this effect only in rats and a few other animals, not in people. A number of related compounds have since been discovered. Tocopherol is the generic name for this entire group of homologous fat-soluble nutrients designated alpha (α)-, beta (β)-, gamma (γ)-, and delta (δ)-tocopherol or tocotrienol. Of these eight, α-tocopherol is the only one significant in human nutrition and thus is used to calculate dietary needs.[4]

rickets a disease of childhood characterized by softening of the bones from an inadequate intake of vitamin D and insufficient exposure to sunlight; also associated with impaired calcium and phosphorus metabolism.

tocopherol the chemical name for vitamin E, which was named by early investigators because their initial work with rats indicated a reproductive function. In people, vitamin E functions as a strong antioxidant that preserves structural membranes such as cell walls.

Functions

The most vital function of α-tocopherol is its antioxidant action in tissues. An antioxidant is a molecule that prevents the modification of cellular structures by free radicals (a process called oxidation).

Antioxidant Function

α-Tocopherol is the body's most abundant fat-soluble antioxidant. The polyunsaturated fatty acids (see Chapter 3) in the phospholipids of cell and organelle membranes are particularly susceptible to free radical oxidation. α-Tocopherol intercepts this oxidation process, protecting the polyunsaturated fatty acids from damage.

Relation to Selenium Metabolism

Selenium is a trace mineral that, as part of the selenium-containing enzyme *glutathione peroxidase*, works with α-tocopherol as an antioxidant. Glutathione peroxidase is the second line of defense in preventing free radical damage to membranes. Glutathione peroxidase spares α-tocopherol from oxidation, thus reducing the dietary requirement for α-tocopherol, just as α-tocopherol spares glutathione peroxidase from oxidation, thus reducing the dietary requirement for selenium.

Requirements

α-Tocopherol requirements are expressed in milligrams per day. The RDA for men and women ages 14 years and older is 15 mg/day, with lesser amounts necessary during childhood. During the first year of infancy no RDA has been determined, but the AI is 4 to 6 mg/day.

Deficiency Disease

Young infants, especially premature infants who missed the final 1 to 2 months of gestation when α-tocopherol stores are normally filled, are particularly vulnerable to the deficiency disease hemolytic anemia. In hemolytic anemia, red blood cell (RBC) membrane phospholipids and proteins are left unprotected and are easily oxidized and degraded, and the continued loss of functioning RBCs leads to anemia (see the Clinical Applications box, "Vitamin E and Premature Infants"). In older children and adults, α-tocopherol deficiency disrupts normal synthesis of *myelin,* the protective phospholipid-rich membrane covering nerve cells. This is especially devastating for the neurons in the brain.[5] The main nerves involved are (1) spinal cord fibers that affect physical activity (e.g., walking), and (2) the retina of the eye that affects vision.

CLINICAL APPLICATIONS

VITAMIN E AND PREMATURE INFANTS

Hemolytic anemia, a medical problem found in infants, especially premature ones, has responded positively to vitamin E therapy.

Anemia is a blood condition characterized by loss of mature, functioning RBCs. Different types of anemia usually are named according to the cause or to the nature of an abnormal nonfunctioning cell produced. The name of this type of anemia comes from its cause. The word hemolysis comes from two roots: *hemo,* referring to blood, and *lysis,* meaning dissolving or breaking. Therefore hemolysis means the bursting or dissolving of RBCs; the resulting condition is hemolytic anemia. Vitamin E can help prevent this destruction of RBCs and the loss of their vital oxygen-carrying hemoglobin because it is one of the body's foremost antioxidants.

An oxidant is a compound or oxygen itself that oxidizes other compounds, thereby breaking them down or changing them. Vitamin E is readily oxidized. When plenty of vitamin E is found among the other compounds exposed to an oxidant, vitamin E can, by its nature, take on the oxidative attack, thus protecting the others. Vitamin E is fat soluble, so it is found among the polyunsaturated fatty acids that compose the core of the cell membranes in body tissues rich in fat. The cell membranes of RBCs are particularly rich in these polyunsaturated lipids and are exposed to concentrated oxygen because they constantly circulate through the lungs. This situation would be destructive to the RBCs if vitamin E was not present. Vitamin E takes the oxygen itself, protecting the polyunsaturated fatty acids and keeping the RBCs intact to continue their life-sustaining journey throughout the body. Thus vitamin E acts as nature's most potent fat-soluble antioxidant.

The protective need of vitamin E is especially great in small, premature infants fed formulas containing iron, which acts as an oxidant, and high concentrations of polyunsaturated fatty acids, which are vulnerable to oxidative breakdown. To avoid this problem and comply with American Academy of Pediatrics recommendations, manufacturers have increased the amount of vitamin E and lowered the iron in formulas for premature infants. The proportions of vitamin E, polyunsaturated fatty acids, and iron in today's improved formulas usually supply enough necessary nutrients, so in most cases supplements are no longer necessary to prevent hemolytic anemia in premature infants.

Toxicity Symptoms

α-Tocopherol from food sources has no known toxic effects in people. Supplemental α-tocopherol intakes exceeding the UL of 1000 mg/day may interfere with vitamin K activity and blood clotting.

Food Sources

The richest sources of α-tocopherol are vegetable oils (e.g., wheat germ, soybean, and safflower oil). Note that vegetable oils also are the richest sources of polyunsaturated fatty acids, which α-tocopherol protects. Other food sources of α-tocopherol include nuts, fortified cereals, and avocado. Table 7-3 provides a list of vitamin E food sources.

Stability

α-Tocopherol is unstable to heat and alkalis.

VITAMIN K

In 1929 Henrik Dam, a biochemist at the University of Copenhagen, discovered a hemorrhagic disease in chicks fed a diet from which all lipids had been removed. Dam hypoth-

TABLE 7-3

FOOD SOURCES OF VITAMIN E AS α-TOCOPHEROL

ITEM	QUANTITY	AMOUNT (mg α-TE)
Bread, Cereal, Rice, Pasta		
Total Whole Grain, General Mill's cereal	1 cup	18.0
Wheat germ, toasted, plain	1 oz	4.53
Fruits		
Avocado	¼ medium	1.04
Mango, raw	½ medium	1.16
Meat, Poultry, Fish, Dry Beans, Eggs, Nuts		
Almonds, dried	1 oz	7.33
Hazelnuts, dried	1 oz	4.26
Sunflower seeds	2 Tbsp	6.21
Fats, Oils, Sugar		
Corn oil	1 Tbsp	2.83
Cottonseed oil	1 Tbsp	4.80
Palm oil	1 Tbsp	2.17
Peanut oil	1 Tbsp	2.12
Safflower oil	1 Tbsp	4.64
Sunflower oil	1 Tbsp	5.59

α-TE, α-Tocopherol equivalents.
Data from the USDA, Agricultural Research Service, Nutrient Data Laboratory: *USDA nutrient database for standard reference, release 20,* www.ars.usda.gov/ba/bhnrc/ndl.

esized that an unidentified lipid factor had been removed from the chicks' feed. Dam called it "koagulations vitamin," or vitamin K, and the letter he assigned is still used today. Dam later succeeded in isolating the agent from alfalfa and identifying it, for which he received the Nobel Prize for physiology and medicine. As with many of the vitamins, not one, but several homologous forms of vitamin K, make up the group. The major form in plants that initially was isolated from alfalfa by Dam is **phylloquinone**. Phylloquinone is the dietary form of vitamin K. *Menaquinone,* a second form, is synthesized by intestinal bacteria. Menaquinone contributes approximately half of our daily supply of vitamin K. *Menadione* is a synthetic precursor of vitamin K, but it has not been used as a dietary supplement since the FDA banned it because of toxicity effects.

Functions

Vitamin K has two well-established functions in the body: blood clotting and bone development.

Blood Clotting

The most well-known and the earliest discovered function of vitamin K is in the blood clotting process. Vitamin K is essential for maintaining normal blood concentrations of four of the 11 blood clotting factors. The first of these vitamin K–dependent blood factors to be identified and characterized was *prothrombin* (clotting factor II). Phylloquinone is an antidote for the effects of excessive anticoagulant drug doses and often is used to control and prevent certain types of hemorrhages. Because this fat-soluble vitamin is more completely absorbed when bile is present, conditions that hinder the release of bile into the small intestine increase the length of time required for blood to clot. When bile salts are given with vitamin K concentrate, the blood clotting time returns to normal.

Bone Development

A more recently discovered function of vitamin K relates to bone development. Synthesis of the second most abundant protein in bone, osteocalcin, requires vitamin K. Vitamin K is involved in modifying the glutamic acid residues of osteocalcin to form calcium-binding gamma-carboxy-glutamic acid residues. Like the blood clotting proteins, osteocalcin binds calcium. Unlike the blood clotting proteins, it forms bone crystals.

phylloquinone a fat-soluble vitamin of the K group found primarily in green plants.

Requirements

Because intestinal bacteria synthesize a form of vitamin K (menaquinone), a constant supply normally is available to support needs. Currently not enough scientific evidence is available to establish an RDA.[6] Therefore the DRIs for vitamin K are AIs. Values gradually increase from birth to adulthood. The AI for men is 120 mcg/day and for women is 90 mcg/day.

Deficiency Disease

Deficiency diseases relating to vitamin K are not usually found in people. A deficiency is unlikely except in clinical conditions related to blood clotting, malabsorption, or lack of intestinal bacteria to synthesize vitamin K. For example, because the intestinal tract of a newborn is sterile, phylloquinone is routinely given to prevent hemorrhaging when the umbilical cord is cut. The vitamin K injection given at birth is commonly phytonadione (AquaMEPHYTON, Mephyton). Patients who have severe malabsorption disorders, such as Crohn's disease, are prescribed low-quality diets after surgery, or are treated with antibiotics that kill intestinal bacteria are susceptible to vitamin K deficiency–induced blood loss.

Toxicity Symptoms

Toxicity from vitamin K—even when large amounts are taken over extended periods—has not been observed. Therefore no UL has been established. (See the Drug-Nutrient Interaction box, "Vitamin K Considerations with Anticoagulant and Antibiotic Medications" for additional information regarding special medication-related considerations with this nutrient.)

Food Sources

Green, leafy vegetables such as spinach, turnip greens, and broccoli are the best dietary sources, providing 40 to 80 mcg of phylloquinone per half cup of raw food. Small amounts of phylloquinone are contributed by milk and dairy products, meats, fortified cereals, fruits, and vegetables (Table 7-4).

Stability

Phylloquinone is fairly stable, although it is sensitive to light and irradiation. Therefore clinical preparations are kept in dark bottles.

Table 7-5 provides a summary of the fat-soluble vitamins.

TABLE 7-4

FOOD SOURCES OF VITAMIN K

ITEM	QUANTITY	AMOUNT (mcg)
Vegetables		
Broccoli, raw	½ cup, chopped	45
Brussels sprouts, cooked, drained	½ cup	109
Kale, raw	½ cup, chopped	273
Mustard greens, raw	½ cup, chopped	139
Spinach, raw	½ cup	72
Turnip greens, raw	½ cup	69

Data from the USDA, Agricultural Research Service, Nutrient Data Laboratory: *USDA nutrient database for standard reference, release 20,* www.ars.usda.gov/ba/bhnrc/ndl.

DRUG-NUTRIENT INTERACTION

VITAMIN K CONSIDERATIONS WITH ANTICOAGULANT AND ANTIBIOTIC MEDICATIONS

Anticoagulation medications such as warfarin act to reduce the overall production of blood clotting factors. Because the primary action of vitamin K is the manufacturing of these same proteins, excessive dietary intake of vitamin K–rich foods during anticoagulation treatment can act antagonistically to the drug. Patients are encouraged to work with a dietitian to achieve a balance between their medication level and desired intake of vitamin K–rich foods.

One form of vitamin K, menaquinone, is synthesized by healthy bacteria in the gut. This source is significant in meeting overall vitamin K needs. Therefore long-term use of medications that destroy GI bacteria, such as antibiotics, also obliterates a valuable source of vitamin K. Patients should be advised to maintain daily intakes of food sources of vitamin K (see Table 7-4).

TABLE 7-5

SUMMARY OF FAT-SOLUBLE VITAMINS

VITAMIN	FUNCTIONS	RECOMMENDED INTAKE (ADULTS)	DEFICIENCY	UL AND TOXICITY	SOURCES
Vitamin A (retinol, retinal, and retinoic acid) Provitamin A (carotene)	Vision cycle: adaptation to light and dark; tissue growth, especially skin and mucous membranes; reproduction; immune function	RDA: men, 900 mcg/day; women, 700 mcg/day	Night blindness; xerosis; xerophthalmia; susceptibility to epithelial infection; dry skin; impaired immunity, growth, and reproduction	UL: 3000 mcg/day Hair loss, irritated skin, bone pain, liver damage, birth defects	Retinol (animal foods): liver, egg yolk, cream, butter or fortified margarine, fortified milk Provitamin A (plant foods): dark-green and deep orange vegetables (e.g., spinach, collards, broccoli, pumpkin, sweet potatoes, carrots)
Vitamin D (cholecalciferol, ergocalciferol)	Absorption of calcium and phosphorus; calcification of bones and teeth; growth	AI: 19-50 yr: 5 mcg/day 51-70 yr: 10 mcg/day 70+: 15 mcg/day	Rickets and growth retardation in children; osteomalacia (soft bones) in adults	UL: 50 mcg/day Calcification of soft tissue, kidney damage, growth retardation	Synthesized in skin with exposure to sunlight; fortified milk, fish oils
Vitamin E (α-tocopherol)	Antioxidant: protection of materials that oxidize easily	RDA: Adults: 15 mg/day	Breakdown of RBCs, anemia, nerve damage, retinopathy	UL: 1000 mg/day (from supplements) Inhibition of vitamin K activity in blood clotting	Vegetable oils, vegetable greens, wheat germ, nuts, seeds
Vitamin K (phylloquinone, menaquinone)	Normal blood clotting and bone development	AI: men, 120 mcg/day; women, 90 mcg/day	Bleeding tendencies, hemorrhagic disease, poor bone growth	UL: Not set Interference with anticoagulation drugs	Synthesis by intestinal bacteria; dark-green, leafy vegetables; soybean oil

SECTION 2 | WATER-SOLUBLE VITAMINS

VITAMIN C (ASCORBIC ACID)

Functions

Vitamin C has several critical functions in the body. It acts as a protective agent (antioxidant) and cofactor of enzymes and plays a role in many metabolic and immunologic activities.

Connective Tissue

Ascorbic acid is necessary to build and maintain strong tissues by its involvement in collagen synthesis. Collagen is especially important in tissues of mesodermal origin, including connective tissues (e.g., ligaments, tendons, bone matrix, and other binding lattices that hold together and give tensile strength to tissues) and other tissues of mesodermal origin that contain connective tissue (e.g., cartilage, tooth dentin, and capillary walls).

Each time proline or lysine is added during collagen synthesis, they are hydroxylated ($-OH$ is added) to form hydroxyproline and hydroxylysine by the ascorbic acid–dependent enzymes prolyl hydroxylase and lysyl hydroxylase. Iron is a cofactor for both enzymes, and ascorbic acid is required to maintain the iron atoms in these enzymes in their active, ferrous (Fe^{2+}) form. Hydroxyproline and hydroxylysine form covalent bonds with other residues, which strengthen collagen's structure. When ascorbic acid is plentiful, collagen, and the connective tissues in which it is integral, quickly develops. Blood vessels are particularly dependent on ascorbic acid's role in collagen synthesis to help their walls resist stretching as blood is forced through them.

General Body Metabolism

The more metabolically active body tissues (e.g., adrenal glands, brain, kidney, liver, pancreas, thymus, and spleen) contain greater concentrations of ascorbic acid. Ascorbic acid in the adrenal glands is drawn upon when the gland is stimulated. This use of ascorbic acid during adrenal stimulation suggests increased need for ascorbic acid during stress. More ascorbic acid is present in a child's actively growing tissues than in adult tissues. Other enzymes requiring ascorbic acid perform such diverse functions as (1) conversion of the neurotransmitter dopamine to the neurotransmitter norepinephrine; (2) the synthesis of carnitine, a mitochondrial fatty acid transporter involved in extracting energy from fatty acids; (3) the catabolism of phenylalanine and tyrosine; and (4) the maturation of some bioactive neural and endocrine peptides. Furthermore, ascorbic acid helps the body absorb nonheme iron by keeping it in its bioactive, reduced ferrous form (Fe^{2+}), making it available for hemoglobin production and thereby helping prevent iron-deficiency anemia. The general clinical needs of ascorbic acid relate to wound healing, fevers and infections, and growth periods.

Antioxidant Function

Similar to vitamin E in function, ascorbic acid is an antioxidant that works to protect the body from free radical damage. Free radicals are associated with increased risks of developing cancer and heart disease.

Requirements

The DRI guidelines for ascorbic acid give an RDA of 75 mg/day for women and 90 mg/day for men, with increases for women during pregnancy and lactation. Because cigarette smoke increases oxidative stress and free radicals in body tissues, the DRI committee recommends an additional 35 mg/day for smokers (see the Clinical Applications box, "Ascorbic Acid Needs in Smokers").

CLINICAL APPLICATIONS

ASCORBIC ACID NEEDS IN SMOKERS

Free radicals are reactive molecules that can disrupt the normal structure of DNA, proteins, carbohydrates, and fatty acids. Such damage is linked to an increased risk of cancer and cardiovascular disease. Cigarette smoke is one environmental source of free radicals. The body fights these free radicals with antioxidants such as vitamins A, E, and C and minerals such as selenium and zinc. Antioxidants destroy free radicals and work to protect the body from free radical damage.

As free radical production increases, antioxidant needs also increase. Cigarette smokers deplete their supply of ascorbic acid more rapidly than nonsmokers because of increased free radical exposure. The vitamin is needed to break down toxic compounds in cigarette smoke. Therefore cigarette smokers are recommended to consume an additional 35 mg of vitamin C per day to meet the increased needs.

Deficiency Disease

Signs of ascorbic acid deficiency include tissue bleeding (e.g., easy bruising, pinpoint skin hemorrhages), bone and joint bleeding, susceptibility to bone fracture, poor wound healing, and soft, bleeding gums with loosened teeth. Extreme deficiency results in the disease scurvy.

Toxicity Symptoms

The UL for ascorbic acid is 2000 mg/day. Although most excessive intake of water-soluble vitamins is efficiently excreted in the urine, levels greater than 2000 mg/day are cleared less efficiently and may result in GI disturbances and osmotic diarrhea. The Institute of Medicine states that further research into the toxic effects of ascorbic acid is warranted because of the popularity of high intake of the vitamin in the United States.[4]

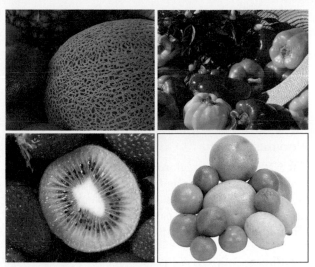

Figure 7-3 Foods high in Vitamin C. (Copyright JupiterImages Corporation.)

Food Sources

The best food sources of ascorbic acid include citrus fruits, red bell peppers, and kiwi (Figure 7-3). Additional good sources include tomatoes, cabbage, berries, melons, green peppers, broccoli, potatoes (white and sweet), and other green and yellow vegetables (Table 7-6).

Stability

Ascorbic acid is readily oxidized on exposure to air and heat. Therefore care must be taken in handling its food sources. Ascorbic acid is not stable in alkaline mediums; thus baking soda, which often is added to foods to preserve color, destroys the ascorbic acid content. Acidic fruits and vegetables retain their ascorbic acid content better than nonacidic foods. The vitamin also is highly soluble in water. The more water added for cooking, the more ascorbic acid leaches out of the fruit or vegetable into the cooking water.

THIAMIN (VITAMIN B₁)
Functions

The name of the vitamin, thiamin, comes from the presence of the thiazole ring in its structure. Thiamin is as a component of a coenzyme *(thiamin pyrophosphate)* involved in energy extraction from glucose and in fat synthesis for energy storage, making energy available to support growth and metabolism. Thiamin is especially necessary for the healthy function of three body systems discussed below.

TABLE 7-6

FOOD SOURCES OF VITAMIN C

ITEM	QUANTITY	AMOUNT (mg)
Vegetables		
Green pepper, raw	½ cup, chopped	60
Peppers, hot chili, red, raw	½ cup, chopped	108
Red pepper, sweet, raw	½ cup, chopped	95
Fruits, Raw		
Kiwi	1 medium	70.5
Lemon juice, fresh	8 fl oz	112
Orange juice, fresh	8 fl oz	124
Orange, navel	1 medium	80
Papaya	½ medium	94
Strawberries	½ cup	49

Data from the USDA, Agricultural Research Service, Nutrient Data Laboratory: *USDA nutrient database for standard reference, release 20,* www.ars.usda.gov/ba/bhnrc/ndl.

ascorbic acid chemical name for vitamin C and named after its ability to cure scurvy.

thiamin chemical name of a major B-complex vitamin; also called vitamin B₁. It was discovered in relation to the classic deficiency disease beriberi and is important in body metabolism as a coenzyme factor in many cell reactions related to energy metabolism.

Gastrointestinal System

Lack of dietary thiamin causes poor appetite, indigestion, constipation, and poor stomach action from lack of muscle tone as well as deficient gastric hydrochloric acid secretion. The cells of smooth muscles and secretory glands must have energy to do their work; thiamin is necessary for producing that energy.

Nervous System

The CNS depends on glucose for energy. Without sufficient thiamin, alertness and reflexes decrease and apathy, fatigue, and irritability result. If the thiamin deficit continues, nerve irritation, pain, and prickly or numbing sensations may eventually progress to paralysis.

Cardiovascular System

Without constant energy, the heart weakens and eventually fails. Blood circulation also is affected when the smooth muscles in the vessel walls weaken. Weakened veins are unable to move blood back toward the heart, so they dilate and fluid accumulates in the lower legs.

Requirements

Thiamin is directly related to energy and carbohydrate metabolism. For healthy persons, the RDAs are based on average energy needs: 1.2 mg/day for men and 1.1 mg/day for women. Children require less. For infants up to age 12 months, no RDA exists; the AI is 0.2 to 0.3 mg/day. Increased thiamin intake is needed during pregnancy and lactation as well as in the treatment of infectious diseases and alcoholism.

Deficiency Disease

Thiamin deficiency is known as beriberi, a paralyzing disease that was especially prevalent in Asian countries. The name describes the disease well; it is Singhalese for "I can't, I can't," because afflicted persons were always too ill to do anything. In industrialized societies thiamin deficiency is largely associated with chronic alcoholism and poor diet. Alcohol inhibits the absorption of thiamin in many ways. Alcohol-induced thiamin deficiency causes a debilitating brain disorder called Wernicke's encephalopathy, which affects mental alertness, short-term memory, and muscle coordination.

Toxicity Symptoms

The kidneys clear excess thiamin; therefore no evidence of toxicity from oral intake and no UL exist.

Food Sources

Although thiamin is widespread in most plant and animal tissues, its content usually is small. Thus thiamin deficiency is a distinct possibility when food intake is markedly curtailed (e.g., in alcoholism or highly inadequate diets). Good food sources of thiamin include wheat germ, lean pork, beef, liver, whole or enriched grains (e.g., flour, bread, cereals), and legumes (Table 7-7). Eggs, fish, and a few vegetables are fair sources.

Stability

Thiamin is a fairly stable vitamin but is destroyed by alkalis and prolonged exposure to high cooking temperatures. Because thiamin is water soluble, little cooking water should be used. As with other water-soluble vitamins, prepared dishes retain more thiamin when their cooking water is used in the dish being prepared rather than being discarded.

RIBOFLAVIN (VITAMIN B$_2$)

Functions

The name riboflavin comes from its chemical nature. It is a yellow-green, fluorescent pigment containing a sugar named *ribose*. Riboflavin is part of two coenzymes involved in both energy production and tissue-protein building—*flavin adenine dinucleotide* and *flavin mono-*

TABLE 7-7

FOOD SOURCES OF THIAMIN

ITEM	QUANTITY	AMOUNT (mg)
Bread, Cereal, Rice, Pasta		
Bran Flakes cereal	1 cup	0.5
Complete, Kellogg's cereal	1 cup	2.08
Product 19, Kellogg's cereal	1 cup	1.5
Quaker Oat Life, Kellogg's cereal	1 cup	0.54
Total Whole Grain, General Mill's cereal	1 cup	2.0
Wheaties, General Mill's cereal	1 cup	0.75
Meat, Poultry, Fish, Dry Beans, Eggs, Nuts		
Ham, sliced, regular (11% fat)	3 oz	0.53
Pork loin, lean, boneless, roasted	3 oz	0.75

Data from the USDA, Agricultural Research Service, Nutrient Data Laboratory: *USDA nutrient database for standard reference, release 20,* www.ars.usda.gov/ba/bhnrc/ndl.

nucleotide. Riboflavin is also an essential factor for glutathione peroxidase, an antioxidant enzyme.

Requirements

Riboflavin needs are related to total energy requirements for age, level of exercise, body size, metabolic rate, and rate of growth. The RDA for adults aged 18 years and older is 1.3 mg/day and 1.1 mg/day for men and women, respectively. The RDA is higher for women during pregnancy (1.4 mg/day) and during lactation (1.6 mg/day). An AI of 0.3 to 0.4 mg/day has been established for infants up to 12 months old.

Deficiency Disease

Signs of riboflavin deficiency include cracked lips and mouth corners; a swollen, red tongue; burning, itching, or tearing eyes caused by extra blood vessels in the cornea; and a scaly, greasy dermatitis in skin folds. Riboflavin deficiency usually occurs with other B vitamin and nutrient deficiencies (e.g., protein malnutrition) rather than by itself. No specific riboflavin deficiency disease is comparable to beriberi. A rare riboflavin deficiency condition has been given the general name *ariboflavinosis.* Its symptoms are tissue inflammation and breakdown and poor wound healing; even minor injuries easily become aggravated and do not heal well.

TABLE 7-8

FOOD SOURCES OF RIBOFLAVIN

ITEM	QUANTITY	AMOUNT (mg)
Bread, Cereal, Rice, Pasta		
Bran Flakes cereal	1 cup	0.57
Complete, Kellogg's cereal	1 cup	2.28
Product 19, Kellogg's cereal	1 cup	1.7
Total Whole Grain, General Mill's cereal	1 cup	2.26
Wheaties, General Mills cereal	1 cup	0.85
Meat, Poultry, Fish, Dry Beans, Eggs, Nuts		
Beef liver, fried	3 oz	2.9
Chicken liver, simmered	3 oz	1.7
Milk, Dairy Products		
Buttermilk, reduced fat	8 fl oz	0.51
Milk, skim or whole	8 fl oz	0.45
Yogurt, low fat	8 fl oz	0.52

Data from the USDA, Agricultural Research Service, Nutrient Data Laboratory: *USDA nutrient database for standard reference, release 20,* www.ars.usda.gov/ba/bhnrc/ndl.

Toxicity Symptoms

No adverse effects from riboflavin intake from food or supplements have been reported. Thus no UL has been determined for riboflavin.

Food Sources

The most important food source of riboflavin is milk. Each serving of milk and milk products contains 0.3 to 0.5 mg of riboflavin. Other good sources include enriched grains and animal protein sources such as meats (especially beef liver), poultry, and fish. Vegetables such as mushrooms, spinach, and avocados are good natural sources. Table 7-8 gives a summary of riboflavin food sources.

Stability

Riboflavin is destroyed by light; therefore milk is now sold and stored in plastic or cardboard cartons, instead of glass containers, to preserve the vitamin.

NIACIN (VITAMIN B$_3$)
Functions

Niacin is part of two coenzymes. The role of one of the niacin-containing coenzymes *(nicotinamide adenine dinucleotide)* is in energy extraction from fat, carbohydrate, and protein (like the coenzymes that contain riboflavin and thiamin). The other niacin-containing coenzyme *(nicotinamide adenine dinucleotide phosphate)* is involved

beriberi a disease of the peripheral nerves caused by a deficiency of thiamin (vitamin B$_1$) characterized by pain (neuritis) and paralysis of legs and arms, cardiovascular changes, and edema. The name is Singhalese for "I can't, I can't."

enriched vitamins and minerals added back to a food after the refining process results in a loss of some nutrients. For example, iron may be lost in the refining process of a grain; therefore the product is enriched with additional iron.

riboflavin chemical name for vitamin B$_2$; discovered in relation to an early vitamin deficiency syndrome called ariboflavinosis that is mainly evidenced in breakdown of skin tissues and resulting infections. It has a role as a coenzyme factor in many cell reactions related to energy and protein metabolism.

niacin chemical name for vitamin B$_3$; discovered in relation to the deficiency disease pellagra, largely a skin disorder. It is important as a coenzyme factor in many cell reactions related to energy and protein metabolism.

in DNA repair and calcium mobilization within the body.

Requirements

Factors such as age, growth, pregnancy and lactation, illness, tissue trauma, body size, and physical activity—all of which affect energy needs—influence niacin requirements. Because the body can make some of its niacin from the essential amino acid *tryptophan*, the total niacin requirement is stated in terms of *niacin equivalents* (NE) to account for both sources. Approximately 60 mg of tryptophan can yield 1 mg of niacin, so 60 mg of tryptophan is designated as 1 NE. The DRI guidelines include an RDA for adults aged 14 and older of 16 mg NE/day for men and 14 mg NE/day for women. The RDA is higher during pregnancy (18 mg NE/day) and lactation (17 mg NE/day). No RDA has been determined for infants up to 12 months old, but the AI is 2 to 4 mg NE/day. Niacin intake generally is adequate in the United States; the recently reported median intake of niacin from food is 28 mg NE/day for men and 18 mg NE/day for women.

Deficiency Disease

Symptoms of general niacin deficiency are weakness, poor appetite, indigestion, and various disorders of the skin and nervous system. Skin areas exposed to sunlight develop a dark, scaly dermatitis. Extended deficiency may result in CNS damage with resulting confusion, apathy, disorientation, and neuritis. Such signs of nervous system damage are seen in chronic alcoholism. The deficiency disease associated with niacin is pellagra, which is characterized by the four Ds: dermatitis, diarrhea, dementia, and death (Figure 7-4). When therapeutic doses of niacin are given, pellagra symptoms improve. Pellagra was common in the United States and parts of Europe in the early twentieth century in regions where corn (which is low in niacin) was the staple food. Between 1900 and 1940 alone, more than 100,000 people living in the southern United States were estimated to have died from pellagra.[7] Although pellagra has virtually disappeared in industrialized countries, it still occurs in India and parts of China and Africa.

Toxicity Symptoms

Excessive niacin intake can produce adverse physical effects, unlike high intakes of thiamin and riboflavin. The UL is 35 mg/day based on skin flushing caused by high intakes.[8] Although no evidence exists of adverse effects from consuming niacin that naturally occurs in foods,

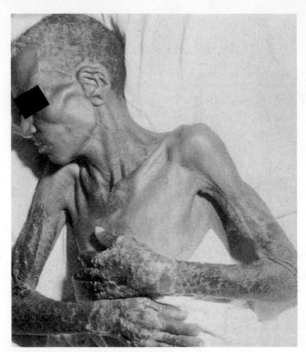

Figure 7-4 Pellagra results from a niacin deficiency. (Reprinted from McLaren DS: *A colour atlas and text of diet-related disorders*, ed 2, London, 1992, Mosby–Year Book.)

evidence does exist of excessive niacin consumption and adverse effects from nonprescription vitamin supplements and fortified foods. The primary reaction is a reddened flush on the skin of the face, arms, and chest accompanied by burning, tingling, and itching. This reaction also occurs in many patients therapeutically treated with niacin (see the Clinical Applications box, "Niacin as a Treatment for High Cholesterol").

Food Sources

Meat is a major source of niacin. Most niacin in diets in the United States is from meat, poultry, fish, or enriched grain products.. In addition, enriched and whole-grain breads and bread products and fortified ready-to-eat cereals have ample niacin. Other good sources of niacin include legumes (e.g., peanuts, dried beans, and peas). Fruits and vegetables are relatively poor sources of niacin. Table 7-9 gives the food sources of niacin.

Stability

Niacin is stable in acidic mediums and in heat but is lost in cooking water unless the water is retained and consumed, as in soup.

CLINICAL APPLICATIONS

NIACIN AS A TREATMENT FOR HIGH CHOLESTEROL

In addition to the many important functions of niacin, researchers have found that supplemental doses of 50 mg/day or greater may improve blood lipid profiles. At high doses, niacin decreases LDL cholesterol and triglyceride levels, both of which are linked with cardiovascular disease. In addition, pharmacologic doses of niacin improve HDL cholesterol, the good cholesterol. When niacin is used in this sense, it is functioning more as a drug than a vitamin and should be used only under medical supervision.

In understanding the potentially beneficial role of niacin at pharmacologic dosing, the potential side effects must be understood. The RDA for niacin in adult men and women is 16 mg/day and 14 mg/day, respectively. The UL for niacin is 35 mg/day. Therefore a long-term dose of 50+ mg/day inevitably has some side effects. Adverse effects from pharmacologic dosing are the same as the toxicity effects: flushing of the skin, tingling sensation in the extremities, nausea, and vomiting. Some individuals may even experience liver damage if long-term use is continued unsupervised for months or years at a time.

TABLE 7-9

FOOD SOURCES OF NIACIN

ITEM	QUANTITY	AMOUNT (mg NE)
Bread, Cereal, Rice, Pasta		
Bran flakes cereal	1 cup	6.7
Complete, Kellogg's cereal	1 cup	26.7
Mueslix Fine Grain, Kellogg's cereal	⅔ cup	5.5
Product 19, Kellogg's cereal	1 cup	20.0
Quaker Oat Life, Kellogg's cereal	1 cup	7.32
Total Whole Grain, General Mills cereal	1 cup	26.6
Wheaties, General Mills cereal	1 cup	9.9
Meat, Poultry, Fish, Dry Beans, Eggs, Nuts*		
Beef liver, fried	3 oz	14.9
Chicken, white meat, boneless, roasted	3 oz	10.6
Chicken liver, simmered	3 oz	9.4
Mackerel, baked	3 oz	5.8
Salmon, cooked, dry heat	3 oz	7.25
Sirloin steak, lean, broiled	3 oz	6.64
Swordfish, cooked, dry heat	3 oz	10.0

*The amino acid tryptophan can be converted to niacin. Therefore foods high in tryptophan also are significant sources of niacin.
Data from the USDA, Agricultural Research Service, Nutrient Data Laboratory: *USDA nutrient database for standard reference, release 20,* www.ars.usda.gov/ba/bhnrc/ndl.

VITAMIN B₆

Functions

Vitamin B_6 collectively refers to a group of six related compounds (pyridoxine, pyridoxal, pyridoxamine, and their respective activated phosphate forms). Two of the phosphorylated compounds are the coenzymes *pyridoxal 5'-phosphate* and *pyridoxamine 5'-phosphate*. The name pyridoxine comes from the *pyridine ring* in its structure. Vitamin B_6 has an essential role in protein metabolism and in many cell reactions involving amino acids. It is involved in neurotransmitter synthesis, and thus in brain and CNS activity. Unlike most water-soluble vitamins, vitamin B_6 is extensively stored in tissues throughout the body, particularly muscle. It participates in amino acid absorption, energy production, synthesis of the heme portion of hemoglobin, and niacin formation from tryptophan. Enzymes using vitamin B_6 coenzymes are also involved in carbohydrate and fat metabolism.

Requirements

Vitamin B_6 is involved in amino acid metabolism; therefore needs vary directly with protein intake. The DRI guidelines set the RDA for healthy men and women up to

pellagra deficiency disease caused by a lack of dietary niacin and an inadequate amount of protein containing the amino acid tryptophan, a precursor of niacin. Pellagra is characterized by skin lesions aggravated by sunlight and by GI, mucosal, neurologic, and mental symptoms. The four Ds often associated with pellagra are dermatitis, diarrhea, dementia, and death.

fortified vitamins and minerals added to foods after processing to improve nutritional value. Such vitamins and minerals may not have been originally present in the food or not in significant quantities. Examples include vitamin A and D fortified milk, calcium-fortified orange juice, and iodine-fortified salt.

pyridoxine the chemical name of vitamin B_6. In its activated phosphate form, B_2PO_4, pyridoxine functions as an important coenzyme factor in many reactions in cell metabolism related to amino acids, glucose, and fatty acids. Clinically pyridoxine deficiency produces a specific anemia and disturbances of the CNS.

age 50 years at 1.3 mg/day. For older adults the RDA is slightly higher at 1.7 mg/day for men and 1.5 mg/day for women. The RDA also is higher during pregnancy (1.9 mg/day) and lactation (2.0 mg/day). The AI for infants up to 12 months old is 0.1 to 0.3 mg/day.

Deficiency Disease

A vitamin B_6 deficiency is unlikely because much more is available in a typical diet than is required. A vitamin B_6 deficiency causes abnormal CNS function with hyperirritability, neuritis, and possible convulsions. Vitamin B_6 deficiency is one cause of microcytic hypochromic anemia because it is required for heme synthesis (part of the RBC protein hemoglobin).

Toxicity Symptoms

High vitamin B_6 intake from food does not result in adverse effects, but large supplemental doses can cause uncoordinated movement and nerve damage. Symptoms improve when supplemental overdosing is discontinued. The UL for adults is 100 mg/day based on studies relating vitamin B_6 dosage to nerve damage.[8]

Food Sources

Vitamin B_6 is widespread in foods. Good sources include grains, enriched cereals, liver and kidney, and other meats. Limited amounts are in milk, eggs, and vegetables. Table 7-10 lists food sources of vitamin B_6.

Stability

Vitamin B_6 is stable to heat but sensitive to light and alkalis.

FOLATE

Functions

The given name *folate* comes from the Latin word *folium*, meaning leaf, because it was originally discovered in dark-green, leafy vegetables. In nutrition the term *folate* refers loosely to a large class of molecules derived from folic acid (*pteroylglutamic acid*) found in plants and animals. Folate also may refer to a specific molecule, the *carboxylate anion* of folic acid. The most stable form of folate is folic acid, which is rarely found in food but is the form usually used in vitamin supplements and fortified food products. In the body folate is converted to and used as the coenzyme *tetrahydrofolate* (THF).

THF participates in DNA synthesis (with the enzyme thymidylate synthetase). THF is involved in the synthesis

TABLE 7-10

FOOD SOURCES OF VITAMIN B_6 (PYRIDOXINE)

ITEM	QUANTITY	AMOUNT (mg)
Bread, Cereal, Rice, Pasta		
Bran flakes cereal	1 cup	0.67
Complete, Kellogg's cereal	1 cup	2.71
Mueslix Fine Grain, Kellogg's cereal	⅔ cup	2.04
Quaker Oat Life, Kellogg's cereal	1 cup	0.73
Total Whole Grain, General Mills cereal	1 cup	2.66
Vegetables		
Potato, baked, with skin	1 medium (173 g)	0.54
Meat, Poultry, Fish, Dry Beans, Eggs, Nuts		
Beef liver, fried	3 oz	0.87
Chicken, white meat, boneless, roasted	3 oz	0.51
Chicken liver, simmered	3 oz	0.64
Sirloin steak, lean, broiled	3 oz	0.52

Data from the USDA, Agricultural Research Service, Nutrient Data Laboratory: *USDA nutrient database for standard reference, release 20,* www.ars.usda.gov/ba/bhnrc/ndl.

of the amino acid glycine, which in turn is required for heme synthesis and thus hemoglobin synthesis (with the enzyme, serine hydroxymethyltransferase).

THF participates in the reduction of *blood homocysteine concentration* and indirectly in *gene expression* (with the enzyme methionine synthase). Blood homocysteine concentrations are high in cardiovascular disease, though whether this contributes to or is merely an effect of cardiovascular disease has not been determined. Nonetheless, adequate dietary folate is important for hyperhomocystinemia prevention.

Requirements

The DRI standards give a general folate RDA for both men and women aged 14 and older of 400 mcg of dietary folate equivalent (DFE) per day. DFE is used because food folate is approximately 50% absorbed compared with approximately 100% of synthetic folic acid. One mcg of DFE equals 1 mcg of food folate, 0.5 mcg of folic acid taken on an empty stomach, or 0.6 mcg of folic acid taken with food. In recognition of folate's role in reducing *neural tube defects*, the DRIs include a new special recommendation that all women capable of becoming pregnant take 400 mcg/day of synthetic folic acid from fortified foods or supplements in addition to natural folate from a varied diet. During pregnancy, the RDA is increased to 600 mcg DFE/day to meet the elevated needs for fetal growth. A lactating mother needs 500 mcg DFE/day. For infants the observed AI is 65 mcg DFE/day during the first 6 months and 80 mcg DFE/day from ages 7 to 12 months. The DRI recommendations are aimed at providing adequate safety allowances that include specific population groups at risk for deficiency, such as pregnant women, adolescents, and older adults.

Deficiency Disease

A primary folate deficiency causes a special type of anemia, *megaloblastic anemia*; pregnant women are particularly susceptible because of increased fetal growth demands. Rapidly growing adolescents, especially those following fad diets and those who smoke, also are susceptible to diminished blood folate concentrations and thus anemia.

In recent years public awareness of and research into the role of adequate folate in reducing the serious public health problem of fetal *neural tube defects* has increased. Neural tube defects, such as spina bifida and anencephaly, are the most common birth defects involving the brain and spinal cord. Incidences vary in countries worldwide from 1 to 9 cases per 1000 births, with the highest rates occurring in Great Britain and Ireland. This defect occurs 21 to 28 days after conception, often before a woman realizes she is pregnant. Additional folic acid intake can significantly improve the folate status of women.[9] Thus increased folic acid intake is recommended for all women who are capable of becoming pregnant.

Toxicity Symptoms

No negative effects have been observed from the consumption of folate from foods. Some evidence, however, shows that excessive folic acid intake from supplements or fortified food products may be problematic. Such high intake of folic acid can mask biochemical indications of vitamin B_{12} deficiency. Prolonged B_{12} deficiency can result in permanent nerve damage; therefore the UL for adults of supplemental folic acid (not DFE) has been set at 1000 mcg/day.

Food Sources

Folate is widely distributed in foods (Table 7-11). Rich sources include green, leafy vegetables, orange juice, dried beans, and liver (Figure 7-5). Consuming a varied, healthy diet containing natural folate is important. Since January 1998, as part of an effort to reduce the occurrences of neural tube defects in infants born in the United States, the FDA has required all manufacturers of certain grain products (e.g., enriched white flour, white rice, corn grits,

TABLE 7-11

FOOD SOURCES OF FOLATE

ITEM	QUANTITY	AMOUNT (mcg)
Bread, Cereal, Rice, Pasta		
Bran flakes cereal	1 cup	133
Mueslix Fine Grain, Kellogg's cereal	⅔ cup	406
Product 19, Kellogg's cereal	1 cup	676
Quaker Oat Life, Kellogg's cereal	1 cup	553
Total Whole Grain, General Mills cereal	1 cup	532
Wheat Flakes, Kellogg's Complete cereal	1 cup	537
Wheaties, General Mills cereal	1 cup	336
Vegetables		
Collard greens, boiled	½ cup	88
Spinach, boiled	½ cup	131
Fruits		
Orange juice, fresh	1 cup, 8 oz	74
Meat, Poultry, Fish, Dry Beans, Eggs, Nuts		
Beef liver, fried	3 oz	221
Black beans, boiled	½ cup	128
Chicken liver, simmered	3 oz	491
Chickpeas (garbanzo beans)	½ cup	141
Kidney beans, boiled	½ cup	115

Data from the USDA, Agricultural Research Service, Nutrient Data Laboratory: *USDA nutrient database for standard reference, release 20,* www.ars.usda.gov/ba/bhnrc/ndl.

cornmeal, noodles, fortified breakfast cereals, bread, rolls, and buns) to fortify them with folic acid. This requirement has successfully reduced the incidence of hospitalization for neural tube defects in the United States by 21%.[10] The special DRI recommendation that women capable of becoming pregnant consume folic acid from supplements or fortified foods is one of only two current RDAs that specifically recommend consuming vitamin sources besides those available in a varied diet of natural foods. (The other supplementation recommendation concerns vitamin B_{12} intake in older persons.)

Stability

Folate is easily destroyed by heat and easily leaches into cooking water, especially when the food is submerged in the water. As much as 50% of food folate may be destroyed during food processing, storage, and preparation.

hyperhomocystinemia **high levels of homocysteine in the blood; a predictor of cardiovascular disease.**

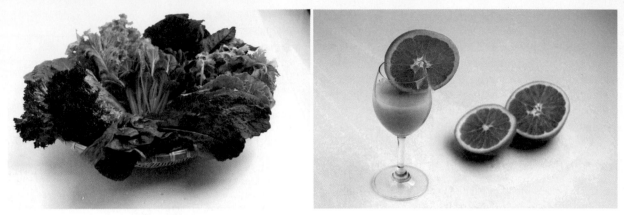

Figure 7-5 Foods high in folate. (Copyright JupiterImages Corporation.)

COBALAMIN (VITAMIN B$_{12}$)

Functions

Vitamin B$_{12}$ is the B vitamin designation of cobalamin. As with folate, vitamin B$_{12}$ may have two meanings, each depending on the context. Vitamin B$_{12}$ originally referred to the synthetic pharmaceutical molecule *cyanocobalamin*. In nutrition, it has become a term for all cobalamin derivatives, including the two biologically active coenzyme derivatives *methylcobalamin* and *deoxyadenosylcobalamin*. Vitamin B$_{12}$ is essential for neural myelin sheath synthesis. The name cobalamin was derived from cobalt, the trace mineral that is the single gray atom at the center of cobalamin's *corrin* ring.

Methylcobalamin is a coenzyme required for the catalytic activity of two of the same enzymes as THF, methionine synthase and serine hydroxymethyltransferase. Thus, like THF, methylcobalamin participates in (1) the reduction of *blood homocysteine concentration* and indirectly in *gene expression* and (2) the synthesis of the amino acid glycine, which in turn is required for heme synthesis and therefore hemoglobin synthesis.

Deoxyadenosylcobalamin is a coenzyme for the mitochondrial enzyme methylmalonyl-coenzyme A mutase, which is involved in the metabolism of fatty acids having an odd (as opposed to even) number of carbon atoms.

Requirements

Although it is essential, the amount of dietary vitamin B$_{12}$ needed for normal human metabolism is quite small, consisting of only a few micrograms per day. The usual mixed diet easily provides this much and more. The DRI guidelines list an RDA for men and women ages 19 years and older of 2.4 mcg/day. The RDA during pregnancy is 2.6 mcg/day and during lactation is 2.8 mcg/day. No RDA is given for infants up to 12 months old. An observed AI during the first year is 0.4 to 0.5 mcg/day. Evidence exists that 10% to 30% of people older than 50 years may poorly absorb vitamin B$_{12}$ from food sources. Therefore the DRIs include a special recommendation that both men and women older than 50 years meet their RDA with vitamin B$_{12}$–fortified foods or supplements.

Deficiency Disease

The search for the agent responsible for *pernicious anemia* led to the discovery of vitamin B$_{12}$. A component of the gastric digestive secretions called *intrinsic factor* is necessary for absorption of vitamin B$_{12}$ by intestinal cells (Figure 7-6). GI disorders that destroy the cells lining the stomach disrupt the secretion of intrinsic factor and hydrochloric acid, both of which are needed for vitamin B$_{12}$ absorption. If vitamin B$_{12}$ cannot be absorbed, pernicious anemia develops. In such cases vitamin B$_{12}$ must be hypodermically injected to bypass the absorption defect. Deficiency in elderly individuals is more commonly caused by a lack of intrinsic factor or hydrochloric acid than by a lack of dietary intake.

The only reported cases of dietary vitamin B$_{12}$ deficiency have been in some vegans (see Chapter 4), for whom cobalamin supplements are recommended to prevent such deficiency.[11] The general symptoms of dietary vitamin B$_{12}$ deficiency include sore mouth and tongue, amenorrhea, neuritis and, if not treated, irreversible nerve damage.

Toxicity Symptoms

Vitamin B$_{12}$ has not been shown to produce adverse effects in healthy individuals when intake from food or supplements exceeds body needs; therefore no UL has been established.

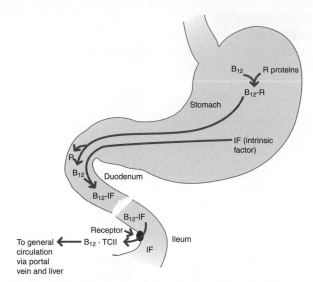

Figure 7-6 Digestion and absorption of vitamin B_{12}. (Reprinted from Mahan LK, Escott-Stump S: *Krause's food & nutrition therapy*, ed 12, Philadelphia, 2008, Saunders.)

Food Sources

Food sources of vitamin B_{12} are mostly animal products. It occurs bound to protein in foods. All dietary vitamin B_{12} originates from bacteria that inhabit the GI tracts of herbivorous animals. Human intestinal bacteria also synthesize B_{12}, but it is not bioavailable. The richest sources are beef and chicken liver, lean meat, clams, oysters, herring, and crab (Table 7-12).

Stability

Vitamin B_{12} is stable in ordinary cooking processes.

PANTOTHENIC ACID

Functions

The name **pantothenic acid** refers to its widespread functions in the body and its widespread availability in foods of all types. The name is based on the Greek word *pantothen*, which means from every side. Pantothenic acid is present in all living things and is essential to all forms of life. Pantothenic acid is part of *coenzyme A* (CoA), a carrier of *acetyl* moieties or larger *acyl* moieties. It is involved in (1) cellular metabolism and (2) protein acetylation and protein acylation.

Acetyl CoA is involved in energy extraction from the fuel molecules: glucose, fatty acids, and amino acids. CoA also is involved in *biosynthesis* of (1) sphingolipids (found in neural tissue); (2) leucine, arginine, and methionine (amino acids); (3) isoprenoid derivatives (e.g., choles-

TABLE 7-12

FOOD SOURCES OF VITAMIN B_{12} (COBALAMIN)

ITEM	QUANTITY	AMOUNT (mcg)
Meat, Poultry, Fish, Dry Beans, Eggs, Nuts		
Beef liver, fried	3 oz	71
Clams, cooked, moist heat	3 oz	84
Mussels, steamed	3 oz	20
Oysters, cooked, moist heat	3 oz	25

Data from the USDA, Agricultural Research Service, Nutrient Data Laboratory: *USDA nutrient database for standard reference, release 20, www.ars.usda.gov/ba/bhnrc/ndl.*

terol, steroid hormones, vitamin A, vitamin D); (4) δ-aminolevulinic acid, the precursor of the porphyrin rings in hemoglobin, the cytochromes of the electron transport chain, and the corrin ring of vitamin B_{12}; (5) the neurotransmitter acetylcholine; and (6) melatonin (a sleep inducer) derived from the neurotransmitter serotonin.

CoA involvement in protein acetylation and protein acylation is beyond the scope of this text.

Requirements

No specific RDA for pantothenic acid is given in the DRI guidelines. The usual intake range of the American diet is 4 to 7 mg/day. The DRI guidelines report an AI for persons aged 14 years and older of 5 mg/day. The AI is slightly higher during pregnancy (6 mg/day) and lactation (7 mg/day). For infants during the first year, the observed AI is 1.7 to 1.8 mg/day.

cobalamin the chemical name for the B-complex vitamin B_{12}; found mainly in animal protein food sources, so deficiencies mostly are seen among vegans. It is closely related to amino acid metabolism and formation of the heme portion of hemoglobin. Absence of its necessary digestion and absorption agents in the gastric secretions, HCl and intrinsic factor, leads to pernicious anemia and degenerative effects on the nervous system, which require monthly cobalamin injections, bypassing the intestinal absorption defect.

pantothenic acid a B-complex vitamin found widely distributed in nature and occurring throughout the body tissues. It is an essential constituent of the body's main activating agent, CoA. This special compound has extensive metabolic responsibility in activating a number of compounds in many tissues; it is a key energy metabolism substance in every cell.

Deficiency Disease

Given its widespread natural occurrence, deficiencies of pantothenic acid are unlikely. The only cases of deficiency are in individuals fed synthetic diets containing virtually no pantothenic acid.

Toxicity Symptoms

No observed adverse effects have been associated with pantothenic acid intake in people or animals. Therefore the DRI guidelines have not established an UL for this vitamin.

Food Sources

Pantothenic acid occurs as widely in foods as in body tissues. It is found in all animal and plant cells and is especially abundant in animal tissues, whole-grain cereals, and legumes (Table 7-13). Smaller amounts are found in milk, vegetables, and fruits.

Stability

Pantothenic acid is stable to acid and heat but is sensitive to alkalis.

BIOTIN
Functions

Biotin is a coenzyme for five *carboxylase* enzymes. Carboxylase enzymes transfer carbon dioxide (CO_2) moieties from one molecule to another in the following biotin enzymes:

1. Alpha-acetyl-CoA carboxylase, involved in fatty acid synthesis.
2. Beta-acetyl-CoA carboxylase, involved in inhibiting fatty acid breakdown within the hours after starch, sucrose, or fructose is consumed.
3. Pyruvate carboxylase, involved in synthesizing glucose during fasting (from glycerol or glucogenic amino acids) or during short bursts of energy (from lactic acid).
4. Methylcrotonyl-CoA carboxylase, involved in the degradation of the amino acid leucine.
5. Propionyl-CoA carboxylase, involved in the breakdown of the 3-carbon fatty acid propionic acid.

Requirements

The amount of biotin needed for metabolism is extremely small, measured in micrograms. The DRI guidelines do not establish an RDA for biotin. An AI has been set based on

TABLE 7-13

FOOD SOURCES OF PANTOTHENIC ACID

ITEM	QUANTITY	AMOUNT (mg)
Bread, Cereal, Rice, Pasta		
All-Bran cereal	1 cup	1.34
Mueslix Fine Grain, Kellogg's cereal	⅔ cup	2.53
Total Whole Grain, General Mills cereal	1 cup	13.3
Wheat Flakes, Kellogg's Complete cereal	1 cup	13.5
Vegetables		
Corn, yellow, boiled	½ cup	0.72
Potato, baked, with skin	1 medium (173 g)	0.65
Portabella mushroom, grilled	½ cup, pieces	0.97
Fruits		
Avocado, raw	¼ medium	0.70
Meat, Poultry, Fish, Dry Beans, Eggs, Nuts		
Beef liver, fried	3 oz	5.90
Chicken liver, simmered	3 oz	5.67
Egg, scrambled	1 large	0.61
Beef, ground, 70% fat, pan browned	3 oz	0.68
Mackerel, baked	3 oz	0.84
Milk, Dairy Products		
Milk, skim	8 fl oz	0.88
Yogurt, low fat	8 fl oz	1.45

Data from the USDA, Agricultural Research Service, Nutrient Data Laboratory: *USDA nutrient database for standard reference, release 20, www.ars.usda.gov/ba/bhnrc/ndl.*

intakes of healthy individuals. The AI for adults aged 18 years and older is 30 mcg/day. For infants during the first 12 months, the observed AI is 5 to 6 mcg/day. The AI during pregnancy also is 30 mcg/day; during lactation it is 35 mcg/day. The intestinal cells also absorb biotin synthesized by the bacteria that normally inhabit the intestine.

Deficiency Disease

Because the potency of biotin is great, despite the tiny microgram quantities present in the body, no known natural deficiency occurs. Biotin is bound by avidin, a protein in uncooked egg whites. Thus consuming raw eggs inhibits biotin absorption. Other induced deficiencies have occurred in patients who received long-term total parenteral nutrition without biotin supplementation. Occasional cases of inborn errors of biotin metabolism also have been discovered.

Toxicity Symptoms

No toxicity effects or other adverse effects from consumption of biotin by people or animals are known. No data currently support setting an UL for biotin.

Food Sources

Biotin is widely distributed in natural foods but is not equally absorbed from all of them. For example, the biotin in corn and soy meal is completely bioavailable (i.e., able to be digested and absorbed by the body). However, almost none of the biotin in wheat is bioavailable. The best food sources of biotin are liver, egg yolk, soy flour, cereals (except bound forms in wheat), meats, tomatoes, and yeast.

Stability

Biotin is a stable vitamin, but it is water soluble. A summary of these water-soluble vitamins is given in Table 7-14.

CHOLINE
Functions

Choline is a water-soluble nutrient associated with the B-complex vitamins. The DRI guidelines include choline but state that human data are insufficient to determine whether choline is essential in the human diet.[8] The human body may be able to synthesize an adequate supply of choline in some stages of life. As a nutrient, choline is important in maintaining the structural integrity of cell membranes as a component of the phospholipid *lecithin* (phosphatidyl choline). Choline is also a component of the neurotransmitter *acetylcholine,* which is involved in involuntary functions, voluntary movement, and long-term memory storage, among other things.

Requirements

Insufficient data exist on which to base an RDA for choline. Therefore the DRI guidelines give an AI of 550 mg/day for men older than 14 years and 425 mg/day for women older than 18 years. During pregnancy, the AI is 450 mg/day; during lactation it is 550 mg/day because an ample amount of choline is secreted into human milk. For infants the observed AI is 125 to 150 mg/day during the first year of life.

Deficiency Disease

A deficiency of choline from food sources can cause liver damage. In clinical settings patients subsisting on total parenteral nutrition solutions that did not include choline also developed liver damage, which was corrected with choline supplementation.

Toxicity Symptoms

Choline has a low toxicity. Adverse effects have only been observed in cases in which choline intake was several times greater than the normal intake from food. Very high doses of supplemental choline have caused lowered blood pressure, fishy body odor, sweating, excessive salivation, and reduced growth rate. The UL for adults is 3.5 g/day.

Food Sources

Choline is found naturally in a wide variety of foods. Milk, eggs, liver, and peanuts are especially rich sources of choline. A normal, varied diet can deliver 1 g of choline per day, and typical dietary intake for adults in the United States has been estimated to be 700 to 1000 mg/day.

Stability

Choline is a stable nutrient and is water soluble, as are all the B-complex vitamins.

SECTION 3 — PHYTOCHEMICALS

Besides the vitamins discussed so far in this chapter, other bioactive molecules with health benefits, called *phytochemicals,* come from the plants we eat. Phytochemicals are organic molecules like the vitamins; however, no specific phytochemical deficiency diseases have been characterized or defined to date. The term *phytochemical* comes from the Greek word *phyton,* meaning plant. Phytochemicals act as either antioxidants (like vitamins E and C) or hormones (like vitamins A and D) in the originating plant or in the person eating it. Some researchers believe

TABLE 7-14

SUMMARY OF VITAMIN C AND THE B-COMPLEX VITAMINS

VITAMIN	FUNCTIONS	RECOMMENDED INTAKE (ADULTS)	DEFICIENCY	UL AND TOXICITY	SOURCES
Vitamin C (ascorbic acid)	Antioxidant; collagen synthesis; helps prepare iron for absorption and release to tissues for red blood cell formation, metabolism	RDA: Men: 90 mg Women: 75 mg Smokers: additional 35 mg/day	Scurvy (deficiency disease); sore gums; hemorrhages, especially around bones and joints; anemia; tendency to bruise easily; impaired wound healing and tissue formation; weakened bones; impaired wound healing	2000 mg; diarrhea	Citrus fruits, kiwi, tomatoes, melons, strawberries, dark leafy vegetables, chili peppers, cabbage, broccoli, chard, green and red peppers, potatoes
Thiamin (vitamin B₁)	Normal growth; coenzyme in carbohydrate metabolism; normal function of heart, nerves, and muscle	RDA: Men: 1.2 mg Women 1.1 mg	Beriberi (deficiency disease); GI: loss of appetite, gastric distress, indigestion, deficient hydrochloric acid; CNS: fatigue, nerve damage, paralysis; CV: heart failure, edema of legs	Not set; unknown	Pork, beef, liver, whole or enriched grains, legumes, wheat germ
Riboflavin	Normal growth and energy; coenzyme in protein and energy metabolism	RDA: Men: 1.3 mg Women: 1.1 mg	Ariboflavinosis; wound aggravation; cracks at corners of mouth, swollen, red tongue; eye irritation; skin eruptions	Not set; unknown	Milk, meats, enriched cereals, green vegetables
Niacin (vitamin B₃, nicotinamide, nicotinic acid)	Coenzyme in energy production; normal growth, health of skin	RDA: Men: 16 mg NE Women: 14 mg NE	Pellagra (deficiency disease); weakness; loss of appetite; diarrhea; scaly dermatitis; neuritis; confusion	35 mg; skin flushing	Wheat germ, legumes, meats, poultry, seafood
Vitamin B₆ (pyridoxine)	Coenzyme in amino acid metabolism: protein synthesis, heme formation, brain activity; carrier for amino acid absorption	RDA: 19-50 yr: 1.3 mg Men >51: 1.7 mg Women >51: 1.5 mg	Anemia; hyperirritability; convulsions; neuritis	100 mg; nerve damage	Liver, green leafy vegetables, legumes, yeast, orange juice (fortified)
Folate (folic acid, folacin)	Coenzyme in DNA and RNA synthesis; amino acid metabolism; RBC maturation	RDA: 400 mcg DFE	Megaloblastic anemia (large, immature RBCs); poor growth; neural tube defects	1000 mcg; mask Vitamin B₁₂ deficiency	Liver, lean meats, fish, seafood
Cobalamin (vitamin B₁₂)	Coenzyme in synthesis of heme for hemoglobin; myelin sheath formation to protect nerves	RDA: 2.4 mcg	Pernicious anemia; poor nerve function	Not set; unknown	Meats, eggs, milk, whole grains, legumes, vegetables
Pantothenic acid	Formation of CoA; fat, cholesterol, protein, and heme formation	AI: 5 mg	Unlikely because of widespread distribution in most foods	Not set; unknown	Liver, egg yolk, soy flour (except bound form in wheat), nuts
Biotin	CoA partner; synthesis of fatty acids, amino acids, purines	AI: 30 mcg	Natural deficiency unknown	Not set; unknown	

CV, Cardiovascular.

that fruits and vegetables provide more than 25,000 phytochemicals, many of which have yet to be identified.

FUNCTION

Multiple studies are exploring the possible link between increased phytochemical intake and reduced risk of developing chronic diseases. What prompted researchers toward investigating phytochemicals were differences between those eating whole fruits and vegetables versus those simply taking vitamin or mineral supplements. Those obtaining their vitamins and minerals from a diet rich in whole grains, fruits, vegetables, legumes, nuts, and seeds benefited far more than those eating mostly refined foods and taking vitamin and mineral supplements.

The beneficial effects of phytochemicals are thought to result from synergistic actions of multiple constituents as opposed to the actions of isolated compounds.[12] Diets high in phytochemicals protect against cardiovascular disease, counteract inflammatory compounds, help prevent cancer, and increase antioxidant status.[13]

RECOMMENDED INTAKE

The National Cancer Institute (NCI) expanded on their *Fruits and Veggies More Matters* program by highlighting the phytochemical content of fruits and vegetables with color in their "Sample the Spectrum" program. Phytochemicals give fruits and vegetables their specific colors and make distinguishing the sources of different phytochemicals easy. The NCI and American Institute for Cancer Research recommend consuming a combined total of five to nine servings of fruits and vegetables daily. At *www.fruitsandveggiesmatter.gov*, the NCI provides recommendations for the number of cups of fruits and vegetables a person should consume daily based on age, gender, and activity level. NCI states that 1 cup of raw or cooked vegetables or vegetable juice or 2 cups of raw, leafy greens are equivalent to 1 cup from the vegetable group. 1 cup of fruit or 100% fruit juice, or half a cup of dried fruit is equivalent to 1 cup from the fruit group.[14] This recom-

mendation is based on the finding that consuming 400 to 600 g/day of fruits and vegetables reduces the risk of developing some forms of cancer. Current reports from the Economic Research Service of the USDA show that only 20% of individuals older than 2 years met the Pyramid's fruit intake recommendations, and only 36% met the Pyramid's vegetable intake recommendations on a daily basis.[15]

FOOD SOURCES

Foods derived from animals and those that have been processed and refined are virtually devoid of phytochemicals. Phytochemicals are found in whole and unrefined foods such as vegetables, fruits, legumes, nuts, seeds, whole grains, and some oils such as olive oil.

The following is a list of seven typical fruit and vegetable colors along with the specific phytochemical (e.g., lycopene) or phytochemical class (e.g., flavonoids) that these fruits and vegetables may contain. The specified phytochemical or phytochemical class is present in fruits or vegetables of other colors, but color is one prominent indicator that a significant quantity of the specified phytochemical or phytochemical class may be present. One specific exception worth noting is flavonoids. Although orange-yellow foods are high sources, other significant sources include purple grapes, black tea, olives, onions, celery, green tea, oregano, and whole wheat—none of which are orange-yellow.

- *Red* foods provide lycopene
- *Yellow-green* foods provide zeaxanthin
- *Red-purple* foods provide anthocyanin
- *Orange* foods provide beta-carotene
- *Orange-yellow* foods provide flavonoids
- *Green* foods provide glucosinolate
- *White-green* foods provide allyl sulfides

By consuming one fruit or vegetable from each of these seven color categories daily, individuals get a variety of phytochemicals. Thousands of other phytochemicals also are widely distributed in fruits, vegetables, grains, soybeans, legumes, and nuts.

SECTION 4 VITAMIN SUPPLEMENTATION

ONGOING DEBATE

The debate between vitamin supplement users and producers and those who believe vitamin supplements have no place in health maintenance continues, fueled by

staunch advocates of both positions. On one hand, conservative health workers may dismiss anyone who suggests a need for vitamin supplements. On the other hand, self-proclaimed and noncredentialed nutrition "experts" may push megadoses of everything from vitamin A to zinc.

Some people believe that all persons should meet the precise DRI recommendations for all essential nutrients. But, as the DRI guidelines emphasize, an RDA is *by definition* a guideline that accommodates 97.5% of a healthy population group over time—not individual needs, which vary widely. Wise practitioners individualize recommendations by using a careful, objective assessment of that person. Not all the ideas expressed in the ongoing debate over vitamin supplementation are valid or have a scientific basis. However, supplementation is and will remain a contested topic because multivitamin and mineral supplements are commonly used throughout the United States.

BIOCHEMICAL INDIVIDUALITY

The term *biochemical individuality* means that each individual, although anatomically, physiologically, and biochemically similar in many aspects, has a unique body. Even within a given individual biochemical changes are associated with the normal life cycle and disease processes. The concept of biochemical individuality cannot be overlooked when individual nutrition needs are assessed because it is influenced by factors such as age, sex, personal habits, work environment, living situation, and health status.

Life Cycle Needs

Vitamin needs fluctuate with age and situation throughout the life cycle.

Pregnancy and Lactation

The DRI guidelines explicitly establish separate recommendations for women during pregnancy and lactation that take into account the increased nutrient requirements. To prevent birth defects early in pregnancy, the DRI committee recommends that women capable of becoming pregnant take folic acid (folate) from supplements in addition to the folate in their diet. Women may find meeting the increased nutrient needs of pregnancy difficult by diet alone because of nutrient bioavailability, tolerances, food preferences, or other factors that can marginalize their diet (i.e., effectively decrease the nutrients their diet provides). Supplements then may become a viable way of ensuring adequate intake to meet the increased nutrient demands.

Infancy

The American Academy of Pediatrics recommends a vitamin K supplement be given at birth to prevent a rare but fatal bleeding disorder called *hemorrhagic disease of the newborn*. Vitamin D is the only other supplement that infants may need if they do not receive sufficient sunlight exposure to produce enough endogenous vitamin D (see Chapter 11).

Children and Adolescents

Rapid growth spurts during childhood and adolescence use more nutrients as a whole, including all vitamins, than slow or nongrowth periods during adulthood. Full growth potential, specifically height, is hindered if inadequate supplies of vitamins are not consumed during these times of rapid growth.

Aging

The aging process may increase the need for some vitamins because of decreased food intake and less-efficient nutrient absorption, storage, and usage (see Chapter 12). Marginal deficiencies of vitamins D and E, ascorbic acid, thiamin, riboflavin, pyridoxine, and cobalamin are common in the geriatric population, even in some individuals taking supplements.

Lifestyle

Personal lifestyle choices and habits also influence individual needs for nutrient supplementation.

Oral Contraceptive Use

Women using oral contraceptives have lower serum concentrations of several B vitamins, including pyridoxine, niacin, and folate, as well as vitamin C. Supplements may be necessary to maintain optimal vitamin status, especially when nutrient intake is marginal. However, poor dietary habits should be addressed before relying on supplements.

Restricted Diets

Persons who habitually follow fad diets may find meeting many of the nutrient intake standards difficult, particularly if their meals provide fewer than 1200 kcal/day. Very restrictive diets are not recommended because they may cause multiple nutrient deficiencies. A wise weight-reduction program should meet all nutrient needs. Persons on strict vegetarian diets need supplements of vitamin B_{12} (cobalamin) because its only natural food sources are of animal origin.

Exercise Programs

Intensive exercise programs (e.g., training for a marathon or endurance bike race) may increase a woman's riboflavin requirement. Combining a restrictive diet with an intensive exercise program increases riboflavin requirement even more and may necessitate a B-complex supplement, especially in women who poorly tolerate milk, the major food source of riboflavin.

Smoking

Smoking cigarettes, especially among women during their childbearing years, adversely affects health in many ways, including reducing the body's vitamin C pool by as much as 30%. If dietary vitamin C intake is marginal and the smoker continues to smoke, a small vitamin C supplement (approximately 100 mg/day) may partially compensate for the smoke-induced vitamin C loss.

Alcohol

Chronic or abusive use of alcohol can interfere with the absorption of B-complex vitamins, especially thiamin, folate, and vitamin B_6. Again, multivitamin supplements rich in B vitamins may partially mitigate the effects of alcohol. But decreased alcohol use must accompany this nutrition therapy to rectify the alcohol-induced deficiency.

Caffeine

In large quantities (four to six cups of coffee a day), caffeine's diuretic effect flushes water-soluble vitamins out of the kidneys faster than they are reabsorbed. Small supplements of B vitamins and ascorbic acid may mitigate caffeine's diuretic effect, but reduced caffeine intake is recommended.

Disease

In states of disease, malnutrition, debilitation, or hypermetabolic demand, each patient requires careful nutrition assessment. In cases of deficiency, nutrition support, including therapeutic supplementation as indicated, is part of the total medical therapy. Increased nutrient needs are particularly evident in cases of acute and chronic illness, especially in the elderly. A dietitian plans dietary and supplemental therapy to meet the patient's clinical requirements.[16,17]

MEGADOSES

Persons taking vitamin megadoses are using them as drugs. At high pharmacologic concentrations, vitamins no longer operate strictly as nutritional agents. Nutrients and drugs (1) participate in or improve physiologic conditions or illnesses, (2) prevent diseases, or (3) relieve symptoms. Many people are, however, ignorant of the implications of the similarities between drugs and vitamins. Most people realize that too much of any drug can be harmful or even fatal and take care to avoid overdosing. However, too many people do not apply this same

logic to nutrients and only realize the dangers of vitamin megadoses when they experience toxic side effects.

Toxic Effects

The liver can store large amounts of fat-soluble vitamins, especially vitamin A. Therefore the potential toxicity of fat-soluble vitamin megadoses, including liver and brain damage in extreme cases, is well known. Many people take megadoses of water-soluble vitamins, believing them to be safe because they are not stored in the body. However, the toxic effects of megadoses of two water-soluble vitamins have been observed. Vitamin B_6 megadoses of up to 5 g/day as long-term therapy for premenstrual syndrome have caused ataxia and, in some cases, severe nerve damage. Ascorbic acid megadoses (more than 2 g/day) have caused GI pain, raised the risk for kidney stone formation, and reduced the bactericidal action of leukocytes (white blood cells). Meanwhile, scientific research has not confirmed that vitamin C megadoses cure colds, lower blood cholesterol concentration, or lower cancer rates—the most common reasons people say they take megadoses.

Artificially Induced Deficiencies

Megadoses of one vitamin can produce toxic effects and lead to a secondary deficiency of another nutrient. Hyperphysiologic levels of one vitamin may increase the need for other nutrients with which it works in the body, effectively inducing a deficiency. Deficiencies also can occur when a person suddenly stops overdosing, known as a rebound effect. For example, infants born to mothers who took ascorbic acid megadoses during pregnancy have developed scurvy after birth when their high doses of ascorbic acid were cut off.

SUPPLEMENTATION PRINCIPLES

The following basic principles may help guide nutrient supplementation decisions:

- *Read the labels carefully.* As labels on dietary supplements become compliant with the Nutrition Labeling and Education Act of 1990, which standardized and defined label terminology on food products, consumers should more easily be able to distinguish between well-founded and unfounded health claims. Consumers can make better informed decisions knowing that a product's ingredients, toxicity levels, potential side effects, and health claims are based on significant evidence.
- *Vitamins, like drugs, can be harmful in large amounts.* The only time larger vitamin doses may be helpful

is when severe deficiency exists or nutrient absorption or metabolism is inefficient.

- *Professionally determined individual needs govern specific supplement usage.* Each person's need should be the basis for supplementing nutrients. This prevents excessive intake, which may have a cumulative effect over time.

- *All nutrients work together to promote good health.* Consuming large amounts of one vitamin often induces deficiencies of other vitamins or nutrients.

- *Food is the best source of nutrients.* Most foods are the best "package deals" in nutrition. Foods provide a wide variety of nutrients in every bite compared with the dozen or so found in a vitamin bottle. And, by itself, a vitamin can do nothing. It is catalytic, so it must have a substrate (e.g., carbohydrate, protein, fat, and their metabolites) on which to work. With careful selection of a wide variety of foods and with good storage techniques, good meal planning, and good preparation techniques, most people can obtain ample amounts of essential nutrients from their diet (see the Cultural Considerations box, "The American Diet"). Furthermore, the evidence still overwhelmingly supports foods as the superior vehicles for delivering nutrients to the body, not supplements.[18,19]

- *Evaluate the information.* The following Web sites offer more detailed information about the safety and efficacy of vitamin supplements and other nutritional supplements: the National Institute of Health Office of Dietary Supplements *(http:// dietary-supplements.info.nih.gov)* and the National Center for Complementary and Alternative Medicine *(http://nccam.nih.gov).*

FUNCTIONAL FOODS

Functional foods include any food or food ingredient that may provide a health benefit beyond its basic nutritional value. Such foods are also referred to as nutraceuticals or designer foods. The position of the American Dietetic Association is that such whole foods, having been fortified, enriched, or enhanced in some way, could be beneficial when regularly consumed as part of a varied diet.[20] The regulation of functional foods is complicated by the fact that they fall under different areas of federal jurisdiction because they include conventional foods, food additives, dietary supplements, medical foods, or foods for special dietary use. One approach given current federal bureaucratic jurisdictions would be to regulate all functional foods based on the FDA-approved health claims criteria that statutorily define the relation between a food and a disease or other health-related condition.

Recommendations for functional food intake have not been established because scientific evidence on which to base such recommendations is insufficient. However, over the past decade much research effort has been focused on determining the clinical efficacy of functional foods. Once efficacy is clearly substantiated and reliable assessments for accurately quantitating active constituents in foods are in place, expert committees will work to establish recommendations for intake. Until recommendations are established, daily intake of foods from all food groups, including functional foods, is the best way to meet macronutrient and micronutrient needs.

CULTURAL CONSIDERATIONS

THE AMERICAN DIET

According to the Economic Research Service of the U.S. Department of Agriculture, Americans are still not meeting the recommended intake for any of the food groups. The six food groups, according to the MyPyramid guidelines, are grains, vegetables, fruit, dairy or dairy substitute, meat or meat substitute, and oils.

By consuming the recommended servings from each group, vitamin and mineral needs should be met. In looking at all individuals ages 2 years and older, 27% of the population consumes the recommended grain servings per day, 36% reach the vegetable recommendations, a mere 20% of the population eats at least two servings of fruit per day, and only 20% and 29% meet the dairy and meat servings per day, respectively. When looking at the statistics by gender, females are no more likely to consume within the recommendations than men at any point throughout the life cycle.*

On evaluation of how close each of the subgroups comes to meeting the recommended servings consumed in each food group, women ages 60 years and older do considerably well for each food group, with the exception of dairy products. Of this subgroup, inadequate consumption of dairy foods, the best source of dietary calcium, is the most prominent problem.

How do you measure up? What about your family and friends? Prevention of deficiency, or any diseases associated with nutrient deficiency, is always better than treatment.

*USDA/Economic Research Service: *Diet and health: food consumption and nutrient intake tables,* www.ers.usda.gov/briefing/dietandhealth/data/foods/ table4.htm, accessed July 2007.

SUMMARY

Vitamins are organic, noncaloric food substances necessary in minute amounts for specific metabolic tasks. The body cannot make vitamins, but a balanced diet usually supplies sufficient vitamins. In individually assessed situations, however, vitamin supplements may be indicated.

The fat-soluble vitamins are A, D, E, and K. They mainly affect body structures (bones, rhodopsin, cell membrane phospholipids, blood clotting proteins). The water-soluble vitamins are vitamin C (ascorbic acid), the eight B-complex vitamins (thiamin, riboflavin, niacin, vitamin B_6, folate, vitamin B_{12}, pantothenic acid, and biotin), and choline. Their major metabolic tasks relate to their roles in coenzyme factors, except for vitamin C, which is a biologic reducing agent that quenches free radicals and aids in collagen synthesis. Little toxicity has been associated with these water-soluble vitamins because excesses are excreted in the urine.

Phytochemicals are compounds found in whole and unrefined foods derived from plants. A diet high in phytochemicals from a variety of sources is associated with a decreased risk of developing chronic diseases.

Vitamin supplementation continues to be a controversial subject in today's society. Megadoses of water-soluble or fat-soluble vitamins can have detrimental effects. The possibility of toxicity is higher for fat-soluble vitamins because the body stores them. Vitamin toxicity is no longer rare because of the prevalence of taking dietary supplements. All water-soluble vitamins, especially vitamin C, are easily oxidized, so care must be taken to minimize exposure of food surfaces to air or other oxidizers during storage and preparation. With few exceptions, all nutrients in foods are more bioavailable and beneficial to the body than nutrients in supplements.

Functional foods are whole foods with added nutrients, such as vitamins, minerals, herbs, fiber, protein, or essential fatty acids that are thought to have beneficial health effects. Functional foods are recognized by the American Dietetic Association as potentially beneficial when consumed in a varied diet.

CRITICAL THINKING QUESTIONS

1. What is a vitamin? Name them and distinguish between fat-soluble and water-soluble vitamins.
2. Describe three general functions of vitamins and give examples of each.
3. How would you advise a friend who was taking self-prescribed vitamin supplements? Give reasons and examples to support your answer.
4. Describe the effects of three vitamins that some persons take in large amounts. What are the risks involved in such megadoses?
5. Describe four situations in which vitamin supplements should be used. Give reasons and examples in each case.
6. What are phytochemicals? How can you incorporate them into your diet?

CHAPTER CHALLENGE QUESTIONS

True-False
Write the correct statement for each statement that is false.
1. *True or False:* A coenzyme acts alone to control a number of different types of reactions.
2. *True or False:* Carotene is preformed vitamin A found in animal food sources.
3. *True or False:* Exposure to sunlight produces vitamin D from cholesterol in the skin.
4. *True or False:* Extra vitamin C is stored in the liver to meet tissue infection demands.
5. *True or False:* Vitamin D and sufficient calcium and phosphorus can prevent rickets.
6. *True or False:* Good sources of vitamin K are found in green, leafy vegetables such as kale and spinach.
7. *True or False:* Dietary supplements are a necessary part of healthy living for all people.

Multiple Choice

1. Vitamin A is fat soluble and formed from carotene in plant foods or consumed as the fully formed vitamin in animal foods. Which of the following supplies the greatest amount of this vitamin?

  a. Oranges
  b. Collard greens
  c. Ground beef
  d. Tomatoes

2. If you wanted to increase the vitamin C content of your diet, which of the following foods would you choose in larger amounts?

  a. Liver, other organ meats, and seafood
  b. Potatoes, enriched cereals, and fortified margarine
  c. Green peppers, tomatoes, and oranges
  d. Milk, cheese, and eggs

3. Which of the following statements is true about the sources of vitamin K?

  a. Vitamin K is found in a wide variety of foods, so no deficiency can occur.
  b. Vitamin K is easily absorbed without assistance, so we absorb all of the nutrient we consume into our circulatory system.
  c. Vitamin K is rarely found in foods, so a natural deficiency can occur.
  d. Most of our vitamin K for metabolic needs is produced by intestinal bacteria.

4. A food with added nutrients through fortification or enrichment is considered a

  a. dietary supplement.
  b. functional food.
  c. phytochemical.
  d. none of the above.

5. One of the primary functions of folate is as a(n)

  a. antioxidant.
  b. coenzyme in protein and energy metabolism.
  c. CoA partner.
  d. coenzyme in DNA and RNA synthesis.

6. Beriberi is the deficiency disorder associated with which vitamin?

  a. Thiamin
  b. Riboflavin
  c. Niacin
  d. Pantothenic acid

7. The formation of prothrombin for normal blood clotting purposes is a primary function of which fat-soluble vitamin?

  a. Vitamin A
  b. Vitamin D
  c. Vitamin E
  d. Vitamin K

---

evolve Please refer to the Students' Resource section of this text's Evolve Web site for additional study resources.

REFERENCES

1. Penniston KL, Tanumihardjo SA: Vitamin A in dietary supplements and fortified foods: too much of a good thing? *J Am Diet Assoc* 103:1185, 2003.

2. Holick MF: High prevalence of vitamin D inadequacy and implications for health, *Mayo Clin Proc* 81(3):353, 2006.

3. Food and Nutrition Board, Institute of Medicine: *Dietary reference intakes for calcium, phosphorous, magnesium, vitamin D, and fluoride,* Washington, DC, 1998, National Academies Press.

4. Food and Nutrition Board, Institute of Medicine: *Dietary reference intakes for vitamin C, vitamin E, selenium, and carotenoids,* Washington, DC, 2000, National Academies Press.

5. Bourre JM: Effects of nutrients (in food) on the structure and function of the nervous system: update on dietary requirements for brain. Part 1: micronutrients, *J Nutr Health Aging* 10(5):377, 2006.

6. Food and Nutrition Board, Institute of Medicine: *Dietary reference intakes for vitamin A, vitamin K, arsenic, boron, chromium, copper, iodine, iron, manganese, molybdenum, nickel, silicon, vanadium, and zinc,* Washington, DC, 2002, National Academies Press.

7. Marks HM: Epidemiologists explain pellagra: gender, race, and political economy in the work of Edgar Sydenstricker, *J Hist Med Allied Sci* 58(1):34, 2003.

8. Food and Nutrition Board, Institute of Medicine: *Dietary reference intakes for thiamin, riboflavin, niacin, vitamin B_6, folate, vitamin B_{12}, pantothenic acid, biotin, and choline,* Washington, DC, 1999, National Academies Press.

9. Dietrich M and others: The effect of folate fortification of cereal-grain products on blood folate status, dietary folate intake, and dietary folate sources among adult non-supplement users in the United States, *J Am Coll Nutr* 24(4):266, 2005.

10. Robbins JM and others: Hospitalizations of newborns with folate-sensitive birth defects before and after fortification of foods with folic acid, *Pediatrics* 118(3):906, 2006.

11. Mangels AR and others: Position of the American Dietetic Association and Dietitians of Canada: vegetarian diets, *J Am Diet Assoc* 103(6):748, 2003.

12. Liu RH: Potential synergy of phytochemicals in cancer prevention: mechanism of action, *J Nutr* 134:3479S, 2004.

13. Heber D: Vegetables, fruits and phytoestrogens in the prevention of diseases, *J Postgrad Med* 50:145, 2004.

14. Centers for Disease Control and Prevention: *What counts as a cup? www.fruitsandveggiesmatter.gov/what/index.html,* accessed July 2007.

15. USDA/Economic Research Service: *Diet and Health: food consumption and nutrient intake tables, www.ers.usda.gov/ briefing/dietandhealth/data/foods/table4.htm*, accessed June 2007.

16. Gariballa S and others: A randomized, double-blind, placebo-controlled trial of nutritional supplementation during acute illness, *Am J Med* 119(8):693, 2006.

17. Lesourd B: Nutritional factors and immunological ageing, *Proc Nutr Soc* 65(3):319, 2006.

18. Lichtenstein AH and Russell RM: Essential nutrients: food or supplements? *JAMA* 294(3):351, 2005.

19. American Dietetic Association: Position of the American Dietetic Association: fortification and nutritional supplements, *J Am Diet Assoc* 105:1300, 2005.

20. Hasler CM and others: Position of the American Dietetic Association: functional foods, *J Am Diet Assoc* 104(5):814, 2004.

FURTHER READING AND RESOURCES

Spina Bifida Association of America: *www.sbaa.org*
    An excellent site for more information on the role of folic acid and neural tube defects.

The following organizations provide current information and guidelines on dietary recommendations for nutrient consumption.

Centers for Disease Control and Prevention, Fruit and Veggies Matter: *www.fruitsandveggiesmatter.gov*

Center for Science in the Public Interest: *www.cspinet.org*

Centers for Disease Control and Prevention: Use of dietary supplements containing folic acid among women of childbearing age—United States, 2005, *MMWR* Sep 30;54(38):955, 2005.

CHAPTER 8

Minerals

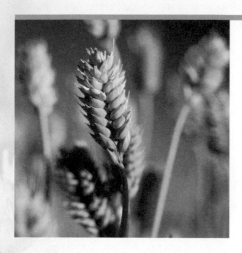

KEY CONCEPTS

- The human body requires a variety of minerals in different amounts to perform numerous metabolic tasks.
- A mixed diet of varied foods and adequate energy value is the best source of the minerals necessary for health.
- Of the total amount of minerals a person consumes, only a relatively limited amount is available to the body.

Over earth's history, shifting oceans and plate tectonics have deposited minerals throughout the earth's crust. These minerals move from rocks to soil to plants to animals and people. Not surprisingly, the mineral content of the human body is quite similar to that of the earth's crust.

In nutrition we focus only on mineral elements, single atoms that are simple when compared with vitamins, which are large, complex, organic compounds. However, minerals perform a wide variety of metabolic tasks essential to human life.

This chapter looks at minerals and shows how they differ from vitamins in the variety of their tasks and in the amounts, ranging from relatively large to exceedingly small, necessary to do those tasks.

NATURE OF BODY MINERALS

Most living matter is composed of four elements—hydrogen, carbon, nitrogen, and oxygen—the building blocks of life. The minerals necessary in human nutrition are elements widely distributed in nature. Of the 117 known elements, 25 are known to be essential to human life. These 25 elements, in varying amounts, perform a variety of metabolic functions.

Classes of Body Minerals

As described in Chapter 7, all vitamins are necessary in minute amounts to do their jobs. However, minerals occur in varying amounts in the body. For example, a relatively large amount (approximately 2%) of the total body weight is calcium, most of which is in the bones. An adult who weighs 150 lb has approximately 3 lb of calcium in the body. Iron, on the other hand, is found in much smaller quantities. The same adult who weighs 150 lb has only approximately 0.11 oz of iron in the body. In both cases the amount of each mineral is specific to its task.

The varying amounts of individual minerals in the body are the basis for classification into two main groups.

Major Minerals

Major describes the amount of a mineral in the body, not its relative importance to human nutrition. Major minerals have a recommended intake of more than 100 mg/day. The seven major minerals are calcium, phosphorus, sodium, potassium, magnesium, chloride, and sulfur. Because the body cannot make any minerals, all minerals must be consumed in the foods we eat.

Trace Minerals

The remaining 18 elements make up the group of trace minerals. These minerals are no less important to human nutrition than are the major minerals; only smaller amounts of them in the body. Trace minerals have a recommended intake of less than 100 mg/day. Trace minerals are essential for their specific vital tasks. Box 8-1 provides a helpful summary of the minerals in human nutrition.

Functions of Minerals

These simple, single elements perform a wide variety of metabolic tasks in the body. They are involved in processes of building tissue and activating, regulating, transmitting, and controlling metabolic processes. For exam-

ple, sodium and potassium are key players in water balance. Calcium and phosphorus are required for osteoclasts to build bone. Iron is critical to the oxygen carrier hemoglobin. Cobalt is at the active site of vitamin B_{12}. Thyroid peroxidase in thyroid cells uses iodine to make thyroid hormone, which in turn regulates the overall rate of body metabolism. Minerals are essential and are involved in most of the body's metabolic processes.

Mineral Metabolism

Mineral metabolism usually is controlled at either the point of intestinal absorption or the points of tissue uptake.

Digestion

Minerals are absorbed and used in the body in their *ionic* (i.e., carrying a positive or negative electric charge) forms. Unlike carbohydrates, proteins, and fat, minerals do not require a great deal of mechanical or chemical digestion before absorption.

Absorption

The following general factors influence how much of a mineral is absorbed into the body from the GI tract. (1) *Food form*—minerals from animal sources usually are more readily absorbed than those from plant sources. (2) *Body need*—more is absorbed if the body is deficient than if the body has enough. (3) *Tissue health*—if the absorbing intestinal surface is affected by disease, its absorptive capacity is greatly diminished.

The absorptive method for each mineral depends on its physical properties. Some minerals require active transport to be absorbed, whereas others enter the intestinal cells by diffusion. Compounds found in foods also may affect the absorptive efficiency of the intestinal cells. For example, the presence of fiber, phytate, or oxalate (found in a variety of whole grains, fruits, and vegetables) can bind certain minerals in the GI tract, inhibiting or limiting their absorption.

BOX 8-1

MAJOR MINERALS AND TRACE MINERALS IN HUMAN NUTRITION

Major Minerals*
Calcium (Ca)
Phosphorus (P)
Sodium (Na)
Potassium (K)
Magnesium (Mg)
Chloride (Cl)
Sulfur (S)

Trace Minerals
Essential†
Iron (Fe)
Iodine (I)
Zinc (Zn)
Selenium (Se)
Fluoride (Fl)
Copper (Cu)
Manganese (Mn)
Chromium (Cr)
Molybdenum (Mo)
Cobalt (Co)
Boron (B)
Vanadium (V)
Nickel (Ni)
Essentiality Unclear
Silicon (Si)
Tin (Sn)
Cadmium (Cd)
Arsenic (As)
Aluminum (Al)

*Required intake more than 100 mg/day.
†Required intake less than 100 mg/day.

---

element a single type of atom. A total of 117 elements have been identified, of which 94 occur naturally on earth. Elements cannot be broken down into smaller substances.

major minerals the group of minerals required by the body in amounts of more than 100 mg/day. The seven major minerals in the body are calcium, phosphorus, sodium, potassium, magnesium, chloride, and sulfur.

trace minerals the group of elements required by the body in smaller amounts of less than 100 mg/day.

Transport

Minerals enter portal blood circulation and travel throughout the body bound to plasma proteins or mineral-specific transport proteins.

Tissue Uptake

Uptake of some minerals into their target tissue is controlled by hormones, and excess minerals are excreted into the urine. For example, thyroid-stimulating hormone (TSH) controls the uptake of iodine from blood by the thyroid gland depending on the amount it needs to make thyroid hormone *(thyroxine)*. When more thyroxine is needed, TSH stimulates the thyroid gland to take up iodine and the kidneys to excrete less iodine into the urine. When thyroxine concentration is normal, less TSH is released from the anterior pituitary gland, resulting in less iodine uptake by the thyroid gland and more excretion of iodine into the urine by the kidneys.

Occurrence in the Body

Body minerals are found in several forms in body tissues related to their functions. The two basic forms in which minerals occur in the body are as (1) *free ions* in body fluids (e.g., sodium in tissue fluids, which influence water balance) and (2) *covalently bound*—minerals may be combined with other minerals (e.g., calcium and phosphorus in hydroxyapatite) or with organic substances (e.g., iron bound to heme and globin to form the organic compound hemoglobin).

MAJOR MINERALS

Calcium

Functions

Most of the U.S. food and nutrition surveys, such as those conducted regularly by the USDA and the National Center for Health Statistics, indicate that calcium is one of the minerals least likely to be consumed in amounts equal to the DRI in a typical American diet.[1] On average, men and boys consume approximately 25% more calcium than do women and girls because men and boys usually eat larger amounts of food. The intestinal absorption of dietary calcium depends on (1) the food form (e.g., plant forms are sometimes bound to oxalate or phytate and are not readily available) and (2) the interaction of three hormones (vitamin D, parathyroid hormone [PTH], and calcitonin [from the thyroid gland]) that directly control calcium's intestinal absorption and utilization, along with indirect control by the estrogens (sex hormones produced primarily by the ovaries). Once absorbed, calcium has four basic functions in the body.

Bone and Tooth Formation. Most of the body's calcium (more than 99%) is found in bones and teeth. Approximately 1% to 2% of normal adult body weight is calcium. When hydroxyapatite is removed from bone, the remaining tissue is a collagen matrix. If dietary calcium is insufficient during childhood growth, initial formation of the fetal skeleton, or the rapid growth of long bones during adolescence, the construction of healthy bones is hindered. Teeth are calcified before they erupt from the gums; thus insufficient dietary calcium later in life does not affect tooth structure as it does bone structure.

Blood Clotting. Calcium is essential for the formation of fibrin, the protein matrix of a blood clot.

Muscle and Nerve Action. Calcium ions are required for muscle contraction and the release of neurotransmitters from neuron synapses.

Metabolic Reactions. Calcium is necessary for many general metabolic functions in the body. Such functions include intestinal absorption of vitamin B_{12}, activation of the fat-splitting enzyme pancreatic lipase, and secretion of insulin by the beta cells of the pancreas, where insulin is synthesized. Calcium also interacts with cell membrane proteins that govern cell membrane permeability to nutrients.

Requirements

As part of the DRIs project, the scientific panel on calcium reviewed all current research and concluded that not enough conclusive scientific data exist regarding calcium requirements through life to establish new specific RDAs. Although calcium is an area of active research, the DRI panel reports that the following are still areas of concern: uncertainties about the nutritional significance of some research data, a lack of firm agreement between observed survey information and experimental laboratory data, and a lack of long-term longitudinal data connecting calcium intake with long-term bone density loss. Therefore the DRI panel set AI levels for calcium instead of a new RDA. The AI amounts should provide sufficient calcium nourishment for the body while recognizing that a lower intake may be adequate for many individuals.

The DRI guidelines give AI levels by age group. For all infants up to 6 months old, the AI level is 210 mg/day; for infants 7 through 12 months of age, the AI is 270 mg/day. Calcium needs increase during the growth years of childhood and adolescence, during which the AIs are as follows: 1 to 3 years, 500 mg/day; 4 to 8 years, 800 mg/day; and 9 to 18 years, 1300 mg/day. For both men and women aged 19 to 50 years, the AI for desirable calcium retention is 1000 mg/day, with a rise to 1200 mg/day for those older than 50 years. During pregnancy and lactation, the AI is currently set equal to the level for the general age group, as follows: 1300 mg/day for up to age 18 years and 1000 mg/day for ages 19 years and older.

Deficiency States

Various bone deformities may occur if insufficient dietary calcium is available during growth years. The deficiency disease *rickets* is related to inadequate vitamin D to support sufficient intestinal absorption of calcium. A decrease of blood calcium concentration, relative to blood phosphorus concentration, results in *tetany,* a condition characterized by muscle spasms. The most common calcium-related clinical issue today is osteoporosis. Osteoporosis is an abnormal decrease in bone density, especially in postmenopausal women, characterized by reduced bone mass, increased bone fragility, and a greater risk for developing bone fractures (Figure 8-1). Such bone fractures are becoming more common in elderly men as well. Each year in the United States more than 1.5 million bone fractures, including 300,000 hip fractures, are linked to osteoporosis.[2]

Osteoporosis is not a primary calcium deficiency disease as such but results from a combination of factors that create chronic calcium deficiency. These factors include (1) inadequate calcium intake, (2) poor intestinal calcium absorption related to deviations in the amounts of hormones that control calcium absorption and metabolism, and (3) a lack of physical activity, which stimulates muscle insertion into bones and determines bone strength, shape, and mass. Insufficient physical activity contributes to the development of osteoporosis, and immobility after injury or disease can cause serious bone loss. Bone is a dynamic tissue, with both new bone formation and resorption constantly occurring. A portion of the skeleton is reabsorbed and replaced with new bone each year; this bone remodeling can affect up to 50% of

total bone mass per year in young children and approximately 5% in adults. Unfortunately, bone resorption often exceeds bone formation in postmenopausal women and in aging men. The interaction of factors in osteoporosis that result in bone calcium resorption outpacing bone calcium deposition are not fully understood. Increased calcium intake alone, be it dietary calcium or supplemental calcium, does not prevent osteoporosis in susceptible adults or successfully treat diagnosed cases of osteoporosis. Therapies that reduce bone loss in osteoporosis include combinations of the various factors involved in building bones: dietary calcium, the active hormonal form of vitamin D, estrogens, and weight-bearing physical activity (see the Cultural Considerations box, "Bone Health in Gender and Ethnic Groups").

Toxicity Symptoms

Toxicity of calcium from food sources is highly unlikely. However, a UL for calcium has been set at 2500 mg/day because of negative effects of excessive calcium supplementation over time. Too much calcium intake is associated with an increased risk of developing kidney stones and decreased intestinal absorption of several other minerals. Calcium can interfere with intestinal absorption of iron, zinc, magnesium, and phosphorus, thus increasing the requirement for these minerals.

Food Sources

Milk and milk products are the most important sources of readily available calcium (Figure 8-2). Milk used in cooking (e.g., in soups, sauces, or puddings) or in milk products such as yogurt, cheese, and ice cream are excellent sources of dietary calcium. Calcium-fortified tofu, fruit juices, and other food products (e.g., cereals, cereal bars) are equally high in bioavailable calcium. Several plants also provide a natural source of this important mineral. Calcium in low-oxalate greens such as Chinese cabbage, broccoli, collards, kale, and turnip greens is well absorbed and can be an important source of calcium for vegetarians. Oxalic acid is a compound found in some plants such as spinach, rhubarb, Swiss chard, beet greens,

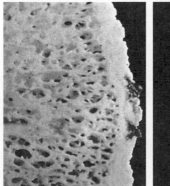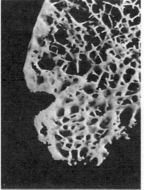

Figure 8-1 Osteoporosis. Normal bone *(left)* versus osteoporotic bone *(right)*. (Reprinted from Mahan LK, Escott-Stump S: *Krause's food & nutrition therapy,* ed 12, Philadelphia, 2008, Saunders.)

thyroid-stimulating hormone (TSH) an anterior pituitary hormone that regulates the activity of the thyroid gland; also known as thyrotropin.

osteoporosis abnormal thinning of the bone, producing a porous, fragile, latticelike bone tissue of enlarged spaces prone to fracture or deformity.

resorption the destruction, loss, or dissolution of a tissue or part of a tissue by biochemical activity, such as the loss of bone or of tooth dentin.

CULTURAL CONSIDERATIONS

BONE HEALTH IN GENDER AND ETHNIC GROUPS

The most recent Surgeon General's report on osteoporosis states that approximately 10 million Americans older than 50 years have osteoporosis and an additional 34 million are at risk.*

Osteoporosis often is thought of as a problem exclusively for older Caucasian women. However, this debilitating bone disease is becoming more and more prevalent in other gender and ethnic groups as well. The National Institute of Health estimates that 6% of all men older than 50 years will have a hip fracture and 5% will have a vertebral fracture as a result of osteoporosis.† The disparity between genders is prevalent, with the experts stating that one out of every two women older than 50 years will have an osteoporosis-related fracture in their lifetime. Among postmenopausal American women, the incidence of osteoporosis is 21% for Caucasians and Asians, 16% for Hispanics, and 10% for African Americans.‡ The reasons for these observed differences by race are unclear; however, ethnicity, gender, and age are all well accepted as important factors in calculating risk for osteoporosis, the most common form of bone disease.

Many factors are involved in bone mineral density and the relative risk for developing fragile bones, including body weight, physical activity, hormonal influences, and dietary intakes of several vitamins and minerals, not just calcium. Nutrition affects bone health by providing the materials needed for tissue deposition, maintenance, and repair. Overall bone strength is determined by bone mineral density and the collagen matrix formation. Collagen, a structural protein, accounts for more than 20% of the dry weight of total bone mass and 90% of the organic bone matrix. Collagen degradation is associated with osteoporosis. As such, the vitamins and minerals critical for strong collagen and bone matrix also are integral to overall bone health. A delicate balance of several nutrients is important for healthy bone building, such as protein; vitamins C, D, and K; calcium; phosphorus; copper; magnesium; manganese; potassium; and zinc.

Osteoporosis is currently costing Americans more than $10 billion annually in direct medical costs. Coupled with the general trends of an aging population, this bone disease is a serious national concern. Because bone mineral density reaches a peak mass by the average age of 30 years, the years before this are vital for developing healthy bones and preventing the onset of osteoporosis. Establishing peak bone mass ensures a greater reserve of bone mineral and collagen so that as age-associated degradation ensues, effects are essentially postponed or abated altogether. A healthy diet, following MyPyramid guidelines, should provide all essential nutrients and is imperative during the first 3 decades of life to establish healthy bones.

*U.S. Department of Health and Human Services: *Bone health and osteoporosis: a report of the surgeon general*, Rockville, MD, 2004, U.S. Department of Health and Human Services.
†National Institute of Health, Department of Health and Human Services: *Osteoporosis in men, www.niams.nih.gov/Health_Info/Bone/Osteoporosis/men.asp*, accessed July 2007.
‡Food and Nutrition Board, Institute of Medicine: *Dietary reference intakes for calcium, phosphorus, magnesium, vitamin D, and fluoride*, Washington, DC, 1998, National Academies Press.

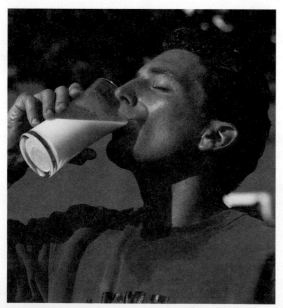

Figure 8-2 Milk is the major food source of calcium. (Copyright PhotoDisc.)

and certain other vegetables and nuts that forms an insoluble salt with calcium (calcium oxalate), interfering with intestinal absorption of calcium. Secondary sources of calcium include grains, legumes, and nuts. Phytate, another plant compound in grains such as wheat, can bind with calcium and interfere with its intestinal absorption. Table 8-1 lists food sources of calcium.

In addition to food sources, calcium intake from supplements is widespread. Surveys show that almost 6% of women in the United States specifically take calcium supplements, whereas 22% of the total population takes a multivitamin and mineral supplement that contains some calcium.[3] The bioavailability of calcium from supplements depends on the dose and whether it is taken with a meal. Calcium is best absorbed in doses of 500 mg or less and when taken with food rather than on an empty stomach (see the For Further Focus box, "Calcium from Food or Supplements: Which Is Better?").

TABLE 8-1

FOOD SOURCES OF CALCIUM

ITEM	QUANTITY	AMOUNT (mg)
Bread, Cereal, Rice, Pasta		
Corn muffin, commercially prepared	1 medium (113 g)	84
Cream of Wheat cereal, cooked	¾ cup	86
English muffin, plain, enriched	1 muffin (57 g)	93
Oatmeal, instant, fortified, prepared with water	¾ cup	98
Whole-grain cereal, Total	¾ cup	1000
Vegetables		
Collards, boiled	¾ cup	140
Spinach, boiled*	¾ cup	122
Fruits		
Orange juice, fortified with calcium and vitamin D	8 fl oz	351
Meat, Poultry, Fish, Dry Beans, Eggs, Nuts		
Salmon, pink, canned, drained solids with bone	3 oz	235
Sardines, canned in oil, solids with bone	3 oz	325
Soybeans, boiled	½ cup	88
Tofu, raw, firm, prepared with calcium sulfate	½ cup	861
Milk, Dairy Products, or Substitute		
Cheese, mozzarella, part skim milk	1 oz	222
Milk, skim	8 fl oz	301
Milk, whole	8 fl oz	276
Soy milk	8 fl oz	93
Soy milk, calcium fortified	8 fl oz	368
Tofu yogurt	8 fl oz	309
Yogurt, plain, low fat	8 fl oz	448

*Low bioavailability.
Data from the USDA, Agricultural Research Service, Nutrient Data Laboratory: *USDA nutrient database for standard reference, release 20, www.ars. usda.gov/ba/bhnrc/ndl.*

Phosphorus

Functions

The phosphorus atom in nature is most commonly found combined with four oxygen atoms to form the phosphate molecule. Phosphorus and calcium (in the form of hydroxyapatite) are used in bone formation. In addition, phosphorus functions in the following metabolic processes.

Bone and Tooth Formation. Calcification of bones and teeth depends on deposition of hydroxyapatite $[Ca_{10}(PO_4)_6(OH)_2]$ by osteoblast in bone's collagen matrix. The ratio of calcium to phosphorus in typical bone is approximately 1.5:1 by weight.

Energy Metabolism. Phosphorus, in the form of phosphate (PO_4^{3-}), is necessary for the controlled oxidation of carbohydrate, fat, and protein to release the energy in their covalent bonds (e.g., as a component of thiamin pyrophosphate) and capture energy for use in the body as a component of adenosine triphosphate.

Phosphate also is involved in protein construction (e.g., as a component of RNA), cell function (e.g., as a component of cell enzymes activated by phosphorylation), and genetic inheritance (as a component of DNA).

Acid-Base Balance. Phosphate is an important chemical buffer that helps maintain pH homeostasis of body fluids. Normal physiologic pH is 7.35.

Requirements

The typical American diet contains enough phosphorus to meet body needs. Surveys indicate that the mean daily phosphorus intake in the United States is approximately 1300 mg/day.[1] The AI level during the first 6 months of life is 100 mg/day, and from ages 7 to 12 months is 275 mg/day. Healthy breastfed infants receive adequate phosphorus. For children, the RDA varies with the stage of growth. For ages 1 to 3 years the RDA is 460 mg/day; for ages 4 to 8 years it is 500 mg/day. For ages 9 to 18 years, a period of rapid bone growth, the RDA is 1250 mg/day. The established RDAs in the DRI guidelines for both men

FOR FURTHER FOCUS

CALCIUM FROM FOOD OR SUPPLEMENTS: WHICH IS BETTER?

If only we could take a supplement to meet all our nutrition needs, then we would not have to bother with eating healthy! Unfortunately that is the type of thinking that fuels the continued search for the "magic pill." Good health is not a simple matter, and our bodies are no simple machines. They require lots of nutrients, which must be provided by the diet, to function properly. One of the major minerals needed by our body is calcium. According to the U.S. Department of Health and Human Services, relatively few Americans meet the AI for calcium through their diet. Men consume more dietary sources of calcium throughout their life span than do women but still fall short of meeting 100% of the AI.* Only 6% of women, who are at higher risk for developing osteoporosis (after age 60), meet the *Dietary Guidelines* for calcium consumption.† The following represents the average calcium intake for females by age group*:

- Younger than 6 years = 785 mg/day
- 6-11 years = 860 mg/day
- 12-19 years = 793 mg/day
- 20-39 years = 797 mg/day
- 40-59 years = 744 mg/day
- 60 years and older = 660 mg/day

A variety of factors influence our dietary intake of calcium. Over the past decade, Americans' food choices have changed in ways that directly affect calcium-rich food consumption. For instance, Americans (1) are replacing milk with soft drinks; (2) are eating out more often at restaurants, where the overall calcium density is lower than meals at home; (3) seem to be perpetually dieting (and dairy products are often one of the first foods to go); and (4) are largely unaware of the healthy link between calcium-rich foods and health.

Health organizations, such as the National Institute of Health, American Dietetic Association, American Medical Association, and National Academy of Sciences, agree that the best source of calcium is from dairy products. The primary reason for this is because, unlike calcium supplements, calcium-rich foods supply the body with other beneficial nutrients as well, including protein; vitamins A, B_{12}, and D (if fortified); magnesium; potassium; riboflavin; niacin; and phosphorus. Some nondairy foods naturally contain calcium, such as salmon with bones, dried beans, turnip greens, mustard greens, kale, tofu, and broccoli. Most individuals find meeting their recommended calcium intake exclusively from nondairy foods difficult because the relative amount of calcium in these foods is significantly less than in dairy products. For example, half a cup of chopped kale has 47 mg calcium, whereas 8 oz of skim milk contains 302 mg. Also, many vegetables contain phytates and oxalates that form insoluble complexes with calcium and decrease their bioavailability to the body.

Calcium-fortified foods are excellent sources of calcium, especially for vegans and individuals who are lactose intolerant. However, as with calcium supplements, the benefits of consuming dairy products rich in many vitamins and minerals may be lost in fortified foods such as orange juice or cereal.

Keller and colleagues analyzed the consumer cost and bioavailability of calcium from all sources. They found Total cereal was the least expensive food source of calcium, with fluid milk and calcium-fortified orange juice the next least expensive.‡ Calcium from supplements may be found in a variety of forms, including calcium carbonate, citrate, phosphate, lactate, and gluconate. The amount of calcium absorbed into the body from these different sources varies considerably. Of the calcium supplements, calcium carbonate, in a chewable form (e.g., Tums) or supplement, provides the least expensive and most bioavailable source of calcium, with a 34% absorption fraction.‡

The best way to improve overall diet is to consume a variety of foods high in calcium, preferably from dairy sources. However, calcium-fortified foods and supplements may be necessary for some individuals to meet their recommended intake of calcium. An individual consuming calcium supplements should be aware of potential side effects such as constipation and drug-nutrient interactions. Also, calcium is best absorbed in doses of 500 mg or less at a single time.

Regardless of where your calcium comes from, take a moment to consider the overall value of your diet and assess if improvements are warranted.

*Ervin RB and others: *Dietary intake selected minerals for the United States population: 1999-2000. Advance data from vital and health statistics; no 341*, Hyattsville, MD, 2004, National Center for Health Statistics.
†USDA/Economic Research Service: *Diet and health: food consumption and nutrient intake tables, www.ers.usda.gov/Briefing/DietAndHealth/data/nutrients/table3.htm*, accessed July 2007.
‡Keller JL and others: The consumer cost of calcium from food and supplements, *J Am Diet Assoc* 102(11):1669, 2002.

and women aged 19 years and older is 700 mg/day, with no additional need for women who are pregnant or lactating.

Deficiency States

Phosphate (the dietary form of phosphorus) is widely distributed in foods; thus a deficiency is rare. A person must be completely deprived of food for an extended period to develop a dietary phosphorus deficiency. The only evidence of deficiency has been among persons who for weeks or months habitually consumed large amounts of antacids containing aluminum hydroxide. The aluminum (Al^{3+}) binds with phosphate, making it unavailable for intestinal absorption. Phosphorus deficiency results in bone loss and is characterized by weakness, loss of appetite, fatigue, and pain.

Toxicity Symptoms

A toxicity of phosphorus from food intake is equally rare. However, if phosphorus intake is significantly higher than calcium intake for a long period, bone resorption may occur. The DRI guidelines list the UL for phosphorus at 4 g/day for persons aged 9 to 70 years.

Food Sources

Phosphorus is part of all living tissue and is found in all animal and plant cells; therefore phosphorus is sufficient in the natural food supply of virtually all animals. High-protein foods are particularly rich in phosphorus, so milk and milk products, meat, fish, and eggs are the primary sources of phosphorus in the average diet. The bioavail-ability of phosphorus from plant seeds (e.g., cereal grains, beans, peas, other legumes, and nuts) is much lower because they contain *phytic acid,* which is a storage form of phosphorus in seeds that human beings cannot directly digest. However, intestinal bacteria can make up to 50% of phosphorus from phytic acid available for intestinal absorption. Table 8-2 outlines some main food sources of phosphorus.

Sodium

Functions

Sodium is one of the most plentiful minerals in the body. Approximately 120 g (4.2 oz) is present in an adult body. The main function of sodium is maintenance of

TABLE 8-2

FOOD SOURCES OF PHOSPHORUS

ITEM	QUANTITY	AMOUNT (mg)
Vegetables		
Potato, baked, with skin	1 medium (173 g)	121
Meat, Poultry, Fish, Dry Beans, Eggs, Nuts		
Almonds, roasted	1 oz (22 nuts)	139
Bacon, fried	3 medium slices	128
Beef, ground, 70% lean, pan browned	3 oz	172
Beef liver, pan fried	3 oz	412
Beef top round, lean, broiled	3oz	173
Chicken, dark meat, roasted, without skin	3 oz	152
Chicken, white meat, roasted, without skin	3 oz	184
Chickpeas (garbanzo beans), boiled	½ cup	138
Clams, cooked, moist heat	3 oz	287
Cod, cooked, dry heat	3 oz	117
Crab, Alaskan king, cooked, moist heat	3 oz	238
Halibut, cooked, dry heat	3 oz	242
Ham, sliced, regular (11% fat)	3 oz	130
Lentils, boiled	½ cup	178
Lobster, cooked, moist heat	3 oz	157
Pinto beans, boiled	½ cup	126
Sirloin steak, lean, broiled	3 oz	184
Soybeans, boiled	½ cup	211
Tofu, raw, firm, prepared with calcium sulfate	½ cup	152
Trout, rainbow, cooked, dry heat	3 oz	226
Tuna, light, canned in water, drained solids	3 oz	139
Milk, Dairy Products		
Cheese, cheddar	1 oz	145
Cheese, mozzarella, part skim milk	1 oz	131
Cottage cheese, 1% milk fat	½ cup	151
Milk, 1% fat	8 fl oz	232
Yogurt, plain, low fat	8 fl oz	353

The food group composed of bread, cereal, rice, and pasta is not an important source of phosphorus. Whole-grain products are higher in phosphorus than are refined grain products, but the phosphorus, in the form of phytate, is not bioavailable to human beings.
Data from the USDA, Agricultural Research Service, Nutrient Data Laboratory: *USDA nutrient database for standard reference, release 20, www.ars. usda.gov/ba/bhnrc/ndl.*

body/water balance, which is further discussed in Chapter 9. Sodium also has important tasks in muscle action and nutrient absorption.

Water Balance. Ionized sodium concentration is the major influence on the volume of body water *outside* the cells (extracellular) (Figure 8-3). Variation in sodium concentration largely controls the movement of water across biologic membranes by *osmosis*. Sodium also is an integral part of the digestive juices secreted into the GI tract, most of which are reabsorbed by the intestinal cells.

Muscle Action. Sodium and potassium ions are necessary for the normal response of stimulated neurons, the transmission of nerve impulses to muscles, and the contraction of muscle fibers.

Nutrient Absorption. Sodium-dependent glucose transporters, an integral part of intestinal cells, allow the passage of glucose and galactose from the intestinal lumen into intestinal cells.

Requirements

The body is able to function on various amounts of dietary sodium through mechanisms designed to conserve or excrete the mineral as needed. For that reason, no specific RDA exists for sodium. Individual sodium needs vary greatly depending on growth stage, sweat loss, and medical conditions (e.g., diarrhea, vomiting). The DRI

standards include an AI for the three major electrolytes needed for maintaining body fluid balance: sodium, chloride, and potassium. A sodium intake of 1.5 g/day should be adequate for healthy persons who are not excessively losing sodium through extended exercise and sweating. Adults ages 50 to 70 years have a slightly reduced AI (1.3 g/day) corresponding to decreased energy intake. The AI for individuals older than 71 years is 1.2 g/day.[4]

Deficiency States

Sodium deficiencies are rare because the body's need is low and intake typically is high. An exception is during heavy sweating, such as by those engaged in heavy labor or strenuous physical exercise in a hot environment for an extended period (greater than 2 hours). Such persons may need fluids with electrolytes to replace heavy sodium losses. Drinking too much plain water during extended strenuous exercise can dilute blood sodium concentration and exacerbate sodium deficiency complications (see Chapter 16). Sodium deficiency can result in acid-base imbalance and muscle cramping.

Commercial sports drinks, which replace sodium, glucose, and fluid, may be useful for athletes participating in endurance events. Most persons do not require these beverages for nonendurance activities (see Chapters 9 and 16).

Toxicity Symptoms

The sodium content of the average American diet, which contains a high amount of processed foods, usually far exceeds the recommended intake range. The National Health and Nutrition Examination Survey of 1999 to 2000 revealed that men consume an average of 3877 mg/day and women average 2896 mg/day of sodium.[1] Excessive sodium intake has been linked to hypertension in individuals who are salt sensitive (approximately 25% of hypertensive patients). However, for most people with healthy kidneys and adequate water intake, the kidneys excrete excess sodium in the urine. Acute excessive intake of sodium chloride (table salt) causes the accumulation of sodium in the extracellular spaces. This sodium can pull water out of cells into the extracellular space by osmosis, causing edema. The current DRIs set the UL for sodium intake at 2.3 g/day but state that some individuals may have a much lower tolerance.[4]

Food Sources

Common table salt, as used in cooking, seasoning, and processing foods, is the main dietary source of sodium. Sodium occurs naturally in foods and generally is most prevalent in foods of animal origin. Enough sodium is found in natural food sources to meet the body's needs. When food manufacturers add salt and other sodium

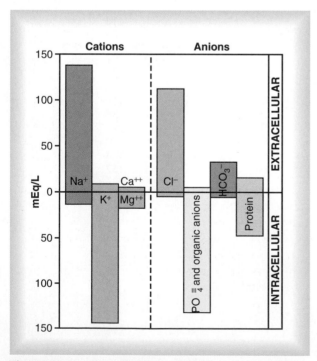

Figure 8-3 Ionic composition of the major body fluid compartments. (Reprinted from Guyton AC, Hall JE: *Textbook of medical physiology*, ed 12, Philadelphia, 2006, Saunders.)

compounds to processed foods, sodium intake dramatically increases. For example, cured ham has approximately 20 times more sodium than does raw pork. Natural, unprocessed food sources of sodium include animal products such as milk, meat, and eggs and vegetables such as carrots, beets, leafy greens, and celery (see Appendix C for the sodium and potassium content of foods and Appendix D for salt-free seasoning guides).

Potassium

Functions

The adult body contains approximately 270 g (9.5 oz) of potassium—nearly twice the amount of sodium. Potassium is involved with sodium in the maintenance of body/water balance and also has many other metabolic functions.

Water Balance. Potassium is the major electrolyte *inside* cells (intracellular). Its osmotic effect holds water inside cells and counterbalances the osmotic effect of sodium, which draws water out of cells into the extracellular fluid (see Figure 8-3).

Metabolic Reactions. Potassium plays a role in the conversion of blood glucose to stored glycogen, the synthesis of muscle protein, and energy production.

Muscle Action. Potassium ions also play a role in nerve-impulse transmission to stimulate muscle action. Along with magnesium and sodium, potassium acts as a muscle relaxant opposing the stimulating effect of calcium, which causes muscle contraction. The heart muscle is sensitive to potassium levels; therefore blood potassium concentration is regulated within narrow tolerances.

Insulin Release. Potassium is necessary for the release of insulin from pancreatic β cells in response to rising blood glucose concentrations.

Blood Pressure. Sodium is one of the main dietary factors associated with hypertension; however, hypertension may be more related to the *sodium/potassium ratio* (a molar ratio as opposed to a mass ratio) than to the amount of dietary sodium alone. A potassium intake equal to sodium intake may prevent the development of hypertension; such is the basis for the Dietary Approaches to Stop Hypertension (DASH) diet (see *www.nhlbi.nih.gov/health/public/heart* for more information).

Requirements

As with sodium, the present DRI guidelines do not have an RDA for potassium, although potassium is essential in the diet. The AI of potassium is approximately 4.7 g/day for all adults.[4] The National Research Council recommends an increase in potassium intake through increased consumption of fruits and vegetables. The average American diet provides significantly less potassium than the established AI, with a median daily intake of 2 to 3 g/day.[1] The *Dietary Guidelines for Americans* committee identified potassium as a key nutrient lacking in the typical American diet, which lead to the recommendation of increasing fruits, vegetables, and dairy servings.[5]

Deficiency States

Symptoms of potassium deficiency are well defined but seldom related to inadequate dietary intake. Potassium deficiency is more likely to develop during clinical situations such as prolonged vomiting or diarrhea, use of diuretics, severe malnutrition, or surgery. Potassium deficiency also is a concern while a person is using antihypertension drugs, particularly diuretics that cause urinary potassium loss. Those who simultaneously take diuretics and excessive doses of drugs that replace potassium also may experience imbalanced blood potassium concentrations. Characteristic symptoms of potassium deficiency include heart muscle weakness with possible cardiac arrest, respiratory muscle weakness with breathing difficulties, poor intestinal muscle tone with resulting bloating, and overall muscle weakness.

Toxicity Symptoms

As with sodium, the kidneys normally excrete excess potassium so that toxicity does not occur. However, if oral potassium intake is excessive or intravenous potassium is given that causes high blood potassium concentration, the heart muscle can weaken to the point at which it stops beating. A UL has not been established for potassium from food sources.

Food Sources

Potassium is an essential part of all living cells; thus it is abundant in natural foods. The richest dietary sources of potassium are unprocessed foods: fruits such as oranges and bananas, vegetables such as broccoli and leafy green vegetables, fresh meats, whole grains, and milk products. Those who eat large amounts of fruits and vegetables have a high potassium intake. Plant sources of potassium are highly water soluble; therefore much of the potassium is lost when fruits and vegetables are boiled or blanched (unless the water is retained). Table 8-3 lists food sources of potassium.

Chloride

Functions

Chloride is the chemical form of chlorine in the human body. Chloride accounts for approximately 3% of the body's total mineral content and is widely distributed

TABLE 8-3

FOOD SOURCES OF POTASSIUM

ITEM	QUANTITY	AMOUNT (mg)
Bread, Cereal, Rice, Pasta		
Wheat germ, toasted cereal	¾ cup	803
Vegetables		
Avocado, raw	¼ medium	244
Brussels sprouts, boiled	½ cup	247
Potato, baked, with skin	1 medium (173 g)	926
Spinach, boiled	½ cup	419
Sweet potato, with skin, baked	1 medium (114 g)	542
Tomato, raw	1 medium	254
Fruits		
Banana	1 medium (118 g)	422
Dates, dried, pitted	¼ cup, chopped	292
Orange juice, fresh	8 fl oz	496
Orange, navel	1 medium (140 g)	232
Prunes, dried, pitted	½ cup (87 g)	637
Prune juice, canned	8 fl oz	707
Raisins, seedless	¼ cup	272
Meat, Poultry, Fish, Dry Beans, Eggs, Nuts		
Beef liver, pan fried	3 oz	298
Beef top round, lean, broiled	3 oz	221
Chickpeas (garbanzo beans), boiled	½ cup	239
Clams, cooked, moist heat	3 oz	534
Crab, blue, cooked, moist heat	3 oz	275
Ground beef, 70% lean, pan browned	3 oz	279
Halibut, cooked, dry heat	3 oz	490
Ham, sliced, 11% fat	3 oz	244
Lentils, boiled	½ cup	365
Lima beans, boiled	½ cup	478
Pinto beans, boiled	½ cup	373
Salmon, cooked, dry heat	3 oz	352
Sirloin steak, lean, broiled	3 oz	348
Soybeans, boiled	½ cup	443
Milk, Dairy Products		
Milk, skim	8 fl oz	382
Milk, whole	8 fl oz	349
Yogurt, plain, low fat	8 fl oz	573
Sugar		
Molasses	1 Tbsp	293

Data from the USDA, Agricultural Research Service, Nutrient Data Laboratory: *USDA nutrient database for standard reference, release 20, www.ars. usda.gov/ba/bhnrc/ndl.*

throughout body tissues. Chloride predominantly is found in the extracellular fluid compartments, where it helps maintain water and acid-base balances (see Figure 8-3). Its two significant functions involve digestion and respiration.

Digestion. Chloride (Cl^-) is one element in the hydrochloric acid (HCl) secreted in gastric juices. The action of gastric enzymes requires that stomach fluids have a specific acid concentration (pH approximately 1.0).

Respiration. Carbon dioxide, a by-product of cellular metabolism, is transported by RBCs to the lungs where it is expelled during respiration. Within RBCs, the enzyme carbonic anhydrase combines carbon dioxide (CO_2) with water (H_2O) to form carbonic acid (H_2CO_3). Carbonic acid then dissociates into bicarbonate ion (HCO_3^-) and a proton (H^+). Bicarbonate ions move out of the RBC into the plasma and chloride ions (Cl^-) move into the RBC out of the plasma, maintaining the balance of negative charges on either side of the RBC membrane. The exchange of a bicarbonate ion with a chloride ion in the plasma is called the *chloride shift* (Figure 8-4).

Requirements

The AI for chloride for young adults is set at 2.3 g/day based on a molecular equivalence to sodium.[4] Similar to sodium's AI, the need for chloride gradually declines after age 50 years.

Deficiency States

A dietary deficiency of chloride does not occur under normal circumstances. Because the normal intake and output of chloride from the body parallels that of sodium, conditions leading to a sodium deficiency also can lead to a chloride deficiency. The primary reason for chloride deficiency is excessive losses through vomiting, which leads to metabolic alkalosis from disturbances in acid-base balance (see in Chapter 9).

Toxicity Symptoms

The only known dietary cause of chloride toxicity is from severe dehydration in which the concentration of chloride is too great. No ULs are established for chloride.

Food Sources

Dietary chloride is almost entirely provided by sodium chloride, the chemical name of ordinary table salt. The kidneys efficiently reabsorb chloride when dietary intake is low.

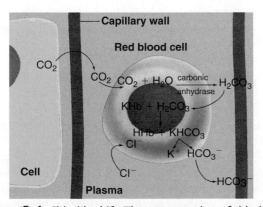

Figure 8-4 Chloride shift. The concentration of chloride ions (Cl^-) in RBCs increases as bicarbonate ions (HCO_3^-) diffuse out of the cell. Bicarbonate ions form as a result of the buffering of carbonic acid by the potassium salt of hemoglobin. (Reprinted from Thibodeau GA, Patton KT: *Anatomy & physiology*, ed 6, St Louis, 2007, Mosby.)

Magnesium

Functions

Magnesium has widespread metabolic functions and is found in all body cells. An adult body contains 25 g of magnesium (a little less than 1 oz) on average. Sixty percent of this magnesium is present in the bones.

General Metabolism. Magnesium is a necessary cofactor for more than 300 enzymes that use nucleotide triphosphates (e.g., ATP) for activation or catalyzing reactions that produce energy, synthesize body compounds, or help transport nutrients across cell membranes.

Protein Synthesis. Magnesium is a cofactor for enzymes that activate amino acids for protein synthesis and that synthesize and maintain DNA. When cells replicate, they must produce new proteins. The cell replication process requires magnesium to function correctly.

Muscle Action. Magnesium ions are involved in conduction of nerve impulses that stimulate muscle contraction as part of magnesium ATP (MgATP). Ca^{++} is pumped out of the myofibrillar spaces into the sarcoplasmic reticulum by pumps that require MgATP for energy.

Basal Metabolic Rate. MgATP is involved in the secretion of thyroid hormone (thyroxine), thus helping the body maintain a normal metabolic rate and adapt to cold temperatures.

Requirements

The DRI guidelines establish RDA amounts by age and gender. For infants, the AI is 30 mg/day during the first 6 months of life and 75 mg/day from ages 7 to 12 months. The RDA is the same for both boys and girls during childhood and early adolescence: 80 mg/day for ages 1 to 3 years, 130 mg/day for ages 4 to 8 years, and 240 mg/day for ages 9 to 13 years. For ages 14 to 18 years, the RDA is 410 mg/day for boys and 360 mg/day for girls. For those 19 to 30 years old, the RDA is 400 mg/day for men and 310 mg/day for women. For adults 31 years of age and older, the RDA is 420 mg/day for men and 320 mg/day for women. The RDA is somewhat higher during pregnancy: 400 mg/day for women 18 years and younger and 350 to 360 mg/day for women 19 years and older. Magnesium is not recommended to be increased during lactation.[6]

Deficiency States

A magnesium deficiency from lack of dietary magnesium is quite rare in persons consuming balanced diets. Symptoms of magnesium deficiency have been observed in clinical situations such as starvation, persistent vomiting or diarrhea with loss of magnesium-rich GI fluids, and surgical trauma. Magnesium depletion also is symptomatic of various diseases involving cardiovascular and neuromuscular function as well as in diabetes mellitus, kidney disease, and alcoholism. Deficiency symptoms include muscle weakness and cramps, hypertension, and blood vessel constriction in the heart and brain.

Toxicity Symptoms

Magnesium from food has not been observed to have adverse effects at high intake levels. Therefore the DRI standards give an UL only for magnesium intake from supplements and pharmaceutical preparations. The UL from nonfood sources is 350 mg/day for persons aged 9 years and older but less for children.[6] Individuals with renal insufficiency are at greater risk for consuming toxic amounts of magnesium if they take dietary supplements. Individuals consuming excessive amounts of magnesium from supplements may experience nausea, vomiting, and diarrhea.

Food Sources

Although magnesium is relatively common in foods, the content is variable. Unprocessed foods have the highest concentrations of magnesium. Major food sources of magnesium include nuts, soybeans, cocoa, seafood, whole grains, dried beans and peas, and green vegetables. Relatively poor sources of magnesium include most fruits (other than bananas), milk, meat, and fish. More than 80% of the magnesium in cereal grains is lost with the removal of the germ and outer layers. Significant amounts of magnesium also may be present in drinking water in regions that have hard water with a fairly high mineral content.

Sulfur

Functions

As part of the amino acids cysteine and methionine, sulfur is an essential part of protein structure and is present in all body cells, participating in widespread metabolic and structural functions. It is also a component of the vitamins thiamin and biotin.

Hair, Skin, and Nails. Disulfide bonds between cysteine residues in the protein keratin are essential to the structure of hair, skin, and nails.

General Metabolic Functions. Sulfhydryl or thiol groups (sulfur covalently bonded to hydrogen) form high-energy bonds that make various metabolic reactions energetically favorable.

Vitamin Structure. Sulfur is a component of two vitamins (thiamin and biotin) that act as coenzymes in cell metabolism.

Collagen Structure. Disulfide bonding of cysteine residues is necessary for collagen superhelix formation and is therefore important in building connective tissue.

Requirements

Dietary requirements for sulfur are not stated as such because sulfur is supplied by protein foods containing the amino acids methionine and cysteine.

Deficiency States

Sulfur deficiency states have not been reported. Such conditions only relate to general protein malnutrition and the deficient intake of the sulfur-containing amino acids.

Toxicity Symptoms

Sulfur is unlikely to reach toxic concentrations in the body from dietary intake; thus no UL has been established.

Food Sources

A diet containing adequate protein contains adequate sulfur. Sulfur is only available to the body as part of the amino acids methionine and cysteine and in the vitamins thiamin and biotin. Thus animal protein foods are the main dietary sources of sulfur. Sulfur is widely available in meat, eggs, milk, cheese, legumes, and nuts.

Table 8-4 provides a summary of the major minerals.

TRACE MINERALS

Iron

Functions

Iron has the longest and best described history of all the micronutrients. Iron is essential for life but toxic in excess. Thus the body has developed exquisite systems for balancing iron intake and excretion and for efficiently transporting iron in and out of cells to maintain health. Iron serves as the functional part of hemoglobin and in the body's general metabolism. The human body contains approximately 45 mg iron/kg body weight.

Hemoglobin Synthesis. Most of the body's iron, approximately 70%, is in hemoglobin within RBCs. Iron is a component of heme, the nonprotein part of hemoglobin. Hemoglobin carries oxygen to the cells, where it is used for oxidation and metabolism. Iron also is part of myoglobin, a protein in muscle cells that is structurally and functionally analogous to the hemoglobin in blood.

General Metabolism. Iron is necessary for glucose metabolism, antibody production, drug detoxification by the liver, collagen and purine synthesis, and the conversion of beta-carotene to active vitamin A. To accomplish these vital functions, precise mechanisms regulate the amount of iron in the body according to the body's need.

TABLE 8-4

SUMMARY OF MAJOR MINERALS

MINERAL	FUNCTIONS	RECOMMENDED INTAKES (ADULTS)	DEFICIENCY	UL AND TOXICITY	SOURCES
Calcium (Ca)	Bone and teeth formation, blood clotting, muscle contraction and relaxation, nerve transmission	AI: 19-50 yr: 1000 mg >51 yr: 1200 mg	Tetany, rickets, osteoporosis	2500 mg; increases risk of kidney stones, constipation; interferes with absorption of other nutrients	Dairy products, fish bones, fortified orange juice and cereals, legumes, green leafy vegetables
Phosphorus (P)	Bone and tooth formation, energy metabolism, DNA and RNA, acid-base balance	RDA: 700 mg	Unlikely, but can cause bone loss, loss of appetite, weakness	4g; bone resorption (loss of calcium)	High-protein foods (meat, dairy) and soft drinks
Sodium (Na)	Major extracellular fluid control, water balance, acid-base balance, muscle action, transmission of nerve impulse and resulting contraction	AI: 19-50 yr: 1.5 g 51-70 yr: 1.3 g >71 yr: 1.2 g	Fluid shifts, acid-base imbalance, cramping	2.3 g; hypertension in salt-sensitive people, edema	Table salt, processed foods (luncheon meats, salty snacks)
Potassium (K)	Major intracellular fluid control, acid-base balance, regulation of nerve impulse and muscle contraction, blood pressure regulation	AI: >14 yr: 4.7 g	Irregular heartbeat, difficulty breathing, muscle weakness	Not set; cardiac arrest	Fresh fruits, vegetables, meats, whole grains
Chloride (Cl)	Acid-base balance (chloride shift), hydrochloric acid (digestion)	AI: 19-50 yr: 2.3 g 51-70 yr: 2.0 g >71 yr: 1.8 g	Hypochloremic alkalosis in prolonged vomiting, diarrhea	Not set; unlikely	Table salt, processed foods
Magnesium (Mg)	Coenzyme in metabolism, muscle and nerve action, aids thyroid hormone secretion	RDA: Men: 400-420 mg Women: 310-320 mg	Tremor, spasm, low serum level after GI losses or renal losses from alcoholism, convulsions	350 mg (from supplements); nausea, vomiting, diarrhea	Whole grains, nuts, legumes, green vegetables, seafood, cocoa
Sulfur (S)	Essential constituent of cell protein, hair, skin, nails, vitamin, and collagen structure; high-energy sulfur bonds in energy metabolism	Diets adequate in protein contain adequate sulfur	Unlikely	Not set; unlikely	Meat, eggs, cheese, milk, nuts, legumes

Requirements

Iron needs vary throughout life depending on growth and development. The DRIs establish recommended intakes of iron for children as follows: the AI for infants up to age 6 months is 0.27 mg/day; for ages 7 to 12 months the RDA is 11 mg/day; for ages 1 to 3 years is 7 mg/day; and for ages 4 to 8 years is 10 mg/day. RDAs for iron from ages 9 years and older are between 8 and 11 mg/day for boys to accommodate for growth spurts and 8 to 18 mg/day for girls.[7] Women require more iron to cover the losses during menstruation and pregnancy. During pregnancy a woman's RDA for iron increases to 27 mg/day. This increase usually requires an iron supplement because neither the usual American diet nor the iron stores of many women can meet the increased iron demands of pregnancy.

Deficiency States

The major condition indicating a deficiency of iron is anemia, characterized by a decrease in the number of RBCs, a drop in the amount of RBC hemoglobin, or both. Iron-deficiency anemia is the most prevalent nutrition problem in the world today. The World Health Organization estimates that iron deficiency is one of the 10 leading risk factors for death in developing and developed countries; women and children are affected more than others.[8] Globally more than 800,000 deaths are attributed to iron-deficiency anemia annually, with 71% of that burden residing in Africa and Asia alone.[9] This iron deficiency, or inability to use iron, may have several causes: (1) inadequate dietary iron; (2) excessive blood loss; (3) inability to form hemoglobin because of a lack of factors such as vitamin B_{12} (i.e., pernicious anemia); (4) lack of gastric hydrochloric acid, which liberates iron for intestinal absorption; (5) inhibitors of iron absorption (e.g., phosphate or phytate); or (6) intestinal mucosal lesions affecting the absorptive surface area.

Toxicity Symptoms

Iron toxicity from a single large dose (20 to 60 mg/kg) can be fatal. In the United States iron overdose from supplements is one of the leading causes of poisoning among young children, with more than 2000 children younger than 6 years exposed annually.[10] Symptoms include nausea, vomiting, and diarrhea. If not immediately treated, several organ systems may be adversely affected, including the cardiovascular system, CNS, kidney, liver, and hematologic system.[7]

Chronically elevated iron intake may impair the absorption of zinc, cause GI upset, and increase the risk for developing heart disease and cancer.[7] The congenital disease *hemochromatosis* is an autosomal recessive disorder that results in iron overload even though iron intake is within the normal range. This disorder affects 1 in 300 individuals of northern European descent. Afflicted individuals absorb excessive amounts of iron from food and, over time, usually between ages 40 to 60 years, the iron accumulation causes widespread organ damage. Treatment involves reducing iron intake and withdrawing blood regularly. The UL for iron is 45 g/day for adults.

Food Sources

The typical Western diet provides an average of 6 mg of iron per 1000 kcal of energy intake. Iron is widely distributed in the U.S. food supply, mainly in meat, eggs, vegetables, and cereals (Figure 8-5). Liver and fortified cereal

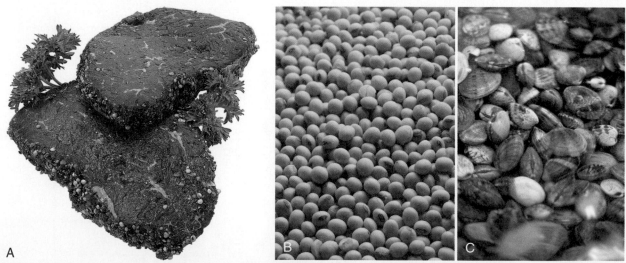

Figure 8-5 Food sources of dietary iron. **A,** Beef. **B,** Black-eyed peas. **C,** Oysters and clams. (Copyright JupiterImages Corporation.)

products are especially good sources. The body absorbs iron more easily when it is taken along with vitamin C. Iron in food occurs in two forms—*heme* and *nonheme*. Heme iron is the most efficiently absorbed form of dietary iron, but it contributes least to total iron intake. Heme iron is found in only 40% of the animal food sources and in no plant foods (Table 8-5). Nonheme iron is less efficiently absorbed because it is more tightly bound in foods, yet most of our food sources—60% of the animal food sources and all the plant food sources—contain nonheme iron. To enhance the absorption and availability of nonheme iron, food sources of vitamin C, moderate amounts of lean meats, and enriched cereal products should be included in the diet. Table 8-6 lists food sources of iron.

Iodine

Functions

The average adult body contains only 20 to 50 mg of iodine. Iodine's basic function is as a component of thyroxine (T4), a hormone synthesized by the thyroid gland that helps control the basal metaboloic rate (BMR). Thyroxine synthesis ultimately is controlled by the hypothalamus and the pituitary gland. The hypothalamus excretes thyrotropin-releasing hormone (TRH). TRH, in turn, stimulates the release of TSH from the anterior pituitary gland. TSH controls the thyroid gland's uptake of iodine from the blood stream and release of T_3 (triiodothyronine) and T_4 into the blood stream (Figure 8-6). Blood T_4 concentration determines how much TRH the hypothalamus releases and how much TSH the pituitary gland releases. As blood T_4 concentration decreases, the hypothalamus and pituitary gland are stimulated to release more TRH and TSH, respectively.

The transport form of iodine in the blood is called serum *protein-bound iodine*. T_3, T_4, and inorganic iodine are eventually disposed of by the liver in bile.

Requirements

The body's need for iodine has been extensively studied. To maintain desirable tissue levels of iodine, the adult body's minimal requirement is 50 to 75 mcg/day; therefore, to provide an extra margin of safety, the RDA is 150 mcg/day for all persons aged 14 years and older. Less is indicated for infants and children. During pregnancy the need increases to 220 mcg/day, and during lactation it increases to 290 mcg/day.[7]

Deficiency States

A lack of iodine in the diet causes several deficiency diseases, as discussed below.

Goiter. A lack of iodine in the diet causes the classic condition goiter, which often occurs in geographic areas where the water and soil contain little iodine (Figure 8-7). Some 5 billion people live in areas with iodine-deficient soils in underdeveloped countries, making goiter a significant health problem. Goiter is characterized by an enlargement of the thyroid gland, sometimes to a tremendous size. When the thyroid gland is starved for iodine, it cannot produce a normal amount of T_4. Because of low blood T_4 concentration, the pituitary gland continues to release more TSH. These large amounts of TSH overstimulate the nonproductive thyroid gland, causing its size to increase greatly. An iodine-starved thyroid gland may weigh 0.45 to 0.67 kg (1 to 1.5 lb) or more. Although the thyroid is one of the larger endocrine glands, it normally is only 10 to 20 g in an adult.

Cretinism. Cretinism is characterized by physical deformity, dwarfism, and mental retardation. This serious condition occurs in children born to mothers who had limited iodine intake during adolescence and pregnancy. During pregnancy, the mother's need for iodine takes precedence over that of the developing child. Thus

TABLE 8-5

CHARACTERISTICS OF HEME AND NONHEME PORTIONS OF DIETARY IRON

	HEME (SMALLEST PORTION)	NONHEME (LARGEST PORTION)
Food sources	None in plant sources; 40% of iron in animal sources	All iron in plant sources; 60% of iron in animal sources
Absorption rate	Rapid; transported and absorbed intact	Slow; tightly bound in organic molecules

anemia blood condition characterized by a decreased number of circulating RBCs, decreased hemoglobin, or both.

thyroxine (T4) an iodine-dependent thyroid gland hormone that regulates the metabolic rate of the body.

thyrotropin-releasing hormone (TRH) a hormone secreted by the hypothalamus that stimulates release of TSH by the pituitary.

goiter an enlarged thyroid gland caused by lack of enough available iodine to produce the thyroid hormone T4.

TABLE 8-6

FOOD SOURCES OF IRON

ITEM	QUANTITY	AMOUNT (mg)
Bread, Cereal, Rice, Pasta		
Bran Flakes cereal	¾ cup	8.1
Bran muffin	1 medium (113 g)	4.75
Cream of Wheat, instant, cooked	¾ cup	8.98
Oatmeal, fortified, instant, prepared with water	¾ cup	7.26
Wheat Bran flakes cereal, Complete	¾ cup	17.98
Fruits and Vegetables		
Prune juice, canned	8 fl oz	3.02
Spinach, boiled, drained	½ cup	3.21
Meat, Poultry, Fish, Dry Beans, Eggs, Nuts		
Beef, ground, 70% lean, pan browned	3 oz	2.11
Beef liver, pan fried	3 oz	5.24
Beef top round, lean, broiled	3 oz	2.78
Chickpeas (garbanzo beans), boiled	½ cup	2.37
Clams, cooked, moist heat	3 oz	23.77
Lentils, boiled	½ cup	3.3
Lima beans, large, boiled	½ cup	6.74
Oysters, cooked, dry heat	3 oz	6.6
Shrimp, cooked, moist heat	3 oz	2.63
Soybeans, boiled	½ cup	4.42
Tofu, raw, firm, prepared with calcium sulfate	½ cup	2.03

Data from the USDA, Agricultural Research Service, Nutrient Data Laboratory: *USDA nutrient database for standard reference, release 20,* www.ars.usda.gov/ba/bhnrc/ndl.

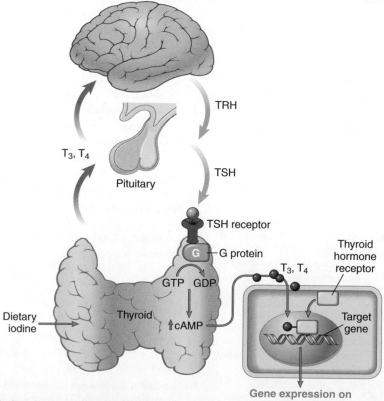

Figure 8-6 Uptake of iodine for T_3 and T_4 production. (Reprinted from Guyton AC, Hall JE: *Textbook of medical physiology,* ed 12, Philadelphia, 2006, Saunders.)

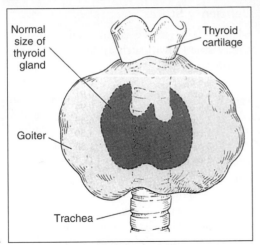
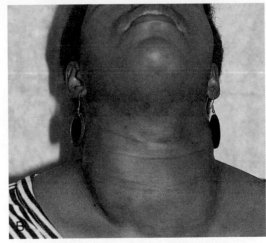

Figure 8-7 **A,** Illustration of a goiter. **B,** The extreme enlargement is a result of extended duration of iodine deficiency. (**B** Reprinted from Swartz MH: *Textbook of physical diagnosis,* ed 5, Philadelphia, 2006, Saunders.)

the fetus suffers from iodine deficiency and continues to do so after birth. The physical and mental development of these children is retarded.

Hypothyroidism. An adult form of hypothyroidism, called *myxedema,* occurs when a poorly functioning thyroid gland does not make enough T_4, greatly reducing the BMR. The symptoms of this condition are thin, coarse hair; dry skin; poor cold tolerance; weight gain; and a low, husky voice.

Hyperthyroidism. Hyperthyroidism is a condition in adults in which the overstimulated thyroid gland releases excessive T_4, greatly increasing the BMR. Hyperthyroidism is known as Graves' disease, or *exophthalmic goiter,* because of its prominent symptom of protruding eyeballs. Other symptoms include weight loss, hand tremors and general nervousness, increased appetite, and intolerance of heat.

Toxicity Symptoms

Incidental intake of iodine through supplementation may result in toxicity for some persons. Excessive iodine intake may result in acnelike skin lesions or may worsen the preexisting acne of adolescents or young adults. Excessive intake also may cause iodine goiter, which can be misdiagnosed as goiter caused by an insufficient iodine intake.

Research has found that (1) moderately excessive iodine intake is relatively harmless in children, (2) persons living in certain regions may be at greater risk of developing goiter, and (3) individual iodine intake varies greatly and may be insufficient (depending on geographic location and food supply).[11] Therefore, although the risk of iodine toxicity exists, continued use of iodized salt is still widely practiced in several countries, including the United States. The UL of iodine in healthy adults is 1100 mcg/day.

Food Sources

The amount of iodine in natural food sources varies considerably depending on the iodine content of the soil in which the food was grown. Seafood consistently provides a good amount of iodine. The major reliable source of iodine in U.S. diets, however, is iodized table salt, with each gram containing 76 mcg of iodine. Salt used in preparation of processed food supplies iodine for those persons who do not use table salt.

Zinc

Functions

Zinc is an essential trace mineral with wide clinical significance. Zinc is especially important during growth periods such as pregnancy, lactation, infancy, childhood, and adolescence. The amount of zinc in the adult body is approximately 1.5 g (0.05 oz) in women and 2.5 g (0.09 oz) in men. Zinc is present in minute quantities in all body organs, tissues, fluids, and secretions. In these tissues, zinc participates in three different types of metabolic functions, as outlined below.

Enzyme Constituent. Zinc's wide tissue distribution reflects its broad metabolic activity as an essential part of certain cell enzyme systems. More than 200 zinc-containing enzymes have been identified. Zinc's role in protein metabolism is associated with wound healing and healthy skin. Zinc greatly influences rapidly growing tissues, including fetal development during gestation.

Immune System. A considerable amount of protein-bound zinc is present in leukocytes (white blood cells). Zinc is integral in the health of the immune system through its role in the synthesis of nucleic acids (DNA and RNA) and protein. Zinc also is needed for lymphocyte transformation. Healthy lymphoid tissue, which gives rise to lymphocytes, is rich in zinc. The leukocytes of patients with leukemia, for example, contain about 10% less zinc than normal.

Other Functions. Zinc stabilizes the prohormone/storage form of insulin in the pancreas. It also is involved in the protection of RBCs from oxidative damage and in taste and smell acuity.

Requirements

The DRIs establish an AI for infants of 2 to 3 mg/day during the first 3 years of life and of 5 mg/day for children ages 4 to 8 years. Zinc requirement continues to rise until adulthood for both genders. Males 14 years and older require 11 mg of zinc per day, whereas females need 8 mg/day, with the exception of 14- to 18-year-old girls, whose needs are slightly higher. Pregnant women require 11 mg/day to meet fetal growth needs and 12 mg/day for lactation. Pregnant or lactating girls younger than 18 years require 2 mg/day more zinc than pregnant women older than 18 years. The zinc content of the typical mixed diet in the United States averages 11.4 mg/day.[1]

Deficiency States

Adequate zinc intake is imperative during periods of rapid tissue growth such as childhood and adolescence. Retarded physical growth (i.e., dwarfism) and retarded sexual maturation, especially in boys, have been observed in some populations in whom dietary zinc intake is low. Impaired taste and smell (i.e., hypogeusia and hyposmia) are improved with increased zinc intake if dietary zinc intake was previously inadequate. Zinc deficiency commonly causes poor wound healing, hair loss, diarrhea, and skin irritation. Patients with poor appetites, subsisting on marginal diets, or who have chronic wounds or illnesses with excessive tissue breakdown may be particularly vulnerable to developing zinc deficiency (see the For Further Focus box, "Zinc Barriers").

Toxicity Symptoms

As with several other minerals, zinc toxicity from food sources is uncommon. However, prolonged supplementation exceeding recommended zinc intake can cause adverse effects such as nausea, vomiting, and decreased immune function. The UL for zinc (40 mg/day) was established based on the negative effect of excess zinc supplementation on copper metabolism. Excessive zinc intake inhibits copper absorption, resulting in a copper deficiency.[7]

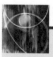

FOR FURTHER FOCUS

ZINC BARRIERS

Are people eating more zinc but absorbing it less? Current trends toward a heart-healthy diet may be the reason why. Some Americans may be at risk for developing zinc deficiency—not because they are avoiding zinc-rich foods, but because they are choosing foods and supplements that reduce its availability for absorption. Following are examples:

- Animal foods, rich in readily available zinc, are consumed less by an increasingly cholesterol-conscious public.
- Dietary fiber may hinder absorption and create a negative zinc balance.
- Food processing may make zinc less available.
- Vitamin-mineral supplements may contain *iron/zinc ratios* greater than 3:1 and provide enough iron to inhibit zinc absorption.

The risk for zinc deficiency is greatest among pregnant and breastfeeding women. Low levels of zinc can reduce the amount of protein available to carry iron and vitamin A to the target tissues and can reduce the mother's appetite and taste for foods. As a result, the fetus is at even greater risk for inadequate growth and development.

The following suggestions may help increase dietary zinc:

- Include some form of animal food (e.g., meat, milk, and eggs) or vegetarian-acceptable fortified food in the diet each day to ensure an adequate intake of zinc.
- Avoid excessive use of alcohol.
- Avoid "crash" diets.

Signs of zinc deficiency are fairly rare in the United States but are becoming more apparent among at-risk persons (e.g., older adults hospitalized with long-term chronic illnesses). There is no need, however, for the general public to take massive supplement doses. These large doses may compete with other minerals, such as iron, and create other deficiency problems. Excess zinc can lead to nausea, abdominal pain, anemia, and immune system impairment. As with all other nutrients, too much of a good thing can sometimes be as bad as, or even worse than, too little.

Food Sources

The greatest source of dietary zinc in the United States is meat, which supplies approximately 70% of the zinc consumed. Seafood, particularly oysters, is another excellent source of zinc. Legumes and whole grains are additional sources of zinc, but the zinc in these foods is less available for intestinal absorption. A balanced diet usually meets adult needs for zinc, but considerable evidence shows that diets high in processed foods may be low in zinc. Strict vegetarians, especially women, may be at risk for developing marginal zinc deficiency. Table 8-7 gives food sources of zinc.

Selenium

Functions

Selenium is present in all body tissues except adipose tissue. The highest concentrations of selenium are in the liver, kidneys, heart, and spleen. Selenium is an essential part of the antioxidant enzyme glutathione peroxidase, which protects the lipids in cell membranes from oxidative damage. An abundance of selenium may spare vitamin E to an extent because they both protect against free radical damage. Selenium also is a component of (1) the protein in the center of teeth, (2) the enzyme that converts thyroid hormone to T_3, and (3) the antioxidant defense system of the body along with vitamin C.

Recent human studies suggest that selenium's antioxidant function may have a protective role against the development of certain cancers.[12-14] The DRI panel on antioxidants reviewed the current scientific research on selenium. The panel concluded that, although selenium intakes higher than the RDA may protect against cancer, further large-scale research is necessary to confirm such an effect.[15]

Requirements

The recommendations for selenium intake are made by age group without specificity to gender. For both men and women ages 14 years and older, the RDA amount is

TABLE 8-7

FOOD SOURCES OF ZINC

ITEM	QUANTITY	AMOUNT (mg)
Bread, Cereal, Rice, Pasta		
Bran Flakes cereal	¾ cup	1.5
Bran muffin	1 medium (113 g)	2.08
Wheat Bran flakes cereal, Complete	¾ cup	15.22
Meat, Poultry, Fish, Dry Beans, Eggs, Nuts		
Almonds, roasted	1 oz	1
Beef, ground, 70% lean, pan browned	3 oz	5.06
Beef liver, pan fried	3 oz	4.45
Beef round top, lean, broiled	3 oz	3.83
Cashews, roasted	1 oz	1.59
Chicken, dark meat only, cooked, without skin	3 oz	1.81
Chickpeas (garbanzo beans), boiled	½ cup	1.25
Clams, cooked, moist heat	3 oz	2.32
Crab, Alaskan king, cooked, moist heat	3 oz	6.48
Ham, sliced, regular (11% fat)	3 oz	1.15
Lentils, boiled	½ cup	1.26
Lima beans, large, boiled	½ cup	2.68
Lobster, cooked, moist heat	3 oz	2.48
Oysters, cooked, dry heat	3 oz	38.4
Shrimp, cooked, moist heat	3 oz	1.33
Sirloin steak, lean, broiled	3 oz	4.84
Tofu, raw, firm, prepared with calcium sulfate	½ cup	1.05
Milk, Dairy Products		
Milk, skim	8 fl oz	1.03
Yogurt, plain, low fat	8 fl oz	2.18

Data from the USDA, Agricultural Research Service, Nutrient Data Laboratory: *USDA nutrient database for standard reference, release 20, www.ars. usda.gov/ba/bhnrc/ndl.*

55 mcg/day. The RDA decreases by age for children: 40 mcg/day for children 9 to 13 years of age, 30 mcg/day for children 4 to 8 years of age, and 20 mcg/day for children 1 to 3 years of age. The DRI does not list an RDA for infants. Based on mean intakes of breastmilk, an infant's observed AI level is 15 mcg/day for the first 6 months of life and 20 mcg/day from ages 7 to 12 months. Selenium compounds in breast milk are more biologically available to infants than the selenium in formula. The recommended selenium intake is 60 mcg/day during pregnancy and 70 mcg/day during lactation.[15]

Deficiency States

Selenium deficiency can significantly compromise the immune system. Mild selenium deficiency may decrease the body's ability to fight infection, whereas severe deficiency may put individuals at risk for developing certain types of cancer. Research indicates that adequate selenium intake plays a role in preventing Keshan disease. Keshan disease, named after the area in China where it was discovered, is a heart muscle disease that primarily affects young children and women of childbearing age and can lead to heart failure from cardiomyopathy (i.e., degeneration of the heart muscle).

Toxicity Symptoms

The most common symptom of selenium toxicity is brittle hair and nails. Other problems include GI upset, skin rash, garlic-like body odor, and nervous system abnormalities. Most known cases of dietary selenium toxicity are in isolated regions of the world where the soil has extremely high levels of selenium. The UL for selenium is 400 mcg/day for persons aged 14 years and older.

Food Sources

Most selenium in food is highly available for intestinal absorption. The amount of selenium in food depends on the quantity of selenium in the soil used to graze animals and grow plants. Seafood, kidney, and liver are consistently good sources of selenium. To a lesser extent other meats also provide selenium. Grains and other seeds have a more variable selenium content. Fruits and vegetables generally contain little selenium. In the United States and Canada the dietary intake of selenium can vary by the geographic region in which the fruits and vegetables are grown, but these local differences are reduced by the national food distribution system.

The following sections briefly review the remaining essential trace minerals.

Fluoride

Fluoride forms a strong bond with calcium; thus it accumulates in calcified body tissues such as bones and teeth. Fluoride's main function in human nutrition is preventing dental caries. Fluoride strengthens the ability of teeth to withstand the erosive effect of bacterial acids. The continued intake of fluoride throughout life maximizes the protective effect of fluoride on teeth and maintains an adequate level of fluoride in tooth enamel. To a great extent the fluoridation of the public water supply (for which the optimal level is 1 mg/L) is responsible for the remarkable decline in dental caries in recent decades. The use of fluoridated toothpaste (0.1%) and improved dental hygiene habits have also benefited dental health.

Because fluoride stimulates new bone formation, it became an experimental drug in the treatment of osteoporosis. Currently no evidence supports fluoride's ability to prevent osteoporosis. According to the DRI guidelines, research data are insufficient about fluoride intake to support a specific RDA. Alternatively, the DRI lists observed AI amounts by age group. For adults ages 19 years and older, the AI is 4 mg/day for men and 3 mg/day for women, with lower intakes for children. It is not recommended that fluoride intake increase during pregnancy and lactation. The DRI guidelines set the UL for fluoride at 10 mg/day for persons ages 9 years and older to avoid dental fluorosis. Fish, fish products, and tea contain the highest concentrations of fluoride. Cooking in fluoridated water raises the fluoride concentration in many foods.

Copper

Copper has frequently been called the "iron twin" because both iron and copper are metabolized in much the same way and both are components of cell enzymes. Both also are involved in energy production and hemoglobin synthesis. Severe copper deficiency is rare and is attributable to individual adaptation to somewhat lower intakes. However, copper depletion sufficient enough to cause low blood copper concentration has been observed during total parenteral nutrition and in anemia. The adult RDA for dietary copper intake is 900 mcg/day. Pregnant and lactating women are recommended to increase their copper intake to 1 mg/day and 1.3 mg/day, respectively. Average daily intake of dietary copper in the United States is 1.2 mg/day.[1] Wilson's disease is a genetic disorder causing an abnormally high storage of copper in the body. Without treatment, Wilson's disease can result in liver and nerve damage. Copper is widely distributed in natural foods. The UL for copper is 10 mg/day to avoid GI upset and liver damage. Organ meats, especially liver, followed by seafood, nuts, and seeds, including legumes and grains, are the richest food sources of copper.

Manganese

The adult body contains approximately 20 mg of manganese, found mainly in the liver, pancreas, pituitary gland, and bones. Although manganese is considered to be essential to the diet, it also is toxic at high intake levels.[7] Manganese functions like many other trace minerals—as a component of cell enzymes. Manganese-dependent enzymes catalyze many important metabolic reactions. In some *magnesium*-dependent enzymes, manganese may serve as a substitute for magnesium depending on the availability of these two minerals. Intestinal absorption and bodily retention of manganese are associated with serum ferritin concentration. Manganese deficiency is rare but has been reported in cases of diabetes and pancreatic insufficiency and in protein-energy malnutrition states such as *kwashiorkor*. Manganese toxicity occurs as an industrial occupation disease known as *inhalation toxicity* in miners and other workers exposed to manganese dust over long periods. The excess manganese accumulates in the liver and CNS, producing severe neuromuscular symptoms similar to those of Parkinson's disease. The UL from dietary sources is 11 mg/day for healthy adults.

The DRIs estimate an AI of 2.3 mg/day for men and 1.8 mg/day for women older than 19 years. Needs gradually increase during and after childhood, and pregnant and lactating women need more magnesium (2.0 mg/day and 2.6 mg/day, respectively). The best food sources of manganese are of plant origin. Whole grains, cereal products, and teas are the richest food sources.

Chromium

The precise amount of chromium present in body tissues is uncertain because analysis is difficult. Although large geographic variations occur, total body chromium is less than 6 mg. Chromium is an essential component of the organic complex *glucose tolerance factor*, which stimulates the action of insulin. Chromium supplements were previously thought to reduce insulin resistance (the cause of impaired glucose tolerance) and improve lipid profiles for at-risk patients. However, a recent randomized, double-blind study examining the effects of chromium supplements in subjects with impaired glucose tolerance did not find significant improvement in glucose tolerance in those who took chromium compared with the control group.[16] For adults, the AI of chromium intake is 35 mcg/day for men and 25 mcg/day for women. Chromium needs gradually rise from infancy to adulthood and then decline after the age of 50 years. Pregnant and lactating women have an increased need of 30 mcg/day and 45 mcg/day, respectively. No UL has been established. Brewer's yeast is a rich source of chromium, and most grains and cereal products contain significant amounts.

Molybdenum

Molybdenum is better absorbed than many minerals, and inadequate dietary intake is unlikely. The amount of molybdenum in the body is exceedingly small; it ranges from 0.1 to 1 mcg per gram of body tissue. Molybdenum is the functional catalytic component in several cell enzymes. For adults, the RDA of molybdenum is 45 mcg/day. Pregnant and lactating women need an additional 5 mcg/day. The National Academy of Sciences did find it necessary to establish an UL at 2000 mcg/day for adults older than 19 years.[7] The amounts of molybdenum in foods vary considerably depending on the soil they are grown in. Food sources include legumes, whole grains, milk, leafy vegetables, and organ meats.

Table 8-8 provides a summary of selected trace minerals.

Other Essential Trace Minerals

RDAs and AIs were not set for the remaining trace minerals: aluminum, arsenic, boron, nickel, silicon, tin, or vanadium. At the time of the 2002 DRIs, not enough data were available to establish such recommendations.[7] Most of these minerals are deemed essential to the nutrition of specific animals and probably are essential in human nutrition as well, although the complete process of their metabolism is not yet fully understood. Because these minerals occur in such small amounts, they are difficult to study and dietary deficiency is highly unlikely.

The available research data about boron, nickel, and vanadium is sufficient to establish a tolerable UL level. The adult UL for both boron and vanadium were set based on data gathered from animal studies: boron 20

fluorosis excess intake of fluoride causing yellowing of teeth, white spots, and pitting or mottling of tooth enamel.

TABLE 8-8
SUMMARY OF SELECTED TRACE ELEMENTS

MINERAL	FUNCTIONS	RECOMMENDED INTAKES (ADULTS)	DEFICIENCY	UL AND TOXICITY	SOURCES
Iron (Fe)	Hemoglobin and myoglobin formation, cellular oxidation of glucose, antibody production	RDA: Men: 8 mg Women: 19-50 yr: 18 mg >50 yr: 8 mg	Anemia, pale skin, impaired immune function	45 mg; nausea, vomiting, diarrhea; liver, kidney, heart, and CNS damage Hemochromatosis: iron overload disease	Liver, meats, egg yolk, whole grains, enriched bread and cereal, dark green vegetables, legumes, nuts
Iodine (I)	Synthesis of T_4, which regulates cell oxidation and BMR	RDA: 150 mcg	Goiter, cretinism, hypothyroidism, hyperthyroidism	1100 mcg; goiter	Iodized salt, seafood
Zinc (Zn)	Essential enzyme constituent, protein metabolism, storage of insulin, immune system, sexual maturation	RDA: Men: 11 mg Women: 8 mg	Impaired wound healing and taste and smell acuity, retarded sexual and physical development	40 mg; nausea, vomiting, decreased immune function, impaired copper absorption	Meat, seafood (especially oysters), eggs, milk, whole grains, legumes
Selenium (Se)	Forms glutathione peroxidase, spares vitamin E as an antioxidant, protects lipids in cell membrane	RDA: 55 mcg	Impaired immune function, Keshan disease, heart muscle failure	400 mcg; brittleness of hair and nails, GI upset	Seafood, kidney, liver, meats, whole grains
Fluoride (Fl)	Constituent of bone and teeth, prevents dental caries	AI: Men: 4 mg Women: 3 mg	Increased dental caries	10 mg; dental fluorosis	Fluoridated water, toothpaste
Copper (Cu)	Associated with iron in energy production, hemoglobin synthesis, absorption and transport of iron, nerve and immune function	RDA: 900 mcg	Anemia, bone abnormalities	10 mg; toxicity disease: Wilson's disease, resulting in liver and nerve conduction damage	Liver, seafood, whole grains, legumes, nuts
Manganese (Mn)	Activates reactions in urea synthesis, energy metabolism, lipoprotein clearance, and synthesis of fatty acids	AI: Men: 2.3 mg Women: 1.8 mg	Clinical deficiency present only in protein-energy malnutrition	11 mg; inhalation toxicity in miners: neuromuscular disturbances	Cereals, whole grains, soybeans, legumes, nuts, tea, vegetables, fruits
Chromium (Cr)	Associated with glucose metabolism	AI: Men: 35 mcg Women: 25 mcg	Impaired glucose metabolism	Not set; unlikely	Whole grains, cereal products, brewer's yeast
Molybdenum (Mo)	Constituent of many enzymes	RDA: 45 mcg	Unlikely	2 mg; unlikely	Organ meats, milk, whole grains, leafy vegetables, legumes

mg/day and vanadium 1.8 mg/day. The adult UL for arsenic was set at 1 mg/day.[7]

MINERAL SUPPLEMENTATION

The same principles in Chapter 7 relating to vitamin supplementation apply to mineral supplementation. Special needs during growth periods and in clinical situations may require specific mineral supplements. According to the Third National Health and Nutrition Examination Survey, approximately 22% of the U.S. population takes a multivitamin/mineral supplement on a regular basis.[3] Before taking supplements, potential nutrient-nutrient interactions and drug-nutrient interactions should be considered. Several situations can occur in which mineral bioavailability may be hindered (see the Drug-Nutrient Interaction box, "Mineral Depletion").

Life Cycle Needs

Mineral supplements may be needed during rapid growth periods throughout the life cycle.

Pregnancy and Lactation

Women require additional magnesium, iron, zinc, selenium, iodine, copper, manganese, chromium, and molybdenum to meet the demands of rapid fetal growth during pregnancy. RDAs remain elevated for several minerals throughout lactation to meet both mother and infant needs.

Adolescence

Rapid bone growth during adolescence requires increased calcium and phosphorus. If an adolescent's diet provides insufficient calcium, the risk for bone density problems (e.g., osteoporosis) in later adult years is increased. Too much dietary phosphorus and too little dietary calcium can result in resorption of calcium from bone to maintain an appropriate blood calcium concentration. With the major increases in soft drink consumption (high in phosphorus) coupled with decreased milk consumption per capita in the United States, concern has increased about poor bone growth during these critical years.

Supplements combining iron with folate may be indicated for adolescent girls as they begin their menstrual cycle.

Adulthood

Healthy adults do not need mineral supplements, but advertisers and others in the media have perpetuated the notion that calcium supplements prevent and treat osteoporosis. Although currently marketed to prevent the loss of bone density, calcium supplements alone have little effect, especially when the overall diet is poor. A well-rounded, varied diet combined with adequate physical activity and exercise maintain optimal bone health in most adults. In addition, an idiopathic (i.e., cause unknown) form of osteoporosis that occurs in young adults does not respond to calcium supplementation. At any adult age calcium supplementation alone neither prevents nor successfully treats

DRUG-NUTRIENT INTERACTION

MINERAL DEPLETION

The use of some prescription and over-the-counter drugs can lead to mineral depletion by either blocking absorption or inducing renal excretion. The following are examples of common drug-nutrient interactions specifically affecting mineral status:

- *Diuretics*: Persons requiring long-term use of diuretic drugs for treatment of hypertension may need to pay special attention to certain minerals that also are lost. Minerals usually excreted with excess water are sodium, potassium, magnesium, and zinc. Increased intake of foods high in these minerals generally is enough to regain homeostasis. Some diuretics, such as spironolactone, are potassium sparing and thus extra potassium does not need to be consumed.
- *Chelating agents*: Penicillamine, a drug used to treat Wilson's disease (the excess accumulation of copper in

the body) and rheumatoid arthritis and to prevent kidney stones, attaches to zinc and copper and can lead to the excretion and thus depletion of these essential minerals.
- *Antacids*: Phosphate deficiency is a concern for individuals chronically abusing over-the-counter antacids. In extreme cases, hypercalcemia may result and damage to soft tissue can form.

Regular use of functional foods with added minerals in addition to a daily multimineral supplement may cause an excess accumulation of certain minerals in the body. Care should be taken to ensure that megadosing of minerals does not occur.

osteoporosis, the cause of which is not clear and involves multiple factors. Calcium supplements may be used as part of a treatment program together with vitamin D, estrogen, and increased physical activity.

Clinical Needs

Persons with certain clinical problems or those at high risk for developing such problems may require mineral supplements.

Iron-Deficiency Anemia

One of the most prevalent health problems encountered in population surveys is iron-deficiency anemia. The need for increased iron intake has long been established for pregnant and breastfeeding women.[7] The following high-risk groups also may need to supplement their diets: adolescent girls and women in their childbearing years who consume poor diets, low-income adolescent boys, athletes, vegetarians, and elderly persons who consume poor diets.

Zinc Deficiency

The increased popularity of vegetarian diets has amplified concern about possible zinc deficiency because of the low zinc content of plant foods. The American Dietetic Association and Dietitians of Canada position statement about vegetarian diets indicates that zinc requirements for individuals who consume high phytate diets may exceed the current DRIs.[17] Concern about children and elderly persons is greatest because their needs are highest and they already are consuming less zinc than recommended.[1] Signs of zinc deficiency are slow growth, impaired taste and smell, poor wound healing, and skin problems, but 3 to 24 weeks pass before symptoms appear. Others at risk for zinc deficiency include alcoholics; persons on long-term, low-calorie diets; and elderly persons in long-term institutional care.

SUMMARY

In nutrition, minerals are elements that are widely distributed in foods. They are absorbed by the intestines and used in building body tissue; activating, regulating, and controlling metabolic processes; and transmitting neurologic messages.

Minerals are classified according to their relative amounts in the body. Major minerals are necessary in larger quantities than trace minerals and make up 60% to 80% of all the inorganic material in the body. *Trace minerals,* which are necessary in quantities as small as a microgram (mcg), make up less than 1% of the body's inorganic material.

RDAs have not been set for all minerals because of the lack of scientific data. However, AIs or ULs have been set for almost all essential minerals without RDAs.

Mineral supplementation, as with vitamin supplementation, continues to be a hot topic of debate. Periods occur throughout the life cycle and specific disease states that may warrant supplementation. However, in most situations a balanced diet (as defined in guidelines such as MyPyramid or *Dietary Guidelines for Americans*) provides an adequate supply of all essential nutrients.

CRITICAL THINKING QUESTIONS

1. List the seven major minerals and describe their functions and the problems created by dietary deficiency or excess.
2. List the trace minerals proved to be essential in human nutrition. Which ones have established RDAs? Which ones have AIs suggested? Why is establishing an RDA for everyone difficult?
3. Considering the normal dietary supply of minerals, would you recommend taking a multimineral dietary supplement? If so, to whom and for what reasons?

CHAPTER CHALLENGE QUESTIONS

True-False

Write the correct statement for each statement that is false.

1. *True or False:* Most of the phosphorus in the diet is absorbed and used by the body for bone formation.

2. *True or False:* Typical adult use of sodium is approximately 10 times the amount the body actually requires for metabolic balance.

3. *True or False:* Potassium is the major electrolyte controlling the water outside cells.

4. *True or False:* Chloride is a necessary component of stomach fluids.

5. *True or False:* Copper has many metabolic functions, the most important of which is its role in T_4 synthesis.

6. *True or False:* A high intake of selenium has been proved to prevent cancer in almost everyone.

7. *True or False:* Iodine is associated with iron functions in the body and is called the "iron twin."

Multiple Choice

1. Overall calcium balance is mostly maintained by which two balanced regulatory agents?

    a. Vitamin A and thyroid hormone
    b. Ascorbic acid and growth hormone
    c. Vitamin D and PTH
    d. Phosphorus and TSH

2. Optimal levels of body iron are controlled at the point of absorption, interrelated with a system of transport and storage. Which of the following statements correctly describes this iron regulating process?

    a. The iron form in foods requires an acid medium to reduce it to the form necessary for absorption.
    b. Most of the iron ingested in food, approximately 70% to 90%, is absorbed.
    c. Vitamin C acts as a binding and carrying agent to transport and store iron.
    d. When RBCs are destroyed, the iron used in making the hemoglobin is excreted.

3. The only known function of fluoride in human nutrition is for dental health. Which of the following statements correctly describes this relation?

    a. Small amounts of fluoride produce mottled, discolored teeth.

    b. Fluoridation of the public water supply in very small amounts helps prevent dental caries.
    c. Topical application of fluoride is not effective on young teeth.
    d. Fluoride works with vitamin A to build strong teeth.

4. Cretinism is a disorder in children born to mothers who had a deficiency of _____ during adolescence and pregnancy.

    a. Calcium
    b. Phosphorus
    c. Iron
    d. Iodine

5. Which mineral has the following functions: blood clotting, muscle and nerve action, and bone and teeth formation?

    a. Calcium
    b. Phosphorus
    c. Magnesium
    d. Chloride

6. Which of the following minerals is a trace mineral?

    a. Potassium
    b. Iron
    c. Chloride
    d. Sulfur

---

evolve Please refer to the Students' Resource section of this text's Evolve Web site for additional study resources.

REFERENCES

1. Ervin RB and others: *Dietary intake of selected minerals for the United States population: 1999-2000. Advance data from vital and health statistics; no 341,* Hyattsville, MD, 2004, National Center for Health Statistics.

2. U.S. Department of Health and Human Services: *Bone health and osteoporosis: a report of the surgeon general,* Rock-ville, MD, 2004, U.S. Department of Health and Human Services.

3. Ervin RB and others: *Prevalence of leading types of dietary supplements used in the third National Health and Nutrition Examination Survey, 1988-94. Advanced data from vital and health statistics; no 349,* Hyattsville, MD, 2004, National Center for Health Statistics.

4. Food and Nutrition Board, Institute of Medicine: *Dietary reference intakes for water, potassium, sodium, chloride, and sulfate,* Washington, DC, 2004, National Academies Press.

5. U.S. Department of Health and Human Services, U.S. Department of Agriculture: *Dietary guidelines for Americans, 2005,* Washington, DC, 2005, USDA.

6. Food and Nutrition Board, Institute of Medicine: *Dietary reference intakes for calcium, phosphorus, magnesium, vitamin D, and fluoride*, Washington, DC, 1997, National Academies Press.

7. Food and Nutrition Board, Institute of Medicine: *Dietary reference intakes for vitamin A, vitamin K, arsenic, boron, chromium, copper, iodine, iron, manganese, molybdenum, nickel, silicon, vanadium, and zinc*, Washington, DC, 2002, National Academies Press.

8. World Health Organization: *World health report 2002: reducing risk, promoting healthy life*, Geneva, 2002, World Health Organization.

9. Stoltzfus RJ: Iron deficiency: global prevalence and consequences, *Food Nutr Bull* 24(4 Suppl):S99, 2003.

10. Watson WA and others: 2003 annual report of the American Association of Poison Control Centers Toxic Exposure Surveillance System, *Am J Emerg Med* 22(5):335, 2004.

11. Zimmermann MB and others: High thyroid volume in children with excess dietary iodine intakes, *Am J Clin Nutr* 81(4):840, 2005.

12. Peters U and others: High serum selenium and reduced risk of advanced colorectal adenoma in a colorectal cancer early detection program, *Cancer Epidemiol Biomarkers Prev* 15(2):315, 2006.

13. Brinkman M and others: Use of selenium in chemoprevention of bladder cancer, *Lancet Oncol* 7(9):766, 2006.

14. Lowe JF, Frazee LA: Update on prostate cancer chemoprevention, *Pharmacotherapy* 26(3):353, 2006.

15. Food and Nutrition Board, Institute of Medicine: *Dietary reference intakes for vitamin C, vitamin E, selenium, and carotenoids*, Washington, DC, 2000, National Academies Press.

16. Gunton JE and others: Chromium supplementation does not improve glucose tolerance, insulin sensitivity, or lipid profile: a randomized, placebo-controlled, double-blind trial of supplementation in subjects with impaired glucose tolerance, *Diabetes Care* 28(3):712, 2005.

17. Mangels AR and others: Position of the American Dietetic Association and Dietitians of Canada: vegetarian diets, *J Am Diet Assoc* 103:748, 2003.

FURTHER READING AND RESOURCES

Medline Plus Health Information: *www.nlm.nih.gov/medlineplus/vitaminandmineralsupplements.html*
> *This Web site provides the most current information about vitamins and minerals, complete with an encyclopedia, drug information, dictionaries, and articles about research and clinical applications of vitamins and minerals.*

The following Web sites are good sources for information on certain minerals in the diets and their role in general health. Go to The National Heart, Lung, and Blood Institute Web site to learn about the role of sodium and heart disease, such as in hypertension, and how to follow a low-sodium diet. Examine the American Dental Association Oral Health Topics for more information on the protective role of fluoride in dental hygiene.

National Osteoporosis Foundation: *www.nof.org*

The National Heart, Lung, and Blood Institute: *www.nhlbi.nih.gov/health/public/heart*

American Dental Association: *www.ada.org/public/topics/index.asp*

National Digestive Diseases Information Clearinghouse, hemochromatosis: *dayigestive.niddk.nih.gov/daydiseases/pubs/hemochromatosis/index.htm*

Franchini M: Hereditary iron overload: update on pathophysiology, diagnosis, and treatment, *Am J Hematol* 81(3):202, 2006.
> *The hereditary autosomal recessive disease hemochromatosis is discussed in terms of the varying forms of the disease, pathophysiology, diagnosis, and management.*

CHAPTER 9

Water Balance

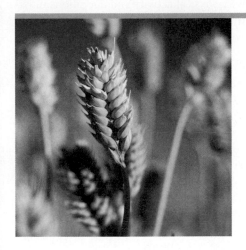

KEY CONCEPTS

- Water compartments inside and outside cells maintain a balanced distribution of total body water.
- The concentration of various solute particles in water determines internal shifts and movement of water.
- A state of dynamic equilibrium among all parts of the body's water balance system sustains life.

Water is the most vital nutrient to human existence. Humans can survive far longer without food than without water. Only the continuous need for air is more demanding.

One of the most basic nutrition tasks is ensuring a balanced distribution of water to all body cells. Water is critical for many physiologic functions necessary to support life. This chapter briefly looks at the finely developed water balance system in the body, how this system works, and the various parts and processes that maintain it.

BODY WATER FUNCTIONS AND REQUIREMENTS

Water: The Fundamental Nutrient

Basic Principles

Three basic principles are essential to an understanding of the balance and uses of water in the human body.

A Unified Whole. The human body forms one continuous body of water contained by a protective envelope of skin. Water moves to all parts, controlled by solvents within the water and membranes separating the compartments. Virtually every space inside and outside cells is filled with water-based body fluids. Within this environment, all processes necessary to life are sustained.

Body Water Compartments. The key word *compartment* generally is used in human physiology to refer to the dynamic areas within the body. Body water can be discussed in terms of total body water as well as in separate individual locations throughout the body (i.e., intracellular or extracellular compartments). *Membranes* separate compartments of water. The body's dynamic mechanisms constantly shift water to places of greatest need and maintain equilibrium with all parts. Specific compartments are discussed later in this chapter.

Particles in the Water Solution. The concentration and distribution of *particles* (e.g., sodium, chloride, calcium, magnesium, phosphate, bicarbonate, and protein) in the water solution determine the internal shifts and balances between compartments within the total body of water.

Homeostasis

The body's state of dynamic balance is called homeostasis. W.B. Cannon, a physiologist, viewed these balance principles as "body wisdom."[1] He applied the term *homeostasis* to the capacity built into the body to maintain its life systems, despite what enters the system from the outside. The body has a great capacity to use numerous, finely balanced, *homeostatic mechanisms* to protect its vital water supply.

Body Water Functions

To serve life-sustaining functions, the body water supply (1) acts as a solvent, (2) serves as a means of transport, (3) regulates temperature control, and (4) provides lubrication for the body.

Solvent. Water provides the basic liquid solvent for all chemical reactions within the body. The polarity of water effectively ionizes and dissolves many substances.

Transport. Water circulates throughout the body in the form of blood and various other secretions and tissue fluids. In this circulating fluid, the many nutrients, secretions, metabolites (products formed from metabolism), and other materials can be carried about to meet the needs of all body cells.

Thermoregulation. Water is necessary to help maintain a stable body temperature. As the body temperature rises, sweat increases and evaporates from the skin, thus cooling the body.

Lubricant. Water also has a lubricating effect on moving parts of the body. For example, fluid within joints (*synovial* fluid) helps provide smooth movement and prevents damage from friction.

Body Water Requirements

The Dietary Reference Intake (DRI) for water, set for the first time by the National Academy of Sciences in 2004, is based on the median *total* water intake reported by participants in the Third National Health and Nutrition Examination Survey, 1988 to 1994. Total water includes water in beverages and food. Set as adequate intakes (AIs,), the DRIs for water are the amounts required to meet the needs of healthy individuals who are relatively sedentary and living in temperate climates.[2] Recommendations primarily are established to prevent harmful effects of dehydration such as metabolic and functional abnormalities. To meet adult fluid needs, and thus be hydrated, the average sedentary woman should consume 2.7 L (91 oz) of *total* water per day. Because approximately 19% of total water intake comes from food, a

woman should aim for 74 fluid ounces (9 cups) of fluids in the form of beverages per day, with the rest provided by food. A sedentary man should consume 3.7 L (125 oz) of *total* water per day.[2] Assuming approximately 0.7 L of water is consumed within food, a man should aim for 101 fluid ounces (3 L) of fluid in the form of beverages per day. However, physical activity and alterations in climate require more fluid to offset losses. Table 9-1 gives the AI of fluid intake for all individuals.

The body's requirement for water varies according to several factors: environment, activity level, functional losses, metabolic needs, age, and other dietary factors.

Surrounding Environment. As the temperature rises in the surrounding environment, body water is lost as sweat in an effort to maintain body temperature. Water intake must accommodate such losses in sweat. This increasing temperature may be caused by the natural climate or the heat produced by physical work. On the opposite end of the spectrum, cold temperatures and altitude result in elevated respiratory water loss, hypoxia- and/or cold-induced diuresis, and increased energy expenditure, all of which increase water needs.[2]

Activity Level. Heavy work or extensive physical activity, such as participation in sports, increases the water requirement for two reasons: (1) more water is lost in sweat and respiration, and (2) more water is necessary for the increased metabolic demand involved in physical activity.

Athletes require a large increase in water intake, especially in hot weather. The American College of Sports Medicine recommends drinking 400 to 600 mL (13.5 to 20 oz) of fluid 2 to 3 hours before exercise, with an additional 150 to 350 mL (5 to 12 oz) of fluid at 15- to 20-minute intervals throughout the duration of exercise.[3]

Functional Losses. When any disease process interferes with the normal functioning of the body, water requirements are affected. For example, with GI problems such as prolonged diarrhea, large amounts of water may be lost. Uncontrolled diabetes mellitus causes an excess loss of water through urine as a result of high glucose levels in the blood. In such cases, replacement of lost water and electrolytes is vital to prevent dehydration.

Metabolic Needs. Body metabolism requires water. A general rule is that roughly 1000 mL of water is necessary for every 1000 kcal in the diet.

Age. Age plays an important role in determining water needs, especially in infants. The average usual intake for infants ages 0 to 6 months and 7 to 12 months is 700 mL and 800 mL *total* water per day from human milk and complementary foods, respectively.[4] Water intake is critical for an infant because of the following: (1) an infant's body content of water is large (approximately 70% to

TABLE 9-1

ADEQUATE INTAKE OF WATER (LITERS PER DAY)

AGE	MALE			FEMALE		
	FROM FOOD	FROM BEVERAGES	TOTAL WATER	FROM FOOD	FROM BEVERAGES	TOTAL WATER
0-6 months	0.0	0.7	**0.7**	0.0	0.7	**0.7**
7-12 months	0.2	0.6	**0.8**	0.2	0.6	**0.8**
1-3 years	0.4	0.9	**1.3**	0.4	0.9	**1.3**
4-8 years	0.5	1.2	**1.7**	0.5	1.2	**1.7**
9-13 years	0.6	1.8	**2.4**	0.5	1.6	**2.1**
14-18 years	0.7	2.6	**3.3**	0.5	1.8	**2.3**
>19 years	0.7	3.0	**3.7**	0.5	2.2	**2.7**
Pregnancy **14-50 years**				0.7	2.3	**3.0**
Lactation **14-50 years**				0.7	3.1	**3.8**

1 L = 33.8 oz; 1 L = 1.06 qt; 1 cup = 8 oz
Data from Food and Nutrition Board, Institute of Medicine: *Dietary reference intakes for water, potassium, sodium, chloride, and sulfate*, Washington, DC, 2004, National Academies Press.

75% of the total body weight), and (2) a relatively large amount of this total body water is outside the cells and thus is more easily lost.

Other Dietary Factors. Certain dietary additives and medications can affect water requirements because of their natural diuretic effect. Several medications contain diuretics specifically for the purpose of reducing overall body fluid, as in the case of antihypertensive medications (e.g., hydrochlorothiazide [Esidrix], furosemide [Lasix], bumetanide [Bumex], torsemide [Demadex]). Individuals on medications promoting water loss should be monitored for dehydration and electrolyte imbalance. Other dietary factors that have long been viewed as diuretics are alcohol and caffeine. However, recent studies evaluating hydration status in individuals consuming caffeinated and noncaffeinated beverages did not differ, indicating that caffeine did not negatively affect total water balance when consumed in moderation.[5,6] Although alcohol does acutely increase urine output after ingestion (within the first 3 hours), the long-term (up to 12 hours) effect is antidiuretic.[7] Thus alcohol intake does not appear to cause total body fluid loss over a 24-hour period (see the Drug-Nutrient Interaction box, "Drug Effects on Water and Electrolyte Balance").

Dehydration

Dehydration is the excessive loss of total body water. Relative severity can be measured in terms of percent total body weight loss with symptoms apparent after 2% of normal weight is lost. Initial symptoms include thirst, headache, decreased urine output, dry mouth, and dizziness. As the condition worsens, symptoms can progress to visual impairment, hypotension, loss of appetite, muscle weakness, kidney failure, and seizures. Chronic or severe dehydration is known to increase resting heart rate; contribute to kidney infections, gallstones, and constipation; and adversely influence cognitive function, exercise performance, and the maintenance of body temperature (thermoregulation).[2,8-12] Dehydration weight loss greater than 20% usually is fatal.

Dehydration presents special concerns in elderly adults. The hypothalamus is the regulatory center for thirst, hunger, body temperature, water balance, and blood pressure. However, physiologic changes in the hypothalamus naturally occur with age and, as a result, elderly individuals exhibit an overall decreased thirst sensation and reduced fluid intake when dehydrated as

---

homeostasis the state of relative dynamic equilibrium within the body's internal environment; a balance achieved through the operation of various interrelated physiologic mechanisms.

polarity interaction between the positively charged end of one molecule to the negative end of another or the same molecule.

diuretic any substance that induces urination and subsequent fluid loss.

DRUG-NUTRIENT INTERACTION

DRUG EFFECTS ON WATER AND ELECTROLYTE BALANCE

Some medications can affect fluid and electrolyte balance. Anticholinergics such as amitriptyline (Elavil) and chlorpromazine (Thorazine) may result in a thickening of the saliva and dry mouth. Individuals using these mediations should be advised to increase fluid intake on a regular basis.

Antidepressants such as lithium carbonate (Lithane, Lithobid, Lithonate, Lithotabs, Eskalith) can cause a metallic taste, nausea, vomiting, and dry mouth. Patients can avoid some of the negative side effects by drinking 2 to 3 L water per day and maintaining a consistent sodium intake.

Corticosteroids such as prednisone, methylprednisolone, and hydrocortisone increase the excretion of several nutrients, including potassium. Patients should be encouraged to increase their daily intake of fluids and foods high in potassium to maintain adequate body balance.

Loop diuretics (Lasix) and *Thiazide diuretics* (hydrochlorothiazide) are both used to treat hypertension by increasing urinary excretion of fluids. Along with fluid excretion, minerals are lost in the urine as well. Patients are recommended to increase fresh fruit and vegetables in the diet as well as other foods that are a good source of potassium. Even though sodium and chloride also are lost in the urine, it is not necessary to increase the intake of these electrolytes as long as the individual is consuming a normal varied diet.

Potassium-sparing diuretics (Triamterene) also work to rid the body of excess fluids, but they do so without wasting potassium in the urine. Therefore patients should be careful not to use potassium-based salt substitutes to avoid hyperkalemia (excessively high potassium in the blood).

---

compared to younger adults.[13] Other physiologic changes, such as diminishing kidney function, accompany the aging process and may cause additional losses of body fluid. The average daily intake of *total* water declines from 3848 mL/day for men ages 31 to 50 years to 2994 mL/day for men older than 71 years (see the Clinical Applications box, "Adverse Effects of Progressive Dehydration").[4]

Water Intoxication

Although not nearly as common, water intoxication from overconsumption can occur. Excessive intake of plain water may result in the dangerous condition of hyponatremia (low serum sodium levels of less than 136 mEq/L). Under normal situations, excess water consumed is lost

CLINICAL APPLICATIONS

ADVERSE EFFECTS OF PROGRESSIVE DEHYDRATION

As little as a 3% loss of total body weight from dehydration can result in impaired physical performance. Physical performance is relative to the individual in question. A runner who is progressively losing body water in the form of sweat, without appropriate fluid replacements, will likely suffer from decreased speed or endurance. However, an elderly person who also has lost 3% of his or her body weight may suffer dramatically more complicated physical impairments, such as a fall.

Individuals with fever, diarrhea, and vomiting can lose body weight in the form of fluids quite rapidly. Likewise, the risk of dehydration increases in hot, humid environments and at altitudes greater than 8200 feet.* The figure shown in this box demonstrates progressive complications associated with total body water loss. Note that the thirst response is not present until approximately 0.5% total body weight loss. This is why solely relying on thirst for an indication of fluid needs is not the most sensitive indicator. By the time you are thirsty, you have already lost precious body water.

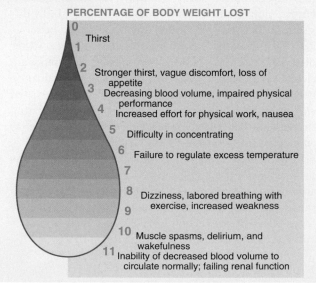

PERCENTAGE OF BODY WEIGHT LOST

0
Thirst
1
2 Stronger thirst, vague discomfort, loss of appetite
3 Decreasing blood volume, impaired physical performance
4 Increased effort for physical work, nausea
5 Difficulty in concentrating
6 Failure to regulate excess temperature
7
8 Dizziness, labored breathing with exercise, increased weakness
9
10 Muscle spasms, delirium, and wakefulness
11 Inability of decreased blood volume to circulate normally; failing renal function

*Food and Nutrition Board, Institute of Medicine: *Dietary reference intakes for water, potassium, sodium, chloride, and sulfate,* Washington, DC, 2004, National Academies Press. Illustration reprinted from Mahan LK, Escott-Stumps: *Krause's food and nutrition therapy,* ed 12, Philadelphia, 2008, Saunders.

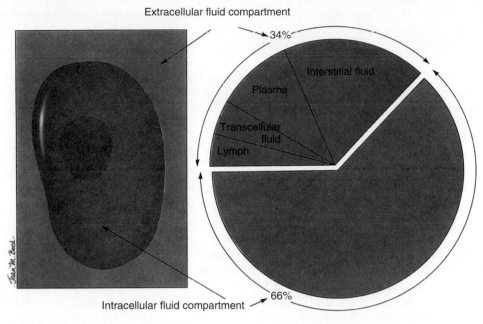

Figure 9-1 Distribution of total body water. (Reprinted from Thibodeau GA, Patton KT: *Anatomy & physiology*, ed 6, St Louis, 2007, Mosby.)

by increased urine output and is not likely to pose a problem for a normal healthy person eating an otherwise typical diet. However, individuals with renal insufficiency or neurologic disorders affecting the thirst mechanism and those participating in heavy endurance exercise may not be able to dilute and/or excrete urine appropriately.

As blood volume is diluted with excess water, the water moves to the intracellular fluid spaces to reestablish equilibrium with sodium concentrations there, thus diluting intracellular fluid as well. This movement causes edema, lung congestion, and muscle weakness. Individuals at risk from hyponatremia from water intoxication are infants (if forced by an adult), psychiatric patients with polydipsia, patients on psychotropic drugs, and individuals participating in prolonged endurance events without fluid and electrolyte replacement.[2]

THE HUMAN WATER BALANCE SYSTEM

Body Water: The Solvent

Amount and Distribution

Normal body water content ranges from 45% to 75% of the total body weight in adults. Men generally have 10% more body water than women, averaging 60% and 50% total body weight, respectively. Differences generally are attributable to a higher ratio of muscle to fat mass in males. Muscle contains significantly more water than does adipose tissue.

Total body water is categorized into two major *compartments* (Figure 9-1).

Extracellular Fluid. The total body water outside the cell is called the *extracellular fluid* (ECF). This water collectively makes up approximately 20% of the total body *weight* and 34% of total body *water*. One fourth of the ECF (4% to 5% of the total body weight) is contained in the blood plasma, or *intravascular*, compartment. The remaining three fourths (15% of the total body *weight*) is composed of the following: (1) water surrounding the cells and bathing the tissues *(interstitial fluid)*, (2) water within the lymphatic circulation, and (3) water moving through the body in various tissue secretions *(transcellular fluid)*. Interstitial fluid circulation helps move materials in and out of body cells. Transcellular fluid is the smallest component of ECF and is 2.5% of total body *water*. Transcellular fluid consists of water within the GI tract, cerebrospinal fluid, ocular and joint fluid, and urine within the bladder.

polydipsia **excessive thirst and drinking.**

Intracellular Fluid. Total body water inside cells is called the *intracellular fluid* (ICF). This water collectively amounts to roughly twice that outside the cells, making up approximately 40% to 45% of the total body *weight* and 66% of total body *water*.

The relative amounts of water in the different body water compartments are compared in Table 9-2.

Overall Water Balance. Water enters and leaves the body by various routes controlled by basic mechanisms such as thirst and hormones. The average adult metabolizes 2.5 to 3 L of water per day in a balance between intake and output.

Water Intake. Water enters the body in three main forms: (1) as preformed water in liquids that are consumed, (2) as preformed water in foods that are eaten, and (3) as a product of cell oxidation when nutrients are burned in the body for energy (i.e., metabolic water or "water of oxidation") (Figure 9-2). The average water intake through fluids of adult men and women are 3 L/day (approximately 13 cups) and 2.2 L/day (approximately 9 cups), respectively.[4] Table 9-3 provides a list of foods with high water content.

Older adults are at higher risk for dehydration because of inadequate intake and physiologic changes associated with aging. As a result, many older persons have dry mouth, xerostomia, caused by severe reduction in the flow of saliva, which in turn affects their food intake. This condition may be associated with the use of certain medi-cations, diseases or conditions, or radiation therapy to the head and neck. Conscious attention to adequate fluid intake (i.e., not less than the recommended minimum of 1500 to 2000 mL/day) is an important part of health maintenance and care. Fluid intake should not depend on thirst because the thirst sensation is an indicator of present dehydration instead of a warning in advance.

Water Output. Water leaves the body through the kidneys, skin, lungs, and feces (see Figure 9-2). Of these output routes, the largest amount of water exits through the kidneys. A certain amount of water must be excreted as urine to rid the body of metabolic waste. This is called *obligatory* water loss because it is compulsory for survival. The kidneys also may put out an additional amount of water each day depending on body activities, needs, and intake. This additional water loss varies according to the climate and physical activity. On average, the daily water output from the body totals approximately 2600 mL, which balances the average intake of water.

Table 9-4 summarizes the comparative intake and output of body water balance.

Solute Particles in Solution

The solutes in body water are a variety of particles in varying concentrations. Two main types of particles control water balance in the body: electrolytes and plasma protein.

TABLE 9-2

VOLUMES OF BODY FLUID COMPARTMENTS*

BODY FLUID	INFANT	ADULT MALE	ADULT FEMALE
ECF			
Plasma	4	4	4
Interstitial fluid	26	16	11
ICF	45	40	35
Total	75	60	50

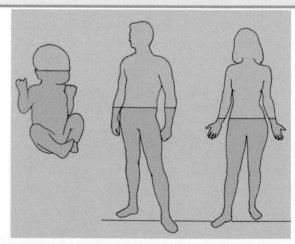

(Copyright JupiterImages Corporation.)

Reprinted from Thibodeau GA, Patton KT: *Anatomy & physiology*, ed 6, St Louis, 2007, Mosby. Illustration copyright Rolin Graphics.
*Percentage of body weight.

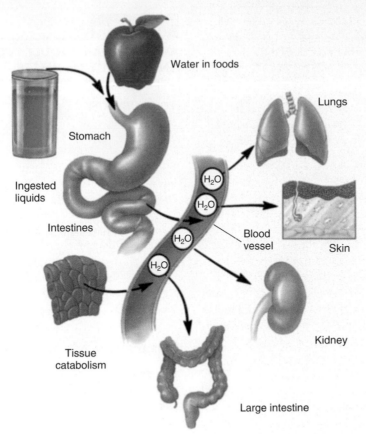

Figure 9-2 Sources of fluid intake and output. (Reprinted from Thibodeau GA, Patton KT: *Anatomy & physiology*, ed 6, St Louis, 2007, Mosby.)

no carbon
positive or
negative electrical
charge

Electrolytes

Electrolytes are small, inorganic substances (i.e., either single-mineral elements or small compounds) that can dissociate or break apart in solution and carry an electrical charge. These charged particles are called *ions*. In any chemical solution, separate particles are constantly in balance between cations and anions to maintain electrical neutrality.

Cations. Cations are ions carrying a positive charge (e.g., sodium [Na^+], potassium [K^+], calcium [Ca^{2+}], and magnesium [Mg^{2+}]).

Anions. Anions are ions carrying a negative charge (e.g., chloride [Cl^-], bicarbonate [HCO_3^-], phosphate [PO_4^{3-}], and sulfate [SO_4^{2-}]).

The constant balance between electrolytes—namely Na^+ and K^+—maintains electrochemical and cell membrane potentials. Because of their small size, electrolytes can freely diffuse across most membranes of the body, thereby maintaining a constant balance between the intracellular and extracellular electrical charge. Fluid and

electrolyte balance is intimately related, so an imbalance in one produces an imbalance in the other.

Electrolyte concentrations in body fluids are measured in terms of *milliequivalents* (mEq). Milliequivalents represent the number of ionic charges or electrovalent bonds in a solution. The number of milliequivalents of an ion in a liter of solution is expressed as mEq/L. Table 9-5 outlines the balance between cations and anions in the ICF and ECF compartments, which are exactly balanced.

Plasma Proteins

Plasma proteins, mainly in the form of albumin and globulin, are organic compounds of large molecular size. They do not move as freely across membranes as electro-

---

xerostomia condition of dry mouth from a lack of saliva. Saliva production can be hindered by certain diseases, such as diabetes or Parkinson's disease, or by some prescription and over-the-counter medications.

TABLE 9-3

WATER CONTENT OF SELECTED FOOD

FOOD	% WATER
Apple, raw	86
Apricot, raw	86
Banana, raw	75
Bread, white	36
Bread, whole wheat	38
Broccoli, cooked	89
Cantaloupe, raw	90
Carrots, raw	88
Cheese, cheddar	37
Cheese, cottage	79
Chicken, roasted	64
Corn, cooked	70
Grapes, raw	81
Lettuce, iceberg	96
Macaroni/spaghetti, cooked	66
Mango, raw	82
Orange, raw	87
Peach, raw	89
Pear, raw	84
Pickle	92
Pineapple, raw	86
Potato, baked	75
Squash, cooked	94
Steak, tenderloin, cooked	50
Sweet potato, boiled	80
Turkey, roasted	62

Modified from Food and Nutrition Board, Institute of Medicine: *Dietary Reference Intakes for water, potassium, sodium, chloride, and sulfate*, Washington, DC, 2004, National Academies Press.

TABLE 9-4

AVERAGE DAILY ADULT INTAKE AND OUTPUT OF WATER

FORM OF WATER	INTAKE (mL/Day)	BODY PART	OUTPUT (mL/Day)
Preformed		Lungs	350
Liquids	1500	Skin	
In foods	700	Diffusion	350
Metabolism	200	Sweat	100
(oxidation		Kidneys	1400
of food)		Feces	1200
Total	2400	Total	2400

Modified from Thibodeau GA, Patton KT: *Anatomy & physiology*, ed 6, St Louis, 2007, Mosby.

Separating Membranes

Two types of membranes separate and contain water throughout the body: the capillary membrane and cell membrane.

Capillary Membrane

The walls of capillaries are thin and porous. Therefore water molecules and small particles can move freely across them. Such small particles, having free passage across capillary walls, include electrolytes and various nutrient materials. However, larger particles such as plasma protein molecules cannot pass through small pores in the capillary membrane. These larger molecules remain in the capillary vessel and exert COP to bring water and small molecules back into the capillary.

Cell Membrane

Cell membranes are specially constructed to protect and nourish the cell contents. Although water is freely permeable, other molecules or ions use channels within the phospholipid bilayer for passage across the membrane. The membrane channels, or tunnels, are highly specific to the molecules allowed to pass. For example, sodium channels only allow Na^+ and chloride channels only allow Cl^- to pass.

Forces Moving Water and Solutes across Membranes

A variety of forces are at work in the cell membrane to allow dynamic equilibrium.

lytes, which are much smaller. Thus plasma protein molecules are retained in blood vessels, controlling water movement in the body and maintaining blood volume by influencing the shift of water in and out of capillaries in balance with the surrounding water. In this function, plasma proteins are called *colloids*, which exert colloidal osmotic pressure (COP) to maintain integrity of the blood volume. Cellular proteins help guard cell water in a similar manner.

Small Organic Compounds

In addition to electrolytes and plasma protein, other small organic compounds are dissolved in body water. However, their concentration ordinarily is too small to influence shifts of water. However, in some instances they are found in abnormally large concentrations and do influence water movement. For example, glucose is a small particle circulating in body fluids, but it can increase water loss from the body, a condition known as polyuria, when it is in abnormally high concentrations (e.g., in uncontrolled diabetes).

TABLE 9-5

BALANCE OF CATION AND ANION CONCENTRATIONS IN ECF AND ICF

ELECTROLYTE	ECF (mEq/L)	ICF (mEq/L)
Cation		
Na^+	142	35
K^+	5	123
Ca^{2+}	5	15
Mg^{2+}	3	2
Total	155	175
Anion		
Cl^-	104	5
PO_4^{3-}	2	80
SO_4^{2-}	1	10
Protein	16	70
CO_3^{2-}	27	10
Organic acids	5	
Total	155	175

This balance maintains electro-neutrality within each compartment.

Osmosis

Osmosis is the movement of water molecules from an area with low solute concentration to an area with high solute concentration. When solutions of different concentrations exist on either side of selectively permeable membranes, the osmotic pressure moves water across the membrane to help equalize the solutions on both sides. Therefore osmosis can be defined as the force that moves water molecules from an area of greater concentration of water molecules (i.e., with fewer particles in solution) to an area of lesser concentration of water molecules (i.e., with more particles in solution). Figure 9-3 illustrates how water will move from the 10% glucose solution across the semipermeable membrane to the 20% glucose solution to equalize the solute concentrations. Because the membrane is permeable to glucose, the amount of glucose also will change on either side of the membrane to establish equilibrium.

Diffusion

As osmosis applies to water molecules, diffusion applies to the particles in solution. Simple diffusion is the force by which these particles move outward in all directions from an area of greater concentration of particles to an area of lesser concentration of particles (see Chapter 5). The relative movement of water molecules and solute particles by osmosis and diffusion effectively balances solution concentrations, and hence pressures, on both sides of the membrane. The two balancing forces of osmosis and diffusion are shown in Figure 9-4.

Facilitated Diffusion

Facilitated diffusion follows the same principles of simple diffusion in that particles passively move down a concentration gradient. The only difference is that with facilitated diffusion membrane transporters assist particles in crossing the membrane. Some molecules, such as glucose, can diffuse across the cell membrane by either simple diffusion or facilitated diffusion but move much faster with the help of a transporter.

Filtration

Water is forced, or filtered, through the pores of membranes when the pressure outside the membrane is different. This difference in pressure results from the differences in the particle concentrations of the two solutions, causing water and small particles to move back and forth between capillaries and cells according to shifting pressures to establish homeostasis.

Active Transport

Particles in solution that are vital to body processes must move across membranes throughout the body at all times, even when the pressures are against their flow. Thus some type of energy-driven active transport is necessary to carry these particles "upstream" across separating membranes. Such active transport mechanisms usually require a carrier to help ferry the particles across the membrane (see Chapter 5).

Pinocytosis

Sometimes larger particles, such as proteins and fats, enter absorbing cells by the process of pinocytosis (Figure 9-5). In this process, larger molecules attach themselves to the thicker cell membrane and are then engulfed by the cell. In this way they are encased in a vacuole, which is a

---

colloidal osmotic pressure (COP) fluid pressure produced by protein molecules in the plasma and cell. Because proteins are large molecules, they do not pass through the separating membranes of the capillary walls. Thus they remain in their respective compartments, exerting a constant osmotic pull that protects vital plasma and cell fluid volumes in these areas.

polyuria excess water loss through urination.

osmosis passage of a solvent, such as water, through a membrane that separates solutions of different concentrations, tending to equalize the concentration pressures of the solutions on either side of the membrane.

osmotic pressure pressure produced as a result of osmosis across a semipermeable membrane.

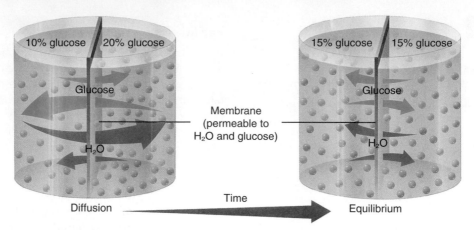

Figure 9-3 Diffusion through a membrane. Note that the membrane separating a 10% glucose solution from a 20% glucose solution allows glucose and water to pass. The container on the *left* shows the two solutions separated by the membrane at the start of diffusion. The container on the *right* shows the result of diffusion after time. (Reprinted from Thibodeau GA, Patton KT: *Anatomy & physiology*, ed 6, St Louis, 2007, Mosby.)

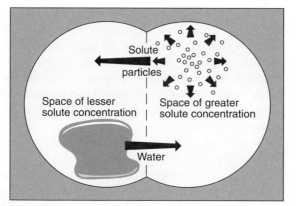

Figure 9-4 Movement of molecules, water, and solutes by osmosis and diffusion.

small space or cavity formed in the protoplasm of the cell. In this small cavity, nutrient particles are carried across the cell membrane and into the cell. Once inside the cell, the vacuole opens and cell enzymes metabolize the particles. Pinocytosis is one of the basic mechanisms by which fat is absorbed from the small intestine.

Tissue Water Circulation: The Capillary Fluid Shift Mechanism

One of the body's most important controls in maintaining overall water balance is the *capillary fluid shift mechanism*. This mechanism operates a balancing act between opposing fluid pressures to nourish the life of the cell.

Purpose

Water and other nutrients constantly circulate through the body tissues by way of blood vessels. However, to nourish cells the water and nutrients must get out of

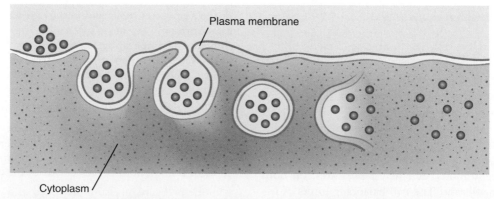

Figure 9-5 Pinocytosis, engulfing a large molecule by the cell.

the blood vessels—the capillaries—and into the cells. Water and cell metabolites, products of metabolism leaving the cell, must then get back into the capillaries to circulate throughout the body. In other words, essential water, nutrients, and oxygen must be pushed out of blood circulation into tissue circulation to distribute their goods throughout the body; then water, cell metabolites, and carbon dioxide must be pulled back into blood circulation to dispose of metabolic wastes through the kidneys or lungs. The body maintains this constant flow of water through the tissues, carrying materials to and from the cells, by means of opposing fluid pressures: (1) *hydrostatic pressure,* an intracapillary blood pressure from the contracting heart muscle pushing blood into circulation; and (2) COP, pressure from the plasma proteins drawing tissue fluids back into ongoing circulation. A *filtration* process operates according to the differences in osmotic pressure on either side of the capillary membrane.

Process

When blood first enters the capillary system from the larger vessels coming from the heart—the arterioles—the greater blood pressure from the heart forces water and small particles (e.g., glucose) into the tissues to bathe and nourish the cells. This force of blood pressure is an example of *hydrostatic* pressure. Plasma protein particles, however, are too large to go through the pores of capillary membranes. When the circulating tissue fluids are ready to reenter the blood capillaries, the initial blood pressure has diminished. The COP of the concentrated protein particles remaining in the capillary vessel is now the greater influence. Colloidal osmotic pressure draws water and its metabolites back into the capillary circulation after having served the cells and carries them to larger vessels—the venules—for blood circulation back to the heart. A small amount of normal turgor pressure from the resisting tissue of the capillary membrane remains the same and operates throughout the system. This fundamental fluid shift mechanism constantly controls water balance through its capillary-tissue circulation to nourish cells all over the body. This vital fluid flow through tissue is maintained by the balance between blood pressure and the osmotic pressure of the plasma protein particles (Figure 9-6).

Organ Systems Involved

In addition to blood circulation, the human water balance system uses two other major organ systems to control the overall water balance of the body: the GI circulation, which supports digestion and absorption of

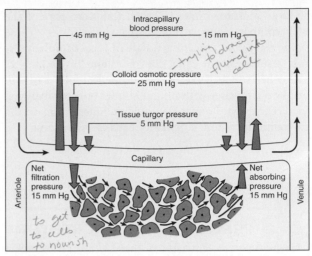

Figure 9-6 The fluid shift mechanism. Note the balance of pressures that controls the flow of fluid.

nutrients, and the renal circulation, which maintains normal blood levels of various nutrients and metabolites.

Gastrointestinal Circulation

Secretions aiding in the process of digestion and absorption include saliva, gastric juice, bile, pancreatic juice, and intestinal juice. Of these secretions, all but bile are predominately water. In the latter portion of the intestine, most of the water and electrolytes are then reabsorbed into the blood to circulate over and over again. This constant movement of a large volume of water and its electrolytes among the blood, cells, and GI tract is called *GI circulation.* The sheer magnitude of this vital GI circulation, as shown in Table 9-6, indicates the seriousness of fluid loss from the upper or lower portion of the GI tract. This circulation is maintained in *isotonicity* with the surrounding extracellular water and carries risk for clinical imbalances.

TABLE 9-6	

APPROXIMATE TOTAL VOLUME OF DIGESTIVE SECRETIONS

SECRETION	VOLUME (mL)
Saliva	1500
Gastric	2500
Bile	500
Pancreatic	700
Intestinal	3000
Total	8200

Produced in 24 hours by an adult of average size.

Law of Isotonicity. The GI fluids are part of the ECF compartments, which also includes blood. These fluids are *isotonic*, meaning a state of equal osmotic pressure resulting from equal concentrations of electrolytes and other solute particles. For example, when a person drinks plain water without any solutes or accompanying food, electrolytes and salts enter the intestine from the surrounding blood supply to equalize pressures. If a concentrated solution of food is ingested, additional water is then drawn into the intestine from the surrounding blood to dilute the intestinal contents. In each instance, water and electrolytes move among the parts of the ECF compartment to maintain solutions that are isotonic in the GI tract with the surrounding fluid (see the Clinical Applications box, "Principles of Oral Rehydration Therapy").

CLINICAL APPLICATIONS

PRINCIPLES OF ORAL REHYDRATION THERAPY

The principles of electrolyte absorption dictate rehydration methods for children with diarrhea. Although diarrhea usually is considered a trivial problem in developed countries, it is responsible for the deaths of one fourth to one half of all children younger than 4 years worldwide. Although 90% of the deaths from diarrhea are associated with fluid loss, the mere provision of water alone can be dangerous.

Intravenous (IV) therapy, developed by Darrow in the 1940s, provided sodium chloride—a base—and potassium in water and proved very successful. Unfortunately, however, IV therapy is not readily available to those who need it most. A large number of isolated, poor, rural families in both developed and developing countries do not have access to health care facilities. Fortunately, though, the World Health Organization has developed a means of oral rehydration therapy that is much less expensive and is being used in the United States as well as in developing countries. If safe drinking water is available, the rehydration solution can be mixed at home under the guidance of a public health worker and administered by a family member. The ingredients are 1 L safe water, 3.5 g sodium chloride (table salt), 2.5 g sodium bicarbonate (baking soda), 1.5 g potassium chloride (or salt substitute such as Diamond Crystal or Morton Salt Substitute), and 20 g glucose (1½ Tbsp sugar). This combination is based on principles of sodium absorption in the small intestine.

A premade formula such as Pedialyte (Abbott Laboratories, Abbott Park, Ill.) also is appropriate.

Transport of Metabolic Compounds
A number of metabolic compounds—principally glucose but also certain amino acids, dipeptides, and disaccharides—depend on sodium to cross the intestinal wall.

Additive Effects
The rate at which sodium is absorbed depends on the presence of substances such as glucose or other protein metabolic products. The more substances present, the better the absorption of sodium.

Water Absorption
The rate of water absorption is enhanced as sodium absorption improves. Thus a solution of sodium and potassium salts plus glucose can be given orally.

In addition to oral rehydration therapy, infants and older children with acute diarrhea should continue to eat well-tolerated foods. Fasting practices were based on the former belief that recovery is more effective if the bowel is allowed to rest and heal. To the contrary, children should be fed their regular age-appropriate diets (e.g., breast milk, formula, or solid foods), allowed to determine the amount of food they need, and given extra food as the diarrhea subsides to recover nutritional deficits. Food choices should be guided by individual tolerances. Use of the BRAT diet (bananas, rice, applesauce, and tea or toast) is not recommended because it does not include typical foods consumed by infants and small children and only worsens the energy-nutrient decline.

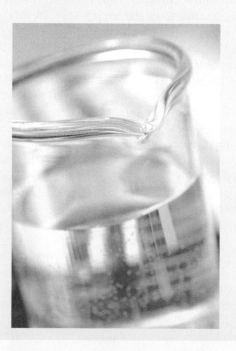

Clinical Applications. Because of the large amounts of water and electrolytes involved, upper and lower GI losses are the most common cause of clinical fluid and electrolyte problems. Such problems exist, for example, in cases of persistent vomiting or prolonged diarrhea, in which large amounts of water and electrolytes are lost. The large concentration of electrolytes involved in the GI circulation is shown in Table 9-7.

Renal Circulation

The kidneys maintain appropriate levels of all constituents of blood by filtering it and then selectively reabsorbing water and needed materials to be carried throughout the body. Through this continual "laundering" of the blood by the millions of nephrons in the kidneys, water balance and the proper solution of blood are maintained. When disease occurs in the kidneys and this filtration process does not operate normally, water imbalances occur (see Chapter 21).

Hormonal Controls

Two basic hormonal controls operate in the kidneys to help maintain constant body water balance.

Antidiuretic Hormone Mechanism. Antidiuretic hormone (ADH), also called *vasopressin,* is synthesized by the hypothalamus and stored in the pituitary gland for release. ADH is water conserving and works on the kidneys' nephrons to induce reabsorption of water. In any stressful situation with threatened or real loss of body water, this hormone is released to conserve body water.

Aldosterone Hormone Mechanism. The hormone *aldosterone* is produced by the adrenal glands, which are located on top of each kidney, in response to a reduced renal filtration rate or decreased sodium level. Aldosterone triggers the kidneys' nephrons to reabsorb sodium. Therefore it primarily is a sodium-conserving mechanism, but it also exerts a secondary control over water reabsorption because water follows sodium. Both ADH and aldosterone may be activated by stressful situations, such as body injury or surgery.

TABLE 9-7

APPROXIMATE CONCENTRATION OF CERTAIN ELECTROLYTES IN DIGESTIVE FLUIDS (mEq/L)

SECRETION	Na$^+$	K$^+$	CL$^-$	HCO
Saliva	10	25	10	15
Gastric	40	10	145	0
Pancreatic	140	5	40	110
Jejunal	135	5	110	30
Bile	140	10	110	40

HUMAN ACID-BASE BALANCE SYSTEM

The optimal degree of acidity or alkalinity must be maintained in body fluids to support human life. This vital balance is achieved by chemical and physiologic buffer systems.

Acids and Bases

The concept of acids and bases relates to *hydrogen* ion concentration. Acidity is expressed in terms of pH. The abbreviation *pH* is derived from a mathematical term that refers to the power of the hydrogen ion concentration. A pH of 7 is the neutral point between an acid and a base. Because pH is a negative mathematical factor, the higher the hydrogen ion concentration (more acid), the lower the pH number; conversely, the lower the hydrogen ion concentration (less acid), the higher the pH number. Substances with a pH *less than* 7 are *acid* and substances with a pH *higher than* 7 are *alkaline.*

Acids

An acid is defined as a compound that has more hydrogen ions—enough to releases extra hydrogen ions when in solution.

Bases

A base is a compound that has fewer hydrogen ions. Thus in solution it accepts hydrogen ions, effectively reducing the solution's acidity.

Acids and bases are a normal by-product of nutrient absorption and metabolism. As such, mechanisms to reestablish equilibrium within the body are constantly at work. Box 9-1 lists various sources of acids and bases.

Acid-Base Buffer System

The body deals with degrees of acidity by maintaining buffer systems to handle an excess of either acid or base. The human body contains many buffer systems because only a relatively narrow range of pH is compatible with life (7.35 to 7.45).

Chemical Buffer System

A chemical buffer system is a mixture of acidic and alkaline components, an acid and a base partner, that together protect a solution from wide variations in its pH, even when strong bases or acids are added to it. For example, if a strong acid is added to a buffered solution, the base partner reacts with the acid to form a weaker acid. If a strong base is added to the solution, the acid partner

BOX 9-1

SOURCES OF ACIDS AND BASES

Acids
Carbonic acid and lactic acid: aerobic and anaerobic metabolism of glucose
Sulfuric acid: oxidation of sulfur-containing amino acids
Phosphoric acid: oxidation of phosphoproteins for energy
Ketone bodies: incomplete oxidation of fat for energy
Minerals: chlorine, sulfur, phosphorus

Bases
Minerals: potassium, calcium, sodium, magnesium
Sodium bicarbonate
Calcium carbonate

combines with the intruder to form a weaker base. The carbonic acid (H_2CO_3)/base bicarbonate ($NaHCO_3$) buffer system is the body's main buffer system for the following reasons.

Available Materials. The raw materials for producing carbonic acid (H_2CO_3) are readily available [water (H_2O) and carbon dioxide (CO_2)].

Base/Acid Ratio. The bicarbonate buffer system is able to maintain this essential degree of acidity in the body fluids because bicarbonate (basic) is approximately 20 times more abundant than carbonic acid. This *20:1 ratio* is maintained even though the absolute amounts of the two partners may fluctuate during adjustment periods. Whether or not added base or acid enters the system, as long as the 20:1 ratio is maintained, over time the ECF pH is held constant.

Physiologic Buffer Systems

When chemical buffers cannot reestablish equilibrium, the respiratory and renal systems will respond.

Respiratory Control of pH. With every breath, CO_2 (an acid), leaves the body. Therefore changes in respiration rates can either increase or decrease the loss of acids. Hyperventilation (increasing the depth and rate of breathing) increases the release of CO_2, thus combating acidosis. Conversely, hypoventilation (slowing down the depth and pace of breathing) retains CO_2, which ultimately increases the acidity of blood to alleviate alkalosis.

Urinary Control of pH. In the event that chemical buffer systems and the respiratory buffer system do not reestablish blood pH, the kidneys can adapt by excreting more or less hydrogen ions. If blood pH is too acidic, the kidneys will accept more hydrogen ions from blood in exchange for a sodium ion. Because sodium ions are basic, blood is losing an acid (H^+) while gaining a base, thus increasing blood pH back to normal.

Chemical and physiologic buffer systems are critical for maintaining the blood pH within an acceptable range for life.

acidosis blood pH less than 7.35. Respiratory acidosis is caused from an accumulation of carbon dioxide (an acid). Metabolic acidosis may be cause by a variety of conditions resulting in excess accumulation of acids in the body or from a significant loss of bicarbonate (base).

alkalosis blood pH greater than 7.45. Respiratory alkalosis is caused from hyperventilation and excess loss of carbon dioxide. Metabolic alkalosis is seen with extensive vomiting in which significant amounts of bicarbonate are secreted (a base).

SUMMARY

The human body is approximately 50% to 60% water. The primary functions of body water are to provide the water environment necessary for cell work, act as a transporter, control body temperature, and lubricate moving parts. Body water is distributed in two collective body water compartments: ICF and ECF. The water inside cells is the larger portion, accounting for approximately 40% to 45% of the total body weight. The water outside cells consists of the fluid in spaces between cells (e.g., interstitial and lymph fluid), blood plasma, secretions in transit (e.g., GI circulation), and a smaller amount of fluid in cartilage and bone.

The overall water balance of the body is maintained by fluid intake and output. Two types of solute particles control the distribution of body water: (1) electrolytes, mainly charged mineral elements, and (2) plasma protein, chiefly albumin. These solute particles influence the movement of water across cell or capillary membranes, allowing tissue circulation to nourish cells.

The acid-base buffer system, which is mainly controlled by the lungs and kidneys, uses electrolytes and hydrogen ions to maintain a normal ECF pH of approximately 7.4. This pH level is necessary to sustain life.

CRITICAL THINKING QUESTIONS

1. If a large amount of dietary sodium were consumed in one day, what effect would that likely have on total body water, and which compartment would be most affected?

2. Define the term *homeostasis*. Give examples of how this state is maintained in the body.

3. Describe five factors that influence water requirements. List and describe four functions of body water.

4. Apply your knowledge of the capillary fluid shift mechanism to account for the gross body edema seen in malnourished individuals.

CHAPTER CHALLENGE QUESTIONS

Matching
Match the terms provided with the corresponding items listed in the following.

DEFINITIONS

1. Chief electrolyte guarding the water outside cells

2. An ion carrying a negative electrical charge

3. Sodium-conserving mechanism or control agent

4. Simple passage of water molecules through a membrane separating solutions of different concentrations from the side of lower concentration of solute particles to that of higher concentration of particles, thus tending to equalize the solutions

5. A substance (element or compound) that, in solution, conducts an electrical current and is dissociated into cations and anions

6. Particles in solution, such as electrolytes and protein

7. State of dynamic equilibrium maintained by an organism among all its parts and controlled by many finely balanced mechanisms

8. Chief electrolyte guarding the water inside cells

9. Major plasma protein that guards and maintains blood volume

10. Fluid located inside the cell wall

11. An ion carrying a positive electrical charge

12. The body's method of maintaining tissue water circulation by opposing fluid pressures

13. Force exerted by a contained fluid (e.g., blood pressure)

14. Movement of particles throughout a solution and across membranes outward from the area of denser concentration of particles to all surrounding spaces

15. A type of fluid outside cells

16. Movement of particles in solution across cell membranes and against normal osmotic pressures, involving a carrier and energy for the work

TERMS

a. Osmosis
b. Solutes
c. Diffusion
d. Cation
e. Interstitial fluid
f. Homeostasis
g. Anion
h. Potassium
i. Albumin
j. Hydrostatic pressure
k. Sodium
l. Electrolyte
m. Active transport
n. Aldosterone
o. Capillary fluid shift mechanism
p. ICF

evolve Please refer to the Students' Resource section of this text's Evolve Web site for additional study resources.

REFERENCES

1. Cannon WB: *The wisdom of the body*, New York, 1932, W.W. Norton.
2. Food and Nutrition Board, Institute of Medicine: *Dietary reference Intakes for water, potassium, sodium, chloride, and sulfate*, Washington, DC, 2004, National Academies Press.
3. Manore MM and others: American College of Sports Medicine, American Dietetic Association, Dietitians of Canada Joint position statement: nutrition and athletic performance, *Med Sci Sports Exerc* 32(12):2130, 2000.
4. U.S. Department of Agriculture, Agricultural Research Service: *Continuing Survey of Food Intakes by Individuals (CSFII)*, 1994-1996, 1998.
5. Millard-Stafford ML and others: Hydration during exercise in warm, humid conditions: effect of a caffeinated sports drink, *Int J Sport Nutr Exerc Metab* 17(2):163, 2007.
6. Grandjean AC and others: The effect of caffeinated, non-caffeinated, caloric and non-caloric beverages on hydration, *J Am Coll Nutr* 19(5):591, 2000.
7. Taivainen H and others: Role of plasma vasopressin in changes of water balance accompanying acute alcohol intoxication, *Alcohol Clin Exp Res* 19(3):759, 1995.
8. Ritz P, Berrut G: The importance of good hydration for day-to-day health, *Nutr Rev* 63(6 Pt 2):S6, 2005.
9. Manz F, Wentz A: The importance of good hydration for the prevention of chronic diseases, *Nutr Rev* 63(6 Pt 2):S2, 2005.
10. Petri NM and others: Effects of voluntary fluid intake deprivation on mental and psychomotor performance, *Croat Med J* 47(6):855, 2006.
11. Baker LB and others: Progressive dehydration causes a progressive decline in basketball skill performance, *Med Sci Sports Exerc* 39(7):1114, 2007.
12. Ebert TR and others: Influence of hydration status on thermoregulation and cycling hill climbing, *Med Sci Sports Exerc* 39(2):323, 2007.
13. Kenney WL, Chiu P: Influence of age on thirst and fluid intake, *Med Sci Sports Exerc* 33(9):1524, 2001.

FURTHER READING AND RESOURCES

The following organizations provide up-to-date recommendations for water and electrolyte balance in addition to a plethora of other health information.

Mayo Clinic, Food and Nutrition: *www.mayoclinic.com/health/water/NU00283*

USDA, Food and Nutrition Information Center: *http://fnic.nal.usda.gov* (use search word "water")

American College of Sports Medicine: *www.acsm.org*

Ritz P, Berrut G: The importance of good hydration for day-to-day health, *Nutr Rev* 63(6 Pt 2):S6, 2005.
   This article discusses the importance of adequate hydration for maintaining health and preventing diseases associated with dehydration.

Ferry M: Strategies for ensuring good hydration in the elderly, *Nutr Rev* 63(6 Pt 2):S22, 2005.
   This article proposes ideas and strategies for ensuring appropriate hydration in the elderly—a population at risk for dehydration.

Robinson JR: Water, the indispensable nutrient, *Nutr Today* 5(1):16, 1970.
   This classic but still current article by a New Zealand physician who is a world authority clearly describes the processes involved in body water balance. This article is filled with excellent charts and diagrams to illustrate key principles.

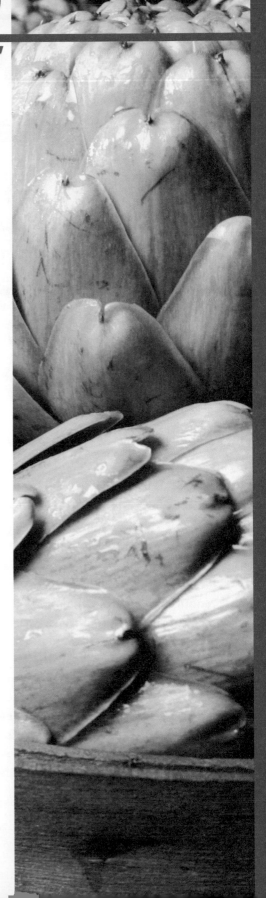

PART 7

Nutrition throughout the Life Cycle

CHAPTER 10

Nutrition during Pregnancy and Lactation

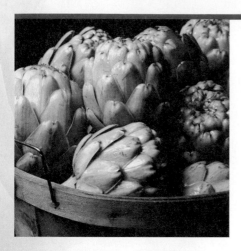

KEY CONCEPTS

- The mother's food habits and nutritional status before conception, as well as during pregnancy, influence the outcome of her pregnancy.
- Pregnancy is a prime example of physiologic synergism in which the mother, fetus, and placenta collaborate to sustain and nurture new life.
- Through the food a pregnant woman eats, she gives her unborn child the nourishment required to begin and support fetal growth and development.
- Through her diet, a breastfeeding mother continues to provide all her nursing baby's nutrition needs.

Healthy body tissues depend directly on essential nutrients in food. This is especially true during pregnancy because a whole new body is being formed. The tremendous growth of a baby from the moment of conception to the time of birth depends entirely on nourishment from the mother. The complex process of rapid human growth demands more nutrients from the mother.

This chapter looks at the beginning of life and how the infant's fetal development and mother's supporting tissues directly relate to the mother's diet. It explores the nutrition needs of pregnancy and the lactation period that follows and recognizes the vital role each plays in producing a healthy infant.

NUTRITIONAL DEMANDS OF PREGNANCY

Not many years ago, traditional practices and diet during pregnancy were highly restrictive in nature, built on assumptions and folklore of the past and having little or no basis in scientific fact. Early obstetricians even supported the notion that semistarvation of the mother during pregnancy was a blessing in disguise because it produced a small, lightweight baby who was easy to deliver. To this end, they used a diet restricted in kilocalories, protein, water, and salt for pregnant women.

Developments in both nutrition and medical science have refuted these ideas and laid a sound base for positive nutrition in current maternal care. However, old dogma dies hard. Shreds of old beliefs are sometimes still evidenced, but it is now known that the mother's and child's health depend on the pregnant woman eating a well-balanced diet with increased amounts of essential nutrients. In fact, women who have always eaten a well-balanced diet are in a good state of nutrition at conception, even before they know they are pregnant. Such women have a better chance of having a healthy baby and remaining in good health than are women who have been undernourished.

The 9 months between conception and the birth of a fully formed baby is a marvelous period of rapid growth and intricate functional development. All these tremendous activities require increased energy and nutrient support to produce a positive, healthy outcome. General guidelines for these increases are provided in the comprehensive DRIs by the National Academy of Sciences.[1-5]

The DRIs are based on general needs for healthy populations. Some women (e.g., those who are poorly nourished when becoming pregnant or those with additional risks) demand more nutrition support. The *Dietary Guidelines for Americans, 2005* also outline specific recommendations for pregnant and lactating women (Box 10-1). This chapter reviews the basic nutrition needs for positive support of a normal pregnancy, with emphasis on critical energy and protein requirements as well as key vitamin and mineral needs. In each case reasons exist for the increased demand, general amount of increase, and food sources to supply it. The following section underscores the importance of sufficient weight gain and the problems facing high-risk mothers and infants.

Energy Needs

Reasons for Increased Need

During pregnancy the mother needs more energy, in the form of kilocalories, for two important reasons: (1) to supply the increased fuel demanded by the metabolic workload for both mother and fetus and (2) to spare protein for the added tissue-building requirements. For these reasons the mother must include more nutrient-dense food into her diet.

Amount of Energy Increase

The national standard recommends an increase of 340 kcal/day during the second trimester and approximately 450 kcal/day during the third trimester of pregnancy.[5] This totals approximately 2200 to 2800 kcal for most women starting with the second trimester of pregnancy, which is approximately a 15% to 20% increase over the energy need of nonpregnant women. Active, large, or nutritionally deficient women may require even more energy. The emphasis always should be on adequate kilocalories to secure nutrient and energy needs of a rapidly growing fetus. Sufficient weight gain is vital to a successful pregnancy; however, excess weight gain can pose risks and should be avoided. Increased complex carbohydrates and protein in the diet are the preferred sources of energy, especially during late pregnancy and lactation.

BOX 10-1

DIETARY GUIDELINES, 2005 FOR SPECIFIC POPULATIONS REGARDING PREGNANCY AND LACTATION

- *Women of childbearing age who may become pregnant:* Eat foods high in heme iron and/or consume iron-rich plant foods or iron-fortified foods with an enhancer of iron absorption, such as vitamin C–rich foods.
- *Women of childbearing age who may become pregnant and those in the first trimester of pregnancy:* Consume adequate synthetic folic acid daily (from fortified foods or supplements) in addition to food forms of folate from a varied diet.
- *Pregnant women:*
  - Ensure appropriate weight gain as specified by a health care provider.
  - In the absence of medical or obstetric complications, incorporate 30 minutes or more of moderate-intensity physical activity on most, if not all, days of the week. Avoid activities with a high risk of falling or abdominal trauma.
- *Breastfeeding women:*
  - Moderate weight reduction is safe and does not compromise weight gain of the nursing infant.
  - Be aware that neither acute nor regular exercise adversely affects the mother's ability to successfully breastfeed.
- *Infants and young children, pregnant women, older adults, and those who are immunocompromised:* Do not eat or drink raw (unpasteurized) milk or any products made from unpasteurized milk, raw or partially cooked eggs or foods containing raw eggs, raw or undercooked meat and poultry, raw or undercooked fish or shellfish, unpasteurized juices, or raw sprouts.
- *Pregnant women, older adults, and those who are immunocompromised:* Only eat certain deli meats and frankfurters that have been reheated to steaming hot.

Reprinted from U.S. Department of Health and Human Services: *Dietary guidelines for Americans, 2005*, Washington, DC, 2005, U.S. Government Printing Office.

Protein Needs

Reasons for Increased Need

Protein serves as the building blocks for the tremendous growth of body tissues during pregnancy, as follows:

- *Rapid growth of the fetus.* The mere increase in size of the fetus from one cell to millions of cells in a 3.2-kg (7-lb) infant in only 9 months indicates the relatively large amount of protein required for such rapid growth.
- *Development of the placenta.* The placenta is the fetus's lifeline to the mother. The mature placenta requires sufficient protein for its complete development as a vital and unique organ to sustain, support, and nourish the fetus during growth.

- *Growth of maternal tissues.* To support pregnancy and lactation, increased development of uterine and breast tissue is required.
- *Increased maternal blood volume.* The mother's blood volume increases 20% to 50% during pregnancy. More circulating blood is necessary to nourish the child and support most of the increased metabolic workload. However, with extra blood volume comes a need for more synthesis of blood components, especially hemoglobin and plasma protein, which are proteins vital to the pregnancy. An increase in hemoglobin helps supply oxygen to the growing number of cells. Meanwhile, plasma protein (albumin) production increases to regulate blood volume through osmotic pressure. Adequate albumin prevents an abnormal accumulation of water in tissues beyond the normal edema of pregnancy.
- *Amniotic fluid.* Amniotic fluid, which contains various proteins, surrounds the fetus during growth and guards it against shock or injury.
- *Storage reserves.* Increased storage reserves of tissue are needed in the mother's body to prepare for the large amount of energy required during labor, delivery, immediate postpartum period, and lactation.

Amount of Protein Increase

Protein intake should increase 25 g/day during pregnancy, on top of nonpregnancy needs.[5] This increase is approximately 50% more than the average adult requirement. However, a large number of high-risk or active pregnant women require even more protein.

Food Sources

The only *complete* protein foods of high biologic value are milk, egg, cheese, soy products, and meat (e.g., beef, poultry, fish, pork). Certain other *incomplete* proteins from plant sources such as legumes and grains contribute additional secondary amounts. Protein-rich foods also contribute other nutrients, such as calcium, iron, and B vitamins. The amount of food from each food group that supplies the needed nutrients is indicated in the sample food plan given in Table 10-1 (see Chapter 4 for a discussion on dietary sources of protein and protein quality).

TABLE 10-1

MyPYRAMID FOOD INTAKE RECOMMENDATIONS FOR WOMEN

| | SINGLE SERVING SIZE EXAMPLES* | CALORIE LEVEL | | | | |
		2400	2600	2800	3000	3200
Fruits	Any fruit or 100% fruit juice counts as part of the fruit group. Fruits may be fresh, canned, frozen, or dried and may be whole, cut up, or pureed. 1 cup of fruit or 100% fruit juice, or ½ cup dried fruit	2 cups/day	2 cups/day	2.5 cups/day	2.5 cups/day	2.5 cups/day
Vegetables, total	Any vegetable or 100% vegetable juice counts as a member of the vegetable group. Vegetables may be raw or cooked; fresh, frozen, canned, or dried/dehydrated; and may be whole, cut up, or mashed 1 cup raw or cooked vegetables or vegetable juice, or 2 cups of raw leafy greens	3 cups/day	3.5 cups/day	3.5 cups/day	4 cups/day	4 cups/day
Specific Recommendations for Each Subgroup of Vegetable, per Week						
Dark-green vegetables	*Examples*: Chinese cabbage, broccoli, collard greens, dark-green leafy, lettuce, kale, mesclun, mustard greens, romaine lettuce, spinach, turnip greens, watercress	3 cups/week	3 cups/week	3 cups/week	3 cups/week	3 cups/week
Orange vegetables	*Examples*: acorn squash, butternut squash, carrots, hubbard squash, pumpkin, sweet potatoes	2 cups/week	2.5 cups/week	2.5 cups/week	2.5 cups/week	2.5 cups/week
Legumes	*Examples*: black beans, black-eyed peas, garbanzo beans (chickpeas), kidney beans, lentils, lima beans (mature), navy beans, pinto beans, soy beans, split peas, tofu (bean curd made from soybeans), white beans	3 cups/week	3.5 cups/week	3.5 cups/week	3.5 cups/week	3.5 cups/week

TABLE 10-1

MyPYRAMID FOOD INTAKE RECOMMENDATIONS FOR WOMEN—*cont'd*

	SINGLE SERVING SIZE EXAMPLES*	2400	2600	2800	3000	3200
Starchy vegetables	*Examples*: corn, green peas, lima beans (green), potatoes	6 cups/week	7 cups/week	7 cups/week	9 cups/week	9 cups/week
Other vegetables	*Examples*: artichokes, asparagus, bean sprouts, beets, Brussels sprouts, cabbage, cauliflower, celery, cucumbers, eggplant, green beans, green or red peppers, iceberg (head) lettuce, mushrooms, okra, onions, parsnips, tomatoes, tomato juice, vegetable juice, turnips, wax beans, zucchini	7 cups/week	8.5 cups/week	8.5 cups/week	10 cups/week	10 cups/week
Grains	Any food made from wheat, rice, oats, cornmeal, barley or another cereal grain is a grain product. *Examples*: bread, pasta, oatmeal, breakfast cereals, tortillas, and grits are examples of grain products.	8 oz/day	9 oz/day	10 oz/day	10 oz/day	10 oz/day
Meat or meat substitute and beans	All foods made from meat, poultry, fish, dry beans or peas, eggs, nuts, and seeds are considered part of this group. Dry beans and peas are part of this group as well as the vegetable group. Most meat and poultry choices should be lean or low fat. Fish, nuts, and seeds contain healthy oils, so choose these foods frequently instead of meat or poultry.	6.5 oz/day	6.5 oz/day	7 oz/day	7 oz/day	7 oz/day
Milk or milk substitute	All fluid milk products and many foods made from milk are considered part of this food group. Foods made from milk that retain their calcium content are part of the group, whereas foods made from milk that have little to no calcium, such as cream cheese, cream, and butter, are not. Most milk group choices should be fat free or low fat.	3 cups/day	3 cups/day	3 cups/day	3 cups/day	3 cups/per day
Oils	Oils are fats that are liquid at room temperature. Healthy oils include plant oils (olive, sunflower, safflower, etc.) and those from fish.	7 tsp/day	8 tsp/day	8 tsp/day	10 tsp/day	11 tsp/day
Discretionary calorie allowance	Remaining amount of calories in a food intake pattern after accounting for the calories needed for all food groups, using forms of foods that are fat free and with no added sugars. Thus these calories can be added to the diet with extra servings from any of the food groups.	362	410	426	512	648

*Specific serving sizes and suggestions can be found at *http://Mypyramid.gov* under "Inside the Pyramid" and then "What counts as a cup or oz?" Modified from Center for Nutrition Policy and Promotion, U.S. Department of Agriculture: *Inside the pyramid, http://mypyramid.gov/pyramid/index.html,* accessed November 2007.

Key Mineral and Vitamin Needs

Increases in several minerals and vitamins are needed during pregnancy to meet the greater structural and metabolic requirements. These increases are indicated in the DRI tables inside this text's front cover. Several of these essential substances have key roles in pregnancy and require special attention.

hemoglobin a conjugated protein in RBCs composed of a compact, rounded mass of polypeptide chains forming globin, the protein portion, and attached to an iron-containing red pigment called heme. It carries oxygen in the blood to cells.

plasma protein any of a number of protein substances carried in the circulating blood. A major one is *albumin,* which maintains the fluid volume of the blood through its colloidal osmotic pressure.

Minerals

Calcium. A good supply of calcium, along with phosphorus, magnesium, and vitamin D, is essential for fetal development of bones and teeth as well as the mother's own body needs. Calcium also is necessary for proper clotting of blood. A diet that includes at least 3 cups of vitamin A– and D–fortified milk daily, plus dairy or dairy substitute products (e.g., calcium-fortified soy products) and generous amounts of green vegetables and enriched or whole grains, usually supplies enough calcium. During pregnancy physiologic changes occur in the mother's absorption capacity to help meet the needs of some nutrients; for example, calcium and zinc are both significantly more bioavailable during pregnancy.[6,7] The body's enhanced capability to absorb and retain these nutrients from the diet during pregnancy helps the mother meet her nutrient needs and those of the growing fetus. Calcium supplements may be indicated in cases of poor maternal intake or pregnancies involving more than one fetus. Because food sources of the two major minerals (calcium and phosphorus) are almost the same, a diet sufficient in calcium also provides enough phosphorus.

Iron, Zinc, and Copper. Particular attention is given to iron intake during pregnancy. Iron is essential for the increased hemoglobin synthesis required for the greater maternal blood volume as well as for the baby's necessary prenatal storage of iron. Because iron occurs in small amounts in food sources, and much of this intake is not in a readily absorbable form, the maternal diet alone rarely meets requirements despite increased absorptive capacity during pregnancy. The current standards recommend a daily iron intake of 27 mg/day, which is significantly more than a woman's normal need of 18 mg/day.[4] Consuming foods high in vitamin C along with dietary sources of iron enhances the body's ability to absorb and use low bioavailable iron. In addition, avoiding foods that inhibit iron absorption, such as whole-grain cereals, unleavened whole-grain breads, legumes, tea, and coffee, within meals that provide significant iron is recommended. Because the increased pregnancy requirement is difficult to meet with the iron content of a typical U.S. diet, daily iron supplements often are recommended.[8] As with most supplemental forms of nutrients, bioavailability is suboptimal compared with food sources; thus encouragement of a balanced diet with ample iron is preferable (see Table 8-6 for a list of foods high in iron).

Although taking supplemental iron may be necessary to ensure good health of both mother and infant, it is also important to be conscientious of zinc and copper intake. The DRIs for both zinc and copper increase during pregnancy; meanwhile, absorption of both minerals is inhibited with high iron intake. A single 60-mg supplemental dose of iron significantly decreases zinc absorption; thus women needing high supplemental forms of iron are encouraged to take zinc supplements as well.[9]

Iodine. Adequate iodine intake is essential for producing more T_4, which is the thyroid hormone needed in greater amounts to control increased BMR during pregnancy. This increased iodine need is easily ensured by the use of iodized salt.

Vitamins

Increased attention to most all vitamins is needed to support a healthy pregnancy. Vitamins A and C are needed in higher amounts during pregnancy because they are both important elements in tissue growth. The need for B vitamins is increased because of their vital role as coenzyme factors in energy production and protein metabolism.

Folate. Folate builds mature RBCs throughout pregnancy and also is particularly needed during the early periconceptional period (i.e., from approximately 2 months before conception to week 6 of gestation) to ensure healthy embryonic tissue development and prevent malformation of the neural tube.[10] This tissue forms during the critical period from 17 to 30 days' gestation and grows into the mature infant's spinal column and its network of nerves. Spina bifida and anencephaly are the two most common forms of neural tube defects, which are defined as any malformation of the embryonic brain or spinal cord. The Centers for Disease Control and Prevention estimates that between 2500 and 3000 infants are born annually with a neural tube defect, and an additional 1500 pregnancies end in miscarriage or stillborn births as a result of this defect.[11] Spina bifida occurs when the lower end of the neural tube fails to close (Figure 10-1). As a result, the spinal cord and backbones do not develop properly. The severity of spina bifida varies with the size and location of the opening in the spine, with disability ranging from mild to severe, with limited movement and function.

Anencephaly occurs when the upper end of the neural tube fails to close. In this case, the brain fails to develop or is entirely absent. Pregnancies affected by anencephaly often end in miscarriages or death soon after delivery.

The current DRIs recommend a daily folate intake of 600 mcg/day during pregnancy and 400 mcg/day for nonpregnant women during child-bearing years.[2] Women who are unable to achieve such dietary recommendations by foods fortified with folate need a dietary supplement. All enriched flour and grain products, as well as fortified cereals, contain a well-absorbed form of dietary folic acid. Other natural sources of folate include liver; dark-green, leafy vegetables; legumes (e.g., pinto beans, black beans,

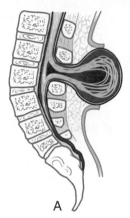
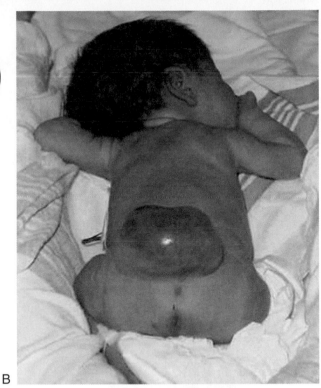

Figure 10-1 A, Myelomeningocele. **B,** Spina bifida in child at birth with cutaneous defect over the lumbar spine. (**B,** Courtesy Dr. Robert C. Dauser, Baylor College of Medicine, Houston, TX.)

and kidney beans); soybeans; wheat germ; orange juice; asparagus; and broccoli.

Vitamin D. Increased vitamin D needs, to ensure absorption and utilization of calcium and phosphorus for fetal bone growth, can be met by the mother's intake of at least 3 cups of fortified milk (or milk substitute) in her daily food plan. Fortified milk contains 10 mcg (400 IU) of cholecalciferol (vitamin D) per quart, which is twice the AI amount. The mother's exposure to sunlight increases endogenous synthesis of vitamin D as well. Lactose-intolerant women or vegetarians can obtain adequate vitamin D from fortified soy or rice milk products.

Registered dietitians are an excellent resource for pregnant women who need help planning a well-accepted balanced diet. DRI tables in the front of this text list all nutrient recommendations for pregnant and lactating women. Many important nutrients are needed in higher quantities during pregnancy. Only the more significant ones have been discussed here.

Weight Gain during Pregnancy

Amount and Quality

The mother's optimal weight gain during pregnancy, sufficient to support and nurture her and the fetus, is essential. Appropriate weight gain should not be viewed negatively. It is a positive reflection of good nutritional status

and contributes to a successful course and outcome of pregnancy and should be individually assessed. The average weight gained is approximately 29 lb (Table 10-2). A report of the National Academy of Sciences, *Nutrition During Pregnancy,* recommends setting weight gain goals together with the pregnant woman according to her pre-pregnancy nutritional status and BMI, as follows[5,12,13]:

- Underweight women (BMI <19.8): 28 to 40 lb
- Normal weight women (BMI 19.8 to 26): 25 to 35 lb
- Overweight women (BMI 26 to 29): 15 to 25 lb
- Obese women (BMI >29): approximately 15 lb
- Teenage girls: 35 to 40 lb (upper end of the recommended range)
- Women carrying twins: 34 to 45 lb
- Women carrying triplets: overall gain of 50 lb

The important consideration in each case is the quantity of weight gain as well as the *quality* of the gain and

spina bifida congenital defects in the embryonic fetal closing of the neural tube to form a portion of the lower spine, leaving the spine unclosed and the spinal cord open in various degrees of exposure and damage.

anencephaly congenital absence of the brain resulting from the incomplete closure of the upper end of the neural tube.

TABLE 10-2

APPROXIMATE WEIGHT GAIN DURING A NORMAL PREGNANCY

PRODUCT	WEIGHT (lb)
Fetus	7.5
Placenta	1.5
Amniotic fluid	2
Uterus (weight increase)	2
Breast tissue (weight increase)	2
Blood volume (weight increase)	3
Maternal stores: fat, protein, water, other nutrients	11
Total	29

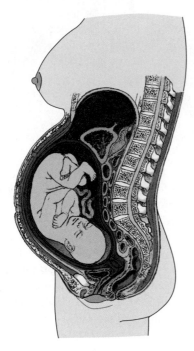

9 Months

Full-term pregnant woman. (Reprinted from Lowdermilk DL, Perry SE: *Maternity & women's health care*, ed 9, St Louis, 2007, Mosby.)

the foods consumed to bring it about. A definite connection exists between high-risk, low-birth-weight babies and inadequate maternal weight gain during the pregnancy.[14] Severe caloric restriction during pregnancy is potentially harmful to the developing fetus and the mother. Such a restricted diet cannot supply all the energy and nutrients essential to the growth process. Thus weight reduction *never* should be undertaken during pregnancy. To the contrary, adequate weight gain, relative to prepregnancy weight recommendations, should be supported with the use of a nourishing, well-balanced diet.

Rate of Weight Gain

Approximately 1 to 2 kg (2 to 4 lb) is the average amount of weight gain during the first trimester (first 3 months) of pregnancy. Thereafter, approximately 0.5 kg (1 lb) a week during the remainder of the pregnancy is usual, although exceptions exist. Only unusual patterns of gain (e.g., a sudden sharp increase in weight after the twentieth week of pregnancy, possibly indicating excessive and abnormal water retention) must be watched. On the other hand, an insufficient or low maternal weight gain in the second or third trimester increases the risk for intrauterine growth restriction (IUGR). A recent study found that maternal weight changes from the first to second trimester were strongly associated with fetal femur and tibia lengths and infant length at birth, indicating a sensitive period during gestation for linear growth.[15] Increased energy demand is normal during late pregnancy and prepares for full infant growth needs and the mother's approaching delivery and lactation. As always, carbohydrates, selected from enriched or whole-grain breads and cereals, fruits, vegetables, and legumes, are the preferred energy sources.

Role of Sodium

Just as with restriction of kilocalories, routine restriction of sodium during pregnancy is physiologically unsound. Maintenance of the increased volume of maternal blood, which is normal during pregnancy to support the increased metabolic work, requires adequate amounts of sodium and protein. A moderate amount (e.g., approximately 2 to 3 g/day) of dietary sodium is needed and can be achieved through the normal use of salt in cooking and seasoning. Extra use of table salt, or excessive consumption of salty processed foods, is not necessary. The typical American diet already contains 3 to 6 g/day, predominantly supplied from processed foods.

Daily Food Plan

General Plan

Ideally some form of a food plan is developed for the pregnant woman on an individual basis to meet her increased nutrition needs. Such a core plan (see Table 10-1) can serve as a guideline, with additional amounts of foods used as needed to meet caloric needs. This core food plan is built on basic foods available in American markets and designed to supply necessary nutrient increases. Energy needs increase as the pregnancy progresses, and the recommended increment of 340 to 450 kcal/day applies to the second and third trimesters.[5] However, adolescent, underweight, or malnourished women need special attention to increased energy needs from the onset of the pregnancy.

Alternative Food Patterns

The core food plan provided here might be only a starting point for women with alternate food patterns. Such food patterns exist among women from different ethnic backgrounds, belief systems, and lifestyles, making individual diet counseling important. Specific *nutrients,* not specific foods, are required for successful pregnancies and may be found in a variety of foods. Wise health care workers encourage pregnant women to use foods that serve both their personal and nutrition needs, whatever such foods may be. Many resources have been developed to serve as guides for a variety of alternative food patterns (e.g., ethnic and vegetarian). If the mother's vegetarian pattern includes dairy products and eggs (lacto-ovo vegetarian), achieving a sound diet to meet pregnancy needs is not a problem. Strict vegans can meet dietary protein needs through the use of soy foods (e.g., tofu, soy milk, soy yogurt, and soybeans) and complementary proteins (see Chapter 4 for additional information and resources for planning a vegetarian diet).

Specific counseling on avoidance of alcohol, caffeine, tobacco, and recreational drug use during pregnancy also is important. Information about the direct effects of poor nutrition on the fetus—especially related to brain development, learning problems, and developmental delays—helps motivate many pregnant women to choose a well-selected diet of optimal nutritional value.

Basic Principles

Whatever the food pattern, two important principles govern the prenatal diet: (1) pregnant women should eat a sufficient *quantity* of high *quality* food, and (2) pregnant women should eat *regular meals and snacks,* avoiding any habit of fasting or skipping meals, especially breakfast.

GENERAL CONCERNS

Functional Gastrointestinal Problems

Nausea and Vomiting

"Morning sickness" in early pregnancy (which actually has nothing to with the morning and can happen at any time throughout the day), usually is mild and only occurs during the first trimester. It is caused by hormonal adaptations in the first weeks and may be increased by stress or anxieties about the pregnancy itself. The following actions usually help relieve symptoms: small frequent meals and snacks that are fairly dry and consist mostly of easily digested energy foods (e.g., carbohydrates) with liquids between, not with, meals. If this sickness becomes severe and prolonged, a condition called *hyperemesis gravidarum,* medical treatment is required. Women with hyperemesis gravidarum, occurring in about 3.5 in 1000 pregnancies, have persistent vomiting throughout the pregnancy that may result in fluid and electrolyte disturbances, weight loss, and nutritional deficiencies.

Constipation

Although usually a minor complaint, constipation may occur in the latter part of pregnancy as a result of the increasing pressure of the enlarging uterus and the muscle-relaxing effect of progesterone on the GI tract, reducing normal peristalsis. Helpful remedies include adequate exercise, increased fluid intake, and high-fiber foods such as whole grains, vegetables, dried fruits (especially prunes and figs), and other fruits and juices. Pregnant women should avoid artificial laxatives.

Hemorrhoids

Hemorrhoids (enlarged veins in the anus, often protruding through the anal sphincter) are a fairly common complaint during the latter part of pregnancy. This vein enlargement usually is caused by the increased weight of the baby and the downward pressure it produces. Hemorrhoids may cause considerable discomfort, burning, and itching and may even rupture and bleed under the pressure of a bowel movement, causing the mother more anxiety. Hemorrhoids usually are controlled by the dietary suggestions given for constipation. Sufficient rest during the latter part of the day also may help relieve some of the downward pressure of the uterus on the lower intestine.

Heartburn

Pregnant women sometimes have heartburn or a "full" feeling. These discomforts occur especially after meals and are caused by the pressure of the enlarging uterus crowding the stomach. Gastric reflux of food may occur in the lower esophagus, causing irritation and a burning sensation. This common symptom has nothing to do with the heart but is called heartburn because of the close proximity of the lower esophagus to the heart. The full feeling comes from general gastric pressure, lack of nor-

intrauterine growth restriction (IUGR) less than 10% of predicted fetal weight for gestational age.

mal space in the area, a large meal, or gas formation. Dividing the day's food intake into a series of small meals and avoiding large meals at any time usually help relieve these issues. Comfort sometimes is improved by wearing loose-fitting clothing.

Effects of Iron Supplements

An iron supplement usually is given during pregnancy to meet the increased iron needs. Effects of added iron include gray or black stools and sometimes nausea, constipation, or diarrhea. To help avoid food-related effects, iron supplements should be taken 1 hour before or 2 hours after a meal with a liquid such as water or orange juice, not milk or tea. Iron absorption in the body is increased with foods high in vitamin C (e.g., orange juice, tomato juice, strawberries, cantaloupe, and broccoli) and decreased with milk, other dairy foods, tea, coffee, whole-grain bread, oatmeal, and cereal.

High-Risk Mothers and Infants

Identifying Risk Factors

Pregnancy-related deaths claimed 495 women in the United States in 2003,[16] and an estimated 500 to 800 additional deaths annually are most likely pregnancy related. Identifying risk factors and addressing them early are critical in promoting a healthy pregnancy. These risk factors are listed in the Clinical Applications box, "Nutritional Risk Factors in Pregnancy."

To avoid the compounding results of poor nutrition during pregnancy, mothers at risk for complications should be identified as soon as possible. These nutrition-related factors are based on clinical evidence of inadequate nutrition. Do not wait for clinical symptoms of poor nutrition to appear. The best approach is to identify poor food patterns and prevent nutrition problems from developing. Three types of dietary patterns that do not support optimal maternal and fetal nutrition are (1) insufficient food intake, (2) poor food selection, and (3) poor food distribution throughout the day.

Teenage Pregnancy

The United States has one of the highest teenage pregnancy rates among industrialized nations.[17] Approximately 1 million teenagers become pregnant each year, of which approximately half end in live births, 3 in 10 end in abortion, and 1 in 7 ends in fetal loss.[17,18] Pregnancy at this early age is physically and emotionally difficult for the teen. From a nutrition standpoint, special care must be given to support adequate growth of both mother and fetus. The current DRIs distinguish specific vitamin and mineral needs for pregnant females younger than 18 years. See the For Further Focus box, "Pregnant Teenagers," for more information on health and nutrition for adolescent mothers.

Recognizing Special Counseling Needs

Every pregnant woman needs personalized care and support during pregnancy. However, women with risk factors such as those listed here have special counseling needs. In each case the clinician must work with the mother in a sensitive and supportive manner to help her develop a healthy food plan that is both practical and nourishing. Dangerous practices, such as fad dieting, extreme macrobiotic diets, or pica, should be identified. *Pica* is the name given to a craving for and consumption of nonfood items (e.g., chalk, laundry starch, or clay), a practice sometimes seen in pregnant or malnourished individuals that frequently is associated with iron-deficiency anemia.[19]

In addition to avoiding dangerous practices, several special needs require sensitive counseling—including those related to age and parity, detrimental lifestyle habits, and socioeconomic problems.

Age and Parity. Pregnancies at either age extreme of the reproductive cycle carry special risks. Adolescent

CLINICAL APPLICATIONS

NUTRITIONAL RISK FACTORS IN PREGNANCY

Risk Factors at the Onset of Pregnancy
- Age: 18 years or younger, 35 years or older
- Frequent pregnancies: three or more during a 2-year period
- Poor obstetric history or poor fetal performance
- Poverty
- Bizarre or trendy food habits
- Abuse of nicotine, alcohol, or drugs
- Therapeutic diet required for a chronic disorder
- Weight: <85% or >120% of ideal weight

Risk Factors during Pregnancy
- Low hemoglobin (<12.0 g) or hematocrit (<34.0 mg/dL)
- Inadequate weight gain: any weight loss or weight gain of <1 kg (2 lb) per month after the first trimester
- Excessive weight gain: >1 kg (2 lb) per week after the first trimester

FOR FURTHER FOCUS

PREGNANT TEENAGERS

Few situations are as life-changing for a single teenage girl and her family as an unintended pregnancy. Depending on how she and her family, as well as her partner, deal with the situation, lifelong consequences may occur for them as well as the broader community. Adolescent pregnancy rates have historically been higher for African Americans than for Caucasians in the United States, but rates are gradually declining in all ethnic groups.* Birth rates for teenagers ages 15 to 19 years are highest in the southern states.

Pregnant teenagers are at high risk for pregnancy complications and poor outcome with increased rates of low birth weight and infant mortality. The following problems contribute to these complications: the physiologic demands of the pregnancy, which compromise the teenager's needs for her own unfinished growth and development; the psychosocial influences of low income; inadequate diet; and the teenage experimentation with alcohol, smoking, and other drugs. Little or no access to appropriate prenatal care also may significantly contribute to a lack of nutrition support for the pregnancy. Early nutrition intervention is essential and can change the course of events and the pregnancy outcome, but it is not an easy task. Changes from the inconsistent, often poor food pattern of teenagers are difficult to achieve, and their care is challenging. Experienced, sensitive health workers in teen clinics emphasize the need for supportive individual and group nutrition counseling. The following suggestions may help secure a positive and healthy environment for the teen.

Know Each Client Personally

All nutrition services must be tailored to the unique needs and characteristics of each pregnant teenager. Many have lower educational levels and even limited reading skills to which educational material must be adapted. Low-income teens lack the financial resources to maintain an adequate diet, and those living at home may have little control over the food available to them. Personal stress over the preg-nancy is paramount, and nutrition concerns often are not a priority. Skipping meals and snacking are common; even dieting is frequent.

Seek Ways to Motivate Clients

Schedule appointments on days that clients are coming in to pick up their WIC food packages. Invite the teen's mother and friends to accompany her to group counseling sessions so they can support the recommendations that are made. Make each recommendation concrete and reasonable. Avoid scare tactics.

Make Appropriate Assessments

Use simple, concrete forms for evaluating dietary intake (e.g., the basic food groups of the MyPyramid Guidelines [see Chapter 1]). This traditional model can be used, with increased amounts indicated for pregnancy, as both an educational and assessment tool.

Make Practical Interventions

Plan short, enjoyable, active learning sessions. Use positive reinforcement liberally. Provide specific suggestions for carrying out changes at home. Review progress in follow-up sessions. Always maintain a positive, supportive atmosphere.

Support the Teenager's Responsibility

Help the teenager learn to be responsible. In the final analysis, pregnant teenagers must take on responsibility, often for the first time, for their own nourishment and the nourishment of others. Helping them in a supportive manner to understand and carry out this responsibility, which ultimately only they can do, is a primary objective of nutrition counseling. Nutrition consultants must be skillful in establishing the kind of rapport and relationship where these responsibilities can develop and grow.

*National Center for Health Statistics: *Health, United States, 2005 with chartbook on trends in the health of Americans,* Hyattsville, MD, 2005, National Center for Health Statistics.

---

pregnancy adds many social and nutritional risks as its social upheaval and physical demands are imposed on an immature teenage girl. Sensitive counseling must involve both information and emotional support with good prenatal care throughout. On the other hand, pregnant women who are more than 35 years old and having their first child also require special attention. These women may be more at risk for high blood pressure and gestational diabetes and need guidance about the rate of weight gain and dietary plan. In addition, women with a high parity rate (i.e., those who have had several pregnancies within a limited number of years) may be at increased risk for poor pregnancy outcomes because they enter each successive pregnancy drained of nutrition resources and usually facing the increasing physical and economic pressures of child care. Such counseling may include discussions of acceptable means of contraception and nutrition information and support.

Alcohol. Alcohol use during pregnancy can lead to the well-documented fetal alcohol syndrome (FAS) or

---

fetal alcohol syndrome (FAS) combination of physical and mental birth defects in infants born to mothers who abused alcohol during pregnancy.

fetal alcohol effects (Figure 10-2), which has become a leading cause of mental retardation and other birth defects in the United States.[20] A recent study comparing risk for FAS in different ethnic and socioeconomic groups of women found that the relative risk for FAS varies between

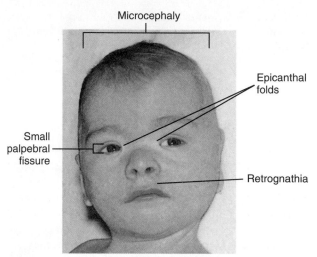

Microcephaly

Epicanthal folds

Small palpebral fissure

Retrognathia

Figure 10-2 Fetal Alcohol Syndrome. (Reprinted from Thibodeau GA, Patton KG: *Anatomy & physiology*, ed 6, St Louis, 2007, Mosby.)

populations and is influenced by environmental and behavioral conditions in addition to prepregnancy BMI and nutrition status, but no ethnic or socioeconomic group is without incidence.[21] The Centers for Disease Control and Prevention estimate that between 1000 and 6000 infants are born annually with FAS, and about three times that amount have fetal alcohol effects.[22]

Nicotine. Cigarette smoking, or exposure to environmental tobacco smoke during pregnancy, is associated with placental abnormalities and fetal damage, including prematurity and low birth weight (see the Clinical Applications box, "Who Will Have the Low-Birth-Weight Baby?").[23-25] The most recent report from the Centers for Disease Control and Prevention noted that 10.7% of all women continue to smoke throughout pregnancy, with a much higher prevalence occurring in American Indian and Alaska Native women than other ethnicities.[16]

Drugs. Drug use, whether medicinal or recreational, poses many problems for both mother and fetus, especially the use of illegal drugs. Self-medication with over-the-counter drugs also may present adverse effects. Drugs cross the placenta and enter the fetal circulation, thus creating a potential addiction in the unborn child. Dangers come from the drug and contaminated needles as well as the impurities contained in street drugs.

 # CLINICAL APPLICATIONS

WHO WILL HAVE THE LOW-BIRTH-WEIGHT BABY?

The number of infants weighing less than 2500 g (5 lb) at birth is still problematic. Perinatal dietitians are aware of the dietary factors, especially poor weight gain during pregnancy, that contribute to this problem. The prevalence of the turn-of-the-century adage to "grow the baby to fit the pelvis" continues to influence some physicians, nurses, and expectant mothers to limit prenatal weight gain to 9 kg (20 lb) or less to avoid obstetric problems at delivery. This practice is harmful and is refuted by current evidence that a weight gain of 25 to 35 lb for average-weight women and 28 to 40 lb for underweight women correlates with a healthy birth weight of more than 2500 g (5 lb).

The obsession with weight control during pregnancy can lead to harmful restrictions of vital energy and nutrients. Weight reduction should never be attempted during pregnancy. Such diets are extremely dangerous to the fetus. Even the common habit of skipping breakfast, especially late in pregnancy, may impair intellectual development by quickly producing a state of pseudostarvation. Increased ketoacidosis from fat breakdown can cause neurologic damage to the fetus.

Nondietary Factors Influencing the Trend toward More Low-Birth-Weight Babies
- Rise in number of older first-time mothers (older than 35 years)

- Number of teenage pregnancies
- Previous induced abortions
- Technologic advances in neonatal care, which keeps premature infants alive longer
- Race: non-Caucasians have higher rates of low birth weight infants than Caucasians.

Reducing the Risk of Low-Birth-Weight Infants
- Explain the reasons for gaining sufficient weight as recommended.
- Help mothers who smoke or drink to stop using cigarettes or alcohol.
- Monitor excessive weight gain and sodium intake in older first-time mothers, who are at risk for hypertensive disorders of pregnancy and obesity.
- Explore the eating habits of teenagers, working with the mother and father, if possible, to include nutrient-dense foods in meals and snacks.
- Stay informed of federal, state, and local supplemental food programs (e.g., WIC; see Chapter 13) that ensure an adequate intake of nutrients in low-income women.
- Encourage regular eating patterns throughout pregnancy.

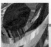

DRUG-NUTRIENT INTERACTION

ACCUTANE

The drug isotretinoin (Accutane) is a known teratogen. It contains high doses of vitamin A compounds that effectively work to reduce and eliminate deep nodular acne. The efficacy rate is high, but the side effects are severe if taken during pregnancy. Besides causing birth defects, Accutane usually causes one or more of the following: dry mouth, cheilitis (lip inflammation), esophagitis, nausea/vomiting, and/or depression.

To minimize these side effects, take Accutane with meals or milk to enhance absorption and swallow with 8 oz of water to decrease GI irritation.

The dosage of Accutane is based on body weight. Ingesting more Accutane than prescribed increases the severity of side effects and may cause unknown side effects. Therefore do not take a vitamin A or beta-carotene supplement and avoid excessive consumption of vitamin A–rich foods when taking this drug. Multivitamins containing vitamin A, or any of its derivatives, are discouraged as well.

Sara Oldroyd

Vitamin abuse from megadosing with basic nutrients such as vitamin A during pregnancy also may cause fetal damage. Drugs made from vitamin A compounds (e.g., retinoids such as tretinoin [Accutane], prescribed for severe acne) have caused spontaneous abortion of malformed fetuses by women who conceived during acne treatment. Thus the use of these drugs without contraception is contraindicated. For further information on Accutane, see the Drug-Nutrient Interaction box, "Accutane."

Caffeine. Caffeine is widely used and can cross the placenta and enter fetal circulation. Average adult consumption of caffeine is 4 mg/kg body weight per day, with pregnant women consuming much less: 1 mg/kg per day. Caffeine stays in the blood stream significantly longer in pregnant women during the third trimester than other adults (average half-life of 10 to 20 hours vs. 2 to 6 hours).[26] Studies have found conflicting results over the years regarding the effects of caffeine on pregnancy outcome, primarily because the majority of women who consume excess caffeine also smoke and use alcohol, both of which are known **teratogens**. On review of the reproductive and developmental risks associated with caffeine consumption, researchers have concluded that when used in extreme excess, caffeine may result in injury to the fetus.[26] Such injuries include low birth weight, smaller head circumference, and congenital malformations. However, toxic doses are not likely to occur under normal conditions. The overall conclusion is that moderate amounts of caffeine (5 to 6 mg/kg per day) throughout the day do not have negative effects on reproduction or fetal health. This is not true when caffeine is used in conjunction with other teratogens, such as alcohol and cigarette smoke. One cup of coffee contains approximately 100 mg of caffeine, and caffeinated soft drinks range between 10 and 50 mg per 12-oz serving. Thus a 60-kg (132-lb) woman should limit caffeine intake to approximately 300 mg/day (3 cups of coffee or six 12-oz sodas). Mothers should be

aware that caffeine stays in the blood stream of a newborn much longer than an adult, with a half-life of 4 days.

Socioeconomic Problems. Special counseling often is needed for women and young girls living in low-income situations. Poverty especially puts pregnant women in grave danger because they need resources for financial assistance and food supplements. Dietitians and social workers on the health care team can provide special counseling and referrals. Community resources include programs such as the WIC, which has helped many low-income mothers have healthy babies (Figure 10-3). WIC also provides nutrition education counseling regarding the mother's nutrition needs as well as their babies.

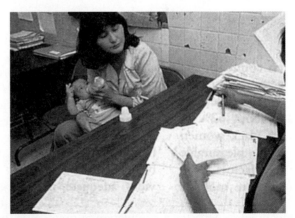

Figure 10-3 This mother is a participant in the U.S. government's WIC program. (From U.S. Department of Agriculture, Washington, DC.)

---

fetal alcohol effects physical and mental birth defects in infants born to mothers who used alcohol during pregnancy. This condition is less severe than FAS, occurs three times more often, but is similar in that no cure exists.

teratogen drug or substance causing birth defect.

Complications of Pregnancy

Anemia

Iron-deficiency anemia is the most common nutritional deficiency worldwide. Although a disproportionate amount occurs in underdeveloped countries, approximately 12% of women ages 12 to 49 years (childbearing years) are iron deficient in the United States. Anemia is more prevalent among poor women, many of whom live on marginal diets lacking iron-rich foods, but is by no means restricted to lower economic groups. A deficiency of iron or folate in the mother's diet can cause nutrition anemia. Dietary intake must be improved and supplements used as necessary. During the second and third trimesters of pregnancy, a low-dose iron supplement of 30 mg of ferrous iron daily can provide the amount of extra iron needed.

Neural Tube Defects

As previously discussed, the DRIs of 400 mcg/day of folate for women who are capable of becoming pregnant is increased to 600 mcg/day during pregnancy.[2] This is especially important when individual dietary adequacy is doubtful or a genetic high risk exists for neural tube defects in the family. Women who do not frequently consume fruit, juices, whole grain or fortified cereals, or green leafy vegetables or take folate supplements are likely to have less than optimal folate intake.

Intrauterine Growth Restriction

IUGR, which is defined as less than 10% of predicted fetal weight for gestational age, affects approximately 100,000 infants born in the United States annually. Children born with IUGR have multiple survival and growth problems. Many factors may contribute to IUGR, but low prepregnancy weight, inadequate weight gain during pregnancy, and the use of cigarettes and/or alcohol are strong factors.

Hypertensive Disorders of Pregnancy

The development of high blood pressure during pregnancy can be fatal for both mother and fetus. If symptoms progress, with the accumulation of proteinuria the condition is referred to as preeclampsia. Complications such as eclamptic convulsions and HELLP syndrome (hemolysis, elevated liver enzymes, and low platelets) require hospitalization and often induced labor.[27] Previous studies have shown that calcium supplementation reduced the risk for hypertension in women who were pregnant for the first time and especially those with low calcium intake to begin with, although the disorder is not thought to be exclusively associated with diet.[28,29] Specific treatment varies according to individual symptoms and needs, but in any case optimal nutrition is important and prompt medical attention is required. Early and consistent prenatal care is imperative to identify risks early in the pregnancy. The only cure for preeclampsia is the termination or delivery of the infant.

Gestational Diabetes

During pregnancy glucose in the urine (*glycosuria*) is not uncommon. In susceptible women it results from the increased metabolic workload during pregnancy and the increased volume of blood with its load of metabolites, including glucose. Some of this extra glucose then spills over into the urine. Gestational diabetes is defined as any degree of glucose intolerance with onset during pregnancy, and the definition applies regardless of whether insulin or only diet modification is used for treatment.[30] The prevalence of gestational diabetes in the United States is approximately 4% of all pregnancies (roughly 135,000) annually. Prenatal clinics routinely screen pregnant women between 24 and 28 weeks' gestation and provide careful follow-up for those who show glucosuria or meet the following diagnostic criteria: have a random blood glucose level greater than 200 mg/dL (11.1 mmol/L) or fasting blood glucose level greater than 126 mg/dL (7.0 mmol/L), or fail to clear glucose from the blood stream within the specified time after an oral glucose tolerance test. Particular attention is given to women at higher risk for developing gestational diabetes, including those age 30 years and older who are overweight (BMI >26) and have a history of any of the following predisposing factors:

- Previous history of gestational diabetes
- Family history of diabetes or ethnicity associated with high incidence of diabetes
- Glucosuria
- Obesity
- Large babies weighing 4.5 kg (10 lb) or more
- Birth of babies with multiple congenital defects

Gestational diabetes occurs more frequently among African Americans, Hispanic/Latino Americans, Asian Americans, Pacific Islanders, and Native Americans. From 20% to 50% of these women subsequently develop type 2 diabetes and are more likely to develop cardiovascular disease at an early age, especially those who also have a family history of type 2 diabetes.[31] Therefore identifying and providing close follow-up testing and treatment with special diet and insulin, as needed, are important interventions. These women are at higher risk for fetal damage, prematurity, or delivery of a very large baby, a complicating condition called *macrosomia* that is associated with survival dangers. Children born to women with gestational diabetes are at greater risk for impaired glucose tolerance, being overweight, and cryptorchidism (abnormal testicular decent in boys).[32,33]

Preexisting Disease

Preexisting clinical conditions, such as hypertension, diabetes, PKU, or other diseases, can cause complications during pregnancy. In each case a woman's pregnancy is managed, usually by a team of specialists, according to the principles of care related to pregnancy and the particular disease involved.

LACTATION

The World Health Organization states that "breastfeeding is an unequalled way of providing ideal food for the healthy growth and development of infants."[34] Breastfeeding is recommended as the exclusive source of nutrition for infants up to 6 months of age. After 6 months, iron-fortified complementary foods should be added to the basic diet of breast milk. The *Healthy People 2010* goals for breastfeeding are as follows[35]:

- 75% of mothers initiate breastfeeding in the early postpartum period
- 50% of mothers continue to breastfeed at 6 months
- 25% of mothers continue to breastfeed at 1 year

Trends

Although the United States has one of the lowest rates of breastfeeding, the number of mothers choosing to breastfeed has been on the rise since the 1960s, with more than 70% mothers currently initiating breastfeeding.[36] The Baby-Friendly Hospital Initiative, launched by the World Health Organization, has contributed to this choice by (1) having a written breastfeeding policy, (2) training staff in the skills needed to implement the policy, (3) informing new mothers about the benefits of breastfeeding, (4) helping new mothers initiate breastfeeding, (5) allowing mothers and infants to remain together 24 hours a day, and (6) fostering the development of support for breastfeeding after mothers leave the hospital.[37] Breastfeeding initiation and continuation are higher among well-educated, older, nonsmoking women of a higher socioeconomic status. The American Academy of Pediatrics recommends breastfeeding for at least the first 12 months postpartum.[38] However, less than 36% of American mothers continue any form of breastfeeding past 6 months postpartum (see the Cultural Considerations box, "Breastfeeding Trends in the United States").[36] Most women report discontinuing breastfeeding because of difficulties such as sore nipples, infant spitting up, and engorged breasts. With proper instruction and a caring environment, many of these difficulties can be overcome. Almost all women who choose to breastfeed their infants can do so. Well-nourished mothers who breastfeed exclusively provide adequate nutrition, with solid foods usually added to the baby's diet at approximately 6 months of age.

Physiologic Process of Lactation

The female breasts are highly specialized secretory organs (Figure 10-4). Throughout pregnancy the mammary glands are preparing for lactation. The mammary glands are capable of extracting certain nutrients from the maternal blood in addition to synthesizing other compounds. The combined effort results in the nutrient-complete breast milk. On delivery, milk production and secretion are stimulated by the two hormones *prolactin* and *oxytocin*.

Stimulation of the nipple from infant suckling sends nerve signals to the brain of the mother (Figure 10-5). This nerve signal then causes the release of prolactin and oxytocin. Prolactin is the milk-producing hormone, and oxytocin is the hormone responsible for the *let-down reflex*. Let-down is the process of the milk moving from the upper milk-producing cells down to the nipple for infant suckling. Milk production is a supply-and-demand procedure. The mammary glands are stimulated to produce milk each time the infant feeds. Therefore the more milk taken from the breast (during breastfeeding and/or pumping), the more milk she produces, thus always meeting the infant's needs. Human milk can meet unique infant needs (Table 10-3), whereas cow's milk is an inappropriate food source for infants younger than 1 year because of high protein and electrolyte levels.

Nutrition Needs

The basic diet followed during pregnancy, as well as the prenatal nutrient supplement used, should be continued through the lactation period. In general, attention to three areas of lactation support is needed.

Diet

Energy and Nutrients. Milk production requires energy for both the process and product. Some of this energy may be met by extra fat stored during pregnancy. The recommendation is 330 kcal/day (plus 170 kcal/day from maternal stores) in the first 6 months and 400 kcal/day in the second 6 months of lactation more than a woman's normal need of approximately 2200 kcal. The need for protein during lactation is 25 g/day more than

CULTURAL CONSIDERATIONS

BREASTFEEDING TRENDS IN THE UNITED STATES

Increasing the prevalence of breastfeeding continues to be a health goal nationally and internationally, as seen in the objectives for *Healthy People 2010* and the World Health Organization. The most recent report from the National Center for Health Statistics shows that the percent of mothers initiating breastfeeding has increased from 54.1% in 1986 to 66.5% in 2001. The percent of mothers who continued to breastfeed past 3 months also increased during this time from 34.6% to 48%.*

In the United Sates breastfeeding is more common in older women, Hispanic or Latino women, and women with higher education (bachelor's degree or higher). A higher prevalence of breastfeeding also is found in the western part of the United States than in other geographic regions (see table below).*

PREVALENCE OF BREASTFEEDING IN THE UNITED STATES

SELECTED CHARACTERISTICS OF MOTHER	PERCENT BREASTFEEDING
Total	66.5
Mother's Age at Baby's Birth	
Younger than 20 years	47.3
20-24 years	59.3
25-29 years	63.5
30-44 years	80.0
Race and Hispanic Origin	
Not Hispanic or Latino	
Caucasian	68.7
Black or African American	45.3
Hispanic or Latino	76.0

Education

No high school diploma or GED	46.6
High school diploma or GED	61.6
Some college, no bachelor's degree	75.6
Bachelor's degree or higher	81.3

Geographic Region

Northwest	66.9
Midwest	61.9
South	60.9
West	78.9

From National Center for Health Statistics: *Health, United States, 2005 with chartbook on trends in the health of Americans,* Hyattsville, MD, 2005, National Center for Health Statistics.

As a health care provider, be sure to note the perceived obstacles to initiation and continuation of breastfeeding so that education and alternatives may be presented at the appropriate time (before delivery). The American Academy of Pediatrics notes the following obstacles†:

- Insufficient prenatal education about breastfeeding
- Disruptive hospital policies and practices
- Inappropriate interruption of breastfeeding
- Early hospital discharge in some populations
- Lack of timely routine follow-up care and postpartum home health visits
- Maternal employment (especially in the absence of workplace facilities that support breastfeeding)
- Lack of family and broad societal support
- Media portrayal of bottle feeding as normative
- Commercial promotion of infant formula through distribution of hospital discharge packs
- Coupons for free or discounted formula
- Misinformation about what medical conditions may be contraindications for breastfeeding
- Lack of guidance and encouragement from health care professionals

---

* From National Center for Health Statistics: *Health, United States, 2005 with chartbook on trends in the health of Americans,* Hyattsville, MD, 2005, National Center for Health Statistics.
†American Academy of Pediatrics: Breastfeeding and the use of human milk, *Pediatrics* 115:496, 2005.

---

a woman's average need of 46 g/day (0.8 g/kg body weight per day), for a total of 71 g/day (or 1.1 g/kg body weight per day).[5] The core food plan for meeting lactation needs (see Table 10-1) includes three servings of milk products (or vegetarian substitute); six to eight ounces of protein foods; one to two servings of dark-green or yellow vegetables; one to two servings of vitamin C–rich fruits and vegetables; two to three servings of other vegetables, fruits, and juices; eight to nine ounces of whole-grain or enriched breads and

cereals; and moderate amounts of butter or fortified margarine.

Fluids. Because milk is a fluid, breastfeeding mothers need ample fluids for adequate milk production (approximately 3 L/day). Water and other sources of fluid such as juices, milk, and soup contribute to the fluid necessary to produce milk. Beverages containing alcohol and caffeine should be limited or avoided because they are secreted to some extent in the mother's milk and can result in dehydration if other fluids are replaced.

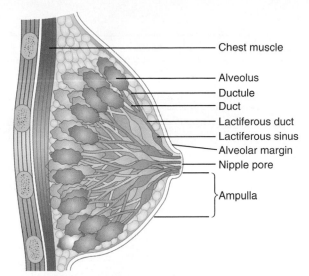

Figure 10-4 Anatomy of the breast. (Reprinted from Mahan LK, Escott-Stump S: *Krause's food & nutrition therapy,* ed 12, Philadelphia, 2008, Saunders.)

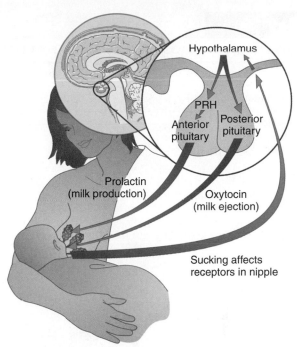

Figure 10-5 Physiology of milk production and the let-down reflex. *PRH,* **Prolactin-releasing hormone.** (Reprinted from Mahan LK, Escott-Stump S: *Krause's food & nutrition therapy,* ed 12, Philadelphia, 2008, Saunders.)

Rest and Relaxation

In addition to the increased diet and adequate fluids, breastfeeding mothers require rest, moderate exercise, and relaxation. Because the production and let-down reflexes of breastfeeding are hormonally controlled, some negative environmental and psychological factors can adversely affect the amount of milk a mother can produce. Such factors are called prolactin inhibitors and include stress, fatigue, prolonged bed rest, medical complications, and irregular breastfeeding. The lactation specialist can help by counseling mothers about their new family situations and helping them develop a plan to meet their personal needs.

Advantages of Breastfeeding

Many physiologic and practical advantages to breastfeeding are gained for both mother and infant, including the following[36]:

1. *Fewer infections* because the mother transfers certain antibodies or immune properties in human milk to her nursing infant.
2. *Fewer allergies and intolerances,* especially in allergy-prone infants (cow's milk contains a number of potentially allergy-causing proteins that human milk does not have); mothers with a family history of allergies are encouraged to breastfeed.
3. *Ease of digestion* because human milk forms a softer curd in the GI tract that is easier for the infant to digest.

4. *Improved cognitive development* in childhood, with a positive relation between the duration of breastfeeding and IQ in the child.
5. *Decreases in the risk of childhood obesity and heart disease.*

Additional benefits for the mother are listed in Box 10-2.

The American Dietetic Association and American Academy of Pediatrics encourage and strongly support breastfeeding for all able mothers for the first 12 months of life and continued thereafter for as long as mutually desired.[38]

BOX 10-2

BENEFITS OF BREASTFEEDING FOR MOTHER

- Promotes faster shrinking of the uterus
- Reduces postpartum bleeding
- Decreases risk of breast and ovarian cancer
- Delays resumption of the menstrual cycle
- Improves glucose profile in those with gestational diabetes
- Strengthens bond with the infant
- Enhances self esteem in the maternal role
- Eliminates the need for preparing and mixing formula
- Saves money not spent on formula

Modified from American Academy of Pediatrics: Breastfeeding and the use of human milk, *Pediatrics* 115:496, 2005.

TABLE 10-3

NUTRITION COMPOSITION OF HUMAN MILK VS. COW'S MILK*

	HUMAN MILK			
NUTRIENT	COLOSTRUM	TRANSITIONAL	MATURE	COW'S MILK
Kilocalories	67	72	74	70
Protein (g)	2.7	1.6	0.9	3.3
Carbohydrate (g)†	5.3	6.6	7.2	4.8
Fat (g)	2.9	3.6	4.5	3.7
Lactalbumin (g)		0.8	0.3	0.4
Fat-Soluble Vitamins				
A (IU)	296	283	240	303
D (IU)			5	4
E (mg)	0.8	1.32	0.2	0.06
K (mcg)			2.3	
Water-Soluble Vitamins				
Thiamin (mg)	0.015	0.006	0.014	0.042
Riboflavin (mg)	0.029	0.033	0.035	0.16
Niacin (mg)	0.075	0.15	0.2	0.085
Pantothenic acid (mg)	0.183	0.288	0.18	0.3
Vitamin C (mg)	4.4	5.4	4.3	0.9
Folate (mcg)	0.05	0.02	0.52	0.23
Minerals				
Calcium (mg)	31	34	30	125
Phosphorus (mg)	14	17	15	96
Iron (mg)	0.09	0.04	0.03	0.04
Zinc (mg)	0.5	0.4	0.16	0.37
Magnesium (mg)	4.2	3.5	4	13
Iodine (mcg)	6		6	11
Electrolytes				
Sodium (mg)	5	19	17	76
Potassium (mg)	74	63	53	152
Chloride (mg)	58	30	37	108

Modified from Mitchell MK: *Nutrition across the life span,* ed 2, Philadelphia, 2003, Saunders.
*Per 100 mL.
†Lactose.

SUMMARY

Pregnancy involves the fundamental interaction of the following three distinct yet unified biologic entities: the fetus, placenta, and mother. Maternal needs also reflect the increasing nutrition needs of the fetus and placenta. Optimal weight gain varies with the normal nutritional status and weight of the woman, with a goal of 25 to 35 lb for a woman of average weight. Sufficient weight gain is important during pregnancy to support the rapid growth taking place. However, the nutritional quality of the diet is as significant as the actual weight gain.

Common problems during pregnancy include first-trimester nausea and vomiting associated with hormonal adaptations and later constipation, hemorrhoids, or heartburn resulting from the pressure of the enlarging uterus. These problems usually are relieved without medication by simple, often temporary, changes in the diet. Unusual or irregular eating habits, age, parity, prepregnancy weight status, and low income are among the many related conditions that put pregnant women at risk for complications.

The ultimate goal of prenatal care is a healthy infant and a healthy mother who can breastfeed her child if she chooses to do so. Breast milk provides essential nutrients in quantities that are uniquely suited for optimal infant growth and development.

CRITICAL THINKING QUESTIONS

1. Which nutrients are required in larger amounts during pregnancy? Plan a 1-day diet that would meet the nutrient needs of a pregnant women in her third trimester.
2. Identify two common GI problems associated with pregnancy and describe the diet management of each.

3. Discuss the major nutritional factors needed to support lactation. What additional, nonnutrition needs does the breastfeeding mother have, and what suggestions can you give to help her meet them?
4. Why is additional fluid needed for lactation?

CHAPTER CHALLENGE QUESTIONS

True-False

Write the correct statement for each statement that is false.

1. *True or False:* The development of the fetus is directly related to the diet of the mother.

2. *True or False:* Strict weight control during pregnancy is necessary to avoid complications.

3. *True or False:* Salt should be removed from the pregnant woman's diet to prevent edema.

4. *True or False:* A higher risk for pregnancy complications occurs in teenagers and older women.

5. *True or False:* A woman's diet before pregnancy has little effect on the outcome of her pregnancy.

6. *True or False:* No woman should ever gain more than 15 to 20 lb during pregnancy.

7. *True or False:* Rapid growth of the fetal skeleton requires increased calcium in the mother's diet.

8. *True or False:* Inadequate vitamin D during pregnancy contributes to faulty skeletal development in the fetus.

9. *True or False:* Anemia is common during pregnancy.

10. *True or False:* Additional kilocalories and fluids are needed during lactation.

Multiple Choice

1. Blood volume during pregnancy
   a. increases.
   b. decreases.
   c. remains unchanged.
   d. fluctuates widely.

2. Pregnant mothers taking high doses of iron supplements are potentially at risk for deficiencies of which of the following minerals because of nutrient interactions?
   a. Sodium
   b. Phosphorus
   c. Selenium
   d. Zinc

3. Which of the following foods has the highest iron content to help meet the need for increased iron during pregnancy?
   a. Lean beef
   b. Liver
   c. Orange juice
   d. Milk

4. The increased need for vitamin A during pregnancy may be met by increased use of foods such as
   a. chicken.
   b. extra egg whites.
   c. citrus fruits.
   d. carrots.

5. Which of the following hormones is responsible for milk let-down during lactation?
   a. Prolactin
   b. Estrogen
   c. Oxytocin
   d. Human growth hormone

6. The World Health Organization and American Academy of Pediatrics recommend breastfeeding for at least
   a. 3 months.
   b. 8 months.
   c. 12 months.
   d. 3 years.

evolve Please refer to the Students' Resource section of this text's Evolve Web site for additional study resources.

REFERENCES

1. Food and Nutrition Board, Institute of Medicine: *Dietary reference intakes for calcium, phosphorous, magnesium, vitamin D, and fluoride,* Washington, DC, 1998, National Academies Press.
2. Food and Nutrition Board, Institute of Medicine: *Dietary reference intakes for thiamin, riboflavin, niacin, vitamin B₆, folate, vitamin B₁₂, pantothenic acid, biotin, and choline,* Washington, DC, 1999, National Academies Press.
3. Food and Nutrition Board, Institute of Medicine: *Dietary reference intakes for vitamin C, vitamin E, selenium, and carotenoids,* Washington, DC, 2000, National Academies Press.
4. Food and Nutrition Board, Institute of Medicine: *Dietary reference intakes for vitamin A, vitamin K, arsenic, boron, chromium, copper, iodine, iron, manganese, molybdenum, nickel, silicon, vanadium, and zinc,* Washington, DC, 2002, National Academies Press.
5. Food and Nutrition Board, Institute of Medicine: *Dietary reference intakes for energy, carbohydrate, fiber, fat, fatty acids, cholesterol, protein, and amino acids,* Washington, DC, 2002, National Academies Press.
6. Vargas Zapata CL and others: Calcium homeostasis during pregnancy and lactation in Brazilian women with low calcium intakes: a longitudinal study, *Am J Clin Nutr* 80(2):417, 2004.
7. Donangelo CM and others: Zinc absorption and kinetics during pregnancy and lactation in Brazilian women, *Am J Clin Nutr* 82(1):118, 2005.
8. Kaiser LL, Allen L: Position of the American Dietetic Association: nutrition and lifestyle for a healthy pregnancy outcome, *J Am Diet Assoc* 102(10):1479, 2002.
9. Chung CS and others: A single 60-mg iron dose decreases zinc absorption in lactating women, *J Nutr* 132(7):1903, 2002.
10. McLone DG: The etiology of neural tube defects: the role of folic acid, *Childs Nerv Syst* 19(7-8):537, 2003.
11. Centers for Disease Control and Prevention: *Folic acid professional resources,* www.cdc.gov/ncbddd/folicacid/health_overview.htm, accessed November 2006.
12. National Academy of Sciences, Committee on Nutritional Status During Pregnancy and Lactation, Food and Nutrition Board: *Nutrition during pregnancy,* Washington, DC, 1990, National Academies Press.
13. Brown JE, Carlson M: Nutrition and multifetal pregnancy, *J Am Diet Assoc* 100:343, 2000.
14. Ehrenberg HM and others: Low maternal weight, failure to thrive in pregnancy, and adverse pregnancy outcomes, *Am J Obstet Gynecol* 189(6):1726, 2003.
15. Neufeld LM and others: Changes in maternal weight from the first to second trimester of pregnancy are associated with fetal growth and infant length at birth, *Am J Clin Nutr* 79:646, 2004.
16. National Center for Health Statistics: *Health, United States, 2006 with chartbook on trends in the health of Americans,* Hyattsville, MD, 2006, National Center for Health Statistics.
17. Centers for Disease Control and Prevention, National Center for Health Statistics: *NCHS data on teenage pregnancy,* www.cdc.gov/nchs/data/factsheets/teenpreg.pdf, accessed July 2007.
18. Hamilton BE and others: Births: preliminary data for 2004, *National Vital Statistics Report* 54(8), 2005.
19. Corbett RW and others: Pica in pregnancy: does it affect pregnancy outcomes? *MCN Am J Matern Child Nurs* 28(3):183, 2003.
20. Krulewitch CJ: Alcohol consumption during pregnancy, *Ann Rev Nurs Res* 23:101, 2005.
21. May PA and others: Alcohol consumption and other maternal risk factors for fetal alcohol syndrome among three distinct samples of women before, during, and after pregnancy: the risk is relative, *Am J Med Genet C Semin Med Genet* 127:10, 2004.
22. Bertrand J and others: *National Task Force on FAS/FAE. Fetal alcohol syndrome: guidelines for referral and diagnosis.* Atlanta, GA, 2004, Centers for Disease Control and Prevention.
23. Hanke W and others: Environmental tobacco smoke exposure among pregnant women: impact on fetal biometry at 20-24 weeks of gestation and newborn child's birth weight, *Int Arch Occup Environ Health* 77:47, 2004.
24. Bailey BA, Byrom AR: Factors predicting birth weight in a low-risk sample: the role of modifiable pregnancy health behaviors, *Matern Child Health J* 11(2):173, 2006.
25. Kharrazi M and others: Environmental tobacco smoke and pregnancy outcome, *Epidemiology* 15(6):660, 2004.
26. Christian MS, Brent RL: Teratogen update: evaluation of the reproductive and developmental risks of caffeine, *Teratology* 64:51, 2001.
27. Yucesoy G and others: Maternal and perinatal outcome in pregnancies complicated with hypertensive disorder of pregnancy: a seven year experience of tertiary care center, *Arch Gynecol Obstet* 273(1):43, 2005.
28. Crowther CA and others: Calcium supplementation in nulliparous women for the prevention of pregnancy-induced hypertension, preeclampsia and preterm birth: an Australian randomized trial. FRACOG and ACT study group, *AUST N Z J Obstet Gynaecol* 39(1):12, 1999.
29. Hofmeyr GJ and others: Calcium supplementation during pregnancy for preventing hypertensive disorders and related problems, *Cochrane Database Syst Rev* 3:CD001059, 2006.
30. American Diabetes Association: Diagnosis and classification of diabetes mellitus, *Diabetes Care* 29(1):S43, 2006.
31. Carr DB and others: Gestational diabetes mellitus increases the risk of cardiovascular disease in women with a family history of type 2 diabetes, *Diabetes Care* 29(9):2078, 2006.
32. Virtanen HE and others: Mild gestational diabetes as a risk factor for congenital cryptorchidism, *J Clin Endocrinol Metab* 91(12):4862, 2006.
33. Malcolm JC and others: Glucose tolerance of offspring of mothers with gestational diabetes mellitus in a low-risk population, *Diabet Med* 23(5):565, 2006.
34. World Health Organization: *Global strategy for infant and young child feeding,* Geneva, 2003, World Health Organization.
35. U.S. Department of Health and Human Services: *Healthy People 2010: understanding and improving health,* Washington, DC, 2000, U.S. Government Printing Office.
36. American Dietetic Association: Position of the American Dietetic Association: promoting and supporting breastfeeding, *J Am Diet Assoc* 105:810, 2005.

37. Suellentrop K and others: Monitoring progress toward achieving Maternal and Infant Healthy People 2010 objectives—19 states, Pregnancy Risk Assessment Monitoring System (PRAMS), 2000-2003, *MMWR Surveill Summ* 55(9):1, 2006.

38. American Academy of Pediatrics: Breastfeeding and the use of human milk, *Pediatrics* 115:496, 2005.

FURTHER READING AND RESOURCES

Each of the following organizations has an earnest interest in the health care of pregnant women and their children. For information on a variety of topics about pregnancy and lactation, explore their Web sites.

American Academy of Pediatrics: *www.aap.org*

Canadian Paediatric Society: *www.cps.ca*

March of Dimes Birth Defects Foundation: *www.modimes.org*

Birth Defect Research for Children, Inc.: www.birthdefects.org

World Health Organization, Breastfeeding: *www.who.int/topics/breastfeeding/en*

La Leche League International, Inc.: *www.lalecheleauge.org*

U.S. Department of Agriculture WIC Program: *www.fns.usda.gov/wic*

The following two articles evaluate energy and micronutrient needs during pregnancy and the relation between micronutrient status in women throughout the life cycle and the risk for adverse pregnancy outcomes and overall health.

Butte NF and others: Energy requirements during pregnancy based on total energy expenditure and energy deposition, *Am J Clin Nutr* 79:1078, 2004.

Bartley KA and others: A life cycle micronutrient perspective for women's health, *Am J Clin Nutr* 81(suppl):1188S, 2005.

Martin JA and others: Births: final data for 2004, *www.cdc.gov/nchs/data/nvsr/nvsr55/nvsr55_01.pdf*
   The National Vital Statistics Reports, provided in part by the Centers for Disease Control and Prevention, can be fully accessed by the Internet. This report gives an in-depth look at teen pregnancy, risk factors, and general health care of births in the United States.

American Academy of Pediatrics: Breastfeeding and the use of human milk, *Pediatrics* 115:496, 2005.
   This article provides the updated and revised recommendations for, and benefits of, breastfeeding.

Nutrition in Infancy, Childhood, and Adolescence

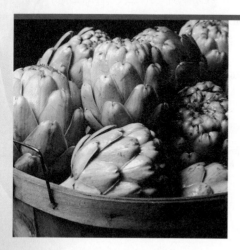

KEY CONCEPTS

- Normal growth of individual children varies within a relatively wide range of measures.
- Human growth and development require both nutritional and psychosocial support.
- A variety of food patterns and habits supply the energy and nutrient requirements of normal growth and development, although basic nutritional needs change with each growth period.

In any culture, food nurtures both the physical and emotional process of "growing up" for each infant, child, and adolescent. Food and eating during these significant years of childhood do not exist apart from the broader overall process of growth and development. The entire process ultimately has a hand in creating and shaping the whole person.

This chapter considers food and feeding in an individual a basic part of growing up. It then relates the various age groups' nutritional needs and food patterns to individual psychosocial development and physical growth.

NUTRITION FOR GROWTH AND DEVELOPMENT

Life Cycle Growth Pattern

The normal human life cycle follows four general stages of overall growth, with individual variation along the way.

Infancy

Growth is rapid during the first year of life, with the rate tapering off somewhat in the latter half of the year. Most infants double their birth weight by the time they are 6 months old and triple it by 1 year of age. Growth in length is not quite as rapid, but on average infants increase their birth length by 50% in the first year and double it by age 4 years.

Childhood

Between infancy and adolescence, the childhood growth rate slows and becomes irregular. Growth occurs in small spurts, during which children have increased appetites and eat accordingly. Appetites usually taper off during periodic plateaus. Parents who recognize the ebb and flow of normal growth patterns in the latent period of childhood can relax and enjoy this time. On the other hand, inexperience or lack of knowledge of this normal flux in growth and appetite can result in stress and battles over food between parents and children.

Adolescence

The onset of puberty begins the second stage of rapid growth, which continues until adult maturity. Growth hormone and sex hormones rise, bringing multiple and often bewildering body changes to young adolescents. During this period long bones grow quickly, sex characteristics develop, and fat and muscle mass increase.

Adulthood

With physical maturity comes the final phase of a normal life cycle. Physical growth levels off during adulthood and then gradually declines during old age. However, mental and psychosocial development lasts a lifetime.

Measuring Childhood Growth

Individual Growth Rates

Children grow at widely varying rates. Therefore the best counsel for parents is that children are *individuals*. A child's growth is not inadequate because the rate does not equal that of another child. General measures of growth in children relate to physical development as well as mental, emotional, social, and cultural growth.

Physical Growth

Growth charts, such as those developed by the National Center for Health Statistics (NCHS) and the Centers for Disease Control and Prevention (CDC), provide an assessment tool for measuring normal growth patterns in infants, children, and adolescents. These charts are based on large numbers of well-nourished children representing the national population. They are used as guides to follow an individual child's pattern of physical growth in relation to the general percentile growth curves of the population. The current charts, published in May 2000, allow the practitioner to plot the growth patterns for height (or length), weight, and head circumference. The body mass index (BMI)-for-age charts for children ages 2 to 20 years can be used continuously from 2 years of age into adulthood. Because BMI in childhood is a determinant of adult BMI, the risk of obesity can be identified early.[1] Specific growth charts have been developed for boys and girls and for infants from birth to age 36 months (Figure 11-1); a separate set of growth charts has been created for children and adolescents from age 2 to 20 years (see the Evolve site for the CDC Growth Charts). An accurate reading depends on using the appropriate growth chart (see the Clinical Applications box, "Use and Interpretation of the CDC Growth Charts").

Individual measures of physical growth for children include weight and height, head circumference, general signs of health, and laboratory tests. Accurate measurement of length (for infants and toddlers), height, weight, and head circumference is critical to the assessment process. Small errors in measurement can easily lead to false alarm about a child's growth pattern.

Psychosocial Development

Various assessments can be used to measure mental, emotional, social, and cultural growth and development. Food is intimately related to these aspects of psychosocial development as well as to physical growth. The growing child does not learn food attitudes and habits in a vacuum, but in close personal and social relationships.

NUTRITIONAL REQUIREMENTS FOR GROWTH

Energy Needs

Kilocalories

The demand for energy, as measured in kilocalories from food, is relatively large during childhood. During the first 3 years of life, children need an average of 90 to 110 kcal/kg body weight per day to support rapid growth. This is significantly higher than adult needs of 30 to 40 kcal/kg per day. Energy needs of premature infants are even greater, ranging from 105 to 130 kcal/kg per day. The DRI values in Table 11-1 present general recommendations for energy and protein needs at different ages. However, specific individual needs vary with age and condition. For example, the total daily caloric intake of an average 5-year-old is spent in the following way:

- Basal metabolism: 50%
- Physical activities: 25%
- Tissue growth: 12%
- Fecal loss: 8%
- Metabolic effect of food: 5%

body mass index (BMI) body weight in kilograms divided by the square of height in meters (kg/m^2). Correlates with body fatness and health risk associated with obesity.

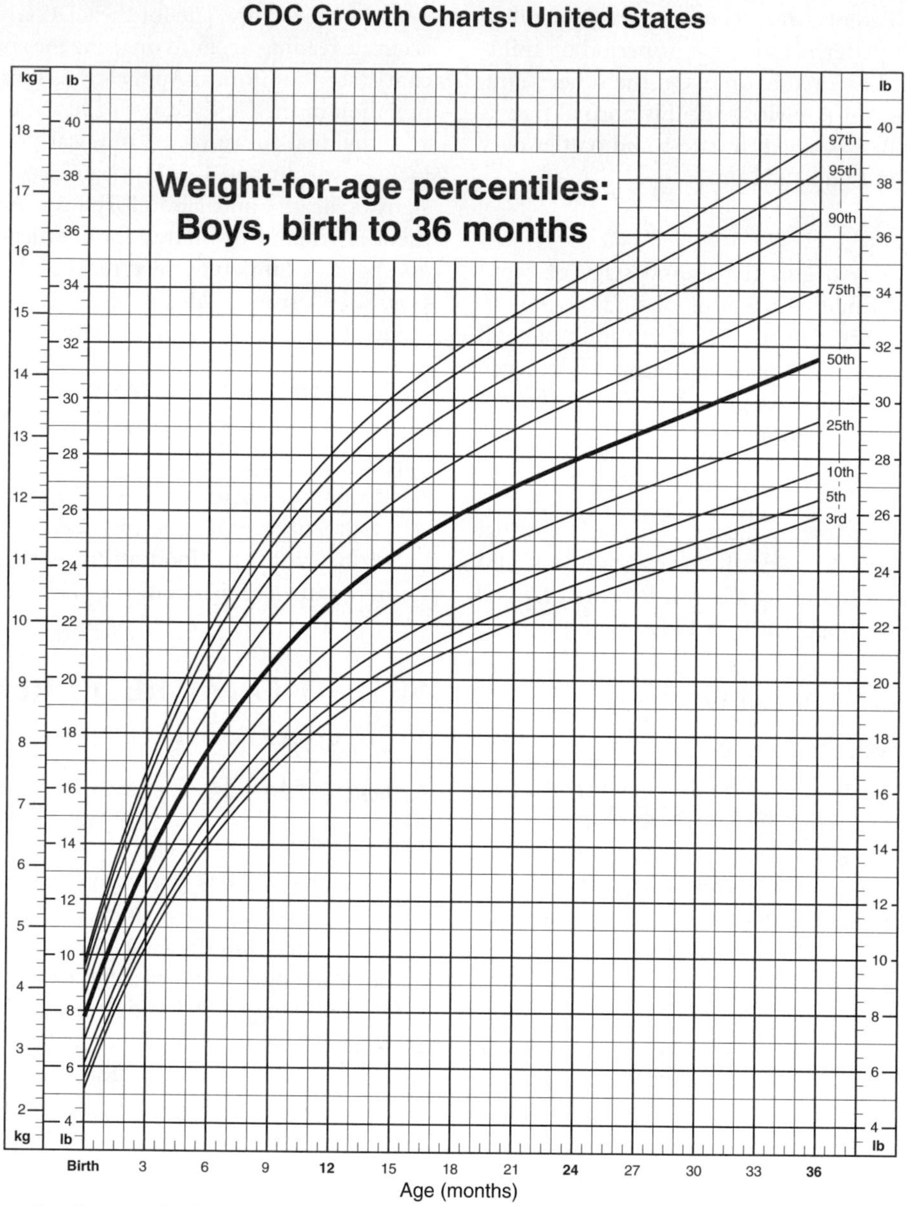

CDC Growth Charts: United States

Figure 11-1 Example of a growth chart produced by the CDC. (Courtesy the National Center for Health Statistics, National Center for Chronic Disease Prevention and Health Promotion, Hyattsville, Md.)

However, some children are more physically active than others and have a higher kilocalorie per kilogram of body weight per day expenditure. Likewise, a child who is growing rapidly has higher tissue growth needs and basal metabolism than a similar child who is not going through a growth spurt.

Macronutrients

Of the total kilocalories, carbohydrates are the main energy source. Carbohydrates also spare protein so that the protein vital for building tissue during childhood growth is not diverted for energy needs. Fat is a backup energy source and supplies *linoleic acid,* an essential fatty acid necessary for growth.

Protein Needs

Protein is the fundamental *tissue-building* substance of the body. It supplies the essential amino acids for tissue growth and maintenance. As a child grows, the protein requirements per unit of body weight gradually decline. For example, for the first 6 months of life the protein re-

USE AND INTERPRETATION OF THE CDC GROWTH CHARTS

Purpose

This guide instructs health care providers on how to use and interpret the CDC growth charts to assess physical growth in children and adolescents. Using these charts, health care providers can compare growth in infants, children, and adolescents with a nationally representative reference based on children of all ages and racial or ethnic groups.

During routine screening, health care providers assess physical growth by using the child's weight, stature, length, and head circumference. Although one measurement plotted on a growth chart can be used to screen children for nutritional risk, it does not provide adequate information to determine the child's growth pattern. When plotted correctly, a series of accurate weights and measurements of stature or length offer important information about a child's growth pattern. Parental stature, for example, is considered before assuming a health or nutrition concern. Other factors, such as the presence of a chronic illness or special health care need, must be considered, and further evaluation may be necessary.

Step 1: Obtain Accurate Weights and Measures

When weighing and measuring children, follow procedures that yield accurate measurements and use equipment that is well maintained.

Step 2: Select the Appropriate Growth Chart

Select the growth chart to use based on the age and gender of the child.

- Enter the child's name and the record number, if appropriate.
- Use the charts listed below when measuring boys and girls in the recumbent position (less than 36 months old): length for age, weight for age, head circumference for age, and weight for length.
- Use the charts listed below when determining the stature (standing height) of boys and girls aged 2 to 20 years: weight for age, stature for age, and BMI for age.

Step 3: Record Data

First record information about factors obtained at the initial visit that influence growth.

- Enter mother's and father's stature as reported.
- Enter the gestational age in weeks.
- Enter the date of birth (omit this step when using growth charts for children aged 2 to 20 years).
- Enter birth weight, length, and head circumference.
- Add notable comments (e.g., breastfeeding).

Record information obtained during the current visit.

- Enter today's date.
- Enter the child's age.
- Enter weight, stature, and head circumference (if appropriate) immediately after taking the measurement.
- Add any notable comments (e.g., was not cooperative).

Step 4: Calculate BMI

BMI is calculated by using weight and stature measurements and is then compared with a child's weight relative to stature with other children of the same age and gender.

- With a calculator, determine BMI with the calculation below.

$$BMI = Weight\ (kg)/Stature\ (cm)/Stature\ (cm) \times 10{,}000$$

or

$$BMI = Weight\ (lb)/Stature\ (in)/Stature\ (in) \times 703$$

Weight and stature measurements must be converted to the appropriate decimal value.

Example: 37 lb 4 oz = 37.25 lb; 41½ in = 41.5 in

Enter BMI to one place after the decimal point (Example: 15.204 = 15.2).

Step 5: Plot Measurements

On the appropriate growth chart, plot the measurements recorded in the data entry table for the current visit.

- Find the child's age on the horizontal axis. When plotting weight for length, find the length on the horizontal axis. Use a straight edge or right-angle ruler to draw a vertical line up from that point.
- Find the appropriate measurement (weight, length, stature, head circumference, or BMI) on the vertical axis. Use a straight edge or right-angle ruler to draw a horizontal line across from that point until it intersects the vertical line.
- Make a small dot where the two lines intersect.

Step 6: Interpret the Plotted Measurements

The curved lines on the growth chart show selected percentiles that indicate the rank of the child's measurement. For example, when the dot is plotted on the 95th percentile line for BMI-for-age, it means that only 5 (5%) of 100 children of the same age and gender in the reference population have a higher BMI-for-age.

1. Determine the percentile rank.
2. Determine if the percentile rank suggests that the anthropometric index is indicative of nutritional risk based on the percentile cutoff value.
3. Compare today's percentile rank with the rank from previous visits to identify any major shifts in the child's growth pattern and the need for further assessment.

ANTHROPOMETRIC INDEX	PERCENTILE CUT-OFF VALUE	NUTRITIONAL STATUS INDICATOR
BMI-for-age	≥95th	Overweight
Weight-for-length	≥95th	
BMI-for-age	≥85th and <95th	At risk of overweight
BMI-for-age		
Weight-for-length	<5th	Underweight
Stature/length-for-age	<5th	Short stature
Head circumference-for-age	<5th->95th	Developmental problems

The training modules are free and can be accessed at *www.cdc.gov/nccdphp/dnpa/growthcharts/training/modules/index.htm.*

Modified from Centers for Disease Control and Prevention: *Use and interpretation of the CDC growth charts, www.cdc.gov/nccdphp/dnpa/growthcharts/resources/growthchart.pdf,* accessed July 2007.

TABLE 11-1

DRIs OF ENERGY AND PROTEIN FROM BIRTH TO 18 YEARS

	AGE	ESTIMATED ENERGY REQUIREMENT	PROTEIN (g)
Infants	0-3 Months	$(89 \times \text{Weight [kg]} - 100) + 175$ kcal	9.1
	4-6 Months	$(89 \times \text{Weight [kg]} - 100) + 56$ kcal	9.1
	7-12 Months	$(89 \times \text{Weight [kg]} - 100) + 22$ kcal	11
	13-36 Months	$(89 \times \text{Weight [kg]} - 100) + 20$ kcal	13
Boys	3-8 Years	$88.5 - (61.9 \times \text{Age [y]} + \text{PA} \times (26.7 \times \text{Weight [kg]} + 903 \times \text{Height [m]}) + 20$ kcal	19
	9-18 Years	$88.5 - (61.9 \times \text{Age [y]}) + \text{PA} \times (26.7 \times \text{Weight [kg]} + 903 \times \text{Height [m]}) + 25$ kcal	34-52
Girls	3-8 Years	$135.3 - (30.8 \times \text{Age [y]} + \text{PA} \times (10.0 \times \text{Weight [kg]} + 934 \times \text{Height [m]}) + 20$ kcal	19
	9-18 Years	$135.3 - (30.8 \times \text{age [y]}) + \text{PA} \times (10.0 \times \text{Weight [kg]} + 934 \times \text{Height [m]}) + 25$ kcal	34-46

PA, Physical activity level.
Data from Food and Nutrition Board, Institute of Medicine: *Dietary reference intakes for energy, carbohydrate, fiber, fat, fatty acids, cholesterol, protein, and amino acids (macronutrients),* Washington, DC, 2002, National Academies Press.

quirements of an infant are 1.52 g/kg of body weight; but the protein needs of a fully grown adult are only 0.8 g/kg.[2] A healthy, active, growing child usually eats enough of a variety of foods to supply the necessary protein and kilocalories for overall growth.

Water Requirements

Water is an essential nutrient, second only to oxygen for life. Metabolic needs, especially during periods of rapid growth, demand adequate fluid intake. For example, compare infant and adult water needs. Infants require more water per unit of body weight than adults do for three important reasons: (1) a greater percentage of the infant's total body weight is composed of water, (2) a larger proportion of the infant's total body water is in extracellular spaces, and (3) infants have a larger proportional body surface area and metabolic rate than do adults. In one day an infant generally consumes an amount of water equivalent to 10% to 15% of body weight, whereas an adult consumes a daily amount equivalent to 2% to 4% of body weight. Table 11-2 provides a summary of the estimated daily fluid needs during growth years.

Mineral and Vitamin Needs

Although yielding no energy themselves, minerals and vitamins have important roles in tissue growth and maintenance as well as in overall energy metabolism. Positive childhood growth depends on adequate amounts of all

TABLE 11-2

APPROXIMATE DAILY FLUID NEEDS DURING GROWTH YEARS

AGE	ml/kg	AGE	ml/kg
0-3 Months	120	4-7 Years	95
3-6 Months	115	7-11 Years	90
6-12 Months	110	11-19 Years	50
1-4 Years	100	>19 Years	30

essential substances. Some nutrients of special interest are discussed below.

Calcium

Calcium needs are critical during the most rapid growth periods of infancy through adolescence. During infancy, mineralization of the skeleton is taking place while bones are growing larger and teeth are forming. Many factors influence bone development in infants and toddlers, including maternal nutritional status during pregnancy, type of infant feeding, calcium and phosphorus content of infant formula or breast milk, introduction of solid foods, and the diet during the toddler and preschool years.[3]

In adolescence, the skeleton grows rapidly to its adult size. Bone density, particularly in long bones and vertebrae, demands adequate calcium, phosphorus, vitamin D, and several other nutrients. In fact, as a preventive measure to reduce the risk for osteoporosis, both research and

CULTURAL CONSIDERATIONS

RACIAL DIFFERENCES IN CALCIUM RETENTION AND PEAK BONE MASS

As discussed in the Cultural Considerations box in Chapter 8, "Bone Health in Gender and Ethnic Groups," noted disparities exist between the genders and ethnic groups regarding bone density. African Americans have significantly higher bone mineral density than their Caucasian counterparts throughout life. Two recent studies involving adolescent girls were able to give insight on the mechanism responsible for racial differences in peak bone mass. Bryant and colleagues found that during the period of peak calcium retention and development of bone mass, African-American girls were able to retain 57% more dietary calcium than Caucasian girls (see figure at right) and had a higher rate of bone formation.*

Authors concluded from this finding that the adult differences of bone mass originate from adolescence, thus making dietary intake of calcium-rich foods throughout the teen years a critical component of lifelong bone health.

Another important finding regarding potential calcium retention was reported by Wigertz and colleagues in their study, "Racial Differences in Calcium Retention in Response to Dietary Salt in Adolescent Girls."† Because adolescence is such a pivotal point for bone health through calcium retention, factors that affect the body's ability to maintain dietary calcium are equally as important. Dietary sodium promotes the loss of calcium through urinary excretion. Wigertz and colleagues were interested in comparing the differences in this effect between African-American and Caucasian girls. They found that "urinary calcium excretion in the adolescent black girls did not increase in response to increased sodium intake to the extent that it increased in the adolescent white girls." This indicates that high intakes of

sodium in Caucasian girls will attenuate the loss of calcium and further weaken potential bone mass.

Health care providers should impress upon adolescent girls, especially Caucasian girls, that high calcium intake with limited sodium consumption will have long-lasting benefits to their bone health.

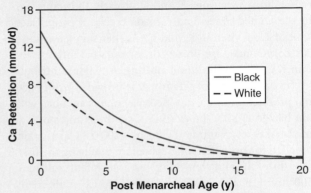

Model for calcium retention, as a function of postmenarcheal age, in African-American and Caucasian girls. *Solid line,* African-American girls; *dashed line,* Caucasian girls. **The cumulative racial difference in bone mass, based on calcium accretion from onset of menarche to 20 years after menarche, is predicted to be 12%.** (Reprinted from Bryant RJ and others: Racial differences in bone turnover and calcium metabolism in adolescent females, *J Clin Endocrinol Metab* 88:1043, 2003.)

*Bryant RJ and others: Racial differences in bone turnover and calcium metabolism in adolescent females, *J Clin Endocrinol Metab* 88:1043, 2003.
†Wigertz K and others: Racial differences in calcium retention in response to dietary salt in adolescent girls, *Am J Clin Nutr* 81:845, 2005.

clinical experience indicate that calcium must be emphasized during adolescence more so than any other time throughout life. Calcium intake during rapid adolescent bone growth is far more effective than the use of more poorly absorbed calcium supplements in older adult years.[4] Furthermore, adolescents taking prednisone or other prescribed steroid therapy have particularly high needs for adequate calcium intake because this line of medication can cause growth stunting and lowered bone density, especially if taken before puberty. A recent study found that race and total sodium intake affected calcium retention in adolescent girls. In this study, African-American girls had significantly higher calcium retention than Caucasian girls, but both races had decreased calcium levels as dietary sodium intake rose (see the Cultural Considerations box, "Racial differences in Calcium Retention and Peak Bone Mass").[5]

Iron

Iron is essential for hemoglobin formation and cognitive development in the early years. Infants of diabetic mothers, growth-restricted newborns, and preterm infants are at greater risk of iron-deficiency anemia regardless of maternal iron stores. The presence of iron deficiency during this critical time can have long-lasting effects on preschool and adolescent children, including poor cognitive, motor, and social-emotional function as well as persisting neurophysiologic differences.[6] The iron content of breast milk is highly absorbable and fully meets the needs of an infant for the first 6 months of life.[7] At that point, the infant's nutrition needs for iron typically exceed that provided exclusively by breast milk, and the addition of solid foods (e.g., enriched cereal, egg yolk, and meat) at approximately 6 months of age helps supply additional iron.

Infants who are not breastfed need iron-fortified formula. Cow's milk, which is very low in iron, should be entirely avoided for the first year of life.

Vitamin Supplements

Much debate has occurred over the years about dietary supplementation of vitamins and minerals for infants. The American Academy of Pediatrics (AAP) recognizes only two vitamins that are potentially needed in supplemental form: vitamins K and D.[8] Nearly all infants born in the United States and Canada receive a prophylactic shot of 1 mg vitamin K, and no further supplementation is recommended for breast- or formula-fed infants. Vitamin K is critical for blood clotting. A major contributor to the daily supply of vitamin K is provided from bacterial production in the gut. Because infants are born without bacterial flora, the vitamin K synthesis and stores are minimal. Oral vitamin D drops (200 IU) are recommended for breastfed infants beginning during the first 2 months of life and continuing until the infant is drinking 500 ml (16 oz) of vitamin D–fortified milk daily.[8] Formula-fed infants do not need an additional supplement of vitamin D because the formula is already fortified.

Excessive supplementation in infants and children is not unheard of and, as with adults, toxicity is a danger. Excess amounts of vitamins A and D, or *hypervitaminosis,* are of special concern in children (see Chapter 7). Excess intake may occur over prolonged periods as a result of ignorance, carelessness, or misunderstanding. Iron toxicity in childhood from overdose of dietary supplements is a leading cause of poison control calls. Parents should provide only the amount directed and no more.

AGE GROUP NEEDS

Infancy

The development of a unique individual begins at birth and continues throughout life. Food is intimately related at each stage of development because physical growth and personal psychosocial development go hand in hand.

Immature Infants

Special care is crucial for tiny, immature babies, who are categorized into two primary groups defined by weight or gestational age.

Weight. Defined by birth weight, low-birth-weight (LBW) infants weigh less than 2500 g (5 lb); very low-birth-weight (VLBW) infants weigh less than 1500 g (3 lb); extremely low-birth-weight (ELBW) babies weigh less than 990 g (2 lb).

Gestational Age. Defined by gestational age, premature infants are born preterm (less than 270 days of gestation) and weigh less than 2500 g (5 lb). Small-for-gestational-age (SGA) infants are born at full term but have had some degree of intrauterine growth failure before birth and have general growth restriction and low weight.

Immature infants are subject to problems with growth and nutrition. Because their bodies are not fully formed, they differ from term infants of normal weight in the following ways: (1) more body water, less protein, and fewer minerals; (2) little subcutaneous fat to maintain body temperature; (3) poorly calcified bones; (4) incomplete nerve and muscle development, making their sucking reflexes weak; (5) limited ability for digestion, absorption, and renal function; and (6) an immature liver lacking developed metabolic enzyme systems or adequate iron stores. To survive, these tiny babies require special feeding.

Type of Milk. Immature infants have grown well on both breast milk (with an added human milk fortifier) and special formulas. Table 11-3 compares these special formulas with standard, term infant formulas and human milk.

Methods of Feeding. Tube feeding and peripheral vein feeding are used in special cases, but both carry hazards and are avoided if possible. For most immature infants bottle feeding or nursing can be successful with much care and support. Infants who have not yet developed the sucking reflex (acquired at approximately 32 weeks' gestation) can still benefit from breast milk, provided the mother is willing and able to pump her breast milk for delivery to the baby by tube feeding.

Term Infants

Mature newborns have more finely developed body systems and grow rapidly, gaining approximately 168 g (6 oz) per week during the first 6 months. The feeding process is an important component of the bonding relationship between parent and child. Mothers may choose to breastfeed or use a formula and then add solid foods at approximately 6 months of age.

Breastfeeding

Human milk is the ideal first food for infants and is the primary recommendation of pediatricians and nutritionists.[9,10] Nutrients in human milk are uniquely adapted to meet the growth needs of infants and are in forms more easily digested, absorbed, and used. Breastfeeding supports early immunity for the baby, helps the mother's uterus quickly return to normal size, and facilitates the important mother-child bonding process. In a recent multicenter cohort study, researchers found that the risk of mortality and morbidity is lower among infants who

TABLE 11-3

NUTRITIONAL VALUE OF SPECIAL FORMULAS AND HUMAN MILK FOR THE PRETERM INFANT

NUTRITIONAL COMPONENT	ADVISABLE INTAKE BY BIRTH WEIGHT		HUMAN MILK		STANDARD FORMULAS*	SPECIAL PREMATURE FORMULAS		
	1.0 kg (2.2 lb)	1.4 kg (3.3 lb)	PRETERM	MATURE	ENFAMIL, SIMILAC, AND SMA	ENFAMIL PREMATURE WITH WHEY	SIMILAC SPECIAL CARE	"PREEMIE" SMA
Kcal/dl			73	73	67	81	81	81
Protein (g/100 Kcal)	3.1	2.7	2.3†	1.5	2.2	3	2.7	2.5
Vitamins, Fat Soluble								
D (IU/120 Kcal/kg/day)	600	600	—	4	70-75	75	180	76
E (IU/120 Kcal/kg/day)	30	30	—	0.3	2-3	2	4	2
Vitamins, Water Soluble								
Folic acid (mcg Kcal/kg/day)	60	60	—	8	9-19	36	45	14
Vitamin C (mg 120 Kcal/kg/day)	60	60	—	7	10	10	45	10
Minerals								
Calcium (mg/100 Kcal)	160	140	40	43	66-78	117	178	92
Phosphorus (mg/100 Kcal)	108	95	18	20	49-66	58	89	49
Sodium (mEq/100 Kcal)	2.7	2.3	1.5‡	0.8	1-1.8	1.7	1.9	1.7

*Enfamil: Mead Johnson Nutritionals, Evansville, Ind.; Similac: Ross Products, Columbus, Ohio; SMA: Wyeth, Philadelphia.
†Range: 1.9-2.8 g/100 kcal.
‡Range: 0.9-2.3 mEq/100 kcal.

are breastfed.[11] Breastfeeding can be successfully started and maintained by most women who try, have support, and consume an appropriate diet for lactation (see Chapter 10). During pregnancy the breasts prepare for lactation and, toward term, produce colostrum. Mature breast milk comes in within the first 3 to 5 days after delivery. As the infant grows, breast milk adapts in composition to match the needs of the developing child. The fat content of breast milk changes from the beginning to the end of a single feeding. *Foremilk,* the first milk to let down, is the lowest in fat content. *Midmilk* has progressively more fat content; and *hindmilk,* the milk coming at the end of the feeding, has the highest fat content. Thus fully emptying each breast at every feeding is important to provide the infant with the energy-dense hindmilk.

The newborn's rooting reflex, oral needs for sucking, and basic hunger usually make breastfeeding simple for healthy, relaxed mothers (Figure 11-2). Working mothers who want to breastfeed their babies can do so by using manual expression or a breast pump while at work as well as freezing and storing milk in sealed plastic baby bottle liners for later use. Childcare facilities provided in some business and industry settings support breastfeeding by employed mothers. Breastfeeding mothers can find support and guidance through local groups of the national La Leche League or professional certified lactation counselors.

Bottle Feeding

If a mother chooses not to breastfeed, or some condition in either the mother or baby prevents it, bottle feeding of an appropriate formula is an acceptable alternative. Sterile procedures in formula preparation, the amount of formula consumed, and weaning from the bottle are some aspects that must be addressed to ensure the health of the child.

Choosing a Formula. Most mothers who bottle feed their infants use a standard commercial formula (see Table 11-3). In some cases of milk allergy or intolerance, a soy-based formula (not soy milk) is used. For infants who are allergic to cow's milk and soy-based formulas, amino acid–based formulas may be medically advised. Examples include Pregestimil and Nutramigen (Mead Johnson Nutritionals, Evansville, Ind.), EleCare and Alimentum (Ross Products, Columbus, Ohio), and Neocate (Nutricia, Gaithersburg, Md.).

Preparing the Formula. Whether preparing a single bottle for each feeding or a day's batch, scrub, rinse, and sterilize all equipment by the *terminal sterilization* method. With any commercial formula, the manufacturer's instructions for mixing concentrated or powdered formula with water should be precisely and consistently followed, and the formula should be refrigerated until use. Throughout the process, scrupulous cleanliness and accurate dilution are essential to prevent infection and illness. A ready-to-feed formula only requires a sterile nipple and bypasses many problems but is more expensive.

Feeding the Formula. Babies usually drink formula either cold or warm; they simply want it to be consistent. Tilting the bottle to keep the nipple full of milk can prevent air swallowing, and the baby's head should be slightly elevated during feeding to facilitate the passage of milk into the stomach. Caregivers should be encouraged to never prop the bottle and leave the baby alone to feed, especially as a pacifier at sleep time. This practice deprives the infant of the cuddling that is a vital part of nurturing and also allows milk to pool in the mouth, causing choking, earache, or *bottle mouth* with early tooth decay. Children should never be put to sleep with a bottle of milk or fruit juice or other caloric liquid capable of pooling in the mouth. Natural bacteria found in the mouth feeds on carbohydrates, producing enamel-damaging acid. Baby bottle tooth decay is a serious and completely avoidable problem resulting from this practice.

Cleaning Bottles and Nipples. Rinse bottles and nipples after each feeding with special bottle and nipple

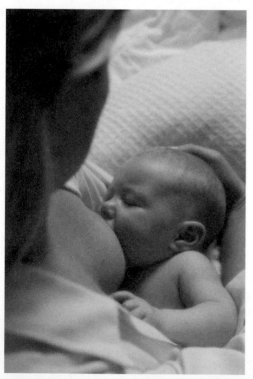

Figure 11-2 Breastfeeding the newborn infant. Note that the mother avoids touching the infant's outer cheek so as not to counteract the infant's natural rooting reflex at the touch of the breast. (Copyright JupiterImages Corporation.)

brushes, forcing water through nipple holes to prevent milk from crusting in them.

Weaning

Throughout the feeding process, observant parents quickly learn to recognize their baby's signs of hunger and satiety and follow the baby's leads. Babies are individuals and set their own particular needs according to age, activity level, growth rate, and metabolic efficiency. A newborn has a very small stomach, holding only 1 to 2 fl oz, but gradually takes more as the stomach capacity enlarges relative to overall body growth. The amounts of increased intake during the first 6 months vary and reflect growth patterns. The following quantities are averages:

- *1 month:* 2 to 3 oz, six to eight feedings, 20 oz total
- *2 months:* 4 to 5 oz, six to seven feedings, 28 oz total
- *3 months:* 6 to 7 oz, five to six feedings, 30 oz total
- *4 months:* 6 to 8 oz, four to five feedings, 30 oz total
- *5 months:* 7 to 8 oz, four to five feedings, 34 oz total
- *6 months:* 7 to 8 oz, four to five feedings, 38 oz total

By 6 to 8 months of age, as increasing amounts of other foods are introduced, weaning from bottle feeding takes place. For some children growing physical capacities and the desire for independence lead to self-weaning, but many children need a little added encouragement from parents.

Cow's Milk

An infant should never be fed cow's milk during the first year of life. Unmodified cow's milk is not suitable for infants; its concentration may cause GI bleeding and provides too heavy a load of solutes for the infant's renal system. Infants and toddlers younger than 2 years also should not be fed reduced-fat cow's milk (e.g., skim or low-fat milk) because (1) *insufficient energy* is provided and (2) *linoleic acid,* the essential fatty acid for growth in the fat portion, is lacking. To meet infant needs during the first year of life, the AAP recommends breast milk, supplemented by vitamin D (if the mother is deficient and the child has inadequate exposure to sunlight), with the gradual addition of iron-fortified foods beginning at approximately 6 months.[10] An alternative formula is appropriate in place of breast milk if the mother chooses.

Solid Food Additions

After critical review of the literature, an expert group on pediatrics stated that the most effective prevention regimen against allergic disease is to provide breast milk and avoid solid foods and cow's milk for at least 4 to 6 months after birth.[12] Because an infant's GI system cannot utilize solid foods well before 6 months, they are not recommended. When solid foods are started, no specific sequence of food additions must be followed. However, some organizations promote the introduction to vegetables, or even meat, before fruits.[13] The root of this recommendation lies in two theories: (1) fruits are much sweeter than vegetables, and infants may develop a preference for a sweet taste first and then not take kindly to the more bitter taste of vegetables (although this theory lacks strong support); and (2) infants given meat before cereal had better zinc intake. Table 11-4 provides a general schedule for introducing solid foods, but individual needs and responses vary and suggestions of individual practitioners should be the guide. Introduce foods one at a time, starting with iron-fortified cereal, and in small amounts so that if an adverse reaction occurs the offending food can easily be identified. Over time, the child is introduced to a variety of foods and comes to enjoy many of them (Figure 11-3). Children's eating behaviors are complex and continue to change with age.

A variety of commercial baby foods are available and are now prepared without added sugar, salt, or monosodium glutamate. Some mothers prefer to prepare their own baby food. Baby food can easily be prepared at home by cooking and straining vegetables and fruits, freezing a batch at a time in ice cube trays, and storing the cubes in plastic bags in the freezer. A single cube can later be reheated for feeding. Throughout the early feeding period, whatever plan is followed, the following basic principles should guide the feeding process: (1) *necessary* nutrients, not any specific food or sequence, are needed; (2) food is a basis of *learning;* and (3) *normal physical development* guides the feeding behavior (see the For Further Focus box, "How Infants Learn to Eat"). Good food habits begin early in life and continue as the child grows. By 8 or 9 months of age, infants should be able to eat table foods (e.g., cooked, chopped, and simply seasoned foods) without needing special infant foods.

---

colostrum a thin, yellow fluid first secreted by the mammary gland a few days after childbirth, preceding the mature breast milk. It contains up to 20% protein, including a large amount of lactalbumin, more minerals, and less lactose and fat than mature milk, as well as immunoglobulins that represent the antibodies found in maternal blood.

weaning to accustom a young child gradually to food other than the mother's milk or a bottle-fed substitute formula as the child's natural need to suckle wanes.

TABLE 11-4

GUIDELINE FOR ADDING SOLID FOODS TO AN INFANT'S DIET DURING THE FIRST YEAR

WHEN TO ADD	FOODS ADDED*
6-8 months	Iron-fortified infant cereal made from rice, barley or oat (offered one at a time) Pureed baby food vegetables or strained fruit
8 months	Whole milk yogurt Pureed baby food meats
8-10 months	Introduce more grain products (one at a time) such as wheat, various crackers and breads, pasta, cereal such as Cheerios Add more vegetables and fruits in various textures (chopped, mashed, cooked, raw) Egg yolk, beans, and additional types of baby food meats Cottage cheese and hard cheeses (cheddar, Colby, Jack)
10-12 months	Infants should be able to tolerate a large variety of grain products and textures Chopped fruits and vegetables Finger foods
12 months	Whole eggs Whole milk

*Semisolid foods should be given immediately before milk feeding. First, 1 or 2 tsp should be given. If food is accepted and tolerated well, the amount should be increased 1 to 2 Tbsp per feeding.

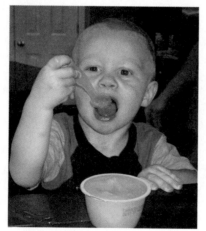
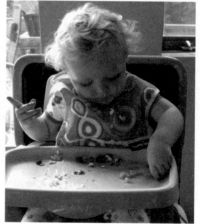

Figure 11-3 Feeding serves as a source of nourishment and facilitates psychosocial and motor skill development.

Summary Guidelines

The Nutrition Committee of the AAP has provided the following recommendations to guide infant feeding:

- *Breastfeeding* provides the ideal first food for the infant, continued for at least the first full year of life, supplemented with a vitamin K shot at birth and daily vitamin D drops (if lifestyle factors indicate a need).
- *Iron-fortified formula* should be used for any infant not breastfeeding or for an infant more than 6 months of age who does not consume a significant portion of his or her kilocalories from added solid foods. Fluoride supplements may be mixed in only if the local water supply is not fluoridated (after 6 months of age).
- *Water and juice* are unnecessary for breastfed infants during the first 6 months.
- *Solid foods* may be introduced at approximately 6 months of age, after the extrusion reflex of early infancy disappears and the ability to swallow solid food is established.
- *Whole cow's milk* may be introduced at the end of the first year if the infant is consuming one third of his or her kilocalories as a balanced mixture of solid foods,

FOR FURTHER FOCUS

HOW INFANTS LEARN TO EAT

Guided by reflexes and the gradual development of muscle control during their first year of life, infants learn many things about living in their particular environment. A basic need is food, which infants obtain through a normal developmental sequence of feeding behaviors in the process of learning to eat.

Age 1 to 3 Months

Rooting, sucking, and swallowing reflexes are present at birth in term infants, along with the tonic neck reflex. Therefore infants secure their first food, milk, with a suckling pattern in which the tongue is projected during a swallow. In the beginning, head control is poor but develops by the third month of life.

Age 4 to 6 Months

The early rooting and biting reflex fades, and the tonic neck reflex has faded by 16 weeks. Infants now change from a suckling pattern with a protruded tongue to a mature, stronger suck with liquids, and a munching pattern begins. Infants are now able to grasp objects with a palmar grip, bringing them to the mouth and biting them.

Age 7 to 9 Months

The gag reflex weakens as infants begin chewing solid foods and develop a normal controlled gag along with control of the choking reflex. A mature munching increases their intake of solid foods while chewing with a rotary motion. These infants can sit alone, secure items, release and re-secure

them, and hold a bottle alone. They begin to develop a pincer grasp to pick up small items between the thumb and forefinger and put them in the mouth.

Age 10 to 12 Months

Older infants can now reach for a spoon. They bite nipples, spoons, and crunchy foods; can grasp a bottle and food and bring them to the mouth; and, with assistance, can drink from a cup. These infants have tongue control to lick food morsels off the lower lip and can finger feed themselves with a refined pincer grasp. These normal developmental behaviors are the basis for the following progressive pattern of introducing semisolid and table foods to older infants:

- *4 to 6 months.* Add iron-fortified, single-grain infant cereals, starting with less-allergenic rice and progressing to wheat and mixed grains.
- *6 to 8 months.* Add strained fruits and vegetables, progressing to strained or finely chopped table meats. Add finger foods (e.g., biscuits or dry toast) that can be secured with a palmar grasp.
- *9 to 12 months.* Gradually delete strained foods and introduce various table foods (e.g., chopped, well-cooked vegetables and meats and chopped, well-cooked or canned fruits). Use smaller finger foods as the pincer grasp develops. Add other well-cooked mashed or chopped table foods, all prepared without added salt or sugar, and help the child drink moderate amounts of juice by cup.

including cereals, vegetables, fruits, and other foods, to supply adequate sources of vitamin C and iron. Reduced-fat or fat-free cow's milk is not recommended until after the age of 2 years.

- Allergens such as wheat, egg white, citrus juice, nuts, and chocolate should not be given as early solid foods but added later, after tolerance has been established through their gradual introduction.
- *Honey* should not be given to an infant younger than 1 year because botulism spores have been reported in honey, and the immune system capacity of the young infant cannot resist this infection.
- *Foods with a high risk for choking* and aspiration, such as hot dogs, nuts, grapes, carrots, popcorn, cherries, peanut butter, and round candy, are best delayed for careful use only with the older child and not given to an infant.

Throughout the first year of life, the requirements for physical growth and psychosocial development are met by human milk or formula, a variety of solid food additions, and a loving, trusting relationship between parents and child.

Childhood

Toddlers (1 to 3 Years)

Once children learn to walk at approximately 1 year of age, these toddlers are off and away, exploring everything and learning new skills. This dawning sense of self, which is a fundamental foundation for ultimate maturity, carries over into many areas, including food. After parents are accustomed to the rapid growth and resulting appetite of the first year of life, they may be concerned when they see their toddler eating less food, and at times having little appetite, while being easily distracted from food to another activity (see the Clinical Applications box, "Feeding Made Simple"). Increasing the variety of foods available helps children develop good food habits. The food

allergens food proteins eliciting an immune system response or allergic reaction. Symptoms may include itching, swelling, hives, diarrhea, and difficulty breathing as well as anaphylaxis in the worst cases.

preferences of young children grow directly from the frequency of a food's use in pleasant surroundings and the increased opportunity to become familiar with a number of foods. Sweets should be reserved for special occasions and not used habitually or as bribes.

Energy and protein needs are still high compared with adult needs (see Table 11-1). Toddlers have a wide range of energy needs during this time directly related to their level of physical activity. Muscle mass, bone structure, and other body tissues continue to grow rapidly and re-

CLINICAL APPLICATIONS

FEEDING MADE SIMPLE

Infants to 2 Years

A study completed in 2002 regarding parental adherence to infant and toddler feeding recommendations (the Feeding Infant and Toddlers Study [FITS]) found that in a random national sample of more than 3000 children, early introduction to solid foods, cow's milk, and juices persists despite recommendations from the AAP to delay the introduction of such foods until infants are developmentally ready (6 months for solid foods and juices and 1 year for cow's milk). The FITS study also found that high-calorie, low-nutrient-density foods such as French fries and soda were consumed on any given day in 10% of children younger than 1 year.* Parents should be reminded that both healthy and unhealthy eating habits develop early, and the nutrient needs of children this young do not allow for empty calories in the diet.

Toddlers 2 to 5 Years

Some parents waste a lot of time coaxing, arguing, begging, and even threatening their 2- to 5-year-olds to eat more than two peas at dinner time. You can help save parents' time, tears, and energy by developing child-feeding strategies based on the normal developmental needs of their children. Parents should be reminded of the following:

- Children are not growing as fast as they did during the first year of life. Consequently, they need less food.
- Children's energy needs are irregular. Note their activity level. Provide food as needed to help their bodies keep up with the many activities planned for each day.

The following suggestions may make feeding children easier:

- *Offer a variety of foods.* After a taste, put new food aside if not taken; then try again later to help develop broad tastes.
- *Serve small portions.* Let children ask for seconds if they are still hungry.
- *Guide children in serving themselves small portions.* Like adults, children's eyes tend to be bigger than their stomachs. Constant, gentle reminders help them learn when to stop.
- *Avoid overseasoning.* Let tastes develop gradually. If a food is too spicy, no amount of cajoling will make them eat it.
- *Do not force foods that the child dislikes.* Individual food dislikes usually do not last long. If the child shuns one

food, offer a similar one if it is available at that meal (e.g., offer a fruit if the child rejects a vegetable) so that little chance of nutrient deficiency occurs.

- *Do not put away the main meal before serving dessert.* Amazing but true: if children are still hungry, some will ask for more food from the main meal after finishing dessert.
- *Keep quick-fix nutritious foods around for off-hour meals.* To keep parents from turning into permanent short-order cooks, keep foods such as fresh and dried fruit, 100% fruit or vegetable juice, cheese, peanut butter, whole-grain bread, and crackers to serve between meals and provide essential nutrients.
- *Enroll the child in a nursery school or preschool program.* Because food is not always available in the classroom, young students learn to eat at regular times. They also tend to try foods they rejected at home, probably because of peer pressure or a desire to impress a new authority figure, the teacher.
- *Be patient.* Remember that although adults may discuss world events over broccoli, toddlers are just now learning how to pick it up with a fork.

Toddlers may take longer. They may not even eat at all. Nevertheless, with flexibility, time, patience, and a sense of humor most parents find that they can get enough nutrients into their children to keep them alive and happy throughout the preschool years. When presented with nutritious food choices, preschoolers tend to self-regulate their intake to meet energy needs without adult intervention.

For more information on typical feeding patterns for children, see the following resources:

- Satter E: *How to get your kid to eat . . . but not too much,* Boulder, CO, 1997, Bull Publishing.
- Satter E: *Child of mine: feeding with love and good sense,* ed 3, Boulder, CO, 2000, Bull Publishing.
- Satter E: *Your child's weight: helping without harming,* Madison, WI, 2005, Kelcy Press.
- Samour PQ, King K: *Handbook of pediatric nutrition,* Sudbury, MA, 2005, Jones and Bartlett.
- Shield J, Mullen M: *The American Dietetic Association guide to healthy eating for kids: how your children can eat smart from five to twelve,* Indianapolis, 2002, Wiley Publishing.
- Ward E: *Healthy foods, healthy kids: a complete guide to nutrition for children from birth to six-year-olds,* Avon, MA, 2002, Adams Media Corporation.

*Briefel RR and others: Feeding infants and toddlers study: improvements needed in meeting infant feeding recommendations, *J Am Diet Assoc* 104(1 Suppl 1):S31, 2004.

quire adequate dietary supply of protein, minerals, and vitamins. The Food and Nutrition Board recommends a daily intake of 19 g of fiber to prevent constipation and promote a healthy GI tract.[2]

Preschool Children (3 to 5 Years)

Physical growth and appetite continue in spurts during this period. Mental capacities develop and the expanding environment is gradually explored. Children continue to form life patterns in attitudes and basic eating habits as a result of social and emotional experiences. These varying experiences frequently lead to food jags (i.e., brief sprees or binges of eating one particular food) that last a few days or weeks but usually are short lived and of no major concern. Again, the key to happy and healthy eating is food variety and relatively small portions. The USDA developed a child-friendly version of MyPyramid, with dietary and physical activity recommendations and messages designed to appeal to young children (Figure 11-4).

Group eating becomes a significant means of socialization (see the Clinical Applications box, "Feeding Made Simple"). For example, during preschool food preferences grow according to what the group is eating. Children in kindergarten also have early learning about healthy eating. The "Five a Day, Let's Eat and Play" program (by the Florida Nutrition Education and Training Program) is designed for preschoolers and allows them to participate in food preparation and then eat their creation. In another program, the Growing Healthy project, the CDC has established 10 content areas focused on the fundamental knowledge of human body biology; principles of health and wellness; and an understanding of health in the larger context of family, community, and the nation (Box 11-1).[13] In such situations a child learns a variety of different food habits and forms new social relationships.

School-Age Children (5 to 12 Years)

The generally slow and irregular growth rate continues in the early school years, and body changes gradually occur. In the year or two before adolescence in particular, reserves are being laid for the rapid growth period ahead. This is the last lull before the storm. By this time, body types are established and growth rates vary widely. Girls' development usually bypasses boys' in the latter part of this period. With the stimulus of school and a variety of learning activities, children experience increasing mental and social maturity, develop the ability to work out problems, and participate in competitive activities. They begin moving from dependence on parental patterns to the standards of peers in preparation for coming independence.

Food preferences are the product of earlier years, but school-age children are increasingly exposed to new stimuli, including television, which influence food habits.[14] The relation between sound nutrition and intellectual learning has long been recognized, establishing breakfast as a particularly important meal for school-age children. The school breakfast and lunch programs provide nourishing meals that meet the Dietary Guidelines recommendations for many children who otherwise would lack balanced meals. The American Dietetic Association has voiced concerns about the lack of such standards with a la carte and competitive foods currently offered at many schools.[15] A report to Congress from the USDA regarding nutrition integrity of school lunch programs stated, "while studies indicate that the school meal programs do contribute to better nutrition and healthier eating behaviors for children who participate, competitive foods undermine the nutrition integrity of the programs and discourage participation."[16] Although such programs (e.g., vending machines, fast food services) can be quite lucrative to schools, the sacrifice to health must be considered.

The classroom also provides positive learning opportunities, particularly when parents provide support at home. An interested and motivated teacher can integrate nutrition into many other learning activities. Community nutrition programs, such as school breakfast and lunch programs, which have a large effect on a child's health, are discussed further in Chapter 13.

Common Nutrition Problems in Childhood

Failure to Thrive. The term *failure to thrive* has been used in pediatrics to describe infants, children, or adolescents who do not grow and develop normally. Failure to thrive most commonly affects young children (1 to

---

school breakfast and lunch programs federally assisted meal programs operating in public and nonprofit private schools and residential child care institutions. They provide nutritionally balanced, low-cost, or free meals to children each school day.

competitive foods any food or beverage served outside federal meal programs, regardless of nutritional value.

nutrition integrity as defined by the School Nutrition Association, "a level of performance that assures all foods and beverages available in schools are consistent with the Dietary Guidelines for Americans, and, when combined with nutrition education, physical activity, and a healthful school environment, contributes to enhanced learning and development of lifelong, healthful eating habits."

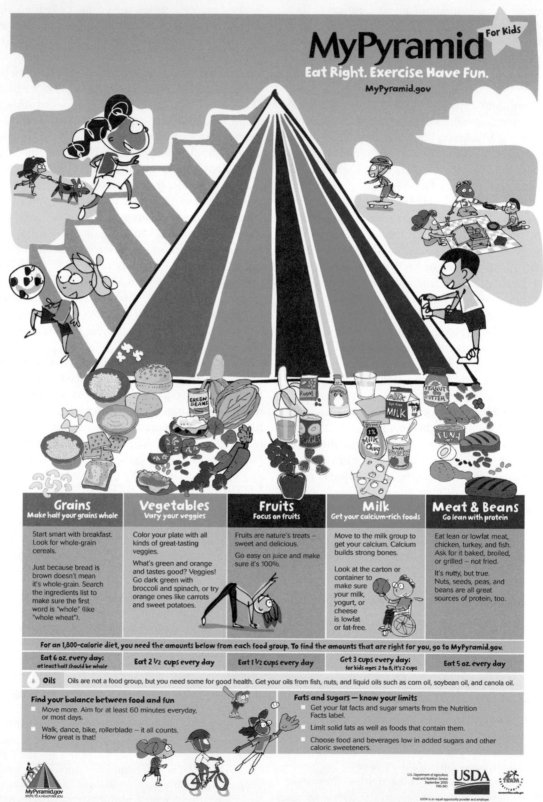

Figure 11-4 MyPyramid for Kids, targeted to meet the needs of children ages 6 to 11 years. (Reprinted from the U.S. Department of Agriculture, Team Nutrition: *MyPyramid for kids: advanced*, Washington, DC, 2005, U.S. Government Printing Office. Available at *teamnutrition.usda.gov/Resources/mpk_poster2.pdf*.)

5 years) of both sexes. Sometimes pediatricians use a brief hospital stay to classify infants who fail to thrive. Careful nutrition assessment is essential for identifying underlying causes of feeding problems. The following factors may be involved:

- *Clinical disease.* CNS disorders (see the Drug-Nutrient Interaction box, "Anticonvulsants and Increased Vitamin Metabolism"), endocrine disease, congenital defects, or partial intestinal obstruction.
- *Neuromotor problems.* Poor sucking or abnormal muscle tone from the retention of primitive reflexes that should have already faded; eating, chewing, and swallowing problems.
- *Dietary practices.* Parental misconceptions or inexperience about what constitutes a normal diet for infants; inappropriate formula feeding or improper dilutions in mixing formula.
- *Unusual nutrient needs or losses.* Adequate diet for growth but inadequate nutrient absorption and thus excessive fecal loss; hypermetabolic state requiring increased dietary intake.
- *Psychosocial problems.* Family environment and relationships resulting in emotional deprivation of the child, requiring medical and nutritional intervention. Similar problems also may occur later (e.g., between 2 and 4 years of age) when parents and children have conflicts about normal changes caused by slowed childhood growth and energy needs that result in changing food patterns, food jags, erratic appetites, reduced milk intake, and disinterest in eating.

Failure to thrive often is caused by a complex of factors, and no easy solutions exist. Careful history taking, supportive nutritional guidance, and warm personal care are necessary to influence growth patterns in these infants. Careful and sensitive correction of the social and environmental issues surrounding the problem is essential.

Anemia. Although fortification of cereals and breads with iron has drastically reduced the cases of iron-deficiency anemia in the United States, it is still a common problem in children with certain eating trends. Children most often deficient in overall iron stores are formula-fed infants who are not receiving iron-fortified formula and older infants (6 months and older) who are not consuming iron-fortified cereals and foods. *Milk anemia* is a term sometimes used for toddlers (older than 1 year) who have excessive consumption of milk, a poor source of iron, that displaces other iron-rich foods. These toddlers and parents are relying on cow's milk for the majority of nutrient intake. Although these children may eat iron-fortified foods, the high calcium intake can inhibit the absorption of iron. Iron-deficiency anemia has been linked to delayed cognitive development in children.[17]

Obesity. Childhood and adolescent obesity has been on the rise for the past 20 years and continues to climb. High blood pressure and type 2 diabetes, health concerns that have historically been associated with older, over-

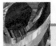

DRUG-NUTRIENT INTERACTION

ANTICONVULSANTS AND INCREASED VITAMIN METABOLISM

Epilepsy is a chronic CNS disorder. The estimated average prevalence is 8.2 per 1000 people in the general population. Medication such as phenobarbital (Luminal), a barbiturate, may be prescribed to treat grand mal and complex partial seizures.

Special diet guidelines should be followed while taking phenobarbital, which increases vitamin D, vitamin K, and folate metabolism, meaning the body uses these vitamins at a faster rate than normal. Therefore an increased intake of these nutrients is warranted and can be accomplished with foods high in the nutrient (e.g., milk for vitamin D and green, leafy vegetables for vitamin K). Women of child-bearing age taking phenobarbital may need as much as 4 mg of folic acid daily; this is an increase from the normal requirement of 0.4 mg/day. Orange juice is the most bioavailable dietary source of folic acid. However, to meet the recommendation of 4 mg/d, a dietary supplement would be necessary. Additional dietary considerations are to avoid caffeine and alcohol; both are contraindicated while taking phenobarbital.*

Sara Oldroyd

*Pronsky ZM: *Food medication interactions*, ed 14, 2006, Birchrunville, PA, Food-Medication Interactions.

weight adults, are increasingly becoming a problem in school-age children. A recently published review of the dynamics and prevalence of early childhood obesity found that African-American race, Hispanic ethnicity, maternal smoking during pregnancy, maternal prepregnancy overweight, and maternal prepregnancy obesity were all positively associated with increased risk of obesity during childhood.[18] Both genetics and environment play major roles in the risk for obesity and are likely covariables. Although overweight parents are more likely to have overweight kids, these families also are self-selecting environments that promote the development of obesity.[19] Such environmental factors include high-fat food selection, or a restrictive feeding practice that ultimately re-

sults in overeating and binging, coupled with low physical activity. Infants and children are quite capable of recognizing satiety and self-regulating energy needs. However, this innate awareness seems to decline between the ages of 3 and 5 years, when "super-sized" meal servings start to influence the amount of food eaten, despite satiety (Box 11-2).[20]

Physical activity is an important part of a healthy lifestyle from birth to death. By developing an appreciation for, and an enjoyment of, regular physical activity during childhood, the risk for obesity may be reduced along with the health problems associated with it. On the other hand, long hours in front of a television, unnecessary snacking, and no involvement in physical activity are

BOX 11-2

CHILDHOOD OVERWEIGHT AND OBESITY FACTS

Overweight is defined as a BMI of greater than the 95th percentile on the CDC 2000 growth charts.

Prevalence

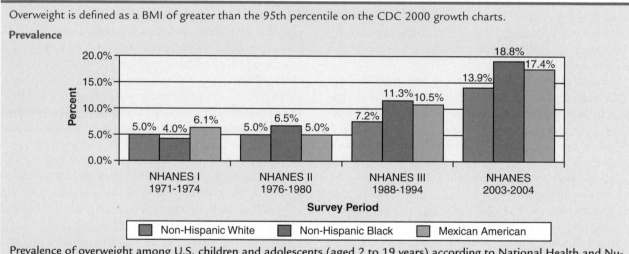

Prevalence of overweight among U.S. children and adolescents (aged 2 to 19 years) according to National Health and Nutrition Examination Surveys. (Reprinted from Centers for Disease Control and Prevention: *Overweight and obesity: childhood overweight*, *www.cdc.gov/nccdphp/dnpa/obesity/childhood/index.htm*, accessed December 2006.)

Contributing Factors
- Genetics
- Behavioral factors
  - Energy intake
  - Physical activity
  - Sedentary behaviors
- Environmental factors
  - Parental role models
  - Positive or negative childcare atmosphere
  - Exposure to health, wellness, and nutrition in the school

Consequences
- Health risk
  - Cardiovascular disease
  - Asthma
  - Hepatic steatosis
  - Sleep apnea
  - Type 2 diabetes
- Psychosocial risk
  - Low self-esteem
  - Social discrimination

The CDC Web site (*www.cdc.gov/nccdphp/dnpa/obesity/childhood/index.htm*) has up-to-date information regarding the prevalence, recommendations, and information about state-based programs to help alleviate the health burden of childhood overweight and obesity.

Data from Centers for Disease Control and Prevention: *Overweight and obesity: childhood overweight*, *www.cdc.gov/nccdphp/dnpa/obesity/childhood/index.htm*, accessed August 2007.

CHAPTER 11 Nutrition in Infancy, Childhood, and Adolescence **205**

habits that start young, die hard, and set the stage for an overweight or obese childhood.

Lead Poisoning. Lead poisoning in children can be extremely harmful to all systems in the body. The CDC estimates that more than 300,000 U.S. children between the ages of 1 and 5 years have health problems associated with lead poisoning each year. Lead exposure in children can cause anemia, kidney damage, colic, muscle weakness, and brain damage, which ultimately can be lethal. The most common method of lead exposure occurs in children living in deteriorating buildings with lead paint. Old, chipped paint results in high levels of lead-contaminated dust. Children explore with their hands and mouths at this age, making oral and inhaled lead highly likely. Lead-based paint was banned in the United States in 1978; however, approximately 24 million homes still contain lead paint. Children living below the poverty line and in older homes are at the greatest risk. The *Healthy People 2010* target is to eliminate lead exposure in children completely.

Adolescence (12 to 18 Years)

Physical Growth

The final growth spurt of childhood occurs with the onset of puberty. This rapid growth is evident in increasing body size and development of sex characteristics in response to hormonal influences. The rate of change varies widely among individual boys and girls, but particularly distinct growth patterns do emerge. Girls store more fat in the abdominal area. As the bony pelvis widens in preparation for future childbearing and subcutaneous fat increases, the size of the hips also increases, causing much anxiety to many figure-conscious young girls. In boys, physical growth is seen more in increased muscle mass and long bone growth. At first a boy's growth spurt is slower than that of a girl, but he soon surpasses her in weight and height.

Researchers have found an association with the timing of sexual maturation and the risk for obesity. Girls who reach sexual maturation early are more likely to become overweight or obese than girls who do not mature until later.[21] However, this association is the opposite for boys. Boys who matured earlier were more likely to be thinner than their counterparts. Racial differences also exist in the timing of maturation; non-Hispanic African-American girls and boys begin the process of sexual maturity before Mexican-American or non-Hispanic Caucasian children.[22] Such differences are specifically important when assessing growth on a growth chart. Age and stage of sexual maturation are associated with body fat and over-

all weight (see the Cultural Considerations box, "Growth Charts: Can You Use Them for All Children?" for more information).

Eating Patterns

Teenagers' eating habits are greatly influenced by their rapid growth as well as self-consciousness and peer pressure; hence their acceptance of popular food fads. Teenagers tend to skip lunch more often than breakfast, derive a great deal of their energy from snacks, eat at fast-food restaurants because these are frequent hangouts, and are likely to eat any kind of food at any time of day. Unfortunately, some teenagers begin to get a significant portion of their total caloric intake in the form of alcohol. Even a mild form of alcohol abuse, when combined with the elevated nutrition demands of adolescence, can easily affect their nutritional status. In general overall nutrition, boys usually fare better than girls. Their larger appetite and sheer volume of food consumed usually ensure an adequate intake of nutrients. On the other hand, under a greater social pressure for thinness, girls may tend to restrict their food and have inadequate nutrient intake.

Eating Disorders

Social, family, and personal pressures concerning figure control strongly influence many young girls and an increasing number of young boys. As a result, they sometimes follow unwise, self-imposed crash diets for weight loss. In some cases self-starvation occurs. Complex eating disorders such as *anorexia nervosa* and *bulimia nervosa* may develop. Psychologists have traditionally identified mothers as the main source of family pressure to remain thin. However, fathers also may contribute to the problem if they are emotionally distant and do not provide important feedback to build self-worth and self-esteem in their young children. Parents must help their children see themselves as loved no matter what they weigh so they are not as vulnerable to social influences that equate extreme thinness with beauty. Eating disorders can have severe effects and involve a distorted body image and a morbid, irrational pursuit of thinness. Such disordered eating often begins in the early adolescent years, when many girls see themselves as fat even though their average weight often is below the normal weight for their height. The longer the duration of the illness, the less likely full recovery will be achieved. Thus early detection and intervention are critical for restoration of overall health.[23] Warning signs, treatment options, and diagnostic criteria are discussed further in Chapter 15.

CULTURAL CONSIDERATIONS

GROWTH CHARTS: CAN YOU USE THEM FOR ALL CHILDREN?

The most recent CDC growth charts, released in May 2000, replaced the previously used charts from 1977. The current set of charts has a new addition, the BMI-for-age charts for both girls and boys aged 2 to 20 years. The current charts also include breastfed infants and are racially and ethnically diverse.

To assess a child's growth accurately, three things are critical: (1) an appropriate growth reference, (2) an accurate measurement, and (3) an accurate calculation of the child's age. Growth charts are not used to identify "short" or "tall" children. They are used as a means of continuous assessment of a child's growth rate. Children are identified with a certain percentile of the population in terms of a specific anthropometric measurement. For example, if a child has a height-for-age at the 70th percentile, then 29% of the children of the same age and gender are taller and 69% are shorter. With adequate nutrition, and in the absence of disease, this child should continue to grow on the 70th percentile curve.

Health professionals use the 5th and 95th percentiles as a cutoff point at which children falling outside this range are screened for potential health- or nutrition-related problems. Children and adolescents with a BMI-for-age above the 85th percentile are at risk for being overweight as adults. The cutoff point of the 95th percentile on the BMI-for-age charts correlates to a BMI of 30 in adults, which is considered obese. Because the BMI-for-age charts correlate with the adult BMI index, they can be used from childhood into adulthood, providing a lifelong assessment tool that indicates risk factors for chronic disease associated with obesity.

Breastfed infants have a slightly different growth curve than formula-fed infants. Breastfed infants grow slightly more rapidly than formula-fed infants in the first 2 months of life; then the rate of growth declines to a rate slower than formula-fed infants. The previous growth charts were predominantly based on formula-fed infants. The new charts use a combined population of both formula-fed and breast-fed infants. However, only approximately one third of the total population was breastfed for more than 3 months. Thus normal growth patterns of breastfed infants may still vary from standardized growth charts.

The World Health Organization (WHO) published a set of international growth charts in April 2006 based on their feeding recommendations, which are to breastfeed for at least 12 months, with solid foods introduced between 4 and 6 months. These growth charts, from birth to 5 years, are specific and appropriate for infants and children who have been exclusively breastfed. The WHO growth charts are available at *www.who.int/childgrowth/en*.

In regard to charting growth patterns of an adolescent, practitioners should be aware of the racial differences in timing of sexual maturation and how that relates to overall weight and body fat. According to a recent study analyzing data from the Third National Health and Nutrition Examination Survey, non-Hispanic African-American girls and boys begin the process of sexual maturity before Mexican-American or non-Hispanic Caucasian children.* The median age at menarche was 12.06 years for the non-Hispanic African-American girls, 12.25 years for the Mexican-American girls, and 12.55 years for the non-Hispanic Caucasian girls, with the median age of 12.43 years for all U.S. girls. The timing of menarche in girls also was assessed in 1973 and, when compared with that data, the average onset of menarche does not appear to have changed over the past 30+ years.† Such differences between racial groups are specifically important when assessing growth on a growth chart because more-mature children are likely to be taller and heavier than their less-mature peers.

Not enough individuals participated in the data collection for the current growth charts to create charts specific to racial or ethnic groups. Therefore the CDC promotes the use of the standard growth charts for all racial and ethnic groups. Future studies will determine if significant differences exist and warrant the development of charts specific to cultural backgrounds.

*Sun SS and others: National estimates of the timing of sexual maturation and racial differences among U.S. children, *Pediatrics* 110(5):911, 2002.
†Sun SS and others: Is sexual maturity occurring earlier among U.S. children? *J Adolesc Health* 37(5):345, 2005.

SUMMARY

Growth and development of healthy children depend on optimal nutrition support. In turn, this good nutrition depends on many social, psychological, cultural, and environmental influences that affect individual growth potential throughout the life cycle.

From birth, the nutrition needs of children change with each unique growth period. *Infants* experience rapid growth. Human milk is the natural first food, with solid foods delayed until approximately 6 months of age, when digestive and physiologic processes have matured. *Toddlers, preschoolers,* and *school-age children* experience slowed and irregular growth. During this period their energy demands are less per kg body weight, but they require a well-balanced diet for continued growth and health. Social and cultural factors influence their developing food habits.

Adolescents undergo a large growth spurt before adulthood. This rapid growth involves both physical and sexual maturation. Boys usually obtain their increased caloric and nutrient demands because they eat larger amounts of food. Girls more often feel social and peer pressure to restrict their food to control their weight, causing some to develop severe eating disorders. This pressure also may prevent them from forming the nutritional reserves necessary for future childbearing.

CRITICAL THINKING QUESTIONS

1. Preterm and term infants have different nutrition needs. Explain why immature infants have special dietary needs.
2. Why is breastfeeding the preferred method of feeding infants? Compare breastfeeding with the commercial formulas available for bottle-fed babies.
3. Outline an appropriate schedule for new parents to use as a guide for adding solid foods to their baby's diet during the first year of life. What foods are not appropriate at this age and why?
4. Compare the changes in growth and development of toddlers, preschoolers, and school-age children. What factors influence their nutrition needs and eating habits?
5. Consider the factors that influence the changing nutrition needs and eating habits of adolescents. Who is usually at greater nutritional risk during this period, boys or girls? Why? What suggestions do you have for reducing the nutritional risk at this vulnerable age?

CHAPTER CHALLENGE QUESTIONS

True-False
Write the correct statement for each statement that is false.
1. *True or False:* A good way to keep infants and toddlers (birth to age 2 years) from being overweight is to use nonfat milk in their diets.
2. *True or False:* A variety of protein foods in a child's diet helps provide all the essential amino acids for growth.
3. *True or False:* Failure to thrive is a condition in some infants and children who do not grow and develop normally and often is associated with parental inexperience.
4. *True or False:* The rooting and sucking reflexes must be learned before a newborn infant can obtain breast milk.
5. *True or False:* A toddler needs the same food variety as an adult, according to the MyPyramid, but with larger serving sizes.

Multiple Choice
1. Fat is needed in the child's diet to supply
   a. minerals.
   b. water-soluble vitamins.
   c. essential amino acids.
   d. essential fatty acids.
2. An iron deficiency in childhood is associated with which of the following diseases?
   a. Scurvy
   b. Rickets
   c. Anemia
   d. Pellagra
3. Growth and development of a school-age child (age 5 to 12 years) are characterized by
   a. a rapid increase in physical growth with increased food requirements.
   b. more rapid growth of girls in the latter part of the period.
   c. food jags and refusal to eat.
   d. increased dependence on parental standards or habits.

evolve Please refer to the Students' Resource section of this text's Evolve Web site for additional study resources.

REFERENCES

1. Centers for Disease Control and Prevention, National Center for Health Statistics: *CDC growth charts: United States,* Atlanta, 2000, CDC. Available at *www.cdc.gov/growthcharts.*
2. Food and Nutrition Board, Institute of Medicine: *Dietary reference intakes for energy, carbohydrate, fiber, fat, fatty acids, cholesterol, protein, and amino acids,* Washington, DC, 2002, National Academies Press.
3. Specker B: Nutrition influences bone development from infancy through toddler years, *J Nutr* 134:691S, 2004.
4. Smith E and others: Does the response of bone mass to calcium supplements depend on calcium absorption efficiency? *Eur J Endocrinol* 151(6):759, 2004.
5. Wigertz K and others: Racial differences in calcium retention in response to dietary salt in adolescent girls, *Am J Clin Nutr* 81:845, 2005.
6. Lozoff B and others: Long-lasting neural and behavioral effects of iron deficiency in infancy, *Nutr Rev* 64:S34, 2006.
7. Food and Nutrition Board, Institute of Medicine: *Dietary reference intakes for vitamin A, vitamin K, arsenic, boron, chromium, copper, iodine, iron, manganese, molybdenum, nickel, silicon, vanadium, and zinc,* Washington, DC, 2002, National Academies Press.
8. American Academy of Pediatrics: Breastfeeding and the use of human milk, *Pediatrics* 115:496, 2005.
9. American Dietetic Association: Position of the American Dietetic Association: promoting and supporting breastfeeding, *J Am Diet Assoc* 105:810, 2005.
10. American Academy of Pediatrics: Breastfeeding and the use of human milk, *Pediatrics* 115:496, 2005.
11. Bahl R and others: Infant feeding patterns and risks of death and hospitalization in the first half of infancy: multicentre cohort study, *Bull World Health Organ* 83(6):418, 2005.
12. Muraro A and others: Dietary prevention of allergic diseases in infants and small children. Part III: critical review of published peer-reviewed observational and interventional studies and final recommendations, *Pediatr Allergy Immunol* 15(4):291, 2004.
13. National Center for Health Education: *Growing healthy, www.nche.org/growinghealthy.htm,* accessed November 2006.
14. Marquis M and others: Does eating while watching television influence children's food-related behaviours? *Can J Diet Pract Res* 66(1):12, 2005.
15. Pilant VB: American Dietetic Association: Position of the American Dietetic Association: local support for nutrition integrity in schools, *J Am Diet Assoc* 106(1):122, 2006.
16. U.S. Department of Agriculture, *Foods sold in competition with USDA school meal programs: a report to Congress, www.fns.usda.gov/cnd/lunch/CompetitiveFoods/report_congress.htm,* accessed July 2007.
17. Walter T: Effect of iron-deficiency anemia on cognitive skills and neuromaturation in infancy and childhood, *Food Nutr Bull* 24(4):S104, 2003.
18. Salsberry PJ, Reagan PB: Dynamics of early childhood overweight, *Pediatrics* 116(6):1329, 2005.
19. Dehghan M and others: Childhood obesity, prevalence and prevention, *Nutr J* 4:24, 2005.
20. Birch LL, Davison KK: Family environmental factors influencing the developing behavioral controls of food intake and childhood overweight, *Pediatr Clin North Am* 48(4):893, 2001.
21. Himes JH and others: Early sexual maturation, body composition, and obesity in African-American girls, *Obes Res* 12:64S, 2004.
22. Sun SS and others: National estimates of the timing of sexual maturation and racial differences among U.S. children, *Pediatrics* 110(5):911, 2002.
23. Rome ES and others: Children and adolescents with eating disorders: the state of the art, *Pediatrics* 111(1):98, 2003.

FURTHER READING AND RESOURCES

KidsHealth: *www.kidshealth.org*

National Center for Education in Maternal and Child Health: *www.ncemch.org*

MyPyramid for kids: *www.mypyramid.gov/kids/index.html*

Food and Nutrition Service: School Meals: *www.fns.usda.gov/cnd*

CDC on lead poisoning in children: *www.cdc.gov/nceh/publications/factsheets/ChildhoodLeadPoisoning.pdf*

WHO child growth standards: *www.who.int/childgrowth/en*

Kidnetic: *www.kidnetic.com*
These Web sites are excellent resources for childhood nutrition information. One of the most important parts of working with parents and children on feeding and health issues is to have access to up-to-date information and ideas. Explore these sites to discover current topics on health and nutrition issues facing youth today.

Salsberry PJ, Reagan PB: Dynamics of early childhood overweight, *Pediatrics* 116(6):1329, 2005.

Dehghan M and others: Childhood obesity, prevalence and prevention, *Nutr J* 4:24, 2005.
These articles explore the many contributing factors to childhood obesity and prevention practices to help alleviate this growing health risk.

Lozoff B and others: Long-lasting neural and behavioral effects of iron deficiency in infancy, *Nutr Rev* 64:S34, 2006.
Iron-deficiency anemia is the most common nutrient disorder worldwide. The authors review the literature regarding iron-deficiency anemia occurring in infancy and the lasting effects observed in early childhood and adolescence. The mechanisms behind such lasting effects are explored in a rat model.

CHAPTER 12

Nutrition for Adults: The Early, Middle, and Later Years

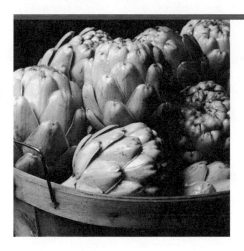

KEY CONCEPTS

- Gradual aging throughout the adult years is an individual process based on genetic heritage and life experience.
- Aging is a total life process, with biologic, nutritional, social, economic, psychological, and spiritual aspects.

The rapid growth and development of adolescence leads to physical maturity as adults. Physical growth in size levels off but continues in the constant cell growth and reproduction necessary to maintain a healthy body. Other aspects of growth and development (e.g., mental, social, psychological, and spiritual) continue for a lifetime.

Food and nutrition continue to provide essential support during the adult aging process. Life expectancy is increasing; thus health promotion and disease prevention are even more important to ensure quality of life throughout the extended years.

This chapter explores the ways in which positive nutrition can help adults lead healthier and happier lives.

ADULTHOOD: CONTINUING HUMAN GROWTH AND DEVELOPMENT

Coming of Age in America

As the pace of modern life becomes faster in the twenty-first century, adults in America are experiencing tremendous change in the composition of the population. The report from the U.S. Department of Health and Human Services, *Healthy People 2010: Understanding and Improving Health,* presents national goals for helping all people make informed decisions about their health.[1] Some of the nutrition goals geared specifically for adults are listed in Box 12-1.

Population and Age Distribution

By the year 2030, according to the U.S. Census Bureau, the total U.S. population will grow to 363.5 million people, up 29.2% from the year 2000.[2] Older segments of the

BOX 12-1

HEALTHY PEOPLE 2010: SELECTED NUTRITION-RELATED OBJECTIVES SPECIFICALLY FOR ADULTS

NUMBER	OBJECTIVE
2-9	Reduce the proportion of adults with osteoporosis.
2-10	Reduce the proportion of adults who are hospitalized for vertebral fractures associated with osteoporosis.
3-12	Increase the proportion of adults who receive a colorectal cancer screening examination.
4-5	Increase the proportion of dialysis patients registered on the waiting list for transplantation.
4-6	Increase the proportion of patients with treated chronic kidney failure who receive a transplant within 3 years of registration on the waiting list.
5-4	Increase the proportion of adults with diabetes whose condition has been diagnosed.
5-12	Increase the proportion of adults with diabetes who have a glycosylated hemoglobin measurement at least once a year.
5-17	Increase the proportion of adults with diabetes who perform self–blood glucose monitoring at least once daily.
10-5	Increase the proportion of consumers who follow key food safety practices.
19-1	Increase the proportion of adults who are at a healthy weight.
19-2	Reduce the proportion of adults who are obese.
21-10	Increase the proportion of children and adults who use the oral health care system each year.
22-1	Reduce the proportion of adults who engage in no leisure-time physical activity.
22-2	Increase the proportion of adults who engage regularly, preferably daily, in moderate physical activity for at least 30 minutes per day.
22-3	Increase the proportion of adults who engage in vigorous physical activity that promotes the development and maintenance of cardiorespiratory fitness 3 or more days per week for 20 or more minutes per occasion.
22-4	Increase the proportion of adults who perform physical activities that enhance and maintain muscular strength and endurance.
22-5	Increase the proportion of adults who perform physical activities that enhance and maintain flexibility.
22-14	Increase the proportion of trips made by walking.
22-15	Increase the proportion of trips made by bicycling.

Modified from the U.S. Department of Health and Human Services: *Healthy people 2010: understanding and improving health,* Washington, DC, 2000, U.S. Government Printing Office.

population will grow significantly during this period; the number of people older than 65 years will more than double, with a large part of that age group older than 85 years (Table 12-1). The median age will increase from 35.3 years to 39 years of age for the total population by 2030. Figure 12-1 shows population growth and projections from 1900 to 2050. Growth rates for various ethnic subgroups continue to rise as well (see the Cultural Considerations box, "Racial and Ethnic Composition of the U.S. Population").

Life Expectancy and Quality of Life

Life expectancy has dramatically increased over the past century, from only 47 years in 1900 to 77.5 years in 2003.[3] By 2010 the average life expectancy is projected to rise to 78 years—74 years for men and 81 years for women. However, notable differences are predicted in life expectancy among various population groups and household incomes. Americans consistently value health-related quality of life—one's personal sense of physical and mental health and ability to act within the environment. Quality of life is a major focus of the *Healthy People 2010* initiative.[1]

Impact on Health Care

Career opportunities in the fields of disease prevention and health promotion are at an all-time high. Community and private classes on healthy lifestyle and nutrition target the prime concerns for a growing adult population. Weight management and diabetes management are two of the most popular topics. Dietitians, nurses, life coaches, personal trainers, psychologists, and other members of the health care team may be involved at various levels in such programs. A dire need exists for the health care system in America to prevent disease development and progression in the adult population instead of having to resort to treatment.

Shaping Influences on Adult Growth and Development

The overall process of human aging begins at birth and lasts a lifetime. Each stage has unique potential for growth and fulfillment. The periods of adulthood—the young, middle, and older years—are no exception. Many indi-

TABLE 12-1

POPULATION PROJECTIONS FOR ADULTS FROM 2000 TO 2030 BY AGE GROUP

AGE (YEARS)	CENSUS 2000	PROJECTION 2030	% INCREASE
20-24	18,964,001	23,136,198	22.0
25-29	19,381,336	22,810,185	17.7
30-34	20,510,388	22,124,671	7.9
35-39	22,706,664	23,399,018	3.0
40-44	22,441,863	23,276,843	3.7
45-49	20,092,404	22,351,985	11.2
50-54	17,585,548	20,550,308	16.9
55-59	13,469,237	19,702,018	46.3
60-64	10,805,447	19,675,860	82.1
65-69	9,533,545	19,980,262	109.6
70-74	8,857,441	17,967,671	102.9
75-79	7,415,813	13,988,906	88.6
80-84	4,945,367	9,913,598	100.5
85+	4,239,587	9,603,034	126.5

Modified from the U.S. Census Bureau, Population Division: *Interim state population projections*, Washington, DC, 2005, U.S. Government Printing Office.

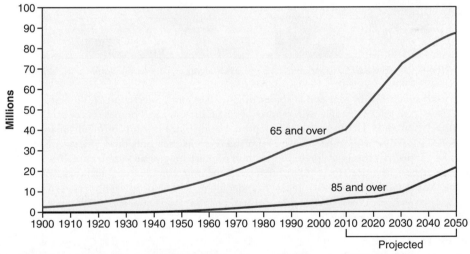

Figure 12-1 Number of people age 65 years and older by age group for the years 1900 to 2000 and projected to 2010 to 2050. Reference population data refer to the resident population. (Reprinted from the Federal Interagency Forum on Aging-Related Statistics: *Older Americans update 2006: key indicators of well being*, Washington, DC, 2006, U.S. Government Printing Office.)

vidual and group events mark the course, but at each stage the four basic areas of adult life—physical, psychosocial, socioeconomic, and nutritional—shape general growth and development.

Physical Growth

Physical maturity is reached in the late teen years, and overall physical growth of the human body, governed by its genetic potential, levels off in the early adult years. Physical growth is no longer a process of increasing numbers of cells and body size but is the vital growth of new cells to replace old ones. Once physical maturity is established, energy requirements decrease. Adjustment to a gradually declining metabolic rate, and thus need for fewer kilocalories, is important for weight management. At older ages, individual vigor reflects the health status of preceding years.

life expectancy the number of years a person of a given age may expect to live; affected by environment, gender, and race.

CULTURAL CONSIDERATIONS

RACIAL AND ETHNIC COMPOSITION OF THE U.S. POPULATION

Shifting racial and ethnic patterns continue to reshape the American population as a whole. The U.S. Census Bureau projects that the proportion of non-Hispanic Caucasians in the population older than 65 years will decline from 82% in 2004 to 61% in 2050. The Hispanic-American population, the fastest growing group in the country, is predicted to grow from 6% of the population to 18%, becoming the second-largest segment of the population. By 2050, African Americans will increase in percentage of the population older than 65 years from 8% to 12% (see figure below).

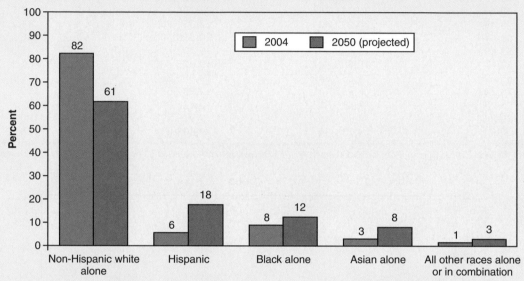

Population age 65 years and older, by race and Hispanic origin, 2004 and projected to 2050. Note: The term "non-Hispanic white alone" is used to refer to people who reported being Caucasian and no other race and who are not Hispanic. The term "black alone" is used to refer to people who reported being black or African American and no other race, and the term "Asian alone" is used to refer to people who reported Asian as their only race. The use of single-race populations in this report does not imply that this is the preferred method of presenting or analyzing data. The U.S. Census Bureau uses a variety of approaches. The race group "All other races alone or in combination" includes American Indian or Alaska Native alone, Native Hawaiian or Other Pacific Islander alone, and all people who reported two or more races. (Reprinted from the Federal Interagency Forum on Aging-Related Statistics: *Older Americans update 2006: key indicators of well being*, Washington, DC, 2006, U.S. Government Printing Office.)

The estimated life expectancy varies among each of these ethnic groups. For example, Caucasians have a life expectancy of 78.3 years, whereas African Americans have a life expectancy of 73.1 years. Living arrangements, household income, educational attainment, type of medical insurance, and many other variables fluctuate among ethnic groups. Health care providers should understand and address the cultural and ethnic needs of an elderly individual when providing nutrition education. All areas of social, socioeconomic, and available health care play significant factors when designing the best care plan. Cookie-cutter meal plans for one ethnic group may not be useful for another culturally diverse population.

Psychosocial Development

Human personality development continues through the adult years. Three unique stages of personal psychosocial growth progress through the young, middle, and older years.

Young Adults (20 to 44 Years). With physical maturity, young adults become increasingly independent. They form many new relationships; adopt new roles; and make many choices concerning continued education, career, jobs,

marriage, and family. Young adults experience considerable stress but also significant personal growth. These are years of professional development, establishing a home, and starting young children on their way through the same life stages—all part of early personal struggles to make one's way in the world. Sometimes health problems relate to these early stress periods. Firm establishment of lifestyle behaviors during this period, such as regular exercise and choosing balanced meals that promote and preserve health, is important for maintaining quality of life long term.

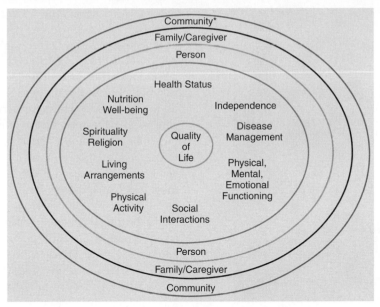

Figure 12-2 Factors that influence quality of life of adults 60 years and older. *Community includes health and supportive services at local, state, and federal levels as well as health professionals and researchers. (Reprinted from the American Dietetic Association: Position paper of the American Dietetic Association: nutrition across the spectrum of aging, *J Am Diet Assoc* 105:616, 2005.)

Middle Adults (45 to 64 Years). The middle years often present an opportunity to expand personal growth. In most cases children have grown and are beginning to make their own lives, and parents may have a sense of "it's my turn now." This also is a time of coming to terms with what life has offered with a refocusing of ideas, life directions, and activities. Early evidence of chronic disease appears in some middle adults. Wellness, health promotion, and reduction of disease risks continue to be a major focus of health care.

Older Adults (65 Years and Older). Adults vary widely in their personal and physical resources to deal with older age. They may have a sense of wholeness and completeness, or they may increasingly withdraw from life. If the outcome of their life experiences is positive, they arrive at an older age as rich persons—rich in the wisdom of their years—and enjoy life and health, enriching the lives of those around them. But some elderly people arrive at these years poorly equipped to deal with adjustments of aging and the health problems that may arise. As this population continues to grow, the subdivision of young-old (65 to 74 years), elderly (75 to 84 years), and old-old (85+ years) has become a popular way to characterize individuals as general health and quality of life continue to improve. Many factors influencing perceived and actual quality of life are integrally associated with nutritional status (Figure 12-2).

Socioeconomic Status

All human beings grow up and live their lives in a social and cultural context. The rapidly changing world currently is experiencing major social and economic shifts. Most adults and their families feel the strain in some way. These pressures directly influence food security and health. As people age, many seniors find themselves under increasing financial pressure. Economic insecurity creates added stress and often leads to the need for food assistance (Figure 12-3). Sometimes social and financial pressures, along with a decreasing sense of acceptance and productivity, cause many elderly persons to feel unwanted and unworthy. Depression is a clinical syndrome, not part of normal aging, and is closely related to poor overall health, poor financial resources, and loneliness.[4,5] Elderly patients with declining health are particularly susceptible to depression, the most common psychiatric condition in the elderly and a leading cause of unintended weight loss. Failure to thrive in the geriatric population, which is generally multifactorial in etiology and caused by a combination of chronic diseases, is associated with impaired physical function, malnutrition, depression, and cognitive impairment.[6] All people need a sense of belonging, achievement, and self-esteem. Instead, many elderly people often are lonely, restless, unhappy, and uncertain.[7]

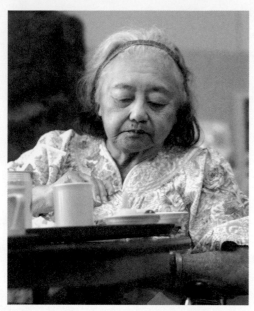

Figure 12-3 Elderly woman assisted by the Food Stamp Program to obtain needed food. (Copyright JupiterImages Corporation.)

Basic needs common to all people are economic security, adequate nutrition, personal effectiveness, suitable housing, constructive and enjoyable activities, satisfying social relationships, and spiritual freedom. An increasing number of healthy, motivated, young-old adults are contributing to the productive workforce and are redefining what being a senior citizen means.

Nutrition Needs

The basic energy and nutrient needs of individual adults in each age group vary according to living and working situations. The DRI standards for healthy adults by age and sex supply most needs, but the aging process influences individual nutritional requirements. Only in the most recent DRIs have scientists distinguished the nutrient needs of the 50- to 70-year-olds from the 71+ years age group. One reason for this was that previously not a large enough population of healthy elderly adults was available to study their nutrient requirements and determine if needs continue to change throughout the life span.

THE AGING PROCESS AND NUTRITION NEEDS

General Physiologic Changes

Biologic Changes

Human biologic growth and decline extend over the entire life span. Throughout life all experiences make their imprint on individual genetic heritage. Everyone ages in different ways depending on individual makeup and resources.

During middle and older adulthood, however, a gradual loss of functioning cells occurs with reduced cell metabolism, starting at approximately age 30 years. As a result, body organ systems gradually lose some capacity to do their jobs and maintain reserves. The rate of this decline accelerates in later life. For example, by age 70 years the kidneys and lungs lose approximately 10% of their former weight, the liver loses 18% of its weight, and skeletal muscle is reduced by 40%. Not all skeletal muscle mass loss is mandatory, however. A major contributing factor in this loss is the lack of physical activity. According to the National Center for Health Statistics (NCHS), a large percent of the adult population is inactive: 35% of adults aged 18 to 44 years, 39% of adults aged 45 to 64 years, and 52% of adults older than 65 years do not participate in any leisure-time activity.[8] The Institute of Medicine, part of the National Academy of Sciences, recommends 60 minutes of moderate exercise every day to maintain a healthy weight.[9] And the *Dietary Guidelines for Americans, 2005* recommend 30 minutes of physical activity per day to reduce the risk of chronic disease and 60 minutes per day to prevent accumulation of excess weight in adulthood (see Chapter 16).[10]

Hormonal changes during the aging process have many repercussions in general health. The common decline in insulin production and/or insulin sensitivity often results in elevated blood glucose levels and diabetes. Decreases in melatonin, the hormone responsible for regulating body rhythms, may interfere with normal sleep cycles. Part of the normal changes in body composition is attributed to decreases in growth hormone and the sex hormones estrogen and testosterone. Menopause, the end of a woman's childbearing years, is marked by the cessation of estrogen and progesterone production by the ovaries. This dramatic change in a woman's life, usually occurring between the ages of 35 and 58 years, represents the most significant hormonal change associated with age. The period of decline in estrogen and progesterone production is accompanied by an increase in body fat, a decrease in lean tissue, and an increase in the risk of chronic disease (specifically heart disease and osteoporosis). Despite these changes, women today are better equipped than ever before with both social and medical support to embrace this period of life and maintain health for many decades to come.

Effect on Food Patterns

Some of the physical changes of aging affect food patterns. For example, secretion of digestive juices and motility of GI muscles gradually diminish, causing decreased absorption and use of nutrients. Decreased taste, smell, and vision also affect appetite and reduce food intake. Several other conditions commonly afflicting the elderly are not so obviously related to food intake but should be considered. For example, decreased hand function, which is especially common in the elderly, can reduce hand-eye coordination and the ability to cook and prepare food. Older persons often have increased concern about body functions, more social stress, personal losses, and fewer social opportunities to maintain self-esteem. All these concerns can affect food intake. Lack of sufficient nourishment is the primary nutrition problem of older adults.

Individuality of the Aging Process

The general process of senescence affects all older adults. Although the biologic changes in aging are general, each person is unique and people show a wide variety of individual responses. Individuals age at different rates and in different ways, depending on their genetic heritage and their health and nutrition resources of past years. Some individuals are in the best shape of their lives *after* retirement. Thus independent needs vary with functional ability.

Nutrition Needs

Kilocalories: Energy

BMR declines an average of 1% to 2% per decade, with a more rapid decline occurring at approximately age 40 years for men and 50 years for women.[9] This correlates to a gradual loss of functioning body cells and reduced physical activity. The current national standard is based on estimates of 5% decreased metabolic activity in middle and older years. The mean energy expenditure for women (with a BMI of 18.5 to 25) ages 51 to 70 years is 2066 kcal/day and for women older than 71 years is 1564 kcal/day. For men of the same ages and BMI, energy expenditure averages 2469 kcal/day and 2238 kcal/day, respectively.[9] These recommendations are based on averages of the population and may vary greatly among individuals. Physical and health status, as well as living situations, influence overall energy and nutrient requirements. Obesity during the adult years has a significant association with chronic illness. One study found that men and women who were obese during their adult years (30 to 49 years) experienced a disability 5 years earlier than did their healthy-weight counterparts.[11] Thus health promotion and disease prevention are important aspects of healthy living throughout the life span, not goals to focus on only during the older years.

The basic fuels necessary to supply these energy needs are primarily carbohydrate, along with moderate fat.

Carbohydrate. Approximately 45% to 65% of total kilocalories should come from carbohydrate foods, with the majority being mostly complex carbohydrates (e.g., whole grains). The National Academy of Sciences has determined that an absolute minimum of 130 g of carbohydrates per day is necessary to maintain normal brain function for children and adults.[9] Easily absorbed sugars (simple sugars in soft drinks, candy, and sweets) also may be used for energy but should be used in limited amounts—no more than 10% of total kilocalorie intake. The prevalence of diabetes and impaired fasting glucose tolerance increases with aging.[12] Decreased glucose tolerance is the prediabetes syndrome in which insulin response to glucose in the bloodstream is inadequate to maintain blood glucose levels within a normal range. Although fasting blood glucose is elevated in individuals with glucose intolerance, it is not high enough for a diagnosis of diabetes. Balanced meals and snacks, including carbohydrates, fat, and protein, can help avoid excessively high blood glucose concentrations and help delay or avoid the onset of diabetes.

Fat. Fats usually contribute approximately 30% of total kilocalories and provide a backup energy source, important fat-soluble vitamins, and essential fatty acids. A reasonable goal is to avoid large quantities of fat and emphasize the quality of the fat used. Fat digestion and absorption may be delayed in elderly persons, but these functions are not greatly disturbed. Sufficient fat for helping food taste better aids appetite and in some cases provides needed kilocalories to prevent excessive weight loss.

Protein. The current national standard recommends an adult protein intake of 0.8 g/kg of body weight, making the total protein need 56 g/day for an average-weight man (154 lb) and 46 g/day for an average-weight woman (127 lb). Protein should provide approximately 10% to 35% of the total kilocalories (see Chapter 4).[9] The need for protein may increase during illness, convalescence, or a wasting disease. In any case, protein needs are related to two basic factors: (1) the protein quality (the quantity and ratio of its amino acids) and (2) adequate total kilocalories in the diet. Healthy adults consuming a balanced diet do not need supplemental amino acid preparations, which are an expensive and inefficient source of available nitrogen.

---

menopause the end of a woman's menstrual activity and capacity to bear children.

senescence the process or condition of growing old.

Vitamins and Minerals

A diet with a variety of foods should supply adequate amounts of most vitamins and minerals for healthy adults. Several of these essential nutrients may need special attention in relation to a few possible health problems in aging.

Osteoporosis. Vitamin D and calcium are essential nutrients for growth and maintenance of healthy bone tissue. Osteoporosis is a disorder in which bone mineral density (BMD) is low and bones become brittle with a high risk of breaking (Figure 12-4). The WHO defines osteoporosis as a BMD value more than 2.5 standard deviations below the mean for normal young Caucasian women. The term osteopenia is used to define low bone mass and increased risk for fracture. Approximately 10 million Americans currently have osteoporosis and an additional 34 million have osteopenia.[13] The prevalence of low bone density and subsequent risk for developing osteoporosis increase significantly with age (Figure 12-5). Race and ethnicity also are determining factors in overall bone health. Risk for fracture is highest among Caucasian women, with African Americans, Hispanics, and Asians having lower incidence rates.[13] Contributing factors for all populations include (1) less use of calcium-rich foods

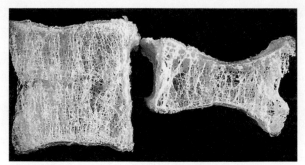

Figure 12-4 Osteoporotic vertebral body *(right)* shortened by compression fractures compared with a normal vertebral body. Note that the osteoporotic vertebra has a characteristic loss of horizontal trabeculae and thickened vertical trabeculae. (Reprinted from Kumar V and others: *Robbins basic pathology*, ed 8, Philadelphia, 2007, Saunders Elsevier.)

such as milk and other dairy products, (2) loss of appetite and lack of adequate body fat, (3) less outdoor physical exercise, (4) decreased estrogen after menopause in women, and (5) decreased capacity of the skin to produce vitamin D with exposure to sunlight. A recently published study also found depression in elderly adults to be positively associated with risk for hip fracture, even after controlling for other known risk factors such as age, gen-

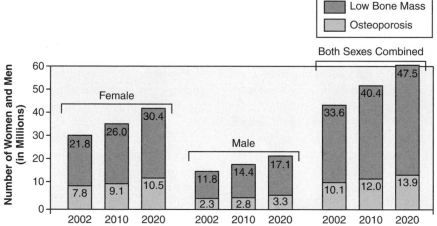

Figure 12-5 Projected prevalence of osteoporosis and/or low bone mass of the hip in women, men, and both sexes, 50 years of age or older. Note: The national Health and Nutrition Examination Survey is conducted by the NCHS, a part of the CDC. This survey is conducted on a nationally representative sample of Americans. As a part of the study BMD of the hip was measured in 14,646 men and women older than 20 years throughout the United States from 1988 until 1994. These values were compared with the WHO definitions to derive the percentage of individuals older than 50 years who have osteoporosis and low bone mass. These percentages were then applied to the total population of men and women older than 50 years to estimate the absolute number of men and women in the United States with osteoporosis and low bone mass. Projections for 2010 and 2020 are based on population forecasts for these years; they are significantly higher than current figures because of the expected growth in the overall population and the expected aging of the population. (Reprinted from the U.S. Department of Health and Human Services: *Bone health and osteoporosis: a report of the surgeon general*, Rockville, MD, 2004, U.S. Department of Health and Human Services.)

der, race, BMI, smoking status, alcohol consumption, and physical activity level.[14]

The DRI standards state the AI level for vitamin D is 10 mcg/day (200 IU) for both men and women age 51 to 70 years and 15 mcg/day (400 IU) for individuals older than 70 years.[15] However, the *Dietary Guidelines for Americans, 2005* recommend a higher level (25 mcg or 1000 IU per day) in light of new research indicating a decreased ability to synthesize vitamin D in the skin of older adults.[10] To meet the dietary recommendation for vitamin D, elderly individuals should consume foods fortified with vitamin D or take a dietary supplement. Chapter 7 discusses food sources of calcium and vitamin D.

Anemia. The poor diet of many older adults lacks sufficient iron to prevent iron-deficiency *anemia*. These individuals need attention and encouragement to help them eat more iron-rich foods along with vitamin C–rich foods for added iron absorption (see Chapter 8).

Box 12-2 outlines Dietary Guidelines specifically targeted to adults.

BOX 12-2

DIETARY GUIDELINES FOR AMERICANS, 2005 PERTAINING TO ADULTS AND THE ELDERLY

- *People over age 50 years.* Consume vitamin B_{12} in its crystalline form (i.e., fortified foods or supplements).
- *Older adults, people with dark skin, and people exposed to insufficient ultraviolet band radiation* (i.e., sunlight). Consume extra vitamin D from vitamin D–fortified foods and/or supplements.
- *Overweight adults and overweight children with chronic diseases and/or on medication.* Consult a health care provider about weight loss strategies before starting a weight-reduction program to ensure appropriate management of other health conditions.
- *Older adults.* Participate in regular physical activity to reduce functional declines associated with aging and achieve the other benefits of physical activity identified for all adults.
- *Individuals with hypertension, African Americans, and middle-aged and older adults.* Aim to consume no more than 1500 mg of sodium per day, and meet the potassium recommendation (4700 mg/day) with food.
- *Pregnant women, older adults, and those who are immunocompromised:* Only eat certain deli meats and hot dogs that have been reheated to steaming hot.

Modified from the U.S. Department of Health and Human Services: *Dietary Guidelines for Americans, 2005*, Washington, DC, 2005, U.S. Government Printing Office.

Nutrient Supplementation

Surveys indicate that 44% of women and 35% of men take vitamin supplements regularly; with higher use in non-Hispanic Caucasians than either non-Hispanic African Americans or Mexican Americans.[16] The use of dietary supplements by elderly adults, usually on a self-prescribed basis, is common. Among all age and gender categories, supplement use is the highest in women older than 80 years (55%).[16] Although such routine use may not be necessary, supplements often are recommended for persons in debilitated states or who have malabsorption conditions. In addition, the DRIs specify that individuals older than 50 years should consume vitamin B_{12} in supplemental form or through fortified foods because of the high risk of deficiency resulting from decreased gastric acid.[17] Hydrochloric acid is secreted from the gastric mucosal cells and is necessary for vitamin B_{12} digestion, along with intrinsic factor. However, as people age the production and secretion of this acid often decreases and may result in inadequate vitamin B_{12} absorption. In this case subcutaneous vitamin B_{12} injections are necessary.

CLINICAL NEEDS

Health Promotion and Disease Prevention

Reduction of Risk for Chronic Disease

The emphasis of adult health care is on reducing individual risks for chronic disease as persons grow older. This approach has always been used for development of the *Dietary Guidelines for Americans* and the national health objectives. These guidelines outline lifestyle changes that people can make to live healthier lives (see Figure 1-2, *Dietary Guidelines for Americans, 2005*). The guidelines emphasize individual needs and good eating habits based on moderation and variety. Health care providers are encouraged to promote healthy lifestyles in all patients and relay the importance of prevention rather than treatment.

osteoporosis a BMD value more than 2.5 standard deviations below the mean 20-year-old sex-matched healthy person average.

osteopenia used to define individuals with low bone mass and increased risk for fracture.

Nutritional Status

Many of the health problems of older adults result from general aging and states of malnutrition (see the Clinical Applications box, "Feeding Older Adults with Sensitivity"). This undernourishment may develop for the following reasons:

- Poor food habits
    - Lack of appetite or loneliness and not wanting to eat alone
    - Lack of food availability because of economic and social issues
- Oral problems, such as poor teeth or poorly fitting dentures
- General GI problems
    - Declining salivary secretions and dry mouth with diminished thirst and taste sensations
    - Less hydrochloric acid secretion in the stomach
    - Decreased enzyme and mucus secretion in the intestines
    - General decline in GI motility

Individual medical symptoms range from vague indigestion or irritable colon to specific diseases such as *peptic ulcer* or *diverticulitis* (see Chapter 18). See Figure 12-6 for the Mini-Nutrition Assessment tool for evaluating nutritional risk.

A recent study that focused on the nutritional status of older adults and their dentition status (number of teeth or dentures) found a positive association between the number of teeth an individual had and his or her overall nutritional status as determined by albumin, hemoglobin, and lymphocyte count.[18] The authors concluded that dental status should be a consideration in evaluating nutritional condition and as a possible cause for malnutrition.

Dehydration, a problem in any age group, is common in the elderly population. Reduced thirst sensation, coupled with declining function of the kidneys, can lead to an overall decline in body water status. Individuals who need assistance with getting water or getting to the bathroom may choose to not drink as much to avoid getting up as often. Water needs, relative to total energy needs, do not decline with age.

Weight Management

Both excessive weight loss and excessive weight gain can be signs of malnutrition. Many of the same depressed living situations and emotional factors that result in unhealthy weight loss also may lead to excessive weight gain. Overeating or undereating becomes a coping mechanism for the conditions encountered by some individuals. Obesity among adults has been on the rise in all subgroups of the adult population (Table 12-2).[8]

CLINICAL APPLICATIONS

FEEDING OLDER ADULTS WITH SENSITIVITY

Many older adults have eating problems and may easily become malnourished. Each person is a unique individual with particular needs and requires sensitive support to meet nutritional and personal requirements. A personal approach, providing assistance for eating when needed, can help meet these needs.

Basic Guidelines

- *Analyze food habits carefully.* Learn about the attitudes, situations, and desires of the older person. Nutrition needs can be met with a variety of foods, so make suggestions in a practical, realistic, and supportive manner.
- *Never moralize.* Never say, "Eat this because it is good for you." This approach has little value for anyone, especially for those struggling to maintain their personal integrity and self-esteem in a youth-oriented, age-fearing culture.
- *Encourage food variety.* Mix new foods with familiar comfort foods. New tastes and seasonings often encour-

age appetite and increase interest in eating. Many people think that a bland diet is best for all elderly persons, but this is not necessarily true. The decreased taste sensitivity of aging necessitates added attention to variety and seasoning. Smaller amounts of food and more frequent meals also may encourage better nutrition.

Assisted Feeding Suggestions

- Make no negative remarks about the food served.
- Identify the food being served.
- Allow the person at least three bites of the same food before going on to another food to allow time for the taste buds to become accustomed to the food.
- Give sufficient time for the person to chew and swallow.
- Give liquids throughout the meal, not just at the beginning and end.

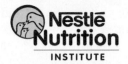

Mini Nutritional Assessment
MNA®

Last name:	First name:	Sex:	Date:

Age:	Weight, kg:	Height, cm:	I.D. Number:

Complete the screen by filling in the boxes with the appropriate numbers.
Add the numbers for the screen. If score is 11 or less, continue with the assessment to gain a Malnutrition Indicator Score.

Screening

A Has food intake declined over the past 3 months due to loss of appetite, digestive problems, chewing or swallowing difficulties?
0 = severe loss of appetite
1 = moderate loss of appetite
2 = no loss of appetite ☐

B Weight loss during last months
0 = weight loss greater than 3 kg (6.6 lbs)
1 = does not know
2 = weight loss between 1 and 3 kg (2.2 and 6.6 lbs)
3 = no weight loss ☐

C Mobility
0 = bed or chair bound
1 = able to get out of bed/chair but does not go out
2 = goes out ☐

D Has suffered psychological stress or acute disease in the past 3 months
0 = yes   2 = no ☐

E Neuropsychological problems
0 = severe dementia or depression
1 = mild dementia
2 = no psychological problems ☐

F Body Mass Index (BMI) (weight in kg) / (height in m)^2
0 = BMI less than 19
1 = BMI 19 to less than 21
2 = BMI 21 to less than 23
3 = BMI 23 or greater ☐

Screening score (subtotal max. 14 points) ☐ ☐

12 points or greater   Normal – not at risk – no need to complete assessment

11 points or below   Possible malnutrition – continue assessment

Assessment

G Lives independently (not in a nursing home or hospital)
0 = no   1 = yes ☐

H Takes more than 3 prescription drugs per day
0 = yes   1 = no ☐

I Pressure sores or skin ulcers
0 = yes   1 = no ☐

J How many full meals does the patient eat daily?
0 = 1 meal
1 = 2 meals
2 = 3 meals ☐

K Selected consumption markers for protein intake
• At least one serving of dairy products (milk, cheese, yogurt) per day?   yes ☐ no ☐
• Two or more servings of legumes or eggs per week?   yes ☐ no ☐
• Meat, fish or poultry every day   yes ☐ no ☐
0.0 = if 0 or 1 yes
0.5 = if 2 yes
1.0 = if 3 yes ☐ ☐

L Consumes two or more servings of fruits or vegetables per day?
0 = no   1 = yes ☐

M How much fluid (water, juice, coffee, tea, milk...) is consumed per day?
0.0 = less than 3 cups
0.5 = 3 to 5 cups
1.0 = more than 5 cups ☐ ☐

N Mode of feeding
0 = unable to eat without assistance
1 = self-fed with some difficulty
2 = self-fed without any problem ☐

O Self view of nutritional status
0 = view self as being malnourished
1 = is uncertain of nutritional state
2 = views self as having no nutritional problem ☐

P In comparison with other people of the same age, how do they consider their health status?
0.0 = not as good
0.5 = does not know
1.0 = as good
2.0 = better ☐.☐

Q Mid-arm circumference (MAC) in cm
0.0 = MAC less than 21
0.5 = MAC 21 to 22
1.0 = MAC 22 or greater ☐.☐

R Calf circumference (CC) in cm
0 = CC less than 31   1 = CC 31 or greater ☐

Assessment (max. 16 points) ☐ ☐.☐

Screening score ☐ ☐

Total Assessment (max. 30 points) ☐ ☐.☐

Malnutrition Indicator Score

17 to 23.5 points	at risk of malnutrition ☐
Less than 17 points	malnourished ☐

08.98 USA

Ref.:   Vellas B, Villars H, Abellan G, et al. Overview of the MNA® - Its History and Challenges. J Nut Health Aging 2006;10:456-465.
Rubenstein LZ, Harker JO, Salva A, Guigoz Y, Vellas B. Screening for Undernutrition in Geriatric Practice: Developing the Short-Form Mini Nutritional Assessment (MNA-SF). J. Geront 2001;56A: M366-377.
Guigoz Y. The Mini-Nutritional Assessment (MNA®) Review of the Literature - What does it tell us? J Nutr Health Aging 2006; 10:466-487.

® Société des Produits Nestlé S.A., Vevey, Switzerland, Trademark Owners.

Figure 12-6 Mini-Nutritional Assessment. (Copyright 2006 Nestle USA, Inc., Glendale, Calif.)

TABLE 12-2

OVERWEIGHT, OBESITY, AND HEALTHY WEIGHT AMONG PERSONS 20 YEARS OF AGE AND OLDER: UNITED STATES, 1988 TO 1994 THROUGH 2001 TO 2004

	PERCENT OF POPULATION	
	1988-1994	2001-2004
Overweight*		
Both sexes	56	66
Men	60.9	70.5
Women	51.4	61.6
Obese†		
Both sexes	22.9	31.4
Men	20.2	29.5
Women	25.5	33.2
Healthy Weight‡		
Both sexes	41.6	32.3
Men	37.9	28.3
Women	45	36.1

*BMI $\geq$25.
†BMI $\geq$30.
‡BMI 18.5-24.9.
Modified from the National Center for Health Statistics: *Health, United States, 2006 with chartbook on trends in the health of Americans,* Hyattsville, MD, 2006, National Center for Health Statistics.

As stated, physical activity is generally lacking in the American adult population. Physical activity is a major factor in weight management and can prevent many of the most debilitating conditions of old age. The American Cancer Society, American Heart Association, American Diabetes Association, and the Department of Health and Human Services all recommend regular physical activity as a means of disease prevention that should be continued throughout life.[19] The *Dietary Guidelines for Americans, 2005* specifically note the long-term benefits of regular cardiovascular and strength training exercises in adults.[10] As the population continues to age, health care facilities are adapting to the increased need for aerobic and stretching classes aimed specifically at older adults who enjoy and benefit from daily exercise (Figure 12-7). Box 12-3 discusses the benefits of physical activity as indicated by the CDC.

Individual Approach

Individual and realistic planning is essential. All personalities and problems are unique, and individual needs vary widely. A malnourished older person needs much personal, sensitive support to build improved eating habits (see the Clinical Applications boxes, "Feeding Older

Adults with Sensitivity" and "Case Study: Situational Problem of an Elderly Woman").

Chronic Diseases of Aging

Chronic diseases of aging (e.g., hypertension, heart disease, stroke, emphysema, diabetes, cancer, arthritis, asthma) may occur in the adult years or at a younger age in the presence of a strong family history. The NCHS reported the percent of persons with any activity limitation caused by chronic conditions rose from 12.5% in adults 45 to 54 years of age to 43.9% in adults older than 75 years.[8] Health experts believe that chronic disease is not an inevitable consequence of aging and estimate that the majority of these cases could have been prevented by lifestyle modifications. The CDC recommends the following lifestyle changes to promote health and prevent chronic disease in adulthood: (1) stop smoking and limit alcohol intake, (2) be moderately physically active for half an hour 5 days or more per week, (3) maintain a healthy weight, and (4) eat a diet low in fat to control cholesterol levels.

Diet Modifications

Diet modifications and nutrition support are an important part of therapy for chronic disease. Details of these modified diets are given in Chapters 17 to 23. In any situation, individual needs and food plans are essential for successful therapy.

BOX 12-3

BENEFITS OF PHYSICAL ACTIVITY FOR SENIOR ADULTS

Physical activity has the following special benefits for older adults:

- Helps maintain the ability to live independently and reduces the risk of falling and fracturing bones.
- Can help reduce blood pressure in some people with hypertension.
- Helps people with chronic, disabling conditions improve stamina and muscle strength.
- Reduces symptoms of anxiety and depression and fosters improved mood and feelings of well-being.
- Helps maintain healthy bones, muscles, and joints.
- Helps control joint swelling and pain associated with arthritis.

Reprinted from the National Center for Chronic Disease Prevention and Health Promotion, Centers for Disease Control and Prevention: Benefits of physical activity for senior adults, *Chronic Disease Notes & Reports* 12(3):11, 1999.

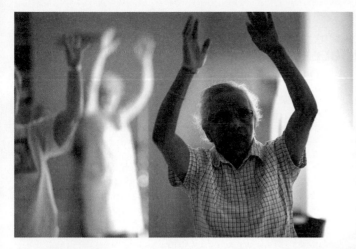

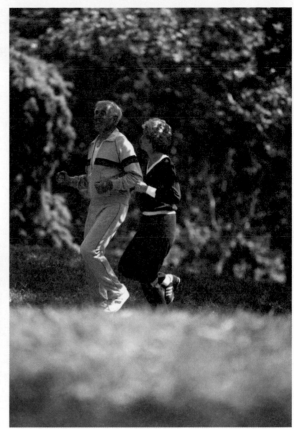

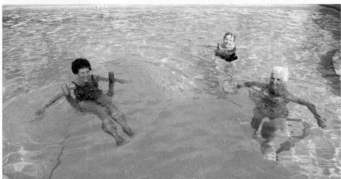

Figure 12-7 Healthy older adults enjoying a variety of physical activities. (Copyright JupiterImages Corporation.)

Medications

Because people are living longer (many with chronic diseases), older adults may be taking as many as eight different prescription drugs for multiple health problems in addition to over-the-counter drugs.[20] **Polypharmacy** can affect overall nutritional status because many drug-nutrient interactions can occur (see Chapter 17). Many of the medications often used by the elderly (e.g., blood pressure medication, antacids, anticoagulation medications, laxatives, diuretics, and decongestants) can directly affect appetite or the absorption and use of nutrients, possibly contributing to malnutrition. When questioning patients about medication use, health care providers should specifically ask about the use of dietary supplements and herbs (see the Drug-Nutrient Interaction box, "St. John's Wort and Depression"). Toxicities from these supplements can be dangerous even though many of these products are considered natural. Each person needs careful evaluation of all drug use and instruction on how to take these medications in relation to food intake (see the Drug-Nutrient Interaction box, "Medication use in the Adult").

COMMUNITY RESOURCES

Government Programs for Older Americans

Poverty has a direct association with prevalence of chronic disease. According to the NCHS, adults living below the national poverty level had a higher incidence of multiple chronic diseases than any other socioeconomic group (Figure 12-8).[8] Health care providers must be aware of community resources and refer when appropriate.

---

polypharmacy use of multiple medications by a patient.

CLINICAL APPLICATIONS

CASE STUDY: SITUATIONAL PROBLEM OF AN ELDERLY WOMAN

Mrs. Johnson, a recently widowed 78-year-old, lives alone in a three-bedroom house in a large city. A fall 1 year ago resulted in a broken hip, and now she depends on a walker for limited mobility. Her only child, a daughter, lives in a distant city and does not want to bear the burden of responsibility for her mother. Mrs. Johnson's only income is a monthly Social Security check for $632. Her monthly property taxes, insurance payments, and utility bills amount to $402.

A recent medical examination revealed that Mrs. Johnson has iron-deficiency anemia and has lost 12 pounds in the past 3 months. Her current weight is 80 pounds; she is 5 feet, 2 inches tall. Mrs. Johnson states that she has not been hungry, and her daily diet is repetitious: broth, a little cottage cheese and canned fruit, saltine crackers, and hot tea. She lacks energy, rarely leaves the house, and appears emaciated and generally distraught.

Questions for Analysis
1. Identify Mrs. Johnson's personal problems and describe how they might be influencing her eating habits. How have her physical problems influenced her food intake?
2. What nutritional improvements could she make in her diet (include food suggestions), and how are these related to her physical needs at this stage of her life?
3. What practical suggestions do you have for helping Mrs. Johnson cope with her physical and social environment? What resources, income sources, food, and companionship can you suggest? How do you think these suggestions would benefit her nutritional status and overall health?

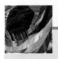

DRUG-NUTRIENT INTERACTION

ST. JOHN'S WORT AND DEPRESSION

Depression is a mental illness that affects 19 million Americans each year. St. John's wort is an herbal supplement commonly used to treat depression and is one of the top-selling supplements in the United States. Clinical trials in the United States and European countries have focused on the efficacy of St. John's wort. Two recent reviews of the literature found conflicting evidence regarding the use of St. John's wort as an alternative for mild to moderate depression.* In several of the randomized controlled trials conducted in patients with mild to moderate depression, it proved just as effective as an antidepressant drug and more effective than placebo. Other trials found only minimal beneficial effects in patients who have major depression.†

Many people do not report herbal supplements when asked about current medications. Unreported herbal supplement use, especially St. John's wort, may result in deleterious side effects when combined with contraindicated medications. St. John's wort interferes with the effectiveness of other antidepressants, drugs to treat HIV infection and AIDS (e.g., indinavir), and drugs to decrease organ transplant rejection (e.g., cyclosporine). Health care providers should specifically ask about dietary supplement use when recording a medication history.

Sara Oldroyd

*Clement K and others: St. John's wort and the treatment of mild to moderate depression: a systematic review, *Holist Nurs Pract* 20(4):197, 2006.
†Linde K and others: St John's wort for depression: meta-analysis of randomized controlled trials, *Br J Psychiatry* 186:99, 2005.

Older Americans Act

The Administration on Aging of the USDHHS administers programs for older adults. Nutrition Services Incentive Programs provide cash and/or commodities to supplement meals. These services include both congregate and home-delivered meals, with related nutrition education and food service components.

Congregate Meals. This program provides older Americans, particularly those with low incomes, with low-cost, nutritionally sound meals in senior centers and other public or private community facilities. In these settings older adults can gather for a hot noon meal and have access to both good food and social support.

Home-Delivered Meals. For those who are ill or disabled and cannot travel to the community centers, meals are delivered by couriers to their homes (Meals on Wheels). This service meets nutrition needs and provides human contact and support. The couriers usually are volunteers concerned about people and their needs. A courier often is the only person a homebound individual may interact with during the day.

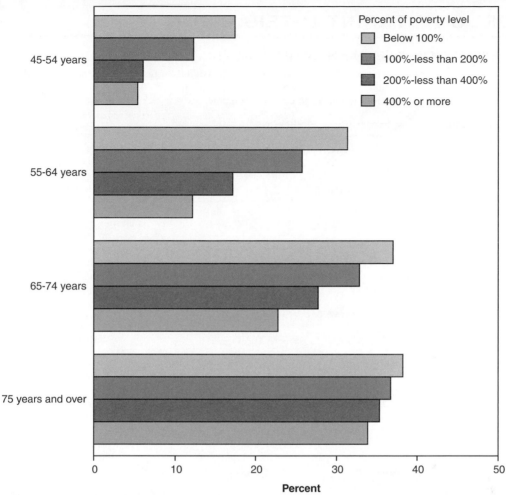

Figure 12-8 Three or more chronic conditions among adults aged 45 years and older, by age and percent of poverty level: United States, 2004. Note: Population is adults who had ever been told by a physician they had three or more of the following conditions: hypertension, heart disease, stroke, emphysema, diabetes, cancer, arthritis and related diseases, or current asthma. Percent of poverty level is based on family income and family size and composition using U.S. Census Bureau poverty thresholds. (Reprinted from the National Center for Health Statistics: *Health, United States, 2006 with chartbook on trends in the health of Americans,* Hyattsville, MD, 2006, National Center for Health Statistics.)

United States Department of Agriculture

The USDA provides both research and services for older adults.

Research Centers. Research centers for studies on aging have been established in various areas of the United States. For example, a Human Nutrition Research Center on Aging was built at Tufts University in Boston and is the largest research facility in the United States specifically authorized by Congress to study the role of nutrition in aging. Studies there involve research on topics such as the protein needs of the aged, the nutritional status of elderly men and women, and the prevention and slowing of osteoporosis through nutrition support. Much more knowledge about the nutritional requirements of older adults is needed to provide better care.

Extension Services. The USDA operates agricultural extension services in state land grant universities, including food and nutrition education services. County home advisors help communities with practical materials and counsel for elderly persons and community workers.

Food Stamp Program. The Food Stamp Program issues electronic benefits transfer cards to the primary care provider in households with a monthly income at or below 130% of the federal poverty line, regardless of age. The

state land grant universities land-grant college or university an institution of higher education that has been designated by the state to receive unique federal support as a result of the Morrill Acts of 1862 and 1890.

DRUG-NUTRIENT INTERACTION

MEDICATION USE IN THE ADULT

Multiple prescription and nonprescription drug use is common in the United States. As the table below indicates, a significant proportion of the population takes at least one prescription medication, and a large percent of the population aged 45 years and older are taking three or more prescription drugs at one time.

Percent of Population Taking Prescription Medication*

AGE GROUP	PERCENT OF POPULATION TAKING AT LEAST ONE PRESCRIPTION DRUG IN THE PAST MONTH	PERCENT OF POPULATION TAKING THREE OR MORE PRESCRIPTION DRUGS IN THE PAST MONTH
18-44 Years	35.9%	8.4%
45-64 Years	64.1%	30.8%
≥65 Years	84.7%	51.6%

In addition to prescription drugs, nonprescription (over-the-counter) medications, dietary supplements (vitamins and minerals), and herbal supplements also are common in this group. The 10 most common medications used by the adult population are listed below per age group.

Top 10 Prescription and Nonprescription Medications Used*

	18-44 YEARS	45-64 YEARS	65-74 YEARS	75+ YEARS
1	Antidepressants	Antidepressants	Hyperlipidemia (high cholesterol)	Hypertension control drugs
2	NSAIDs (pain relief)	Hyperlipidemia (high cholesterol)	Hypertension control drugs	Diuretic (high blood pressure, heart disease)
3	Antihistamines (allergies)	NSAIDs (pain relief)	Blood glucose/sugar regulators (diabetes)	Hyperlipidemia (high cholesterol)
4	Narcotic analgesics (pain relief)	Hypertension control drugs	Nonnarcotic analgesics (pain relief)	Nonnarcotic analgesics (pain relief)
5	Antiasthmatics/ bronchodilators (asthma, breathing)	Blood glucose/sugar regulators (diabetes)	NSAIDs (pain relief)	ACE inhibitors (high blood pressure, heart disease)
6	Vitamins/minerals supplements	Acid/peptic disorders (GI reflux, ulcers)	Acid/peptic disorders (GI reflux, ulcers)	β-blockers (high blood pressure, heart disease)
7	Acid/peptic disorders (GI reflux, ulcers)	Antiasthmatics/ bronchodilator (asthma, breathing)	ACE inhibitors (high blood pressure, heart disease)	Acid/peptic disorders (GI reflux, ulcers)
8	Erythromycins/ lincosamides (infections)	Nonnarcotic analgesics (pain relief)	Diuretic (high blood pressure, heart disease)	Blood glucose/sugar regulators (diabetes)
9	Nonnarcotic analgesics (pain relief)	Narcotic analgesics (pain relief)	β-blockers (high blood pressure, heart disease)	NSAIDs (pain relief)
10	Antitussives/ expectorants (cough and cold, congestion)	ACE inhibitors (high blood pressure, heart disease)	Calcium channel blockers (high blood pressure, heart disease)	Vitamins/minerals supplements

NSAIDs, Nonsteroidal antiinflammatory drugs; *ACE,* angiotensin-converting enzyme.

Several potential drug-nutrient interactions may occur with the most commonly used medications (antidepressants, antihyperlipidemics, hypertensive medication, NSAIDs, and antihistamines). Foods and/or nutrients that should be avoided with these medications are listed on p. 225.

DRUG-NUTRIENT INTERACTION

MEDICATION USE IN THE ADULT—cont'd

DRUG CLASS	FOOD/NUTRIENT	HOW TO AVOID AN ADVERSE REACTION
Certain antidepressants (Nardil and Parnate)	Alcohol and foods containing tyramine	Avoid beer, red wine Avoid tyramine-containing foods: cheese, yogurt, sour cream, liver, cured meats, caviar, dried fish, avocado, banana, raisins, soy sauce, miso soup, ginseng, caffeine-containing products
	Fluids	Drink 2-3 L water per day and take with food; keep sodium intake consistent
Antihyperlipidemics	Take with meal and without alcohol	Take with evening meal and avoid large amounts of alcohol
	Fat-soluble vitamins, folate, B_{12}, and iron	Include rich sources of these vitamins and minerals in diet
Antihypertensives	Licorice and tyramine-rich foods	Avoid licorice and tyramine-containing foods listed above
	Grapefruit juice	Avoid taking with grapefruit juice
NSAIDs	Alcohol	Limit alcohol intake
	Vitamin C, folate, vitamin K	Increase intake of foods high in these vitamins and minerals Take with water
Antihistamines	Alcohol	Avoid alcohol
	Grapefruit juice	Avoid taking with grapefruit juice

*Modified from the National Center for Health Statistics Health, *United States, 2006 with chartbook on trends in the health of Americans,* Hyattsville, MD, 2006, National Center for Health Statistics.

cards are similar to debit cards and can be used at authorized food retail outlets to purchase eligible food items. Currently 17% of participants have an elderly person in the household, and slightly more than 26 million low-income people benefit from the Food Stamp Program every month. The Food Stamp Nutrition Education program promotes the consumption of fruits; vegetables; whole grains; fat-free or low-fat milk products; and lean meats, poultry, and fish.

Commodity Supplemental Food Program. Individuals older than 60 years with a household income at or below 130% of the federal poverty line are eligible for assistance in the form of food packages. The food packages are not intended to provide a complete diet but to supplement the diet with foods high in nutrients typically lacking in the diet of an elderly person.[21]

Senior Farmers Market Nutrition Program. This is a grants-based program that provides low-income older adults with coupons in exchange for fresh fruits, vegetables, and herbs obtained from farmers markets, community-supported agriculture programs, and roadside stands. This program has increased the average servings of fruits and vegetables in participants and provides nutrition education.

Public Health Service

The Public Health Service is a major division of the USDHHS. Skilled health professionals work in the community through local and state public health departments. Public health nutritionists are important members of this health care team, providing nutrition counseling and education and helping various food assistance programs.

Professional Organizations and Resources

National Groups

The American Geriatric Society and The American Gerontological Society are national professional organizations of physicians, nurses, dietitians, and other interested health care workers. These societies publish journals and promote community and government efforts to meet the needs of aging persons.

Community Groups

Local medical societies, nursing organizations, and dietetic associations sponsor various programs to help meet the needs of elderly people. An increasing number of qualified registered dietitians also are in private practice in most communities and can supply a variety of individual and group services. Senior centers in local communities also are valuable resources.

Volunteer Organizations

Many activities of volunteer health organizations (e.g., the American Heart Association and the American Diabetes Association) relate to the needs of older persons and may serve as both a rewarding opportunity for young-old adults and an important source of health-sustaining activities and information for old-old adults.

Chapter 13, Community Food Supply and Health, covers additional resources for nutritional assistance.

ALTERNATIVE LIVING ARRANGEMENTS

A multitude of alternative living arrangements exist for seniors. Independent living facilities, for example, are for independently functioning individuals who do not need medical attention but enjoy recreational and social events with other seniors. Other housing options provide more services, may be staffed with health care workers, and provide different levels of care according to needs. Examples include congregate care, continuing care retirement communities, and assisted living facilities. Nursing homes are fully staffed with medical professionals and are able to provide most medical needs in the absence of an acute episode requiring hospitalization. This text discusses only the types of alternative living arrangements that provide food and health care, not independent living facilities. Several organizations that provide helpful information on alternative living arrangements for seniors are listed under the Further Reading and Resources section of this chapter.

Congregate Care Arrangements

Congregate care arrangements are focused on keeping the elderly living in their own homes for as long as possible with outside assistance for specific needs. Some congregate care arrangements are discussed above: congregate community meals, nutrition education through extension services, and home-delivered meals. Other services include personal care aides, adult day services, transportation, respite care, and more. Personal care aides may shop for groceries, cook, and even help with feeding if necessary.

The emphasis on modified diets in such settings varies. Congregate meals and home-delivered meals are not likely to be specific to diets for individuals with highly particular needs. For example, individuals who precisely count carbohydrates, those with intolerances or allergies, or those who have difficulty swallowing certain food consistencies (dysphagia) may need additional assistance. Most congregate care programs are regulated at the state level. Public programs (congregate meals and home-delivered meals) are required to offer meals that meet the *Dietary Guidelines for Americans, 2005*, and each meal should provide one third of the DRIs.

Continuing Care Retirement Communities

Continuing care retirement communities provide a continuum of residential long-term care from independent living with community-organized events to nursing care facilities. Dietary assistance varies by the needs of the residence. Seniors can move into the community as independent living residences, participating in community activities and meals as they choose. When functional status indicates, seniors receive more care. Continuing care retirement communities usually have assisted living facilities and nursing homes in a campus-style setting. Nutritional involvement within these facilities is discussed below and applies within this continuum of care approach as well.

Assisted Living Facilities

Assisted living facilities can go by several names, including board and care, domiciliary care, sheltered housing, residential care, or personal care. Assisted living arrangements also may exist within continuing care communities. Individual state governments regulate licensure for assisted living facilities. Most assisted living facilities provide all meals and snacks; housekeeping; laundry; and help with dressing, bathing, and personal hygiene. Some facilities provide social activities, limited transportation, and basic medication administration but do not provide medical or nursing care. Living areas vary from full apartments with kitchens to studio-type apartments with small kitchenettes to rooms with baths. Functional status of the individual helps determine the most appropriate setting.

Meals generally are served in a cafeteria or restaurant setting. Some provide menus with several options at each meal, and others serve a set menu for all residences with attention to special needs. Most assisted care facilities cater to basic dietary requests and therapeutic diet needs of their residents. States vary widely in regulations and standards for nutrition policy and services. Some states require that a registered dietitian review meal plans.

Nursing Homes

Nursing homes, or long-term care facilities, provide the most medical, nursing, and nutrition support of the alternative living arrangements. In 2004, 1.44 million people resided in nursing homes in the United States.[8] Nursing homes also provide a residential rehabilitation site outside a hospital for patients to recover from injuries, acute illnesses, and operations. Most patients in nursing homes need help with activities of daily living (bathing, toileting, transferring, etc.), and half of all residents need assistance with eating. Approximately 51% of residents are older than 85 years. A shortage of nursing staff currently exists in the United States, which presents challenges for meeting the needs of all nursing home patients.

Nursing homes do have dietitians on staff and are able to meet specific dietary requirements. However, much less emphasis on modified or therapeutic diets is given for this population. Recent studies have found that family-style eating arrangements (cafeteria with a server) benefit individuals at high risk for malnutrition, especially those with cognitive impairment and below-optimal BMI.[22] Researchers believe that the social interaction and feel of autonomy of family-style eating versus plated tray delivery contribute to the significant increase in energy and nutrient intake. Many of these factors are depicted in Figure 12-2, which stresses how such issues relate to overall quality of life.

SUMMARY

Meeting the nutrition needs of adults—especially older adults—is a challenge for several reasons. Current and past social, economic, and psychological factors influence needs, and the biologic process of aging differs widely in individuals. As average life expectancy continues to increase, research and recommendations on the needs of an aging population are slowly discovered.

Many illnesses in older adults result from malnutrition, not from the effects of aging. Health promotion and disease prevention are key elements in early adulthood to sustain functionality throughout the later years. When working with older people, food habits must be carefully analyzed and approached with encouragement to make positive changes. Individual supportive guidance and patience are necessary using all appropriate nutrition resources. A variety of assisted living arrangements and nutrition services are available for seniors of all functional levels.

CRITICAL THINKING QUESTIONS

1. Mr. Jones is a healthy, active 82-year-old man. He exercises regularly and enjoys a variety of foods. Recently he has started gaining weight. He says he eats exactly the same amount of food he ate when he was 30 years younger. How would you explain to Mr. Jones his weight gain, and what suggestions would you make to prevent any additional unwanted weight gain?

2. Identify and describe three major factors contributing to malnutrition in older adults. How do these factors influence the nutrition counseling process?

3. Your client is on a limited budget and has poor vision and shaky hands. Knowing that fresh fruit and vegetables often are expensive and require washing and cutting, what suggestions would you make for your client to meet the suggested servings of five fruits and vegetables per day?

CHAPTER CHALLENGE QUESTIONS

True-False
Write the correct statement for each statement that is false.

1. *True or False:* Total energy needs slowly decline with age, but water needs decline rapidly.

2. *True or False:* Beginning at approximately 30 years of age, a gradual increase occurs in the performance capacity of most organ systems that lasts throughout adulthood.

3. *True or False:* An extensive research base of knowledge currently exists about the nutrition needs of elderly persons and provides specific energy and nutrient requirements.

4. *True or False:* The simplest basis for judging the adequacy of kilocalorie intake is the maintenance of normal weight.

5. *True or False:* Protein requirement increases with age.

6. *True or False:* Exercise is not recommended for elderly individuals.

Multiple Choice

1. The basic biologic changes of old age include
  a. an increase in the number of cells.
  b. a decreasing need for water.
  c. an increased basal metabolic rate.
  d. a gradual loss of functioning cells and reduced cell metabolism.

2. The Mini-Nutrition Assessment is designed to identify signs of
  a. physical fitness.
  b. emotional stability.
  c. malnutrition.
  d. specific vitamin deficiencies.

3. Which of the following is an example of a physiologic change in aging? *(Circle all that apply.)*
  a. Increased cell metabolism to meet increased aging needs
  b. Decreased GI motility
  c. A gradual increase in the body's muscle mass
  d. Decreased digestive secretions

4. Which of the following actions would help elderly persons find solutions to health problems? *(Circle all that apply.)*
  a. Carefully analyze the individual living situation and food habits
  b. Reinforce good habits, leave harmless ones alone, and suggest needed changes that are practical within the living situation
  c. Encourage variety in foods and seasonings
  d. Explore and use available community resources for assistance

evolve Please refer to the Students' Resource section of this text's Evolve Web site for additional study resources.

REFERENCES

1. U.S. Department of Health and Human Services: *Healthy people 2010. understanding and improving health,* Washington, DC, 2000, U.S. Government Printing Office.
2. U.S. Census Bureau, Population Division: *Interim state population projections,* Washington, DC, 2005, U.S. Government Printing Office.
3. Hoyert DL and others: *Deaths: final data for 2003. National vital statistics reports,* vol. 54, no. 13, Hyattsville, MD, 2006, National Center for Health Statistics.
4. Borg C and others: Life satisfaction among older people (65+) with reduced self-care capacity: the relationship to social, health and financial aspects, *J Clin Nurs* 15(5):607, 2006.
5. Ekwall AK and others: Loneliness as a predictor of quality of life among older caregivers, *J Adv Nurs* 49(1):23, 2005.
6. Robertson RG, Montagnini M: Geriatric failure to thrive, *Am Fam Physician* 70(2):343, 2004.
7. Serby M, Yu M: Overview: depression in the elderly, *Mt Sinai J Med* 70(1):38, 2003.
8. National Center for Health Statistics: *Health, United States, 2006 with chartbook on trends in the health of Americans,* Hyattsville, MD, 2006, National Center for Health Statistics.
9. Food and Nutrition Board, Institute of Medicine: *Dietary reference intakes for energy, carbohydrate, fiber, fat, fatty acids, cholesterol, protein, and amino acids,* Washington, DC, 2002, National Academies Press.
10. U.S. Department of Health and Human Services: *Dietary guidelines for Americans 2005,* Washington, DC, 2005, U.S. Government Printing Office.
11. Peeters A and others: Adult obesity and the burden of disability throughout life, *Obes Res* 12(7):1145, 2004.
12. Cowie CC and others: Prevalence of diabetes and impaired fasting glucose in adults in the U.S. population: National Health and Nutrition Examination Survey 1999-2002, *Diabetes Care* 29(6):1263, 2006.
13. U.S. Department of Health and Human Services: *Bone health and osteoporosis: a report of the surgeon general,* Rockville, MD, 2004, U.S. Department of Health and Human Services.
14. Mussolino ME: Depression and hip fracture risk: the NHANES I epidemiologic follow-up study, *Public Health Rep* 120(1):71, 2005.

15. Food and Nutrition Board, Institute of Medicine: *Dietary reference intakes for calcium, phosphorus, magnesium, vitamin D, and fluoride*, Washington, DC, 1997, National Academies Press.

16. National Center for Health Statistics, Centers for Disease Control and Prevention, U.S. Department of Health and Human Services: *National Health and Nutrition Examination Survey: use of dietary supplements, www.cdc.gov/nchs/data/nhanes/databriefs/dietary.pdf*, accessed December 2006.

17. Food and Nutrition Board, Institute of Medicine: *Dietary reference intakes for thiamin, riboflavin, niacin, vitamin B_6, folate, vitamin B_{12}, pantothenic acid, biotin, and choline*, Washington, DC, 1999, National Academies Press.

18. Chai J and others: Influence of dental status on nutritional status of geriatric patients in a convalescent and rehabilitation hospital, *Int J Prosthodont* 19(3):244, 2006.

19. Kushi LH and others: American Cancer Society guidelines on nutrition and physical activity for cancer prevention: reducing the risk of cancer with healthy food choices and physical activity, *CA Cancer J Clin* 56(5):310, 2006.

20. Steinman MA and others: Polypharmacy and prescription quality in older people, *J Am Geriatr Soc* 54(10):1516, 2006.

21. U.S. Department of Agriculture, Food and Nutrition Service: *Commodity Supplemental Food Program, www.fns.usda.gov/fdd/programs/csfp/about-csfp.htm*, accessed August 2007.

22. Desai J and others: Changes in type of foodservice and dining room environment preferentially benefit institutionalized seniors with low body mass indexes, *J Am Diet Assoc* 107(5):808, 2007.

FURTHER READING AND RESOURCES

Administration on Aging: *www.aoa.dhhs.gov*

Centers for Medicare & Medicaid Services: *www.cms.hhs.gov*

National Institute on Aging: *www.nia.nih.gov*

American Society on Aging: *www.asaging.org*

The Gerontological Society of America: *www.geron.org*

National Osteoporosis Foundation: *www.nof.org*

National Council on the Aging: *www.ncoa.org*

USDA, Food and Nutrition Service, Commodity Supplemental Food Program: *www.fns.usda.gov/fdd/programs/csfp/about-csfp.htm*

CDC, Trends in Healthy Aging: *www.cdc.gov/nchs/agingact.htm*

American Association of Homes and Services for the Aging: *www.aahsa.org*

Assisted Living Federation of America: *www.alfa.org*

USDHHS Eldercare Locator: *www.eldercare.gov/eldercare/Public/Home.asp*
These organizations are excellent sources of information on nutrition, health, and community services for the elderly.

American Dietetic Association: Position paper of the American Dietetic Association: nutrition across the spectrum of aging, *J Am Diet Assoc* 105:616, 2005.

Johnson MA: Nutrition and aging—practical advice for healthy eating, *J Am Med Womens Assoc* 59(4):262, 2004.

McDermott AY, Mernitz H: Exercise and older patients: prescribing guidelines, *Am Fam Physician* 74(3):437, 2006.
The authors discuss the benefits and recommendations for exercising and healthy eating throughout adulthood.

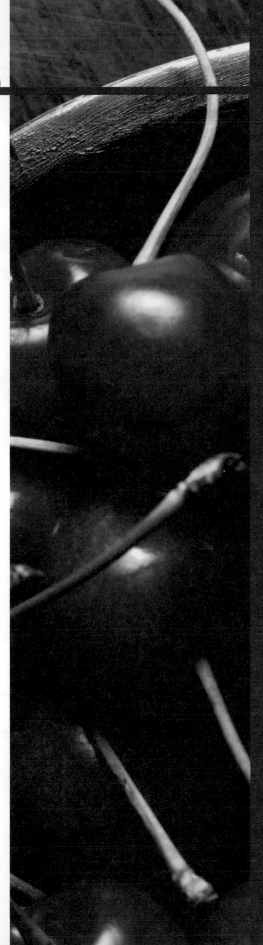

PART 3

Community Nutrition and Health Care

Community Food Supply and Health

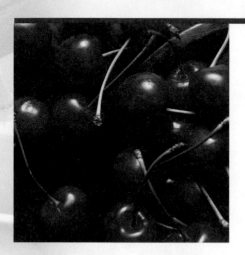

KEY CONCEPTS

- Modern food production, processing, and marketing have both positive and negative influences on food safety.
- Many organisms in contaminated food transmit disease.
- Poverty often prevents individuals and families from having adequate access to their community food supply.

The health of a community largely depends on the safety of its available food and water supply. The American system of government control agencies and regulations, along with local and state public health officials, works diligently to maintain a safe food supply. The food supply in the United States has undergone dramatic changes over the past few decades.

This chapter explores factors that influence the safety of food. America's bountiful food supply is accompanied by certain hazards. Potential health problems related to the food supply can arise from several sources, such as lack of sanitation, food-borne disease, and poverty.

FOOD SAFETY AND HEALTH PROMOTION

Government Control Agencies

The food supply in the United States has exploded in recent years. Keeping the food supply safe is no small task. Several federal agencies now help control food safety and quality. The FDA is the primary governing body of the American food supply, with the exception of meat and poultry. The *USDA Food Safety and Inspection Service* is responsible for food safety of both domestic and imported meat and poultry (Figure 13-1). The *National Marine Fisheries Service* governs the safety of seafood and fisheries. The *Environmental Protection Agency* regulates the use of pesticides and other chemicals and ensures the safety of public drinking water. Regulation of advertising

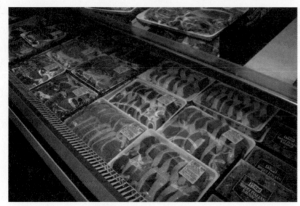

Figure 13-1 Food safety of pork and other meat products is the responsibility of the USDA and the Food Safety and Inspection Service. (Courtesy Ken Hammond, Agricultural Research Service, USDA, Washington, DC.)

and truthful marketing of food products is a large job and is the duty of the *Federal Trade Commission*. The CDC monitors and investigates cases of food-borne illness and is proactive in education and prevention. Multiple other federal, state, and local agencies participate in education and research to promote safety in the food supply.

Food and Drug Administration

Enforcement of Federal Food Safety Regulations. The FDA is a law enforcement agency charged by the U.S. Congress to ensure, among other things, that America's food supply is safe, pure, and wholesome. The agency enforces federal food safety regulations through various activities, including (1) enforcing food sanitation and quality control, (2) controlling food additives, (3) regulating the movement of foods across state lines, (4) maintaining the nutrition labeling of foods, (5) ensuring the safety of public food service, and (6) ensuring the safety of most food products. The agency's methods of enforcement are recall, seizure, injunction, and prosecution. The use of recalls is the most common method, followed by seizures of contaminated food. Injunction involves a court order to stop the sale and/or production of a food item. This procedure is not common and generally is in response to a claim that a food item is potentially harmful or has not undergone appropriate testing or acquired adequate approval for sale. One example of this is the court-ordered halt of the sale of genetically engineered alfalfa in March 2007. The Center for Food Safety filed a case against the USDA for not conducting an Environmental Impact Statement before approving sale of the alfalfa.

Consumer Education. The FDA's division of consumer education conducts an active program of protection through consumer education and general public information. Special attention is given to nutrition misinformation. Materials are prepared and distributed to individuals, students, and community groups. Consumer specialists work in all FDA district offices.

Research. Along with the USDA's Agricultural Research Service, FDA scientists continually evaluate foods and food components through their own research. For a more health-conscious public and a changing marketplace, the FDA is developing nutrition guidelines for a variety of food products, including main dishes, meat substitutes, fruit juices and fruit drinks, and snack foods. The FDA has a long history of food safety activities, research, programs, and initiatives. For information on past research and programs by the FDA that have positively promoted change, the National Food Safety Programs Historical Background Web site is frequently updated *(www.foodsafety.gov/~dms/fs-toc2.html).*

Development of Food Labels

Early Development of Label Regulations

In the mid-1960s the FDA established "truth in packaging" regulations that dealt mainly with food standards. As food processing developed and the number of items grew, the labels included more nutrition information. Both types of label information are important to consumers.

Food Standards. The basic *standard of identity* requires that labels on foods not having an established reference standard must list all the ingredients in the order of amount found in the product. Other food standard information on labels relates to food quality, fill of container, and enrichment.

Nutrition Information. Under regulations adopted in 1973, the FDA began developing a labeling system that describes a food's nutritional value. Some producers began to add limited information on their own to meet this increasing market demand. Many people became concerned that nutrition labeling was inadequate, but the real problem was what and how much were being labeled and in what format. Information about nutrients and food constituents that consumer groups believed should be listed on labels included the amount of macronutrients (carbohydrate, protein, fat) and their total energy value (calories), key micronutrients (e.g., calcium, iron, vitamin A), sodium, cholesterol, trans fat, and saturated fat. Concerned public and professional groups also want nutrients to be identified in terms of percentages of the current DRI standard per defined portion. Surveys indicate that 60% to 80% of shoppers consult the food label before purchasing a new product and that 30% to 40% of that group make their decision to buy on the basis of the information provided.[1]

Background of Present Food and Drug Administration Label Regulations

Over the past 10 years two factors have fueled rapid progress toward better food labels: (1) an increase in the variety of food products entering the U.S. marketplace and (2) changing patterns of American eating habits. Both factors led many health-conscious consumers and professionals alike to rely increasingly on nutrition labeling to help meet health goals. A number of labeling prob-lems, including lack of uniformity, misleading health claims, and imprecise terms such as "natural" and "light" persisted.

These problems indicated a need to reorganize and coordinate the entire food-labeling system. This need had been reinforced by three previous landmark reports relating nutrition and diet to national health goals: *The Surgeon General's Report on Nutrition and Health,* the National Research Council's *Diet and Health,* and the Public Health Service's national health goals and objectives to be reached by the year 2000, *Healthy People 2000.* (These goals were reached and thus not repeated in the *Healthy People 2010* report.) On the basis of these reports, the Institute of Medicine of the National Academy of Sciences established a Committee on the Nutrition Components of Food Labeling to study and report on the scientific issues and practical needs involved in food labeling reform. The report of this committee provided basic guidelines for the rule-making process conducted by the

FDA, USDA, and the USDHHS for submission to Congress to achieve the needed reforms (see the For Further Focus box, "Nutrition Labeling: Recommendations for a New Century"). Three areas of concern formed the basis of recommendations from the Institute of Medicine: (1) foods for mandatory regulations, (2) the format of label information, and (3) education of consumers. This report became the basic guideline for the final law and regulations enacted by the U.S. Congress in 1994.

Current Food Label Format

Nutrition Facts Label. The food label format that is so familiar now is quite different from the one used in the 1970s and 1980s. The title *Nutrition Facts* is printed in bold, eye-catching letters (Figure 13-2). Manufacturers of processed foods may choose to include additional information, such as calories from saturated fat, polyunsaturated fat, monounsaturated fat, potassium, soluble and insoluble fiber, sugar alcohol (e.g., sorbitol), other carbohydrates, or other vitamins and minerals.

Another key term is *percent daily value* (%DV). The FDA set 2000 calories as the reference amount for calculating the %DV, although individuals may vary greatly in their specific needs. As a reference tool, the %DVs can be used to determine the overall value for a specific nutrient in the food (see the For Further Focus box, "Glossary of Terms for Current Labels"). For example, if the %DV for

FOR FURTHER FOCUS

NUTRITION LABELING: RECOMMENDATIONS FOR A NEW CENTURY

The U.S. government is committed by law to the food labeling reform mandated by a health-conscious public. A proliferation of new health-related food products and concerned health professionals have created a demand for accurate information on foods sold in the United States. Nutrition "sells" in today's consumer market.

The initial report and recommendations of the Institute of Medicine's Committee on the Nutrition Components of Food Labeling formed the foundation for final implementation of the Nutrition Labeling and Education Act (NLEA). This baseline focus resulted from a 1-year study requested by the USDHHS and the USDA. The committee made several recommendations, which are embodied in NLEA law.

Foods Covered by Nutrition Labeling
- Nutrition labeling should be mandatory on most packaged foods.
- Nutrition labeling should be provided at the point of purchase for produce, seafood, meats, and poultry.
- Restaurants should make the nutrient content of menu items available to customers on request.

Label Presentation
- The FDA and USDA should set standardized serving sizes.
- More complete ingredient listings should be provided on all foods.
- A modified regulatory scheme should be established for the development and approval of lower fat alternative foods that currently have standards of identity.

Educating Consumers
- A well-designed nutrition labeling program should be fashioned as one part of a comprehensive education program, concurrent with the adoption of regulations on the labeling of nutrition content and format, to help consumers make wise dietary choices.

From the beginning of the process, Congress wanted to develop legislative proposals to clarify the legal basis for reforms. The food industry, health professionals, and consumer groups wanted to promote changes in nutrition labeling that reflect the current DRIs and related product development. These recommendations of the committee have provided a helpful foundation for all concerned.

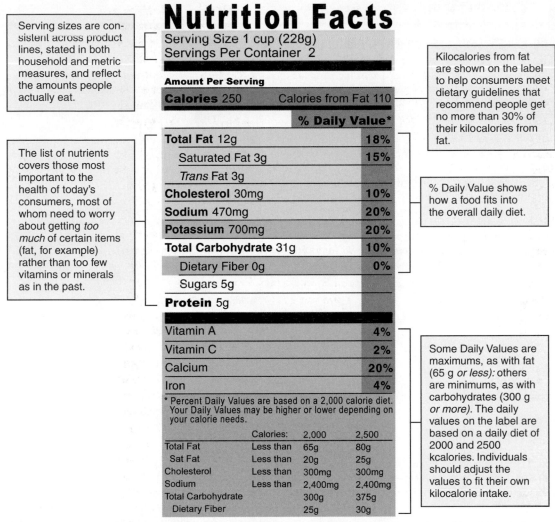

Figure 13-2 Example of a food product label showing the detailed Nutrition Facts box of nutrition information mandated by the FDA under the Nutrition Labeling and Education Act. (Courtesy the FDA, Washington, DC.)

total fat in one serving of potato chips is 25%, a person eating the chips uses one quarter of the recommended total fat allowance for his or her entire day.

In addition, the serving size (i.e., the amount of the food customarily consumed at one time) must be given and expressed in household measures, followed by the metric weight in parentheses and the total number of servings per container.[2]

Health Claims. Health claims that link nutrients or food groups with risk for disease are strictly regulated. To make an association between a food product and a specific disease, the FDA must approve the claim, the food must meet the criteria set forth for that specific claim, and the wording used on the package must be approved. A list of nutrients currently approved for use in the United States and the specific diseases they are associated

with is given in the For Further Focus box, "Glossary of Terms for Current Labels." An example of such a health claim would be the link between a diet low in saturated fat and cholesterol and a reduced risk of coronary heart disease. For a food to carry this label it must be low in saturated fat, low in cholesterol, and low in total fat. If the food is fish or game meat, it must be deemed "extra lean." The specific wording of this example claim must include the following: *saturated fat and cholesterol, coronary heart disease,* or *heart disease,* and a physician statement of the claim defining high or normal total cholesterol. The FDA also provides model claim statements that food producers may choose from. For this specific claim the model statement is, "although many factors affect heart disease, diets low in saturated fat and cholesterol may reduce the risk of this disease."[3]

FOR FURTHER FOCUS

GLOSSARY OF TERMS FOR CURRENT LABELS

To improve communication between producers and consumers, all producers must use standard wording supplied by the FDA. Whether these terms are used in the Nutrition Facts box or elsewhere as part of the manufacturer's product description, they all must use commonly accepted terms. The following is a sampling.

Nutrition Facts Box
Daily Values
DVs are reference values that relate the nutrition information to a total daily diet of 2000 kcal, which is appropriate for most women and teenage girls and some sedentary men. The footnote indicates the daily values for a 2500-kcal diet, which meets the needs of most men, teenage boys, and active women. To help consumers determine how a food fits into a healthy diet, the following nutrients, in the order given, must be listed as %DV:

- Total fat
- Saturated fat
- Trans fat
- Cholesterol
- Sodium
- Total carbohydrate
- Dietary fiber
- Vitamins A and C
- Calcium and iron

Daily Reference Value
As part of the DVs listed, the Daily Reference Values (DRVs) are a set of dietary standards for the following nine nutrients: total fat, saturated fat, trans fat, cholesterol, total carbohydrate, dietary fiber, protein, potassium, and sodium. DRVs do not appear on the label because they are part of a food's DV.

Reference Daily Intake
As part of the DVs listed, the RDIs are a set of dietary standards for essential vitamins, minerals, and protein. RDIs are based on the actual RDAs, when available, or the AIs. This replaced the old term "US RDA," which was developed by food manufacturers as an estimate based on old RDAs. RDIs do not appear on the label because they are part of a food's DV.

Descriptive Terms on Products
The FDA has specifically defined many terms that manufacturers must follow if they use the term on their product. The following are examples:

- *Fat free:* Less than 0.5 g of fat per serving.
- *Low cholesterol:* 20 mg of cholesterol or less per serving and per 100 g; 2 g saturated fat or less per serving. Any label claim about low cholesterol is prohibited for all foods that contain more than 2 g of saturated fat per serving.
- *Light* or *Lite:* At least a one-third reduction in kilocalories. If fat contributes 50% or more of total kilocalories, fat content must be reduced by 50% compared with the reference food.
- *Less sodium:* At least a 25% reduction; 140 mg or less per reference amount per serving.
- *High:* 20% or more of the DV per serving.
- *Reduced saturated fat:* At least 25% less saturated fat than an appropriate reference food.
- *Lean:* Applied to meat, poultry, and seafood; less than 10 g of fat, 4 g of saturated fat, and 95 mg of cholesterol per serving.
- *Extra lean:* Applied to meat, poultry, and seafood; less than 5 g of fat, 2 g of saturated fat, and 95 mg of cholesterol per serving.

For more information, refer to *A Food Labeling Guide—Appendix A,* from the Center for Food Safety and Applied Nutrition, at *www.cfsan.fda.gov/~dms/flg-6a.html.*

Health Claims
The FDA guidelines indicate that any health claim on a label must be supported by substantial scientific evidence. The following claims meet this test:

- Low sodium and the prevention of hypertension
- Calcium and the prevention of osteoporosis
- Low dietary fat and a reduced risk of cancer
- Low dietary cholesterol and saturated fat and reduced coronary heart disease risk
- Fiber-containing grain products, fruits, and vegetables and a reduced cancer risk
- Grain products and fruits and vegetables that contain fiber, especially soluble fiber, and the prevention of coronary heart disease
- Fruits and vegetables rich in vitamins A or C and lowered cancer risk
- Folate and the prevention of neural tube defects
- For more information, refer to *A Food Labeling Guide—Appendix C,* from the Center for Food Safety and Applied Nutrition, at *www.fda.gov/fdac/special/foodlabel/health.html.*

FOOD TECHNOLOGY

The character of America's food supply has radically changed over the years. These changes, which have swept the food marketing system, are rooted in widespread social changes and scientific advances. The agricultural and food processing industries have developed various chemicals to increase and preserve the food supply. However, critics voice concerns about how these changes have affected food safety and the overall environment. Such concerns usually are focused on pesticide use and food additives.

Agricultural Pesticides

Reasons for Use

Large American agricultural corporations as well as individual farmers use a number of chemicals to improve crop yields. These materials have made possible advances in food production necessary to feed a growing population. For example, farmers use certain chemicals to control a wide variety of destructive insects that reduce crop yield (Figure 13-3).

Problems

Concerns and confusion continue about the use and effects of these chemicals. Problems have developed in four main areas: (1) pesticide residues on foods, (2) gradual leaching of the chemicals into groundwater and surrounding wells, (3) increased exposure of farm workers to these strong chemicals, and (4) increased amount of chemicals necessary as insects develop tolerance. Over time, use of these chemicals has created a pesticide dilemma: What do we do in the face of conflicting interests? Thousands of pesticides are in use, and assessing the risks of specific pesticides in use is an important but difficult task.

Alternative Agriculture

An increasing number of concerned farmers, with help from soil scientists, are turning from heavy pesticide use to alternative agricultural methods.

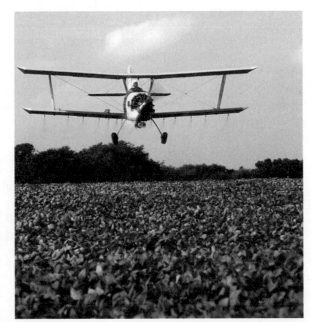

Figure 13-3 A farmer applies insecticide to a corn crop. (Courtesy Ken Hammond, Agricultural Research Service, USDA, Washington, DC.)

Organic Farming. Organic plant foods are grown without synthetic pesticides, fertilizers, sewage sludge, bioengineering, or ionizing radiation. Organic meat, poultry, eggs, and dairy products are from animals raised without antibiotics or growth hormones. In October 2002 the USDA enacted a set of nationally recognized standards to identify certified organic food. For a food to carry the USDA Organic Seal (Figure 13-4), the farm and processing plant where the food was grown and packaged must have undergone government inspections and have met the strict USDA organic standards (see the For Further Focus box, "Organic Food Standards"). All foods produced organically are not required to use the organic label; it is a voluntary program. However, companies using the label on their food without certification face a fine of up to $10,000.[4] Sales of organic foods are rapidly growing and an increasing number of farmers, especially in California, the major supplier of U.S. fruits and vegetables, are using organic farming.

Certified organic foods are not recognized as being more safe or nutritious than conventionally produced foods. Organic farmers can still use natural pesticides and

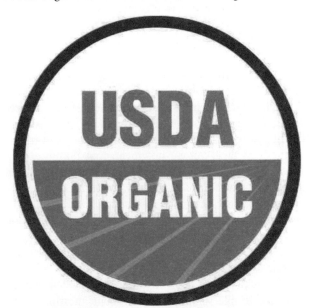

Figure 13-4 Official USDA organic seal, available at *www.ams.usda.gov/nop/Consumers/Seal.html*. (Courtesy The National Organic Program, Agricultural Marketing Service, USDA, Washington, DC.)

organic farming farming methods that use natural means of pest control and meet the standards set by the USDA National Organic Program. Organic foods are grown or produced without the use of synthetic pesticides or fertilizers, sewage sludge, bioengineering, or ionizing radiation.

FOR FURTHER FOCUS

ORGANIC FOOD STANDARDS

The National Organic Program, a constituent of the USDA, was established to ensure standards for organic foods. In response to the growing market, the National Organic Program has set strict standards for the growth, production, and labeling of organic foods. Although many methods prohibited by the organic standards, such as irradiation and genetic modifications, are deemed safe by the USDA, these methods of farming have been banned in certified organic foods because of public concern.

Organic foods have four labeling categories with specific guidelines for each, as follows:

1. *100% Organic:* Products carrying this label must be made or produced exclusively with certified organic ingredients and must have passed a government inspection. These products may use the USDA Organic Seal on their label and advertisements.
2. *Organic:* Products labeled as organic must contain 95% to 100% organic ingredients and also must have passed a government inspection. The National Organic Program must approve all other ingredients for use as nonagricultural substances or products not commercially available in organic form. These products also may use the USDA Organic Seal with the percent of organic ingredients listed.
3. *70% Organic ingredients:* Products made with at least 70% certified organic ingredients may state on the product label "made with organic ingredients" and list up to three ingredients or food groups. These foods also must meet the National Organic Program guidelines for growth or production without synthetic pesticides, fertilizers, sewage sludge, bioengineering, or ionizing radiation. The USDA Organic Seal may not be displayed on these products or used in advertising.
4. *Less than 70% organic ingredients:* Foods made with less than 70% certified organic ingredients may not use the USDA Organic Seal or make any organic claims on the front panel of the package. They can list the specific organic ingredients on the side panel of the package.

All food products with at least 70% organic ingredients also must supply the name and address of the government-approved certifying agent on the product.

For more information on the USDA organic standards, visit the National Organic Program Web site at *www.ams. usda.gov/nop,* call the National Organic Program at 202-720-3252, or write to USDA-AMS-TM-NOP, Room 4008 S. Bldg., Ag Stop 0268, 1400 Independence SW, Washington, DC 20250.

---

fertilizers and therefore are not producing pesticide-free foods. Other common points of confusion are in the use of the following terms: natural, hormone free, and free range. These terms are not synonymous with organic. Truthful terms about the production of a food can appear on the food label but do not mean that the product is organic. The term "natural" may be used on products that contain no artificial ingredients, such as coloring or chemical preservatives, and the product and its ingredients are not more than minimally processed. The Food Safety and Inspection Service of the USDA does not approve the terms *hormone free* or *antibiotic free.* Instead, the phrases "*raised without added hormones*" and "*raised without added antibiotics*" are allowed, provided that the producer is able to supply an affidavit attesting to the production practices used to support the claim. One important note about the use of hormones is that they are approved for use only in beef cattle and lamb production. Therefore any such claim on a chicken product would be allowed only if it were immediately followed with the statement, "federal regulations prohibit the use of hormones in poultry."

Organic farming is safer for the soil, water, agricultural workers, and birds. However, when compared with conventional farming, organic farming is less efficient. Without synthetic pesticides and fertilizers, crops are smaller and require more land. As a result, the products are more expensive.

Genetic Modification. Plant physiologists are developing strains of genetically modified (GM) foods that reduce the need for toxic pesticides and herbicides. Genetic manipulation in various forms has been used to improve crops for thousands of years, but most U.S. consumers are unaware of the extent to which these foods have entered the marketplace. In the United States, 87% of soybean crop acreage, and a steadily increasing percentage of corn crops, are GM herbicide-tolerant varieties (Figure 13-5).[5] Most people in the United States have consumed some form of GM foods at some point, such as seedless oranges or watermelons. An example of biotechnology in today's agriculture is the use of GM corn that expresses a specific protein that ultimately serves as an insecticide. Organic farmers have used this type of biotechnology for more than 40 years. Approved genetic modifications currently are used to protect against virus infections and insects on tomatoes, potatoes, squash, and papayas, among other crops. GM crops are extensively tested regarding composition, safety, and environmental effects. The National Institute of Health, Animal Plant Health Inspection Service of the USDA, FDA, and the Environmental Protection Agency are all involved in the strict regulation of GM foods in commercial use, which are the most heavily regulated new foods.

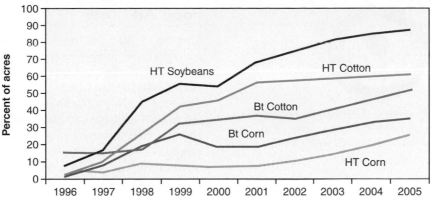

Figure 13-5 Adoption of GM crops grows steadily in the United States. Data for each crop category include varieties with both herbicide-tolerant and Bt (stacked) traits. (Reprinted from Fernandez-Cornejo J and others: The first decade of genetically engineered crops in the United States, *Economic Information Bulletin* [11] 2006.)

The benefits of genetic modifications are not limited to benefits to the producer. Technology is advancing to the point of engineering food to increase its nutritional value, medicinal properties, taste, and aesthetic appeal. Plants are produced with increased fiber, antioxidants, and essential amino acids, all of which are beneficial to the consumer and may have positive effects on human nutrition worldwide. More than 50 biotechnology crop products are approved for commercialization in the United States (Figure 13-6).

Such forms of agriculture remain controversial around the world because of many unknown factors regarding long-term effects on the environment and overall human health. Current testing procedures are unable to determine potential problems from long-term use, such as carcinogenicity or neurotoxicity. Research completed with soybeans revealed that wild-type and GM soybean varieties have exactly the same allergenicity; thus genetic modification did not increase the likelihood of allergies in this crop.[6] This type of research will be important for all types of GM crops to ensure safety and improve consumer acceptability.

Irradiation. Irradiation can kill bacteria and parasites on the food after harvest. Irradiation helps prevent food-borne illness caused by *Escherichia coli, Salmonella, Campylobacter, Listeria, Cyclospora, Shigella,* and *Salmonella.*[7] Three different methods of irradiation are used, all of which are approved by the WHO, CDC, USDA, and FDA. The use of irradiation is not a new science; wheat flour and white potatoes were approved for irradiation in the early 1960s. In addition to reducing or eliminating disease-causing germs, irradiation can be used to increase the shelf life of produce. Foods that are irradiated (1) have essentially unaltered nutritional value, (2) are not radioactive, (3) have no harmful substances introduced as a result of irradiation, but (4) may taste slightly different.[7] A variety of foods have been approved for irradiation in the United States, including meat, poultry, grains, some seafood, fruits, vegetables, herbs, and spices. The FDA requires all irradiated foods be appropriately labeled with either the radura symbol for irradiation (Figure 13-7) or by a written description stating the food has been exposed to irradiation.

Consumer rejection in the United States and around the world mainly is the result of altered taste and fear of unknown long-term affects on human health. Irradiation also introduces trans fats in meats, a known health risk. The U.S. government continues to support the use and safety of such foods, but without consumer acceptance companies using such procedures have limited success.

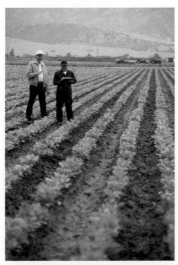

Figure 13-6 A geneticist and technician evaluate sugar beet breeding in California. (Courtesy Scott Bauer, Agricultural Research Service, USDA, Washington, DC.)

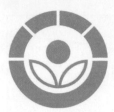

Figure 13-7 Radura symbol of irradiation, available at *www.fsis.usda.gov/news_&_events/FSIS_Images/index.asp*. (Courtesy the Food Safety and Inspection Service, USDA, Washington, DC.)

Food Additives

The use of *food additives* (i.e., chemicals intentionally added to foods to prevent spoilage and extend shelf life) is not new to the food industry either. Table 13-1 lists examples of food additives. The two most common additives are sugar and salt, although consumers often do not recognize these basic ingredients as food additives. Some additives have been used for centuries as preservatives, especially salt in cured meats. The term "generally recognized as safe" is used to define additives that have been used in foods and do not need FDA approval.

TABLE 13-1

EXAMPLES OF FOOD ADDITIVES

FUNCTION	CHEMICAL COMPOUND	COMMON FOOD USES
Acid, alkalis, buffers	Sodium bicarbonate	Baking powder
	Tartaric acid	Fruit sherbets, cheese spreads
Antibiotics	Chlortetracycline	Dip for dressed poultry
Anticaking agents	Aluminum calcium silicate	Table salt
Antimycotics	Calcium propionate	Bread
	Sodium propionate	Bread
	Sorbic acid	Cheese
Antioxidants	Butylated hydroxyanisole	Fats
	Butylated hydroxytoluene	Fats
Bleaching agents	Benzoyl peroxide	Wheat flour
	Chlorine dioxide	
	Oxides of nitrogen	
Color preservative	Sodium benzoate	Green peas, maraschino cherries
Coloring agents	Annatto	Butter, margarine
	Carotene	
Emulsifiers	Lecithin	Bakery goods
	Monoglycerides and diglycerides	Dairy products
	Propylene glycol alginate	Confections
Flavoring agents	Amyl acetate	Soft drinks
	Benzaldehyde	Bakery goods
	Methyl salicylate	Candy, ice cream
	Essential oils, natural extractives	Canned meats
	Monosodium glutamate	Meat, vegetables, sauces
Nonnutritive sweeteners	Saccharin	Diet canned fruit
	Aspartame	Low-calorie soft drinks
Nutrient supplements	Potassium iodide	Iodized salt
	Vitamin C	Fruit juices
	Vitamin D	Milk
	Vitamin A	Margarine
	B vitamins, iron	Bread, cereal
Sequestrants	Sodium citrate	Dairy products
	Calcium pyrophosphoric acid	
Stabilizers and thickeners	Pectin	Jellies
	Vegetable gums (carob bean, carrageenan, guar)	Dairy desserts, chocolate milk
	Gelatin	Confections
	Agar-agar	"Low-calorie" salad dressings
Yeast foods and dough conditioners	Ammonium chloride	Bread, rolls
	Calcium sulfate	
	Calcium phosphate	

Over the past few decades the number and variety of food additives have increased in the food supply. The current variety of food market items would be impossible without them. Scientific advances have created processed food products, and the changing society has created the market demand. The expanding population, larger workforce, and more complex family life have increased the desire for more variety and convenience in foods as well as better safety and quality. Food additives help achieve these needs and serve many purposes. For example, additives (1) enrich foods with added nutrients; (2) produce uniform qualities (e.g., color, flavor, aroma, texture, and general appearance); (3) standardize many functional factors (e.g., thickening or stabilization [keeping parts from separating]); (4) preserve foods by preventing oxidation; and (5) control acidity or alkalinity to improve flavor, texture, and the cooked product. A number of micronutrients and antioxidants are used as additives in processed foods—not for their ability to increase nutrient content, but for their technical effects either during processing or in the final product.

FOOD-BORNE DISEASE

Prevalence

Many disease-bearing organisms inhabit the environment and can contaminate food and water. The Public Health Service estimates 76 million Americans become sick from food-borne illness annually, with a resulting 325,000 hospitalizations.[8] Much has been learned in the past decade about the pathogens that commonly contaminate food and water and ways to prevent food-borne illness outbreaks. However, lapses in control still occur, resulting in high incidences of illness and death as well as economic burden. The estimated annual incidence of food-borne illness has been on the decline for most pathogens in recent years.[9] Microbiologic diseases (bacterial and viral) represent the majority of these outbreaks nationwide, with a large range of costs associated with each type of infection. *Salmonella, Campylobacter, Shigella,* and *Cryptosporidium* are the most common infections in home and community outbreaks.[9]

Food Sanitation

Buying and Storing Food

Control of food-borne disease focuses on strict sanitation measures and rigid personal hygiene. First, the food itself should be of good quality and not defective or diseased. Second, dry or cold storage should protect it from deterioration or decay, which is especially important for products such as refrigerated convenience foods, the fast-est growing segment of the convenience food market and potentially the most dangerous because they are not sterile. These vacuum-packaged or modified-atmosphere chilled food products are only minimally processed, not sterilized, and are at risk of temperature abuse. Home refrigerator temperatures should be held at 40° F or lower. At temperatures greater than 45° F, any precooked or leftover foods are potential reservoirs for bacteria that survive cooking and can recontaminate cooked food. Food safety depends on the following critical actions (Figure 13-8)[10]:

- *Clean:* Wash hands and surfaces often.
- *Separate:* Do not cross-contaminate.
- *Cook:* Cook to proper temperatures.
- *Chill:* Refrigerate promptly.

All food preparation areas must be scrupulously clean, and foods must be washed or cleaned well. Cooking procedures and temperatures must be followed as directed. All utensils, dishes, and anything else that comes in contact with food must be clean. Leftover food should be stored and reheated appropriately or discarded (Table 13-2). Food does *not* need to be cooled to room temperature before refrigerating. This practice allows food to sit in the perfect temperature range for bacterial growth. Garbage must be contained and disposed of in a sanitary manner. Safe methods of food handling, cooking, and storage are simple and mostly common sense; they often are neglected, however, which leads to food-borne illness.

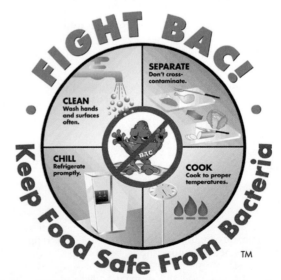

Figure 13-8 The Partnership for Food Safety Education developed the Fight BAC! (bacteria) campaign to prevent food-borne illness. Campaign graphics are available at *www.fightbac.org.* (Courtesy Partnership for Food Safety Education, Washington, DC.)

TABLE 13-2

COLD STORAGE CHART

PRODUCT	REFRIGERATOR (40° F)	FREEZER (0° F)
Eggs		
Fresh, in shell	3 to 5 weeks	Do not freeze
Raw yolks and whites	2 to 4 days	1 year
Hard cooked	1 week	Does not freeze well
Liquid Pasteurized Eggs, Egg Substitutes		
Opened	3 days	Does not freeze well
Unopened	10 days	1 year
Mayonnaise, Commercial: Refrigerate after Opening	2 months	Do not freeze
Frozen Dinners and Entrees: Keep Frozen until Ready to Heat	—	3 to 4 months
Deli and Vacuum-Packed Products: Store-Prepared (or Homemade) Egg, Chicken, Ham, Tuna, and Macaroni Salads	3 to 5 days	Does not freeze well
Hot Dogs		
Opened package	1 week	1 to 2 months
Unopened package	2 weeks	1 to 2 months
Luncheon Meat		
Opened package	3 to 5 days	1 to 2 months
Unopened package	2 weeks	1 to 2 months
Bacon and Sausage		
Bacon	7 days	1 month
Sausage, raw: chicken, turkey, pork, beef	1 to 2 days	1 to 2 months
Smoked breakfast links, patties	7 days	1 to 2 months
Hard sausage: pepperoni, jerky sticks	2 to 3 weeks	1 to 2 months
Summer Sausage, Labeled "Keep Refrigerated"		
Opened	3 weeks	1 to 2 months
Unopened	3 months	1 to 2 months
Corned beef, in pouch with pickling juices	5 to 7 days	Drained, 1 month
Ham, Canned, Labeled "Keep Refrigerated"		
Opened	3 to 5 days	1 to 2 months
Unopened	6 to 9 months	Do not freeze
Ham, Fully Cooked		
Vacuum sealed at plant, undated, unopened	2 weeks	1 to 2 months
Vacuum sealed at plant, dated, unopened	"Use by" date on package	1 to 2 months
Whole	7 days	1 to 2 months
Half	3 to 5 days	1 to 2 months
Slices	3 to 4 days	1 to 2 months
Hamburger and stew meat	1 to 2 days	3 to 4 months
Ground Turkey, Veal, Pork, Lamb, and Mixtures	1 to 2 days	3 to 4 months
Fresh Beef, Veal, Lamb, Pork		
Steaks	3 to 5 days	6 to 12 months
Chops	3 to 5 days	4 to 6 months
Roasts	3 to 5 days	4 to 12 months
Variety meats: tongue, liver, heart, kidneys, chitterlings	1 to 2 days	3 to 4 months
Prestuffed, uncooked pork chops, lamb chops, or chicken breasts stuffed with dressing	1 day	Does not freeze well
Soups and stews, vegetable or meat added	3 to 4 days	2 to 3 months
Fresh Poultry		
Chicken or turkey, whole	1 to 2 days	1 year
Chicken or turkey, pieces	1 to 2 days	9 months
Giblets	1 to 2 days	3 to 4 months

Reprinted from Food Safety and Inspection Service: *Safe food handling: basics for handling food safely*, www.fsis.usda.gov/Fact_Sheets/Basics_for_Handling_Food_Safely/index.asp, accessed July 2007.

TABLE 13-2

COLD STORAGE CHART—cont'd

PRODUCT	REFRIGERATOR (40° F)	FREEZER (0° F)
Cooked Meat and Poultry Leftovers		
Cooked meat and meat casseroles	3 to 4 days	2 to 3 months
Gravy and meat broth	1 to 2 days	2 to 3 months
Fried chicken	3 to 4 days	4 months
Cooked poultry casseroles	3 to 4 days	4 to 6 months
Poultry pieces, plain	3 to 4 days	4 months
Poultry pieces in broth, gravy	1 to 2 days	6 months
Chicken nuggets, patties	1 to 2 days	1 to 3 months
Other Cooked Leftovers		
Pizza, cooked	3 to 4 days	1 to 2 months
Stuffing, cooked	3 to 4 days	1 month

Food safety publications for all types of foods and populations can be found at the Food Safety and Inspection Service Web site at: *www.fsis.usda.gov/Fact_Sheets/index.asp.*

Preparing and Serving Food

All persons handling food, especially those working in public food services, should follow strict measures to prevent contamination. For example, simple handwashing and clean clothing and aprons are imperative. Basic rules of hygiene should apply to all persons handling food, whether they work in food processing and packaging plants, process and package foods in markets, or prepare and serve food in restaurants. In addition, persons with an infectious disease should have limited access to direct food handling.

Following are minimal internal temperatures for various foods:

- Ground beef, hamburgers: 160° F
- Chicken breast: 170° F
- Whole chicken: 180° F
- Egg dishes: 160° F
- Fish: 145° F
- Pork :160° F
- Steaks and roast: 145° F

The Hazard Analysis and Critical Control Point (HACCP) food safety system focuses on preventing food-borne illness through identifying critical points and eliminating hazards. Many organizations, including the USDA and FDA, use HACCP standards. The USDA has developed specific standards for a variety of food products. For more information on HACCP, visit *www.cfsan.fda.gov/~lrd/haccp.html.*

Food Contamination

Food-borne illness usually presents itself as flulike symptoms but can advance to a lethal illness. Not all bacteria found in foods are harmful; some are even beneficial, such as the bacteria in yogurt. Bacteria that are harmful to people are referred to as *pathogens.* Certain subgroups of the population are at higher risk for developing food-borne illness because of age and physical condition. Groups at the highest risk are young children, pregnant women, elderly individuals, and people with compromised immune systems.

Bacterial Food Infections

Bacterial food infections result from eating food contaminated by large colonies of different types of bacteria. Specific diseases result from specific bacteria (e.g., salmonellosis, shigellosis, and listeriosis).

Salmonellosis. Salmonellosis is caused by *Salmonella,* a bacterium named for the American veterinarian pathologist Daniel Salmon (1850–1914), who first isolated and identified the species that commonly causes food-borne infections: *S. typhi* and *S. paratyphi.* Approximately 40,000 cases of salmonellosis are reported in the United States each year, although thousands of other cases are suspected to go unreported.[11] These organisms readily grow in common foods such as milk, custard, egg dishes, salad dressing, and sandwich fillings. Seafood from polluted waters, especially shellfish such as oysters and clams, also may be a source of infection. Unsanitary handling of foods and utensils can spread the bacteria. Resulting cases of gastroenteritis may vary from mild to severe diarrhea. Immunization, pasteurization, and sanitary regulations involving community water and food supplies, as well as food handlers, help control such outbreaks. Because incubation and multiplication of the bacteria take time (after the food is eaten), symptoms of food infection develop relatively slow (up to 72 hours later). Symptoms include diarrhea, fever, vomiting, and abdominal cramps. The illness usually lasts 4 to 7 days, with most affected individuals recovering completely. Severe dehydration from diarrhea and vomiting may require intravenous fluids.

Shigellosis. Shigellosis is caused by the bacteria *Shigella,* named for the Japanese physician Kiyoshi Shiga (1870–1957), who first discovered a main species of the organism, *S. dysenteriae,* during a dysentery epidemic in Japan in 1898. Approximately 18,000 cases are reported annually, but because many cases are not diagnosed the CDC estimates the actual number of cases may be as much as 20 times higher.[12] Shigellosis usually is confined to the large intestine and may vary from a mild, transient intestinal disturbance in adults to fatal dysentery in young children. The bacteria grow easily in foods, especially milk, which is a common vehicle of transmission to infants and children. The boiling of water or pasteurization of milk kills the organisms, but the food or milk may easily be reinfected through unsanitary handling. The disease is spread similarly to how salmonella is transmitted (e.g., by feces, fingers, flies, milk, and food and articles handled by unsanitary carriers). Shigellosis, similar to salmonellosis, is more common in the summer and most commonly occurs in young children.[12] Symptoms appear within 12 to 50 hours and include cramps, diarrhea, fever, vomiting, and blood or mucus in stools.

Listeriosis. Listeriosis is caused by the bacteria *Listeria,* which was named for the English surgeon Baron Joseph Lister (1827–1912), who first applied knowledge of bacterial infection to the principles of antiseptic surgery in a benchmark 1867 publication that led to "clean" operations and the development of modern surgery. However, only within the past 20 years has knowledge of bacteria's role as a direct cause of food-borne illness increased and the major species causing human illness, *L. monocytogenes,* been identified. Before 1981 *Listeria* was thought to be only an organism of animal disease transmitted to people by direct contact with infected animals. However, this organism widely occurs in the environment and in high-risk individuals, such as elderly persons, pregnant women, infants, and patients with suppressed immune systems, and can produce a rare but often fatal illness with severe symptoms such as diarrhea, flulike fever and headache, pneumonia, sepsis, meningitis, and endocarditis. Approximately one third of all listeriosis cases occur in pregnant women.[13] Food-borne disease has been traced to a variety of foods, including soft cheese, poultry, seafood, raw milk, refrigerated raw liquid whole eggs, and meat products (e.g., pâté).

Bacterial Food Poisoning

Food poisoning is caused by the ingestion of bacterial toxins that have been produced in food by the growth of specific kinds of bacteria before the food is eaten. The powerful toxin is directly ingested, so symptoms of food poisoning develop rapidly. Two types of bacterial food poisoning, staphylococcal and clostridial, are most commonly responsible.

Staphylococcal Food Poisoning. *Staphylococcal* food poisoning was named for the causative organism, which is mainly *Staphylococcus aureus,* a round bacteria forming masses of cells. *S. aureus* is the most common form of bacterial food poisoning in the United States. Powerful preformed toxins in the contaminated food rapidly produce illness (1 to 6 hours after ingestion). The symptoms suddenly appear and include severe cramping and abdominal pain with nausea, vomiting, and diarrhea, usually accompanied by sweating, headache, fever, and sometimes prostration and shock. However, recovery is fairly rapid and symptoms subside within 24 hours (see the Clinical Applications box, "Case Study: A Community Food Poisoning Incident"). The amount of toxin ingested and the susceptibility of the individual eating it determine the degree of severity. The source of the contamination usually is a staphylococcal infection on the hand of a worker preparing the food. This infection often is minor and considered harmless or is even unnoticed by the food handler. Foods that are particularly effective carriers for staphylococci and their toxins include custard or cream-filled bakery goods, processed meats, ham, tongue, cheese, ice cream, potato salad, sauces, chicken and ham salads, and combination dishes such as spaghetti and casseroles. The toxin causes no change in the normal appearance, odor, or taste of the food, so the victim has no warning. A careful food history helps determine the source of the poisoning, and portions of the food are obtained for examination if possible. Few bacteria may be found because heating kills the organisms but does not destroy the toxins produced.

Clostridial Food Poisoning. *Clostridial* food poisoning was named for the spore-forming, rod-shaped bacteria, mainly *Clostridium perfringens* and *C. botulinum,* which also can form powerful toxins in infected foods. *C. perfringens* spores are widespread in the environment (in soil, water, dust, refuse, and many other places). This organism multiplies in cooked meat and meat dishes and develops its toxin in foods held at warm or room temperatures for extended periods. A number of

CLINICAL APPLICATIONS

CASE STUDY: A COMMUNITY FOOD POISONING INCIDENT

John and Eva Wesson agreed that their lodge dinner had been the best they had ever had, especially the dessert, custard-filled cream puffs, John's favorite. He had eaten two of them despite Eva's protests. Maybe that was why he began to feel ill shortly after they arrived home. Eva's stomach felt a little upset too, so they both took some antacid pills, thinking their "stomach aches" were from eating more rich food than they were accustomed to. They went to bed early.

However, by 11:00 PM Eva woke up alarmed. John was vomiting and having diarrhea and increasingly severe stomach cramps. He complained of a headache, and his pajamas were wet with sweat. He had a fever and appeared to be in shock. Eva began to have similar pains and symptoms, although they were not as severe as John's.

One of their friends who had been at the lodge dinner then telephoned. She and her husband also had the same symptoms.

By now John was prostrate, unable to move. Eva immediately called 911 and they were both taken to the hospital. After treatment in the emergency department for shock, followed by observational care and rest the following day, John's symptoms had subsided and he was allowed to go home. The physician advised them to eat lightly for a few days and get more rest and said that he would investigate the cause in the meantime. During the next few days, John and Eva learned that almost all their friends who had been at the lodge dinner had had an experience similar to theirs.

The physician contacted the public health department to report the incident. His was one of several similar calls, a public health officer said, and the department was already investigating.

The following week the officer returned the physician's call to report his findings. The cream puffs that the lodge restaurant served that evening had been purchased from a local bakery. At the bakery health officials had located a worker with an infected cut on his little finger—"a small thing," the worker said. He could not understand what all the fuss was about.

The health officials also located the delivery truck driver, who had started out at midmorning to make his rounds and take the cream puffs to the restaurant. On questioning the driver, however, they learned that the truck had broken down during the afternoon deliveries before he reached the restaurant. The driver said that he had been irritated by a 3-hour wait at the garage while the truck was being fixed. But he still got the order to the restaurant in time for the dinner.

At the restaurant, the chef said that everyone was so busy with the dinner that when the cream puffs finally arrived, no one had time to give much notice to them. They had decided not to put the cream puffs in the refrigerator because they were about to be served.

When John and Eva's physician called them afterward to report the story, John and Eva decided they would not eat at that restaurant again. Besides, by then John had lost his taste for cream puffs.

Questions for Analysis

1. Why is control of the community's food supply an important responsibility of the health department?
2. Which disease agents may be carried by food or water?
3. What agent caused John and Eva's illness? Was this a food infection or a food poisoning? Why?
4. While the investigation was occurring and before John and Eva learned the real cause of their illness, John thought it must have been caused by "those things farmers and food processors put into food these days." What substances did John mean? Give some examples.
5. Why are these materials used for growing and processing food?
6. What controls are in place for their use?
7. What are some ways in which food is protected from its point of production to the table? How can food be preserved for later use?
8. Which agency controls food safety and quality? How does it do so?

outbreaks from food eaten in restaurants, college dining rooms, and school cafeterias have been reported. In most cases cooked meat is improperly prepared or refrigerated. Control depends on careful preparation and adequate cooking of meats, prompt service, and immediate refrigeration at sufficiently low temperatures. The bacteria *C. botulinum* causes a far more serious, often fatal food poisoning, *botulism,* from ingestion of food containing its powerful toxin. Depending on the dose of toxin taken and the individual response, the illness may vary from mild discomfort to death within 24 hours. Mortality rates are high. Nausea, vomiting, weakness, and dizziness are initial symptoms. The toxin progressively irritates motor nerve cells and blocks transmission of neural impulses at the nerve terminals, causing gradual paralysis. Sudden respiratory paralysis with airway obstruction is the major cause of death. *C. botulinum* spores are widespread in soil throughout the world and may be carried on harvested food to the canning process. Like all *clostridia*, this species is **anaerobic**, or nearly so. The relatively air-free can and the canning temperatures (greater than 27° C [80° F])

---

anaerobic a microorganism that can live and grow in an oxygen-free environment.

provide good conditions for toxin production. The development of high standards in the commercial canning industry has eliminated this source of botulism but cases still result each year, mainly from ingestion of home-canned foods. Because boiling for 10 minutes destroys the toxin (not the spore), all home-canned food, no matter how well preserved it is considered to be, should be boiled for at least 10 minutes before it is eaten. Within the United States, Alaska and Washington have the highest incidence of botulism, with Alaska having by far the greater number of cases because of native habits of eating uncooked or partially cooked meat that has been fermented, dried, or frozen. Table 13-3 summarizes examples of bacterial sources of food contamination.

Viruses

Illnesses produced by viral contamination of food are few when compared with those produced by bacterial sources. These include upper respiratory infections (e.g., colds and influenza) and viral infectious hepatitis. Explosive epidemics of infectious hepatitis have occurred in schools, towns, and other communities after fecal contamination of water, milk, or food. Contaminated shellfish from polluted waters also have caused several outbreaks. Again, stringent control of community water and food supplies, as well as personal hygiene and sanitary practices of food handlers, is essential for prevention of disease.

TABLE 13-3

EXAMPLES OF BACTERIAL FOOD-BORNE DISEASE

FOOD-BORNE DISEASE	CAUSATIVE ORGANISMS (GENUS, SPECIES)	FOOD SOURCE	SYMPTOMS AND COURSE
Bacterial Food Infections			
Salmonellosis	*Salmonella typhi, S. paratyphi*	Milk, custards, egg dishes, salad dressings, sandwich fillings, polluted shellfish	Mild to severe diarrhea, cramps, vomiting; appearance 12-24 hours or more after eating; duration of 1-7 days
Shigellosis	*Shigella dysenteriae*	Milk and milk products, seafood, salads	Mild diarrhea to fatal dysentery (especially in young children); appearance 7-36 hours after eating; duration of 3-14 days
Listeriosis	*Listeria monocytogenes*	Soft cheese, poultry, seafood, raw milk, meat products (e.g., pâté)	Severe diarrhea, fever, headache, pneumonia, meningitis, endocarditis; symptoms appearing after 3-21 days
Bacterial Food Poisoning (Enterotoxins)			
Staphylococcal	*Staphylococcus aureus*	Custards, cream fillings, processed meats, ham, cheese, ice cream, potato salad, sauces, casseroles	Severe abdominal pain, cramps, vomiting, diarrhea, sweating, headache, fever, prostration; sudden appearance 1-6 hours after eating; symptoms generally subsiding within 24 hours
Clostridial perfringens enteritis	*Clostridium perfringens*	Cooked meat, meat dishes held at warm temperature	Mild diarrhea, vomiting; appearance 8-24 hours after eating; duration of 1 day or less
Botulism	*C. botulinum*	Improperly home canned foods; smoked and salted fish, ham, sausage, shellfish	Symptoms ranging from mild discomfort to death within 24 hours; initial nausea, vomiting, weakness, and dizziness progressing to motor and sometimes fatal breathing paralysis
E. coli infection	*Escherichia coli* 0157:H7	Meats; raw vegetables; unpasteurized milk, water, apple juice, and cider; person-to-person contact	Severe diarrhea and stomach cramps, dehydration, stroke; appearance within a few days after eating; duration of approximately 8 days

CULTURAL CONSIDERATIONS

THE CONTINUED BURDEN OF LEAD POISONING

Exposure to lead continues to be a problem in the United States. One of the *Healthy People 2010* goals is to eliminate blood lead levels (BLL) of ≥10 mcg/dl in children. Although the National Health and Nutrition Examination Surveys continue to indicate that BLLs are declining, much work is still needed to reach the goal for 2010.

Among all age groups, children ages 1 to 5 years have the highest risk for elevated BLL, and among ethnic groups non-Hispanic African Americans have the highest occurrence rates. Following are rates per ethnicity, including all age groups*:

- Non-Hispanic African American: 1.4%
- Mexican American: 1.5%
- Non-Hispanic Caucasian: 0.5%
- Total U.S. population: 0.7%

Subpopulation classification shows that non-Hispanic African Americans aged 1 to 5 years and older than 60 years have the highest prevalence of elevated BLLs, 3.1% and 3.4%, respectively.

The figure to the right depicts BLLs of children per ethnicity over the last three survey periods.

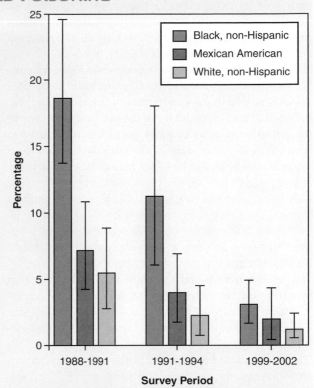

Percentage of children aged 1 to 5 years with blood lead levels of ≥10 mcg/dl, by race or ethnicity and survey period: National Health and Nutrition Examination Surveys, United States, 1988-1991, 1991-1994, and 1999-2002.* 95% confidence interval. (Reprinted from Centers for Disease Control and Prevention: Blood lead levels—United States, 1999-2002, *MMWR Morb Mortal Wkly Rep* 54(20):513, 2005.)

*Centers for Disease Control and Prevention: Blood lead levels—United States, 1999-2002, *MMWR Morb Mortal Wkly Rep* 54(20):513, 2005.

Parasites

The following two types of worms are of serious concern in relation to food: (1) roundworms, such as the *trichina (Trichinella spiralis)* worm found in pork; and (2) flatworms, such as the common tapeworms of beef and pork. The following control measures are essential: (1) laws controlling hog and cattle food sources and pastures to prevent transmission of the parasites to the meat produced for market and (2) avoidance of rare beef or undercooked pork as an added personal precaution.

Environmental Food Contaminants

Heavy metals such as lead and mercury also may contaminate food and water as well as the air and environmental objects. Although lead poisoning in the United

States has dramatically declined since the removal of lead from gasoline, it remains to plague certain subgroups of the population (see the Cultural Considerations box, "The Continued Burden of Lead Poisoning"). The overall prevalence of high blood lead levels in the United States

---

hepatitis inflammation of liver cells. Symptoms of cute hepatitis (less than 6 months) include flu-like symptoms, muscle and joint aches, fever, feeling sick or vomiting, diarrhea and headache, dark urine, and yellowing of the eyes and skin. Symptoms of chronic hepatits (longer than 6 months) include jaundice, abdominal swelling and sensitivity, low-grade fever, and fluid retention (ascites).

population is 0.7%, with the highest prevalence occurring in children aged 1 to 5 years (1.6%).[14] Children are especially vulnerable to lead poisoning, particularly those of poor families living in older homes, rental housing, or other impoverished areas with peeling lead paint.[15] Eliminating blood lead levels of ≥10 mcg/dl or greater in children is one of the goals of *Healthy People 2010*.[16]

Of all sources of lead, paint is the chief source of contamination. An estimated 38 million homes in the United States have lead in paint surfaces. Children living in these homes face lead exposure by eating paint chips or breathing airborne particles of paint dust from abrasive paint removal before remodeling. Drinking water may be a major source of lead in high-risk households whose water comes through lead service pipes or plumbing joints that have been sealed with lead solder. Current Environmental Protection Agency rules for public drinking water, however, have lowered the controlled lead exposure levels even further. Children with prolonged elevated blood lead levels may incur permanent neurological damage.[17,18] Studies also have found this same high-risk population group to be deficient in iron, a condition that can increase lead absorption four- to five-fold, has a similar deleterious effect on neurology, and can thus further complicating lead toxicity.[19]

Natural toxins produced by plants or microorganisms also contaminate the food and water supply. Mercury, found naturally in the environment in addition to human production, is converted to methyl mercury by bacteria. Methyl mercury is a toxin contaminating large bodies of water and the fish within that water. This contamination can pass through the food chain to people regularly consuming large, fatty fish. Aflatoxin, another natural toxin, is produced by fungi and may contaminate foods such as peanuts, tree nuts, corn, and animal feed.

Other food contaminants and pollutants that may pose a risk to human health come from a variety of sources (e.g., factories, sewage, and fertilizers) but end up leaching out into the ground, contaminating food production areas and the water supply.

FOOD NEEDS AND COSTS

Hunger and Malnutrition

Worldwide Malnutrition

Hunger, even famine and death, exist in many countries of the world today. Lack of sanitation, cultural inequality, overpopulation, and economic and political structures that do not appropriately use resources are all factors that may contribute to malnutrition. Chronic food or nutrient shortages within a population perpetuate the cycle of

malnutrition, in which undernourished, pregnant women give birth to LBW infants. These infants are then more susceptible to infant death or growth retardation during childhood. When high-nutrient needs throughout childhood and adolescence are not met, the incidence of malnourished or growth-stunted adults with shorter life expectancy and reduced work capacity continues to rise. Malnutrition may result from total kilocalorie deficiency or single-nutrient deficiencies. The most common deficiencies in the world today are protein-energy malnutrition, vitamin A deficiency, iodine deficiency, and iron deficiency. Figure 13-9 shows the complicated interaction of many factors leading to malnutrition.

The United Nations Committee on World Food Security, the World Food Summit, was formed to address the 840 million people worldwide who do not have enough food to meet basic nutritional requirements. The long-term goal of this committee is to eliminate world hunger and establish a sustainable food supply for all people by 2015.[20] The plan is composed of six commitments focused on stabilizing social, economic, and environmental production and distribution of nutritionally adequate food. The committee is responsible for monitoring, evaluating, and consulting on the international food security situation with follow-up reports. Information and updates on the progress of this committee can be found at *www.fao.org/monitoringprogress/index_en.html*.

Malnutrition in America

Hunger does not stop at the U.S. border. In the United States, one of the wealthiest countries on earth, studies continue to document hunger and malnutrition among the poor. More than 11 million households in the United States have food insecurity, which is defined as "limited or uncertain availability of nutritionally adequate and safe foods or limited or uncertain ability to acquire acceptable foods in socially acceptable ways."[21] Individuals at highest risk of food insecurity within the United States are African Americans, Hispanics, single mothers, and households in central city and nonmetropolitan areas.[21] At both the government and personal levels of any society, food availability and use involve money and politics. Various factors are implicated, such as land management practices, water distribution, food production and distribution policies, and food assistance programs for individuals and families in need.

Food Assistance Programs

In situations of economic stress and natural disasters, individuals and families need financial help. Many people in the United States experience hunger every day. Dieti-

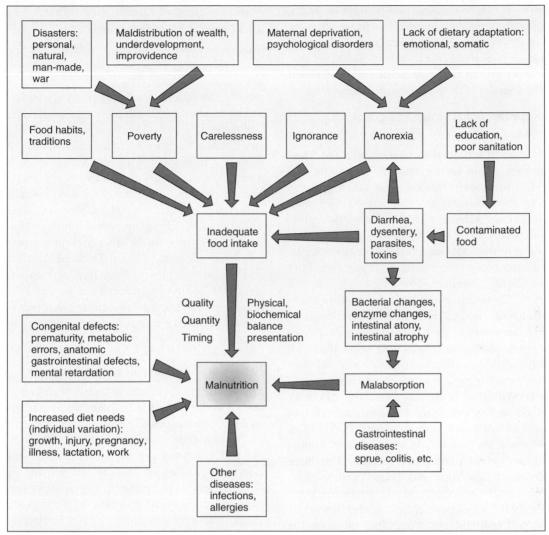

Figure 13-9 Multiple causes of malnutrition. (Modified from Williams CD: Malnutrition, *Lancet* 2:342, 1962.)

tians may need to discuss available food assistance programs and make appropriate referrals.

Commodity Supplemental Food Program

Under the Commodity Supplemental Food Program (CSFP), the USDA purchases food items that are good sources of nutrients often lacking in the diets of the target population (low-income pregnant and breastfeeding women, other new mothers up to 1 year postpartum, infants, children to age 5 years, and elderly people at least 60 years old). The USDA then distributes the food to state agencies and tribal organizations. From there, the food is dispersed to local agencies for public allocation. Local agencies, such as the departments of Health, Social Services, Education, or Agriculture, are responsible for evaluating eligibility, providing nutrition education, and dis-

persing food. This program is not currently available in every state. Information about CSFP can be found at *www.fns.usda.gov/fdd/programs/csfp/default.htm*.

Food Stamp Program

The Food Stamp Program began in the late depression years of the 1930s and was expanded in the 1960s and 1970s. This program has helped many poor persons purchase needed food, although federal cuts in the 1980s curtailed its help to many persons in need. The USDA estimated that 25.7 million people received food stamps in the United States each month in 2005, the majority of whom were children and the elderly.[22] Under this program, the person or "household" is issued coupons, or food stamps, that are supposed to supplement the household's food needs for 1 month. Households must have a monthly income below the program's eligible poverty limit to qualify. The Food Stamp Program is in operation in the 50 states, the District of Columbia, Guam, and the U.S. Virgin Islands and is administered at the local level. More information about this program can be found at the USDA's Food and Nutrition Service Web site at *www.fns.usda.gov/fsp.*

Special Supplemental Food Program for Women, Infants, and Children

WIC provides nutrition supplementation, education, and counseling in addition to referrals for health care and social services to women who are pregnant or postpartum and to their infants and children younger than 5 years. WIC has established criteria for participation, and each applicant must be income eligible and determined to be at nutritional risk. The food is either distributed free or purchased with vouchers. The average food cost per participant, as reported for FY 2007, was $39.14 per month.[23] The vouchers are good for foods such as milk, eggs, cheese, juice, fortified cereals, and infant formulas. These foods supplement the diet with rich sources of protein, iron, and certain vitamins to help reduce risk factors such as poor growth patterns, low birth weight or prematurity, preeclampsia, miscarriage, and anemia.

WIC was established in 1972 and currently has more than 8 million participants. WIC offices are established in every state, the District of Columbia, Guam, Puerto Rico, American Samoa, and the U.S. Virgin Islands. A disproportionate amount of participants are found in three states: California, New York, and Texas.[23] Figure 13-10 displays the distribution of individuals enrolled in WIC. Approximately half of all participants are children ages 1 to 5 years, and non-Hispanic Caucasians make up the largest race and ethnic percentage. More information can be found at *www.fns.usda.gov/wic/default.htm.*

National School Lunch, Breakfast, and Special Milk Programs

The national School Lunch, Breakfast, and Special Milk programs enable schools to provide nutritious meals to low-income students. The USDA offsets the cost of the program by donating large quantities of a variety of foods to public schools. Children eat free or at reduced rates, and these meals often are their main food intake of the day. The lunches provided must fulfill approximately one third of a child's RDA for protein, vitamin A, vitamin C, iron, calcium, and calories and meet the *Dietary Guidelines for Americans,* which call for diets lower in total fat and contain more fruits, vegetables, and whole grains. The Special Milk Program provides milk to children who do not have access to the other meal programs. More information about the National School Lunch, Breakfast, and Special Milk programs can be found at *www.fns.usda. gov/cnd.* A National Summer Food Service Program also is available for low-income children that provides nutritionally balanced meals during the summer months when school is not in session.

Nutrition Services Incentive Program

The Nutrition Services Incentive Program, formerly known as the Nutrition Program for the Elderly, is operated through the USDHHS Administration on Aging.

This program provides cash or commodities from the USDA for the delivery of nutritious meals to the elderly. Regardless of income, all persons older than 60 years can eat hot lunches at a community center under the Congregate Meals Program or, if they are ill or disabled, receive meals at home under the Home-Delivered Meals Program. The act specifies that economically and socially needy persons be given priority. Both programs accept voluntary contributions for meals. More information can be found at *www.fns.usda.gov/fdd/programs/ nsip.*

Food Buying and Handling Practices

For many American families, the problem is spending their limited food dollars wisely. Even on a low-cost plan for food purchasing, an average family of four can expect to spend approximately $630 to $738 per month on food alone.[24] Shopping for food can be complicated, especially when each item in a supermarket's overabundant supply shouts, "Buy me!" Food marketing is big business, and producers compete for prize placement and shelf space. A large supermarket may stock 10,000 or more different food items. A single food item may be marketed a dozen different ways at as many different prices. In diet counsel-

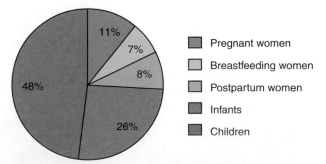

Figure 13-10 Distribution of individuals participating in the WIC program. (Modified from the Food and Nutrition Service, USDA, Washington, DC, 2006.)

ing, clients and families typically express their greatest need as help with buying food. The following wise shopping and handling practices help provide healthy foods as well as control food costs.

Planning Ahead

Use sales circulars in newspapers, plan general menus, and keep a checklist of basic pantry supplies. Make a list ahead of time according to the location of items in a regularly used grocery store. Such planning controls impulse buying and reduces extra trips.

Buying Wisely

Understanding the packaging, carefully reading labels, and watching for sale items help improve purchasing power. Only buy in quantity if it results in real savings and the food can be adequately stored or used. Be cautious in selecting so-called convenience foods. The time saved may not be worth the added cost. For fresh foods, also try alternative food sources such as farmers' markets, consumer cooperatives, and gardens.

Storing Food Safely

Control food waste and prevent illness from food spoilage or contamination. Conserve food by storing items according to their nature and use. Use dry storage, covered containers, and correct temperature refrigeration as needed. Keep opened and partly used food items at the front of the shelf for timely use. Avoid waste by preparing only the amount needed. Use leftovers in creative ways.

Cooking Food Well

Use cooking processes that retain maximal food value and maintain food safety. Cooking vegetables for shorter periods (e.g., stir frying, steaming) and with as little water as possible helps retain vitamin and mineral nutritive quality. Prepare food with imagination and good sense. Give zest and appeal to dishes with a variety of seasonings, combinations, and serving arrangements. No matter how much they know about nutrition and health, people usually eat because they are hungry and the food looks and tastes good, not necessarily because it is healthy.

SUMMARY

Common public concerns about the safety of the community food supply center on the use of chemicals such as pesticides and food additives. These substances have produced an abundant food supply but also have brought concerns and require control. The FDA is the main government agency established to maintain this control and conducts activities related to areas such as food safety, food labeling, food standards, consumer education, and research.

Numerous organisms such as bacteria, viruses, and parasites that can contaminate food may cause food-borne disease. Rigorous public health measures control sanitation of food areas and personal hygiene of food handlers. The same standards should apply to home food preparation and storage.

Families under economic stress may benefit from counseling about financial assistance. Various U.S. food assistance programs help families in need, and referrals can be made to appropriate agencies. Families also may need assistance buying and using food.

CRITICAL THINKING QUESTIONS

1. What is the basis of concern about food additives and pesticide residues?
2. What are some ways agriculture is changing to reduce the use of pesticides and their danger to workers as well as to protect the land?
3. Describe ways that various organisms may contaminate food. What standards of food preparation and handling should be used to keep food safe?
4. Kaycee is a single mother with two children and is working part time making minimum wage. During the school year, her children receive free breakfast and lunch at school. She is concerned for her children's nutritional well-being during the summer months. For what assistance may Kaycee and her children qualify? What suggestions would you make to help establish a well-balanced diet for this family?
5. According to the food buying and handling practices described in this chapter, evaluate your own habits and describe potential hazardous points for food-borne illness contamination and ways to improve your food buying practices.

CHAPTER CHALLENGE QUESTIONS

True-False

Write the correct statement for each statement that is false.

1. *True or False:* U.S. surveys reveal little or no real malnutrition in the population.

2. *True or False:* The politics of a region or country is not involved in the nutritional status of the people.

3. *True or False:* The number of new processed food items that use food additives has declined in recent years because of public pressure and concern.

4. *True or False:* The use of pesticides on farm crops and food additives in processed foods is controlled by the USDA and FDA.

5. *True or False:* Food poisoning is always caused by viral contamination of food.

6. *True or False:* The WIC program buys agricultural food surpluses to support market prices of food and distributes these goods to needy persons.

7. *True or False:* The Nutrition Services Incentive Program provides group meals for all persons older than 60 years, regardless of their income.

Multiple Choice

1. Food additives are used in processed food items to do which of the following? *(Circle all that apply.)*

   a. Preserve food and lengthen its market life
   b. Enrich food with added nutrients
   c. Improve flavor, texture, and appearance
   d. Enhance or improve some physical property of the food

2. The use of food additives in food products is controlled by the

   a. U.S. Public Health Service.
   b. USDA.
   c. FDA.
   d. Federal Trade Commission.

---

evolve **Please refer to the Students' Resource section of this text's Evolve Web site for additional study resources.**

REFERENCES

1. Philipson T: Government perspective: food labeling, *Am J Clin Nutr* 82(suppl):262S, 2005.

2. Center for Food Safety and Applied Nutrition, U.S. Food and Drug Administration: *How to understand and use the nutrition facts label,* vm.cfsan.fda.gov/~dms/foodlab.html, accessed January 2007.

3. Center for Food Safety and Applied Nutrition, U.S. Food and Drug Administration: *A food labeling guide—appendix C,* www.cfsan.fda.gov/~dms/flg-6c.html, accessed January 2007.

4. The National Organic Program: *Organic food standards and labels: the facts,* www.ams.usda.gov/nop/Consumers/brochure.html, accessed January 2007.

5. Fernandez-Cornejo J and others: The first decade of genetically engineered crops in the United States, *Economic Information Bulletin* (11), 2006.

6. Kim SH and others: Evaluating the allergic risk of genetically modified soybean, *Yonsei Med J* 47:505, 2006.

7. National Center for Infectious Disease, Centers for Disease Control and Prevention: *Food irradiation,* www.cdc.gov/ncidod/dbmd/diseaseinfo/foodirradiation.htm, accessed January 2007.

8. FDA Center for Food Safety and Applied Nutrition, Food Safety and Inspection Service, U.S. Department of Agriculture: *Foodborne illness,* www.cdc.gov/ncidod/dbmd/diseaseinfo/foodborneinfections_g.htm, accessed January 2007.

9. Centers for Disease Control and Prevention: Preliminary FoodNet data on the incidence of infection with pathogens transmitted commonly through food—10 states, United States, 2005, *MMWR Morb Mortal Wkly Rep* 55(14):392, 2006.

10. Food Safety Inspection Service, U.S. Department of Agriculture: *Basics for handling food safely,* www.fsis.usda.gov/Fact_Sheets/Basics_for_Handling_Food_Safely/index.asp, accessed January 2007.

11. National Center for Infectious Diseases, Centers for Disease Control and Prevention: *Salmonellosis,* www.cdc.gov/ncidod/dbmd/diseaseinfo/salmonellosis_g.htm, accessed January 2007.

12. National Center for Infectious Diseases, Centers for Disease Control and Prevention: *Shigellosis,* www.cdc.gov/ncidod/dbmd/diseaseinfo/shigellosis_g.htm, accessed January 2007.

13. National Center for Infectious Diseases, Centers for Disease Control and Prevention: *Listeriosis,* www.cdc.gov/ncidod/dbmd/diseaseinfo/listeriosis_g.htm, accessed January 2007.

14. Centers for Disease Control and Prevention: Blood lead levels—United States, 1999-2002, *MMWR Morb Mortal Wkly Rep* 54(20):513, 2005.

15. Lanphear BP and others: Screening housing to prevent lead toxicity in children, *Public Health Rep* 120(3):305, 2005.

16. U.S. Department of Health and Human Services: *Healthy People 2010: understanding and improving health,* Washington, DC, 2000, U.S. Government Printing Office.

17. Yuan W and others: The impact of early childhood lead exposure on brain organization: a functional magnetic resonance imaging study of language function, *Pediatrics* 118(3):971, 2006.

18. Kordas K and others: Blood lead, anemia, and short stature are independently associated with cognitive performance in Mexican school children, *J Nutr* 134(2):363, 2004.

19. Wright RO and others: Association between iron deficiency and blood lead level in a longitudinal analysis of children followed in an urban primary care clinic, *J Pediatr* 142(1):9, 2003.

20. Food and Agriculture Organization and Economic and Social Department: *The state of food insecurity in the world*, Rome, 2005, Food and Agriculture Organization of the United Nations.

21. Olson CM, Holben DH: Position of the American Dietetic Association: domestic food and nutrition security, *J Am Diet Assoc* 102(12):1840, 2003.

22. Food and Nutrition Service, Office of Analysis, Nutrition and Evaluation, U.S. Department of Agriculture: *Characteristics of food stamp households: fiscal year 2005*, Washington, DC, 2006.

23. Food and Nutrition Service, Office of Analysis, Nutrition and Evaluation, U.S. Department of Agriculture: *WIC program data, www.fns.usda.gov/wic,* accessed February 2008.

24. Center for Nutrition Policy and Promotion, U.S. Department of Agriculture: *Official USDA food plans: cost of food at home at four levels, U.S. average, January 2008, www.cnpp. usda.gov/Publications/FoodPlans/2008/CostofFoodJan08.pdf,* accessed March 2008.

FURTHER READING AND RESOURCES

ADA; *Home Food Safety: www.homefoodsafety.org/index.jsp*

CDC; *Food-Related Diseases: www.cdc.gov/ncidod/diseases/food/index.htm*

FDA; *Biotechnology in Animals and Feeds: www.fda.gov/cvm/bio-engineered.html*

FDA; Center for Food Safety & Applied Nutrition: *www.cfsan.fda.gov*

FDA; Center for Food Safety & Applied Nutrition: *Food Labeling and Nutrition, www.cfsan.fda.gov/label.html*

USDA; Agricultural Marketing Service, The National Organic Program: *Organic Food Standards and Labels: The Facts: www.ams.usda.gov/nop/Consumers/brochure.html*

USDA; Cooperative State Research, Education, and Extension Service: *www.csrees.usda.gov*

USDA and FDA Food Safety Information Center: *foodsafety.nal.usda.gov/nal_display/index.php?info_center=16&tax_level=1*

USDA Food Safety and Inspection Service food safety publications: *www.fsis.usda.gov/Fact_Sheets/index.asp*

National Restaurant Association Educational Foundation: *www.nraef.org*
  Explore these Web sites for current information and regulations on food safety, food-borne illness, and food labeling standards.

Stang J and others: Position of the American Dietetic Association: child and adolescent food and nutrition programs, *J Am Diet Assoc* 106(9):1467, 2006.
  The ADA addresses the need for and usefulness of food assistance programs geared toward children and adolescents. The role of the dietitian in such programs also is discussed.

CHAPTER 14

Food Habits and Cultural Patterns

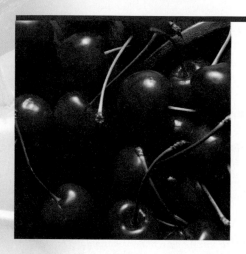

KEY CONCEPTS

- Personal food habits develop as part of a person's social and cultural heritage as well as individual lifestyle and environment.
- Social and economic change usually results in alterations in food patterns.
- American eating patterns are influenced by many different cultures.

W hy do people eat what they eat? Food is necessary to sustain life and health, but people eat certain foods for many other reasons—not necessarily for good health and nutrition, although these are important factors. As stated in Chapter 13, the broader food environment from which we have to choose is often influenced by factors such as politics and poverty, which limit personal control and choice.

A variety of connotations are attached to food. All food habits are intimately related to people's entire way of life—their values, beliefs, and situations. However, sometimes these food patterns change over time with an increase in exposure to other cultural patterns.

SOCIAL, PSYCHOLOGICAL, AND ECONOMIC INFLUENCES ON FOOD HABITS

Social Influences

Social Structure

Human group behavior reveals many activities, processes, and structures that comprise social life. In any society social groups are largely formed by factors such as economic status, education, residence, occupation, and family. Values and habits differ among groups. Subgroups also develop on the basis of region, religion, age, gender, social class, health issues, special interests, ethnic backgrounds, politics, and other common concerns. All various group affiliations influence habitual patterns, including food attitudes and choices.

Food and Social Factors

Food is a symbol of acceptance, warmth, and friendliness in social relationships. People tend to accept food or food advice more readily from friends or acquaintances or from persons they view as trusted authorities. These influences are especially strong in family relationships. Food habits that are closely associated with family sentiments stay with people throughout life. During adulthood, certain foods may trigger a flood of childhood memories and are valued for reasons apart from any nutritional importance.

Psychological Influences

Understanding Diet Patterns

Understanding dietary patterns begins with recognition of the psychological influences involved. Food is a basic enjoyment, and necessity, of life. Social relationships, in turn, affect individual behavior. Many of these psychological factors are rooted in childhood experiences. For example, when a child is hurt or disappointed, parents may offer a sweet food to help the child feel better. Then, when adults feel hurt, they turn to similar sweets to help them feel good again. Certain foods, especially sweets and other pleasurable tastes, stimulate "feel good" body chemicals in the brain called *endorphins* that give a mild "high" or help relieve pain.

Food and Psychosocial Development

Because food is so fundamental to physical survival, it also closely relates to psychosocial development as individuals. From infancy to old age, emotional maturity grows along with physical development. At each stage of human growth, food habits are part of both physical and psychosocial development. For example, when 2-year-old toddlers struggle with their first steps toward eventual independence from their parents, they learn that they can control their parents through food and often become picky eaters, refusing to eat any new foods. Psychologists now believe that another normal developmental factor is involved, which they call *food neophobia,* or fear of unfamiliar foods. This universal trait may be an instinct from the evolutionary past that protected children from eating harmful foods when they were just becoming independent from their mothers.

Marketing and Environmental Influences

Food habits also are manipulated by television, radio, magazines, and other media messages. Influences from peers, convenience items, marketing at the local grocery store, and many other factors of persuasion may dictate the decision-making process for food choices throughout life. Some organizations have even suggested additional taxation and/or banning of advertising of selected foods with little or no nutritional quality.[1] Marketing trends and media also share a strong influence in what a culture

views as beautiful. In the United States a very thin figure is heavily valued, and such influences sway food choices.

Economic Influences

Family Income and Food Habits

Most American families live under socioeconomic pressures, especially in periods of recession and inflation. The problems of middle-income families differ in relative terms, but low-income families—especially those in poverty situations—suffer extreme needs. These families often lack adequate housing and may have little or no access to educational opportunities. As a result, they are poorly prepared for jobs and often only make a day-to-day living at low-paying work or are unemployed. Approximately 12.6% of Americans live with an income below the federal poverty level, with a higher burden on African-American and Hispanic families than Caucasian families.[2] It is not surprising that people with low incomes bear the greater burden of unnecessary illness and malnutrition.

CULTURAL DEVELOPMENT OF FOOD HABITS

Food habits, like any other form of human behavior, do not develop in a vacuum. They grow from many personal, cultural, social, economic, and psychological influences. For each person, these factors are interwoven.

Strength of Personal Culture

Culture involves much more than the major and historic aspects of a person's communal life (e.g., language, religion, politics, and technology); it also develops from all the habits of everyday living and family relationships, such as preparing and serving food. In a gradual process of conscious and unconscious learning, cultural values, attitudes, habits, and practices become a deep part of individual lives. Although part of this heritage may be revised or rejected as adults, people are ultimately responsible for shaping their own lives and passing traditions on to following generations. Americans have a broad range of food habits influenced by a world of cultural diversity.

Food in a Culture

Food habits are among the oldest and most deeply rooted aspects of many cultures. Food availability, economics, and personal food meanings and beliefs are the primary factors of influence. Cultural background largely determines what is eaten as well as when and how it is eaten, but much variation exists. All types of customs, whether rational or irrational, beneficial or injurious, are found in every part of the world. Many foods take on symbolic meanings related to major life experiences (e.g., birth, death, religion, politics, and general social organization). From ancient times, ceremonies and religious rites involving food have surrounded certain events and seasons. Food gathering, preparing, and serving have followed specific customs, many of which remain intact today.

Traditional Cultural Food Patterns

The United States has been called a melting pot of ethnic and racial groups. In more recent years, however, this image no longer seems appropriate. America's diversity has come to be recognized and even celebrated as a basis for national strength. This recognition is especially strong in the diversity of America's cultural food patterns. Pockets of ethnic groups where native lifestyles are somewhat retained are apparent in many American cities.

Many different cultural food patterns are part of American family and community life. These patterns have contributed special dishes or modes of cooking to American eating habits. In turn, many of these cultural food habits have been Americanized. Older members of the family use traditional foods more regularly, with younger members of the family using them mainly on special occasions or holidays. Nevertheless, traditional foods have strong meanings and bind families and cultural communities in close fellowship. A few representative cultural food patterns are briefly reviewed in this chapter. Individual tastes and geographic patterns may vary, but food patterns are connected with culture and have a strong influence on how people eat.

Religious Dietary Laws

The dietary practices within Christianity (Catholic, Protestant, and Eastern Orthodox churches), Judaism, Hinduism, Buddhism, and Islam fluctuate according to each follower's independent understanding and interpretation of what constitutes a healthy and proper diet. Such dietary laws may apply to what, how, and when specific foods are allowed or avoided. Some dietary laws are applicable at all times (no pork at any time for Islamic followers), whereas other laws apply only during religious ceremonies (e.g., Lent for Roman Catholics). Following are examples of two such religions and their dietary laws.

Jewish

Basic Food Pattern. All Jewish festivals are religious in nature and have historic significance, but the observance of Jewish food laws differs among the three basic groups within Judaism: (1) orthodox, with strict observance; (2) conservative, with less strict observance; and (3) reform, with less ceremonial emphasis and minimal general use. The basic body of dietary laws is called the *Rules of Kashruth.* Foods selected and prepared according to these rules are called *kosher,* from the Hebrew word meaning "fit, proper." These laws originally had special ritual significance. Current Jewish dietary laws apply this significance to laws governing the slaughter, preparation, and serving of meat; the combining of meat and milk; and the use of fish and eggs. The following are various food restrictions:

- *Meat.* Appropriate meats should come from animals that chew their cud and have cloven hooves. Pork and birds of prey are avoided at all times. All forms of meat are rigidly cleansed of blood.
- *Meat and milk.* Meat and milk products are both part of the kosher Jewish diet; however, they are not to be eaten at the same meal or prepared using the same dishes. Orthodox homes maintain two sets of regular dishes, one for serving meat and the other for meals using dairy products. An additional two sets of dishes are maintained especially for use during Passover.
- *Fish.* Only fish with fins and scales are allowed. These may be eaten with either meat or dairy meals. Shellfish and crustaceans are avoided.
- *Eggs.* No egg with a blood spot may be eaten. Eggs may be used with either meat or dairy meals.

Influence of Festivals. Many traditional Jewish foods relate to festivals of the Jewish calendar that commemorate significant events in Jewish history. Special Sabbath foods often are used. A few representative foods, mostly of Eastern European influence, include the following:

- *Bagels:* doughnut-shaped, hard yeast rolls
- *Blintzes:* thin, filled, rolled pancakes
- *Borscht (borsch):* soup of meat stock, beaten egg or sour cream, beets, cabbage, or spinach; served hot or cold
- *Challah:* Sabbath loaf of white bread, shaped as a twist or coil, used at the beginning of the meal after the Kiddush, the blessing over wine (Figure 14-1)
- *Gefullte (gefilte) fish:* from a German word meaning "stuffed fish"; usually the first course of Sabbath evening meal; made of chopped and seasoned fish filet, stuffed back into the skin or rolled into balls
- *Kasha:* buckwheat groats (hulled kernels), used as a cooked cereal or as a potato substitute with gravy
- *Knishes:* pastry filled with ground meat or cheese
- *Lox:* smoked, salted salmon
- *Matzo:* flat, unleavened bread
- *Strudel:* thin pastry filled with fruit and nuts, rolled, and baked

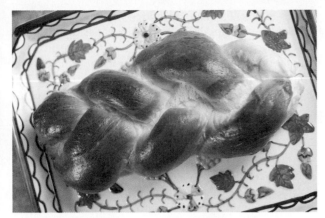

Figure 14-1 Challah, a traditional Jewish bread. (Copyright JupiterImages Corporation.)

Muslim

Basic Food Pattern. Muslim dietary laws are based on the restriction or prohibition of some foods and the promotion of others and are derived from Islamic teachings in the Koran. The laws are binding and must be followed at all times, even during pregnancy, hospitalization, and travel. These laws also are binding to visitors in the host Muslim country. Most all foods are permitted unless specifically conditioned or prohibited, as follows:

- *Milk products:* permitted at all times.
- *Fruits and vegetables:* permitted except if fermented or poisonous.
- *Breads and cereals:* permitted unless contaminated or harmful.
- *Meats:* seafood (including fish, shellfish, eels, and sea animals) and land animals (except swine) are permitted; pork is strictly prohibited. Muslims typically eat kosher meats because the blood of the animal is not to be eaten. Halal meat is the equivalent of kosher meat.
- *Alcohol:* strictly prohibited.

All food combinations are consumed as long as no prohibited items are included. Milk and meat may be eaten together, in contrast to Jewish kosher laws. The Koran mentions certain foods as being of special value, such as figs, olives, dates, honey, milk, and buttermilk. Prohibited foods by the Muslim dietary laws may be eaten when no other sources of food are available.

Representative Foods. Following are a number of favorite foods and dishes used as appetizers, main dishes, snacks, or salads:

- *Bulgur (or burghel):* partially cooked and dried cracked wheat, available in coarse grind as a base for pilaf or fine grind for use in tabouli and kibbeh

- *Falafel:* a "fast food" made from a seasoned paste of ground, soaked beans formed into shapes and fried
- *Fatayeh:* snack or appetizer similar to a small pizza, with toppings of cheese, meat, or spinach
- *Kibbeh:* meat dish made of cracked wheat shell filled with small pieces of lamb and fried in oil
- *Pilaf:* sautéed, seasoned bulgur or rice steamed in a bouillon, sometimes with poultry, meat, or shellfish
- *Pita:* flat circular bread, torn or cut into pieces, stuffed with sandwich fillings (Figure 14-2) or used as scoops for a dip such as *hummus,* which is made from chickpeas
- *Tabouli:* salad made from soaked bulgur combined with chopped tomatoes, parsley, mint, and green onion and mixed with olive oil and lemon juice

Influence of Festivals. The fourth pillar of Islam commanded by the Koran is fasting. Among the Muslim people, a 30-day period of daylight fasting is required during Ramadan, the ninth month of the Islamic lunar calendar. Ramadan was chosen for the sacred fast because that was when Mohammed received the first of the revelations that were subsequently compiled to form the Koran, and it also is the month when his followers first drove their enemies from Mecca in 624 AD. During the month of Ramadan, Muslims all over the world observe daily fasting, taking no food or drink from dawn to sunset. However, nights often are spent in special feasts. First, an appetizer is served, such as dates or a fruit drink, followed by the family's "evening breakfast," the *iftar.* At the end of Ramadan, a traditional feast lasting up to 3 days climaxes the observance. Special dishes, with delicacies such as thin pancakes dipped in powdered sugar,

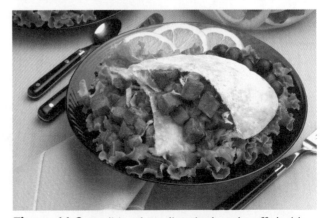

Figure 14-2 Traditional Muslim pita bread stuffed with sandwich fillings. (Copyright JupiterImages Corporation.)

Ramadan the ninth month of the Muslim year, a period of daily fasting from sunrise to sunset.

savory buns, and dried fruits, mark this occasion (see the Cultural Considerations box, "Id al-Fitr: The Post-Ramadan Festival").

All Muslims, regardless of medical condition, observe the fast of Ramadan. Individuals with diabetes, who are on certain medications, or who are pregnant or breast-feeding may have complications during this time. Health care professionals must be sensitive to such religious practices when counseling patients.

Spanish and Native American Influences

Mexican

The food habits of the early Spanish settlers and Native American nations form the basis of the current food patterns for persons of Mexican heritage who now live in the United States, chiefly in the Southwest. The following three foods are basic to this pattern: dried beans, chili peppers, and corn. Variations and additions may be found in different places or among those of different income levels. Relatively small amounts of meat are used, and eggs occasionally are eaten. Fruit (e.g., mango and papaya) is consumed in varying amounts, depending on availability and price. For centuries corn has been the basic grain used for bread in the form of tortillas, which are flat cakes baked on a hot surface or griddle. Wheat also is used in making tortillas, and rice and oats are added cereals. Coffee is a popular beverage. Major seasonings are chili peppers, onions, and garlic; the basic fat is lard.

Puerto Rican

The Puerto Rican people share a common heritage with many Hispanic Caribbean countries, so much of their food patterns are similar (Figure 14-3).[3] Puerto Ricans, however, add tropical fruits and vegetables, many of which are available in their neighborhood markets in the United States. *Viandas,* which are starchy vegetables and fruits such as plantain and green bananas, are popular foods (Figure 14-4). Two other basic foods are rice and beans. Milk, meat, yellow and green vegetables, and other fruits are used in limited quantities; dried codfish is a staple. Coffee also is a well-liked beverage among Puerto Ricans. The main cooking fat usually is lard.

Native American

The Native American population—Indian and Alaska Natives—is mainly composed of more than 500 federally recognized diverse groups living on reservations, in small rural communities, and in metropolitan cities. Despite their individual diversity, the various groups share a spiritual attachment to the land and a determination to retain their culture. Food has great religious and social significance. Serving food is an integral part of celebrations, ceremonies, and everyday hospitality. Foods may be prepared and used in different ways from region to region. Variation reflects what can be grown locally, harvested or hunted on the land or fished from its rivers, or is available in food markets.

Among the American Indian groups of the Southwest United States, the food pattern of the Navajo people, whose reservation extends over a 25,000-square-mile area at the junction of three states (New Mexico, Arizona, and Utah), is one example. The Navajos learned farming from the early Pueblo people, establishing corn and other crops as staples. They later learned herding from the Spaniards, making sheep and goats available for food and wool. Some families also raise chickens, pigs, and cattle. Today, American Indian food habits combine traditional dietary staples with modern food products from available supermarkets and fast-food restaurants (Figure 14-5). Meat (e.g., fresh mutton [Figure 14-6], beef, pork, chicken, or smoked or processed meat) is eaten daily. Other staples include bread (tortillas or fry bread, blue corn bread, and

CULTURAL CONSIDERATIONS

ID AL-FITR: THE POST-RAMADAN FESTIVAL

At the conclusion of Ramadan, Islam's holy month of prayer and fasting, wealthy merchants and princes in Muslim countries traditionally hold public feasts for the needy, known as the festival of Id al-Fitr.

Over the years, many delicacies have been served to symbolize the joy of returning from fasting and the heightened sense of unity, brotherhood, and charity that the fasting experience has brought to the people. Among the foods served are chicken or veal sautéed with eggplant and onions, then simmered slowly in pomegranate juice and spiced with turmeric and cardamom seeds. The highlight of the meal usually is kharuf mahshi, which is a whole lamb (symbol of sacrifice) stuffed with a rich dressing made of dried fruits, cracked wheat, pine nuts, almonds, and onions and seasoned with ginger and coriander. The stuffed lamb is baked in hot ashes for many hours so that it is tender enough to be pulled apart and eaten with the fingers.

At the conclusion of the meal, rich pastries and candies are served. These may be flavored with spices or flower petals. Some of the sweets are taken home and savored as long as possible as a reminder of the festival.

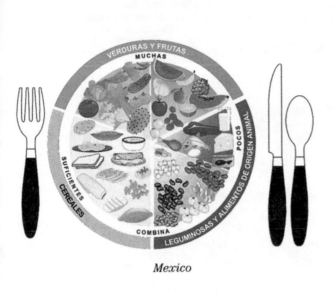

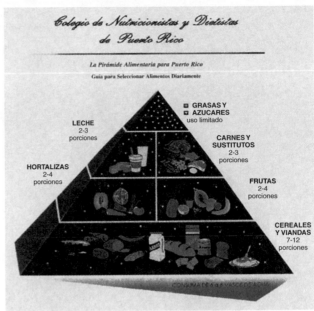

Figure 14-3 National food guides for Mexico and Puerto Rico. (Reprinted from Painter J and others: Comparison of international food guide pictorial representations, *J Am Diet Assoc* 102:483, 2002, with permission from the American Dietetic Association.)

cornmeal mush), beverages (coffee, soft drinks, and other fruit-flavored sweet drinks), eggs, vegetables (corn, potatoes, green beans, and tomatoes), and some fresh or canned fruit. Frying is a common method of food preparation; lard and shortening are the main cooking fats. Some health concerns are growing, however, about an

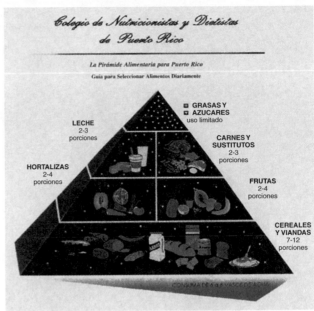

Figure 14-4 Plantain, a popular fruit in Puerto Rico. (Copyright JupiterImages Corporation.)

increased use of modern convenience or snack foods that are high in fat, sugar, calories, and sodium, especially among children and teenagers (see the Cultural Considerations box, "Acculturation to an American Diet").

Other Native American tribes in the United States have their own heritages and distinct dietary habits relative to custom and the regions where they live.

Influences of the Southern United States

African Americans

African-American populations, especially in the Southern states, have contributed a rich heritage to American food patterns, particularly to Southern cooking as a whole. Similar to the moving music styles (e.g., spirituals, blues, gospel, and jazz), the food patterns of Southern African Americans were born of hard times and developed through a creative ability to turn any basic staples at hand into memorable food. Although regional differences occur, as with any basic food pattern, the representative use of foods from basic food groups is evident, as follows:

- *Breads and cereals.* Traditional breads include hot breads such as biscuits, spoon bread (i.e., a souffle-like dish of cornmeal mush with beaten eggs), cornmeal muffins, and skillet cornbread. Cooked cereals such as cornmeal mush, hominy grits (ground corn), and oatmeal are commonly used.

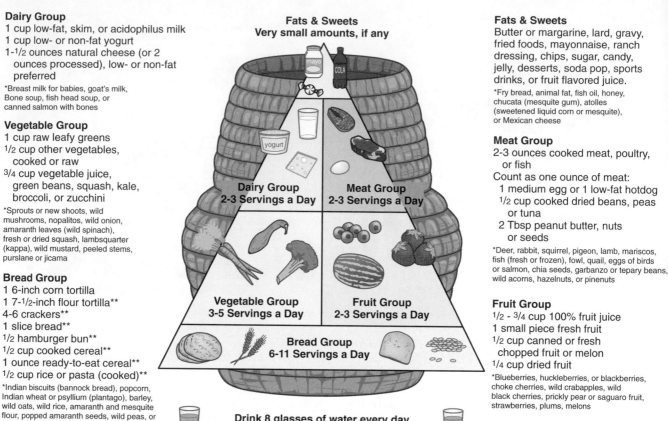

Dairy Group
1 cup low-fat, skim, or acidophilus milk
1 cup low- or non-fat yogurt
1-1/2 ounces natural cheese (or 2
  ounces processed), low- or non-fat
  preferred

*Breast milk for babies, goat's milk,
Bone soup, fish head soup, or
canned salmon with bones

Vegetable Group
1 cup raw leafy greens
1/2 cup other vegetables,
  cooked or raw
3/4 cup vegetable juice,
  green beans, squash, kale,
  broccoli, or zucchini

*Sprouts or new shoots, wild
mushrooms, nopalitos, wild onion,
amaranth leaves (wild spinach),
fresh or dried squash, lambsquarter
(kappa), wild mustard, peeled stems,
purslane or jicama

Bread Group
1 6-inch corn tortilla
1 7-1/2-inch flour tortilla**
4-6 crackers**
1 slice bread**
1/2 hamburger bun**
1/2 cup cooked cereal**
1 ounce ready-to-eat cereal**
1/2 cup rice or pasta (cooked)**

*Indian biscuits (bannock bread), popcorn,
Indian wheat or psyllium (plantago), barley,
wild oats, wild rice, amaranth and mesquite
flour, popped amaranth seeds, wild peas, or
corn (fresh, frozen or cooked)

Fats & Sweets
Very small amounts, if any

Dairy Group
2-3 Servings a Day

Meat Group
2-3 Servings a Day

Vegetable Group
3-5 Servings a Day

Fruit Group
2-3 Servings a Day

Bread Group
6-11 Servings a Day

**Drink 8 glasses of water every day
unless your doctor has advised limited fluids.**

Fats & Sweets
Butter or margarine, lard, gravy,
fried foods, mayonnaise, ranch
dressing, chips, sugar, candy,
jelly, desserts, soda pop, sports
drinks, or fruit flavored juice.

*Fry bread, animal fat, fish oil, honey,
chucata (mesquite gum), atolles
(sweetened liquid corn or mesquite),
or Mexican cheese

Meat Group
2-3 ounces cooked meat, poultry,
  or fish
Count as one ounce of meat:
  1 medium egg or 1 low-fat hotdog
  1/2 cup cooked dried beans, peas
    or tuna
  2 Tbsp peanut butter, nuts
    or seeds

*Deer, rabbit, squirrel, pigeon, lamb, mariscos,
fish (fresh or frozen), fowl, quail, eggs of birds
or salmon, chia seeds, garbanzo or tepary beans,
wild acorns, hazelnuts, or pinenuts

Fruit Group
1/2 - 3/4 cup 100% fruit juice
1 small piece fresh fruit
1/2 cup canned or fresh
  chopped fruit or melon
1/4 cup dried fruit

*Blueberries, huckleberries, or blackberries,
choke cherries, wild crabapples, wild
black cherries, prickly pear or saguaro fruit,
strawberries, plums, melons

Figure 14-5 Southern Arizona American Indian Food Guide: Choices for a Healthy Life. *Traditional foods. **Whole grain products recommended. (Osterkamp LK, Longstaff L: Development of a dietary teaching tool for American Indians and Alaskan Natives in Southern Arizona, *Nutr Educ Behav* 36:272, 2004.)

■ *Eggs and dairy products.* Eggs and some cheese but little milk are used, probably because of the greater prevalence of lactose intolerance among African Americans.

■ *Vegetables.* Leafy greens, such as turnip greens, collards, mustard greens, and spinach, frequently are used and usually are cooked with bacon or salt pork. Cabbage is boiled or chopped raw with a salad dressing (e.g., coleslaw). Other vegetables used include okra (coated with cornmeal and fried), sweet potatoes (baked whole or sliced and "candied" with added sugar), green beans, tomatoes, potatoes, corn, butter beans, and dried beans such as black-eyed peas and red or pinto beans cooked with smoked ham hocks and served over rice. Black-eyed peas served over rice comprise a dish called "hoppin' John" that is traditionally served on New Year's Day to bring good luck for the new year.

■ *Fruits.* Commonly eaten fruits include apples, peaches, berries, oranges, bananas, and juices.

■ *Meat.* Pork is a common meat, including fresh cuts of ribs, sausage, and smoked ham. Some beef is eaten, mainly ground for meat loaf or hamburgers. Poultry is frequently consumed, mainly as fried chicken and baked holiday turkey. Organ meats, such as liver, heart, intestines (chitterlings), or poultry giblets (gizzard and heart), are consumed. Fish, including catfish, some flounder, and shellfish (e.g., crab and shrimp) are eaten when available. Frying is a common method of cooking; lard, shortening, or vegetable oils are fats used.

■ *Desserts.* Favorites include pies (e.g., pecan, sweet potato, and pumpkin) and deep-dish peach or berry cobblers, cakes (e.g., coconut and chocolate), and bread pudding to use up leftover bread.

■ *Beverages.* Coffee, apple cider, fruit juices, lemonade, iced sweet tea, carbonated soft drinks, and buttermilk (which is a more easily tolerated, cultured form of milk) are consumed.

French Americans

The Cajun people, concentrated in the southwestern coastal waterways of southern Louisiana, have contributed a unique cuisine and food pattern to America's rich and varied fare. This pattern continues to provide a unique model for rapidly expanding forms of American

CULTURAL CONSIDERATIONS

ACCULTURATION TO AN AMERICAN DIET

Immigration from one part of the world to another usually is accompanied by changes in dietary intake, lifestyle, and disease risk to match the new culture—a phenomenon referred to as *acculturation.* Several studies have evaluated the changes occurring over time, specifically with Hispanic immigrants, because this population encompasses the fastest growing ethnic group in the United States. One such study evaluated the relations of ethnicity, acculturation, and fruit and vegetable intake among older Hispanic adults. When compared with non-Hispanic Caucasians in the United States, the Hispanic elderly consumed more fruits and vegetables. However, an inverse relation was found with acculturation and fruit and vegetable intake among Hispanic adults and a positive association with fat intake.* As more acculturation takes place for the immigrants to their new environment, the poorer their dietary choices are.

One of the most notable negative effects of acculturation seems to be with the Native American populations. Recent studies have noted a dramatic increase in the prevalence of diabetes, obesity, and cardiovascular disease among this population.† According to the CDC, the prevalence of death from diabetes among Native Americans currently is close to twice that of the total population.‡ Researchers believe the increase in disease risk is directly associated with dietary and lifestyle adaptations to the typical American diet and a more sedentary lifestyle.

For more information on acculturation, see the "Dietary Acculturation: Applications to Nutrition Research and Dietetics" article referenced in the Further Reading and Resources section at the end of the chapter.

*Neuhouser ML and others: Vegetable intakes are associated with greater acculturation among Mexicans living in Washington state, *J Am Diet Assoc* 104:51, 2004.
†Denny CH and others: Surveillance for health behaviors of American Indians and Alaska Natives. Findings from the Behavioral Risk Factor Surveillance System, 1997-2000, *MMWR Surveill Summ* 52(7):1, 2003.
‡Centers for Disease Control and Prevention: *The burden of chronic diseases and their risk factors: national and state perspectives,* www.cdc.gov/nccdphp/burdenbook2004/pdf/burden_book2004.pdf, accessed February 2008.

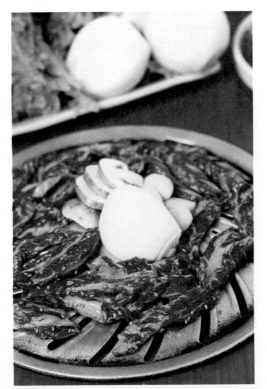

Figure 14-6 Mutton, the meat of sheep or goats. (Copyright JupiterImages Corporation.)

ethnic food. The Cajuns are descendants of the early French colonists of Acadia, a peninsula on the eastern coast of Canada now known as Nova Scotia. In the pre-Revolutionary wars between France and Britain, both countries contended for the area of Acadia. But after Britain finally won control of Canada, fear of an Acadian revolt led to a forcible deportation of the French colonists in 1755. After a long and difficult journey down the Atlantic coast, then westward along the Gulf of Mexico, a group of the impoverished Acadians finally settled along the bayou country of what is now Louisiana. To support themselves, they developed their unique food pattern from the seafood at hand and what they could grow and harvest. Over time, Cajuns blended their own French culinary background with the Creole cooking they found in their new homeland around New Orleans.

The unique Cajun food pattern of the Southern United States represents an ethnic blending of cultures using basic

> **Cajun** a group of people with an enduring tradition whose French-Catholic ancestors established permanent communities in the southern Louisiana coastal waterways after being expelled from Acadia (now Nova Scotia, Canada) by the reigning English in the late eighteenth century; developed unique food pattern from a blend of native French influence and a mix of Creole cooking found in the new land.

foods available in the area. Cajun foods are strong flavored and spicy, with the abundant seafood as a base, and usually cooked as a stew and served over rice. The well-known hot chili sauce, made of crushed and fermented red chili peppers blended with spices and vinegar and sold all over the world under the trade name Tabasco, is still made by generations of a Cajun family on Avery Island on the coastal waterway of southern Louisiana. The most popular shellfish native to the region is the crawfish, which is now grown commercially in the fertile rice paddies of the bayou areas. Catfish, red snapper, shrimp, blue crab, and oysters are some of the other popular seafood used. Popular vegetables include onions, bell peppers, okra, parsley, shallots, and tomatoes; seasonings are Cayenne (red) pepper, hot pepper sauce (Tabasco), crushed black pepper, white pepper, bay leaves, thyme, and filé powder. Some typical Cajun dishes include seafood or chicken gumbo, jambalaya, red beans and rice, blackened catfish or red snapper, barbecued shrimp, breaded catfish with Creole sauce, and boiled crawfish. Breads and starches include French bread, hush puppies (fried cornbread-mixture balls), cornbread muf-

fins, cush-cush (cornmeal mush cooked with milk), grits (ground white corn), rice, and yams. Desserts include ambrosia (fresh peeled orange segments and juice with sliced bananas and freshly grated coconut), sweet potato pie, pecan pie, berry pie, bread pudding, and pecan pralines.

Asian Food Patterns

Chinese

Chinese cooks believe that refrigeration diminishes natural flavors, so they select the freshest foods possible, hold them the shortest time possible, and cook them quickly at a high temperature in a *wok* (a basic round-bottom pan) with small amounts of fat and liquid. The wok allows heat to be controlled in a quick stir-frying method that preserves natural flavor, color, and texture. Vegetables cooked just before serving are still crisp and flavorful when served. Meat is used more in small amounts in combined dishes than as a single main entree. Little milk is used, but eggs and soybean products (e.g., tofu) add other sources

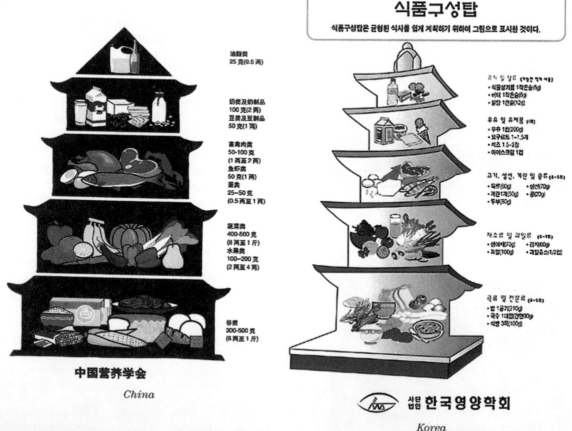

Figure 14-7 National food guides for China and Korea. (Reprinted from Painter J and others: Comparison of international food guide pictorial representations, *J Am Diet Assoc* 102(4):483, 2002, with permission of the American Dietetic Association.)

of protein. Foods that have been dried, salted, pickled, spiced, candied, or canned may be added as garnishes or relishes to mask some flavors or textures or enhance others. Fruits usually are eaten fresh. Rice is the staple grain used at most meals. The traditional beverage is unsweetened green tea. Seasonings include soy sauce, ginger, almonds, and sesame seed. Peanut oil is the main cooking fat. Chinese dietary patterns generally include less total fat and saturated fat than the dietary patterns of African Americans, Caucasians, Hispanics, or Japanese. Figure 14-7 illustrates the official food guides for China and Korea.

Japanese

In some ways Japanese food patterns are similar to those of the Chinese. Rice is a basic grain at meals, soy sauce is used for seasoning, and tea is the main beverage. The Japanese diet contains more seafood, especially in the form of sushi, than the Chinese diet does (Figure 14-8). Many varieties of fish and shellfish are used. The term *sushi* does not necessarily mean raw fish. Some sushi is prepared with only vegetables or with cooked fish. Vegetables usually are steamed; pickled vegetables also are used. Fresh fruit is eaten in season; a tray of fruit is a regular course at main meals. The overall Japanese diet is high in sodium content and low in milk products because of the high prevalence of lactose intolerance.

Southeast Asian

Since 1971, in the wake of the Vietnam War, more than 340,000 Southeast Asians have come to the United States as refugees. The largest groups of refugees are Vietnamese, but others have come from the adjacent war-torn countries of Laos and Cambodia. They mainly have settled in California, with other groups in Florida, Texas, Illinois, and Pennsylvania. As a whole, their food patterns are similar and have an effect on American diet and agriculture. Asian grocery stores throughout the country stock many traditional Asian food items. Rice, both long grain and glutinous, forms the basis of the Indonesian food pattern and is eaten at most meals. The Vietnamese usually eat their rice plain in a separate rice bowl, not mixed with other foods, whereas other Southeast Asians may eat rice in mixed dishes.

Soups also are commonly used at meals. Many fresh fruits and vegetables are eaten along with fresh herbs and other seasonings such as chives, spring onions, chili peppers, ginger root, coriander, turmeric, and fish sauce. Many kinds of seafood (fish and shellfish) are included in the diet, as well as chicken, duck, and pork. Red meat usually is eaten only once or twice per month and in small quantities. Stir-frying in a wok with a small amount of lard or peanut oil is a common method of cooking. A variety of vegetables and seasonings are used, with small amounts of seafood or meat added. In a traditional Asian diet, nuts and legumes are the primary sources of protein.

Since coming to the United States, the Vietnamese have made some dietary changes that reflect American influence. These changes include the use of more eggs, beef, pork, candy and other sweet snacks, bread, fast foods, soft drinks, butter and margarine, and coffee.

Mediterranean Influences

Italian

The sharing of food is an important part of Italian life. Meals are associated with warmth and fellowship, and special occasions are shared with families and friends. Bread and pasta are the basic ingredients in most meals. Milk, seldom used alone, typically is mixed with coffee in equal portions. Cheese is a favorite food, with many popular varieties available. Meats, poultry, and fish are used in many ways, and the varied Italian sausages and cold cuts are famous worldwide. Vegetables are used alone, in mixed main dishes or soups, sauces, and salads. Seasonings include herbs and spices, garlic, wine, olive oil, tomato puree, and salted pork. Main dishes are prepared by initially browning vegetables and seasonings in olive oil; adding meat or fish; covering with such liquids as wine, broth, or tomato sauce; and simmering slowly on low heat for several hours. Fresh fruit often is eaten as dessert or a snack.

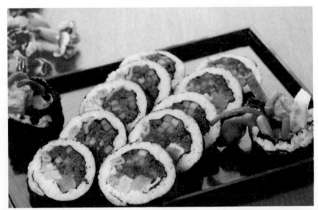

Figure 14-8 Sushi, a traditional Japanese cuisine. (Copyright JupiterImages Corporation.).

filé powder substance made from ground sassafras leaves; seasons and thickens the dish being made.

jambalaya a dish of Creole origin combining rice, chicken, ham, pork, sausage, broth, vegetables, and seasonings.

Greek

Everyday meals are simple, but Greek holiday meals are occasions for serving many delicacies. Bread is always the center of every meal, with other foods considered accompaniments. Milk is seldom used as a beverage but instead in the cultured form of yogurt. Cheese is a favorite food, especially *feta,* a white cheese made from sheep's milk and preserved in brine. Lamb is the preferred meat, but others, especially fish, also are eaten. Eggs are sometimes a main dish but never a breakfast food. Many vegetables are used, often as a main entree, cooked with broth, tomato sauce, onions, olive oil, and parsley. A typical salad of thinly-sliced raw vegetables and feta cheese, dressed with olive oil and vinegar, often is served with meals. The traditional Greek salad also is a favorite at many American restaurants. Rice is a main grain in many dishes. Fruit is an everyday dessert, but rich pastries, such as *baklava,* are served on special occasions. Figure 14-9 illustrates the Mediterranean Diet Pyramid (see Appendix H for more information on traditional foods in various cultures).

CHANGES IN AMERICAN FOOD HABITS

Personal Food Choices

Basic Determinants

As has been shown, universal factors determining personal food choices arise from physical, social, and psychological needs. Box 14-1 lists some of these factors. Changing personal eating patterns is difficult enough; helping clients and patients make needed changes for positive health reasons is even more difficult. Such teaching requires a culturally sensitive and flexible understanding of the complex factors involved.

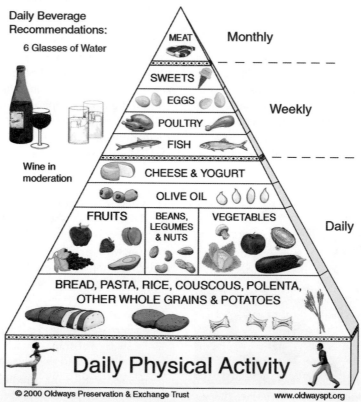

Figure 14-9 Mediterranean Diet Pyramid. (Copyright 2000, Oldways Preservation & Exchange Trust, Boston, *www.oldwayspt.org.*)

BOX 14-1

FACTORS DETERMINING FOOD CHOICES

Physical Features
Food supply available
Food technology
Geography, agriculture, distribution
Sanitation, housing
Season, climate
Storage and cooking facilities

Social and Economic Factors
Advertising
Culture
General education and nutrition education
Income
Political and economic policies
Religion and social class
Social problems, poverty, alcoholism

Physiologic Factors
Allergies
Disability
Health and disease status
Heredity
Nutrient and energy needs
Therapeutic diets

Psychological Factors
Habit
Preference
Emotions
Cravings
Positive or negative experiences and associations
Personal food acceptance

Factors Influencing Change

Ethnic patterns and regional cultural habits are strong influences. They establish early food habits and make changing those habits difficult. On the other hand, the changing society puts the old in conflict with the new. Some of the following newer factors influence changes in food habits:

- *Income.* The generally improved economic situation of society provides sufficient income in most cases to give people more choice and time.
- *Technology.* Expansion in the fields of science and technology increases the number and variety of food items available.
- *Environment.* America's rapidly changing environment results in concerns about food and health.
- *Access to food.* Grocery store and farmers' market locations and fast food availability.
- *Vision.* America's expanding mass media, especially television, stimulates many options for new items and changes expectations and desires. A recent study published in the *New England Journal of Medicine* reported that "marketing strongly influences children's food

preferences, requests, and consumption"—a fact that has not necessarily benefited the youth.[4]

Changing American Food Patterns

The stereotype of the all-American family of parents and two children eating three meals a day with no snacks in between is no longer the norm. Far-reaching changes have occurred in Americans' way of living and, subsequently, their food habits.

Households

American households are increasing in number and changing in nature. Most new households are groups of unrelated persons or persons living together. The U.S. Census Bureau projections are that from 2000 to 2010 the number of nonfamily households will increase 17%, whereas family households will only increase 9%.[5] The average size of American households is projected to decline from 2.59 persons in 2000 to 2.53 persons by 2010. Married couple households from 2000 to 2010 will decline from 54% to 52% of all households.[5] These changes reflect a rapidly changing society.

Working Women

The number of women in the workforce continues to increase rapidly and is not likely to reverse. This trend is not restricted to any social, economic, or ethnic group. Women of all racial and ethnic groups are major entrants into the U.S. labor market, holding half of all management and professional positions. The U.S. Department of Labor reports that women increased their labor force participation from 43% to 59% between 1970 and 2004.[6] This is a widespread change in society. Working parents increasingly rely on food items and cooking methods that save time, space, and labor.

Family Meals

Family meals, as they have been known, have changed. Breakfasts and lunches are seldom eaten in a family setting. Even though frequent family meals are positively associated with improved dietary quality, beneficial developmental assets, and inversely related to high-risk behaviors among adolescents, family mealtime as a group is on the decline.[7,8] In addition, more Americans eat at restaurants at a higher frequency than in years past and choose to eat more food with higher energy density.[9,10]

Meals and Snacks

Americans' habits have changed with regard to when they eat and whether they eat with their families. Mid-morning and midafternoon breaks at work usually involve food or beverages. Evening television snacks and midnight refrigerator raids are common. Nutrition hardliners of the old school may denounce this snacking behavior, but they are few and far between. Americans are moving toward a concept of *balanced days* instead of *balanced meals*. They are increasing the number of times a day they eat to as many as 11 "eating occasions," a pattern recently termed *grazing*. This shift is not necessarily bad, depending on the nature of the periodic snacking or more constant grazing. In fact, studies indicate that frequent small meals are better for the body than three larger meals per day, especially when healthy snacking and grazing contribute to needed nutrient and energy intake (see the For Further Focus box, "Snacking: An All-American Food Habit").

Health and Fitness

Americans' interest in health and fitness is increasing, which has affected food buying in several ways, with more nutrition awareness, weight concern, and interest in gourmet or specialty foods. New lines of low-fat, fat-free, sugar-free, high-protein, and similar foods are available.

Economical Buying

More Americans are making diet changes to save money. No-frills grocery stores are becoming more and more popular across the country. With a warehouse-type store, the cost of overhead is significantly reduced and storeowners can pass that savings on to consumers. Many Americans also are members of bulk-food chains such as Costco and Sam's Club. Buying in bulk (economy size or family size) can save money, but only if the quantity can be efficiently used. No savings is incurred if food is not properly stored or eaten before it goes bad. Grocery stores also provide cost-per-unit pricing on the shelves to make comparing the prices of similar foods in different-size containers or packages easier for the consumer. Because the lowest cost per unit is the best buy, this is beneficial for money-conscious shoppers.

Fast Foods

Most Americans have eaten in a fast-food restaurant at least once. From McDonald's modest beginning in 1955 in Des Plaines, Ill., the fast-food business has grown into a multibillion-dollar enterprise that now captures almost half of the money spent on meals away from home. As family income rises, so does the consumption of fast foods, especially among the middle class. A recent article in the *Journal of the American Dietetic Association* compared portion sizes of selected foods from the year they were introduced to the sizes commonly found today. For example, a *regular* order of French fries from Burger King in 1954 was 2.6 oz. Today, a *medium* order of Burger King fries averages 4.1 oz. Similarly, in 1955 the only size fries McDonald's had to offer was a 2.4-oz portion. Today, the McDonald's portions range from small (2.4 oz) to super-size (7.1 oz). Such sizes dwarf the standard serving sizes on the USDA MyPyramid food guide. A standard serving of soda according to MyPyramid is 12 fl oz. However, the average size soda served at a fast-food outlet is 23 fl oz.[11] Some researchers believe the expanding portion sizes in America's most popular restaurants are closely linked with America's expanding weight problem. The USDHHS created an interesting Portion Distortion Quiz depicting serving size changes over the past 20 years (*http://hp2010.nhlbihin.net/portion/index.htm*).

Tempting advertisements often lure consumers into ordering more food than they need. Deals such as "two for one" or "value meals" could be a great bargain but often supply more food than is necessary for one person. In today's fast-food market, a variety of options are available outside the customary hamburger and fries. Many fast-food chains offer grilled or baked chicken, turkey, or fish; fresh deli sandwiches with vegetables;

FOR FURTHER FOCUS

SNACKING: AN ALL-AMERICAN FOOD HABIT

The snack market in the United States continues to grow. Consumer spending for all foods has increased, with a greater portion of the increase being spent for snacks, mainly salty snacks, cookies, and crackers. Other popular snacks include soft drinks, candies, gum, fresh fruit, bakery items, milk, and chips.

Snacking is said to "ruin your appetite," and perhaps the consumption of excess soft drinks does, but is snacking all together bad? Not necessarily. Surveys have shown a direct association between more complete nutrition and an increase in snacking. Those who snack more show higher nutrient percentages in the "adequate" range of the DRI and RDA standards. Many people snack on foods that are not empty extras, but essential contributions to total nutritional adequacy (e.g., fruit, cheese, eggs, bread, and crackers).

Snacking, or grazing as some persons do, with more frequent nibbling, clearly is a significant component of food behavior. Rather than rule against the practice, dietitians should promote snack foods that enhance nutritional well-being.

side orders of salads or steamed vegetables; soup; and frozen yogurt. A well-balanced meal can be selected at almost any restaurant, provided the consumer is astute in selecting the healthier choice. As with foods from any ethnic or cultural background, "all foods fit in moderation."

SUMMARY

All people grow up and live in a social setting. Each person inherits a culture and particular social structure, complete with its food habits and attitudes about eating. The effects on health associated with major social and economic shifts should be understood, as well as the current social forces (including cultural, religious, and psychological), to best help persons make dietary changes to benefit their health.

Food patterns of Americans are changing. They increasingly rely on new forms of food in fast, complex lives. More women are working, households are getting smaller, more people are living alone, and meal patterns are evolving. People search for less-fancy, lower cost food items and also cook creatively. People generally are more nutrition and health conscious, and this consciousness is influencing the social patterns of eating from food choices at fast-food outlets to the number of times people eat per day.

CRITICAL THINKING QUESTIONS

1. What is the meaning of culture? How does it affect food patterns?
2. This chapter outlines the dietary laws of two religious groups. What other dietary laws are you familiar with? Using the Internet for a reference, compare the dietary practices of another religious group with the ones given in the text. Could any practices be problematic for children, the elderly, or sick individuals?
3. What social and psychological factors influence food habits? Give examples of personal meanings related to food.
4. What are current trends in American food habits? Discuss their implications for nutrition and health.

CHAPTER CHALLENGE QUESTIONS

True-False
Write the correct statement for each statement that is false.
1. *True or False:* Food habits result from instinctive behavioral responses throughout life.
2. *True or False:* The structure of American social classes largely is determined by occupation, income, education, and residence.
3. *True or False:* Lifestyles and eating habits are modified in response to changes in society's values.
4. *True or False:* From the time of birth, eating is a social act built on social relationships.
5. *True or False:* Very few differences exist between various cultural eating and food patterns that would influence how a health care professional would counsel a patient.

Multiple Choice
1. A healthy body requires
   a. specific foods to control specific functions.
   b. certain food combinations to achieve specific physiologic effects.
   c. natural foods to prevent disease.
   d. specific nutrients in various foods to perform specific body functions.
2. Food habits in a given culture largely are based on which of the following? *(Circle all that apply.)*
   a. Food availability
   b. Genetic differences in food tastes
   c. Food economics, market practices, and food distribution
   d. Symbolic meanings attached to certain foods
3. In the Jewish food pattern, the word *kosher* refers to food prepared by which of the following? *(Circle all that apply.)*
   a. Ritual slaughter of allowed animals for maximal blood drainage
   b. Avoiding the combination of meat and milk in the same meal

c. Special seasoning to avoid the use of salt
d. Special cooking of food combinations to ensure purity and digestibility

4. The basic grain used in the Mexican food pattern is
   a. rice.
   b. corn.
   c. wheat.
   d. oat.

5. Stir-frying is a basic cooking method used in the food pattern of
   a. Mexicans.
   b. Jews.
   c. Chinese.
   d. Greeks.

---

evolve Please refer to the Students' Resource section of this text's Evolve Web site for additional study resources.

REFERENCES

1. Davey RC: The obesity epidemic: too much food for thought? *Br J Sports Med* 38:360, 2004.
2. DeNavas-Walt C and others: *U.S. Census Bureau, current population reports, P60-231, income, poverty, and health insurance coverage in the United States: 2005,* Washington, DC, 2006, U.S. Government Printing Office.
3. Painter J and others: Comparison of international food guide pictorial representations, *J Am Diet Assoc* 102:483, 2002.
4. Nestle M: Food marketing and childhood obesity—a matter of policy, *N Engl J Med* 354:2527, 2006.
5. U.S. Census Bureau, U.S. Department of Commerce: *Statistical abstract of the United States 1999,* ed 119, Washington, DC, 1999, U.S. Department of Commerce/Government Printing Office.
6. U.S. Department of Labor, Bureau of Labor Statistics: *Women in the labor force: a databook,* www.bls.gov/cps/wlf-databook2005.htm, accessed August 2007.
7. Fulkerson JA and others: Family dinner meal frequency and adolescent development: relationships with developmental assets and high-risk behaviors, *J Adolesc Health* 39:337, 2006.
8. Neumark-Sztainer D and others: Family meal patterns: associations with sociodemographic characteristics and improved dietary intake among adolescents, *J Am Diet Assoc* 103:317, 2003.
9. Kant AK, Graubard BI: Eating out in America, 1987-2000: trends and nutritional correlates, *Prev Med* 38:243, 2004.
10. Kant AK, Graubard BI: Secular trends in patterns of self-reported food consumption of adult Americans: NHANES 1971-1975 to NHANES 1999-2002, *Am J Clin Nutr* 84:1215, 2006.
11. Young LR, Nestle M: Expanding portion sizes in the U.S. marketplace: implications for nutrition counseling, *J Am Diet Assoc* 103:231, 2003.

FURTHER READING AND RESOURCES

Satia-Abouta J and others: Dietary acculturation: applications to nutrition research and dietetics, *J Am Diet Assoc* 102:1105, 2002.

> This article explores dietary acculturation by immigrants—the process of adopting the dietary practices of a new culture—in the United States and links specific practices with disease risk. The authors take an important look at the public health issues facing the U.S. immigrant population and how health care professionals can play a role in maintaining the healthiest combination of dietary practices.

Kant AK, Graubard BI: Secular trends in patterns of self-reported food consumption of adult Americans: NHANES 1971-1975 to NHANES 1999-2002, *Am J Clin Nutr* 84:1215, 2006.

> The authors explore an interesting trend in food consumption patterns and the correlation to obesity in the United States over a 30-year period.

CHAPTER 15

Weight Management

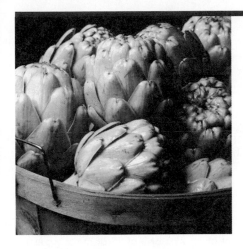

KEY CONCEPTS

- Underlying causes of obesity include a host of various genetic, environmental, and psychological factors.
- Short-term food patterns, or fads, often stem from food misinformation that appeals to some human psychological need but does not necessarily meet physiologic needs.
- Realistic weight management focuses on individual needs and health promotion, including meal pattern planning and regular physical activity.
- America's obsession with thinness carries social, physiologic, and biologic costs.

Currently 66% of adults ages 20 to 74 years in the United States are overweight, with 32% meeting the criteria for obese.[1] This epidemic, contributed in large part by poor diet, physical inactivity, and genetics, is not limited to adults. The NCHS reported that 17% to 19% of children and adolescents also are overweight.[1] Weight loss "diets" are abundant and do not lack in variety regarding philosophy of methods to lose unwanted pounds. Use of these diets seems to increase daily, with new diet books constantly appearing in the public press. Despite this obsession and the fact that weight loss is big business, Americans continue to grow in undesirable directions (Figure 15-1). This chapter examines the problem of weight management and seeks a more positive and realistic health model that recognizes personal needs and sound weight goals.

OBESITY AND WEIGHT CONTROL

Body Weight and Body Fat

Definitions

Obesity develops from many interwoven factors—including personal, physical, psychological, and genetic—and is difficult to define. As used in the traditional medical sense, *obesity* is a clinical term for excess body fat generally applied to persons who are at least 20% above a desired weight for height. The terms *overweight* and *obesity* often are used interchangeably but technically have different meanings. *Overweight* denotes a body weight above a population weight-for-height standard. However, the word *obesity* is a more specific term that refers to the *degree of fatness* (i.e., the relative excess amount of fat in the total body composition), which is the real health problem. Over the past 4 decades the percentage of overweight adults (body mass index [BMI] of 25 or greater)

---

body composition the relative sizes of the four body compartments that make up the total body: lean body mass (muscle mass), fat, water, and bone.

body mass index (BMI) body weight in kilograms divided by the square of height in meters, (kg/m²).

Obesity
4X increase since 1960's

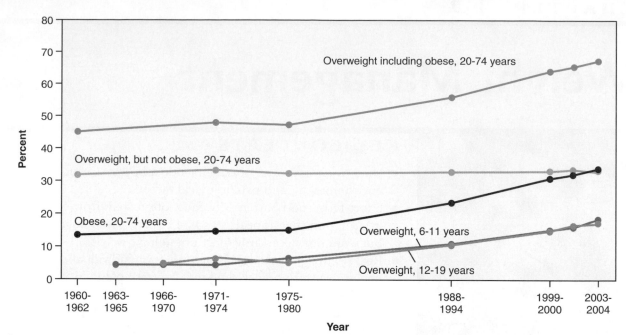

Figure 15–1 Overweight and obesity, by age: United States, 1960-2004. Estimates for adults are age adjusted. For adults: overweight, including obese, is defined as a BMI of 25 or greater; overweight but not obese as a BMI of 25 or more but less than 30; and obese as a BMI of 30 or more. For children: overweight is defined as a BMI at or above the sex- and age-specific 95th percentile BMI cut points from the 2000 CDC Growth Charts: United States. Obese is not defined for children. (Reprinted from National Center for Health Statistics: *Health, United States, 2006, with chartbook on trends in the health of Americans,* Hyattsville, MD, 2006, U.S. Government Printing Office.)

ages 20 to 74 years has increased from 44.8% to 66%. The increase in persons meeting the criteria for clinical obesity (BMI of 30 or greater) has increased even more dramatically, from 13.3% of the population in 1960 to 32.1% in 2004.[1]

BMI can be tracked from childhood to adulthood with CDC growth charts. BMI is a reliable method of predicting the relative risk of becoming an overweight adult based on the presence or absence of excess weight at various times during childhood. Studies show that children who were ever overweight during preschool or elementary school were five times more likely to be overweight at age 12 years.[2]

Every person is different, and *normal* values in healthy persons vary. Until recently, the important factor of *age* in setting a reasonable body weight for adults had been overlooked. With advancing age, body weight usually increases until approximately age 50 years for men and age 70 years for women, and then declines.

The exclusive use of BMI to define obesity has undergone criticism because it does not measure body fat, per se, but total body weight. This method classifies some individuals as obese when they do not have excessive body fat. For example, a football player in peak condition can be extremely "overweight" according to standard height/weight charts. That is, he can weigh considerably

more than the average man of the same height, but much more of his weight is lean muscle mass, not excess fat (Figure 15-2).

Body Composition

Body composition measurements provide a better evaluation of overall health relative to weight. Health professionals can measure body fatness by a variety of methods.

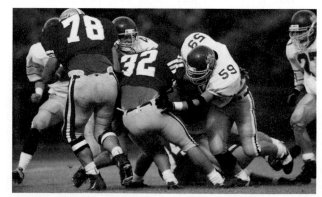

Figure 15–2 According to standard height/weight charts, some football players would be considered overweight. These charts should be used with discretion. (Copyright PhotoDisc.)

Body fat calipers measure the width of skin folds at precise body sites because most of the body fat is deposited in layers just under the skin. These measures are then used in specific formulas to calculate an estimated body fat composition (Figure 15-3). Calipers are an easy, portable, cheap, noninvasive way to measure body fat. However, reliability of the test depends on the skill of the technician and can vary greatly.

Hydrostatic weighing, a more precise method, often is used in athletic programs and research studies. Hydrostatic weighing requires complete submersion of an individual in water. The person must exhale as much air as possible and stay underwater for a few seconds to get an accurate reading. Although this method is more accurate it is not easy, portable, or cheap, and many patients are not willing or able to perform the test.

Bioelectrical impedance analysis is an easy, portable, inexpensive, and noninvasive body composition measurement tool. One type, a foot-to-foot analyzer, requires that the person stand on a modified scale with bare feet while an unnoticeable electrical current travels through the body (Figure 15-4). The analyzer determines body fat percentage on the basis of gender, age, height, weight, total body water, and the rate at which the electrical current travels. Fat impedes the current; therefore a lower total body fat composition results in a faster travel time of the electrical current. Such analyzers have both a standard adult and athletic setting. Although this method does not require any special skill on either the client or technician's part, discrepancies in some people have been noted between total body fat percentages when measured by bioelectrical impedance versus hydrostatic weighing.

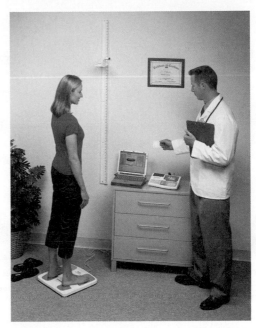

Figure 15–4 Tanita bioelectrical impedance body composition measurement tool. (Courtesy Tanita Corporation, Arlington Heights, Ill.)

Bioelectrical impedance machines that use a multiple-frequency bioelectrical impedance analysis with eight-point tactile electrodes have the least error and the highest correspondence to reference amounts of body fat.[3]

Dual energy x-ray absorptiometry, a much more accurate way of assessing body fat, uses radiation to distinguish bone, muscle, water, and fat density. Although this method is much less intimidating than hydrostatic weighing, it is quite expensive.

Air displacement plethysmography, using the BOD POD (Life Measurement, Inc., Concord, Calif.), may prove to be a reliable method for assessing body composition that does not rely on technical expertise or radiation (Figure 15-5). However, it also is expensive and not easily portable. The BOD POD calculates percent body fat using weight, body volume, thoracic lung volume, and body density. Current studies indicate that the BOD POD is a reliable measurement tool for most subgroups of the population, but discrepancies may arise when measuring athletes, the elderly, and children.[4-6] It does, however, offer a reliable means of assessing body fat percentage in overweight and obese populations, whereas other methods often are not reliable.[7]

A body fat content within the range of 11% to 17% of total body weight is associated with the lowest risk of chronic disease for men aged 18 years and older. For women it is somewhat higher: 19% to 22%. Acceptable

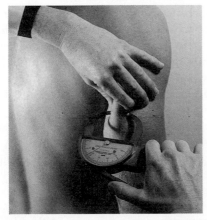

Figure 15–3 Assessment tools include skinfold calipers, which measure the relative amount of subcutaneous fat tissue at various body sites. (Reprinted from Mahan LK, Escott-Stump S: *Krause's food & nutrition therapy,* ed 12, Philadelphia, 2008, Saunders.)

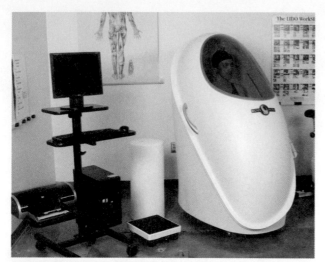

Figure 15–5 The BOD POD uses air displacement technology to measure body composition. (Courtesy Life Measurements, Inc., Concord, Calif.)

body fat percentages are lower for elite athletes, with a minimum of 4% for men and 12% for women in any sport. Health risks associated with too little or too much body fat rise as the percentage of body fat exceeds these ranges in either direction (Table 15-1).

Measures of Weight Maintenance Goals

Standard Height/Weight Tables

Height/weight tables are tools, or general population guides, and should be regarded only as such. Individual needs must be considered. One of the standard tables used in the United States is the Metropolitan Life Insurance Company's ideal weight-for-height charts. These charts are based on life expectancy information gathered since the 1930s from the company's population of life insurance policyholders. Many people have questioned how well these tables represent the total current population because the data are based on such a select group of

individuals (most of whom were Caucasian, middle- to upper-class men for the first few decades of gathering data) and may not consider the wide variety of individuals found within a diverse community.

More recent height/weight tables rely on BMI calculations and are based on the National Research Council data on weight and health, the current *Dietary Guidelines for Americans,* and recent medical studies.[8] These more realistic guides relate height and weight ranges to relative risks for chronic diseases (Table 15-2). Of note, studies show health risks are as great, if not greater, for very underweight persons as for the extremely obese. Within each age group both extremely thin (especially the elderly) and extremely overweight persons have higher mortality rates.[9,10]

Healthy Weight Range

Following are general calculations for determining healthy, or *ideal,* weight goals:

- *Men:* 106 lb for the first 5 feet, then add or subtract 6 lb for each inch above or below 5 feet, respectively. A range is then taken by adding and subtracting 10% to account for small and large body frames.
- *Women:* 100 lb for the first 5 feet, then add or subtract 5 lb for each inch above or below 5 feet, respectively. A range is then taken by adding and subtracting 10% to account for small and large body frames.

Example: A 5-foot, 3-inch woman would have an ideal body weight range of:

$$100 \text{ lb} + (3 \text{ in} \times 5 \text{ lb}) = 115 \pm 10\%$$

Therefore her ideal body weight *range* is 103.5 to 126.5 lb.

Similar to BMI, this calculation does not account for acceptable changes associated with age (loss of stature and slight increases in weight) or for individuals with very high lean body weight. A person's ideal weight may give him or her a ballpark figure for a healthy weight goal. However, two important considerations must be taken into account when relying on ideal body weight calculations.

Individual Variation. Ideal weight varies with time and circumstance throughout the lifespan. A person's ideal weight depends on many factors, including gender, age, body shape, metabolic rate, genetics, and physical activity. Specific individual situations govern needs.

Necessity of Body Fat. Some body fat is essential for survival. Every cell membrane in the body has fat molecules within it. Fat is used for insulation, temperature regulation, cushioning for vital organs, and many other functions. For mere survival, men require 3% to 5% body fat and women require 8% to 12%. Menstruation

TABLE 15-1

CLASSIFICATIONS FOR PERCENT BODY FAT

BODY TYPE	MEN	WOMEN
Athlete	<10%	<17%
Lean	10%-15%	17%-22%
Normal	15%-18%	22%-25%
Above average	18%-20%	25%-29%
Overweight	20%-25%	29%-35%
Obese	25%+	35%+

TABLE 15-2

BMI TABLE

	HEALTHY WEIGHT						OVERWEIGHT					OBESE					
BMI	19	20	21	22	23	24	25	26	27	28	29	30	31	32	33	34	35
HEIGHT							BODY WEIGHT (POUNDS)										
4'10"	91	96	100	105	110	115	119	124	129	134	138	143	148	153	158	162	167
4'11"	94	99	104	109	114	119	124	128	133	138	143	148	153	158	163	168	173
5'	97	102	107	112	118	123	128	133	138	143	148	153	158	163	168	174	179
5'1"	100	106	111	116	122	127	132	137	143	148	153	158	164	169	174	180	185
5'2"	104	109	115	120	126	131	136	142	147	153	158	164	169	175	180	186	191
5'3"	107	113	118	124	130	135	141	146	152	158	163	169	175	180	186	191	197
5'4"	110	116	122	128	134	140	145	151	157	163	169	174	180	186	192	197	204
5'5"	114	120	126	132	138	144	150	156	162	168	174	180	186	192	198	204	210
5'6"	118	124	130	136	142	148	155	161	167	173	179	186	192	198	204	210	216
5'7"	121	127	134	140	146	153	159	166	172	178	185	191	198	204	211	217	223
5'8"	125	131	138	144	151	158	164	171	177	184	190	197	203	210	216	223	230
5'9"	128	135	142	149	155	162	169	176	182	189	196	203	209	216	223	230	236
5'10"	132	139	146	153	160	167	174	181	188	195	202	209	216	222	229	236	243
5'11"	135	143	150	157	165	172	179	186	193	200	208	215	222	229	236	243	250
6'	140	147	154	162	169	177	184	191	199	206	213	221	228	235	242	250	258
6'1"	144	151	159	166	174	182	189	197	204	212	219	227	235	242	250	257	265
6'2"	148	155	163	171	179	186	194	202	210	218	225	233	241	249	256	264	272
6'3"	152	160	168	176	184	192	200	208	216	224	232	240	248	256	264	272	279

Locate the height of interest in the leftmost column and read across the row for that height to the weight of interest. Follow the column of the weight up to the top row that lists the BMI. BMI of 18.5 to 24.9 is the healthy weight range; BMI of 25 to 29.9 is the overweight range; and BMI of 30 and above is the obese range.
Modified from National Institutes of Health, National Heart, Lung, and Blood Institute: *Evidence report of clinical guidelines on the identification, evaluation, and treatment of overweight and obesity in adults*, Bethesda, MD, 1998, National Institutes of Health.

begins when girls reach approximately 20% body fat. This is the amount needed to ovulate and support a healthy pregnancy. Some women dropping below the critical body fat percentage experience amenorrhea because of a decrease in hormone levels.[11]

Obesity and Health

Weight Extremes

Clinically severe or significant obesity is a health hazard in itself and creates other medical problems by placing strain on all body systems. Both extremes of weight, fatness and thinness, pose health problems.

Overweight and Health Problems

The most recent National Health and Examination Survey (2006) data indicated a marked increase in the prevalence of overweight persons in the United States.[1] Experts have estimated that more than 60 million American adults are *obese*, which increases their risk of related conditions such as hypertension; type 2 diabetes; heart disease[12]; sleep apnea; gallbladder disease; stroke; osteoarthritis; and breast, endometrial, and colon cancers.[13]

Weight loss can reduce elevated blood glucose levels and blood pressure in obese persons.[14,15] In turn, these improvements reduce risks related to heart disease.

Causes of Obesity

Basic Energy Balance

How does a person become overweight? Although some persons have congenital obesity, a major cause of obesity in Americans is a *lack of physical activity*. In fact, one study found that a simple, well-defined walking program can help reduce total body weight, percent body fat, and BMI in overweight persons even without any noticeable changes in dietary intake.[16] Regular exercise alone has a significant effect on increasing lean body mass and reducing risk of chronic diseases associated with obesity.

amenorrhea absence of a menstrual period in a women of reproductive age.

clinically severe or significant obesity BMI of 40 or greater or a BMI of 35 to 39 with at least one obesity-related disorder.

The overall energy imbalance (i.e., more energy intake from food than energy output through physical activity and basal metabolic needs) is the primary cause for excess weight. Excess intake is stored in the body as fat. Approximately 3500 kcal is the equivalent of 1 lb (0.45 kg) of body fat (Box 15-1). A minor daily imbalance in which energy intake exceeds output by a mere 100 kcal can result in a significant weight gain in 1 year, as follows:

$$100 \text{ kcal/day} \times 365 \text{ days/year} = 36,500 \text{ extra kcal/year}$$
$$36,500 \text{ kcal/}3500 \text{ kcal/lb} = 10.4 \text{ lb/year (4.7 kg)}$$

However, some overweight persons only eat moderate amounts of food and some persons of average weight eat much more but never seem to gain unwanted pounds. Because many individual differences exist, more factors than energy balance are involved in maintaining a healthy weight.

Hormonal Control

Leptin. A research group at Rockefeller University first reported the "obesity gene" in an overweight strain of laboratory mice. Soon thereafter these researchers located the human equivalent of the same gene.[17] This gene encodes for a hormone released primarily from adipose tissue and is believed to play a role in determining a person's set point for fat storage. The researchers named the hormone *leptin,* from the Greek word *leptos,* meaning thin or slender. Leptin production was first understood to control satiety in people by serving as a negative feedback mechanism against overconsumption of total energy. Plasma leptin levels rise after weight gain and drop after weight loss.[18] At one point, scientists thought that obese individuals were resistant to leptin's negative feedback because the hormone did not cross the blood-brain barrier. However, recent studies indicate that leptin also is produced in the brain and is influenced by the amount of adiposity and gender, with women producing more.[19] With the discovery of leptin production in the brain, the

theory of leptin resistance has been refuted as a primary cause of obesity. Some individuals have been identified as having severe early-onset obesity and lack the leptin receptor, thus receiving no negative feedback regarding energy intake.[20] Even so, such incidence was found in only 3% of individuals with early-onset obesity. The exact role leptin plays in the neurobiology of human obesity remains unclear but is being extensively researched.

Ghrelin. The counterpart to leptin is the enteric peptide ghrelin. Ghrelin is an appetite stimulant secreted from the stomach to activate the appetite-regulating network. When administered peripherally, ghrelin increases appetite and promotes adiposity.[21] Such a discovery has lead to investigations using a ghrelin antagonist to fight obesity.[22] Many questions remain unanswered regarding the dysregulation of leptin and ghrelin and how some individuals do not respond to fluctuations in plasma levels.

Genetic and Family Factors   *Set Point Theory*

Genetic inheritance probably influences a person's chances of becoming fat more than any other factor. Family food patterns provide an environment that allows this genetic trait to present itself.

Genetic Control. Up to 70% of the predisposition to obesity is from heritability factors, thus making certain people highly susceptible to becoming obese in an environment that allows for such a genetic expression (see the Cultural Considerations box, "Genetics and the Predisposition for Obesity").[23] In these types of obesity, genetic metabolic controls regulate the amount of body fat an individual has the potential to carry.[24] A person then eats to regain or lose whatever amount of fat the body is naturally set or programmed for, according to the weight below or above this internally regulated point *(set point).* Thus persons who have unnaturally lost body fat below their programmed level will eat to regain to their genetic set point when food is again available. Similarly, persons with lower programmed fat levels who have gained excess body fat will lose this weight when they resume their regular food intake. This is not to say that a person has no control over his or her own body weight. A genetic influence is the *predisposing* factor, not the *determining* factor. The daily life, environment, and habits a person chooses influence the expression of this genetic trait (Figure 15-6). In one thorough review of environmental and genetic influences on obesity, Speakman[25] states that "although we might say that obesity has a large genetic component to it, this doesn't mean that the obese have somehow miraculously deposited enormous quantities of body fat without eating too much food, or expending too little energy, or doing both." In other words, the genetic predis-

BOX 15-1

KILOCALORIE ADJUSTMENT NECESSARY FOR WEIGHT LOSS

To lose 454 g (1 lb) a week = 500 fewer kcal daily
  Basis of estimation:
1 lb body fat = 454 g
1 g pure fat = 9 kcal
1 g body fat = 7.7 kcal (some water in fat cells)
454 g × 9 kcal/g = 4086 kcal/454 g fat (pure fat)
454 g × 7.7 kcal/g = 3496 kcal/454 g body fat (or 3500 kcal)
500 kcal × 7 days = 3500 kcal = 454 g body fat

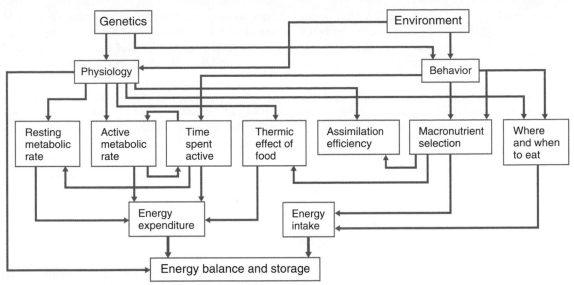

Figure 15–6 The major causal links among genetics, environmental effects, physiology, behavior, and energy balance. (Reprinted from Speakman JR: Obesity: the integrated roles of environment and genetics, *J Nutr* 134[8 suppl]:2090S, 2004.)

CULTURAL CONSIDERATIONS

GENETICS AND THE PREDISPOSITION FOR OBESITY

When comparing the prevalence of obesity in various racial and ethnic groups in the United States, researchers have found a strong genetic influence, specifically in women.* Few differences are seen between racial and ethnic groups among men. According to the NCHS, the prevalence of adult obesity for racial/ethnic groups is as follows:

- Women:
  - Non-Hispanic Caucasian: 31.2%
  - Non-Hispanic African American: 51.1%
  - Mexican American: 38.5%
- Men:
  - Non-Hispanic Caucasian: 30.5%
  - Non-Hispanic African American: 30.7%
  - Mexican American: 27.8%

Thus non-Hispanic African-American women have a disproportionately high level of obesity when compared with other racial and ethnic groups. The exact cause of this dif-ference is not clearly defined; it most likely is a combination of genetics and environmental factors.

An even more dramatic trend noted throughout the NCHS data over the past few decades is the significant increase in obesity in both genders. Summarized below are the findings from these surveys, which include all racial and ethnic groups. The percentages are the prevalence of obesity in both genders (ages 20 to 74 years) as a percent of the population, as follows*:

- 1960 to 1962: 13.3%
- 1971 to 1974: 14.6%
- 1976 to 1980: 15.1%
- 1988 to 1994: 23.3%
- 2001 to 2004: 32.1%

Although genetics does play a role in the prevalence and predisposition to obesity, such influences cannot explain such an increase in obesity for the entire population.

*National Center for Health Statistics: *Health, United States, 2006, with chartbook on trends in the health of Americans,* Hyattsville, MD, 2006, U.S. Government Printing Office.

position may exist but cannot express itself without an environment that supports it.

Family Reinforcement. An individual's genetic predisposition for increased body fat is reinforced by inappropriate family food patterns. Studies show that that the greatest risk for overweight is a history of being overweight.[2,26] In addition to genetic influence, families also exert social pressure and teach children habits and attitudes toward food. Thus developing healthy eating habits during childhood and teenage years, with fat- and calorie-controlled cooking and family meal times, is highly encouraged to establish balanced food patterns.[27]

Physiologic Factors. The amount of body fat a person carries is related to the number and size of fat cells in the body. Critical periods for becoming obese occur

Fat Cell Theory

early-onset obesity a genetically associated obesity occurring in early childhood.

appetite-regulating network a hormonally controlled system of appetite stimulus and suppression.

during early growth periods, when cells are multiplying rapidly in childhood and adolescence. Once the body has added extra fat cells for more fuel storage, these cells remain and can store varying amounts of fat. Middle-aged and older adults tend to store more fat because of a decrease in BMR, physical activity, and lean muscle mass. Women also store more fat during pregnancy and after menopause in response to hormonal changes.

Psychological Factors. Work, family, and social environments may cultivate emotional stress, which many persons respond to by eating for comfort. Social pressures, especially on women, to maintain the cultural "ideal" thin body type contribute to the strain of constant dieting, which in turn can perpetuate the chronic dieters' dilemma of yo-yo dieting (weight loss followed by weight gain) and cause reductions in metabolic rate and lean body mass.

Other Environmental Factors. Many environmental factors add to the ever-increasing problem of obesity in the United States. The following are only a few: increase in food availability, fast and convenient foods, increase in portion sizes, decrease in food preparation time and skills, decrease in physical activity, increase in screen time (e.g., television, computer, video games), and decreased physical requirements of household chores (e.g., domestic appliances such as washing machines, vacuum cleaners, dishwashers, and central heating).

Individual Differences and Extreme Practices

Individual Energy Balance Levels

Several factors influence a person's individual point of energy balance. Some persons have more genetic-based metabolic efficiency (i.e., the ability to "burn" food more readily than others do). Also, when calculating a person's energy intake, the figures indicate only an *estimated* value. Reported food values represent averages of many samples of that food tested. Many factors (e.g., BMR, body size, lean body mass, age, gender, and physical activity) influence total daily expenditure as well. However, these calculations provide useful general information and indicate areas of individual needs and goals.

Extreme Practices

Desperate attempts to lose weight may drive people to extreme measures, which sometimes worsen health risks.

Fad Diets. A constant array of diet books and weight loss supplements promising to "melt the fat away" continue to flood the American market. These books and supplements usually sell briefly and then fade away, largely because their quick fixes do not work (Table 15-3).

Such a complex problem has no simple answers. Most of the fad diets fail on the following two counts:

1. *Scientific inaccuracies and misinformation.* Fad diets and supplements often are nutritionally inadequate.
2. *Failure to address the necessity of changing long-term habits and behaviors.* People often are set up for failure regarding maintenance of a healthy weight once it is achieved. The basic behavioral problem involved in changing food and exercise habits for life, thereby developing a new lifestyle, is unrecognized.

In some diets the degree of energy restriction is impossible to maintain. Many fad dieters find themselves caught in a vicious cycle of chronic dieting syndrome and its harmful physical and psychological effects.

Fasting. This drastic approach takes many forms, from literal fasting to the use of very low calorie diets (800 kilocalories or less per day). Possible effects of a semistarvation diet include acidosis, low blood pressure, electrolyte loss, tissue protein loss, and decreased BMR. Such programs cannot be maintained long term without deleterious effects on health.

Specific Macronutrient Restrictions. Avoiding any food group or macronutrient (carbohydrates, fats, or proteins) as the means for weight loss is unfounded. Such diets as that advocated by Dean Ornish (very low fat) or Robert Atkins (extremely low carbohydrate) are too restrictive to maintain for extended periods and carry health risks.

Clothing and Body Wraps. Special "sauna suits" or body wrapping has claimed to help weight loss in certain body areas or clear up *cellulite* tissue. Some persons endure mummylike body wrapping in an attempt to reduce body size. The resulting small weight loss, however, is caused only by temporary water loss. The only way to lose weight is to burn more energy than is consumed.

Drugs. Various amphetamine compounds, commonly called "speed," were once popular in the medical treatment of obesity but are no longer used because of their danger to health. Common over-the-counter drugs have included phenylpropylamine (Dexatrim), a stimulant similar to amphetamine. Dexatrim has been linked to increased blood pressure and damage to blood vessels in the brain, which can lead to CNS disorders such as confusion, stroke, hallucination, and psychotic behavior. No diuretics or hormones (e.g., thyroid hormone or steroids) should ever be used to alter body weight or leanness without strict medical indication and supervision.

A pair of related weight loss drugs, fenfluramine and phentermine, were produced and prescribed to be used together in the popular fen-phen combination for weight reduction. Shortly thereafter physicians found that one in eight patients using fen-phen developed valvular regurgitation, a sometimes fatal condition.[28] The FDA, with the support of the medical community, quickly removed these drugs from the market. Although the pursuit of pharmacotherapy for the treatment of obesity is intense, few options currently are available. Drugs used to treat obesity generally work in one of the following four ways:

1. Reducing energy intake by suppressing the appetite
2. Increasing energy expenditure by stimulating the BMR
3. Reducing absorption of food in the gut
4. Altering lipogenesis and lipolysis

The FDA has approved two medications, sibutramine (Meridia) and orlistat (Xenical), for treatment of clinically significant obesity.[29,30] Sibutramine works by increasing the heart rate and thus increasing energy expenditure; orlistat inhibits dietary fat absorption. Both medications have been successful with weight loss, but reports indicate that maximal benefits occur only when combined with lifestyle changes that induce negative energy balance.[29,30] As with many medications, unpleasant side effects are associated with these medications.

Surgery. Surgical techniques usually are reserved for the medical treatment of clinically severe obesity in patients who have not had success with other methods of long-term weight loss. Although surgery historically has been the most successful method of permanent weight loss in severe obesity, it is not without risk and complications. A recent study monitored patients for 16 years after weight loss surgery and found significant and sustained weight loss and a reduced relative risk of death by 89% through a decrease in several conditions and diseases associated with obesity.[31]

Two types of surgical procedures are performed for weight loss: gastric restriction and malabsorptive procedures (e.g., gastric bypass). Gastric restriction involves the creation of a small stomach pouch designed to reduce the space for food in the stomach, thus limiting appetite and eating (Figure 15-7, A and B).[32] Adjustable gastric bands can be placed by laparoscopic surgery. The band is subcutaneously adjusted as needed by a small port. Malabsorptive procedures rearrange the small intestine to decrease the length and efficiency of the gut for nutrient absorption (Figure 15-7, C, D, and E). Weight loss surgeries require a skilled team of specialists, nutrition care, careful patient selection, and continuous follow-up in partnership with the patient and family. Inherent risk of surgery and postsurgical malnutrition are critical issues that should be thoroughly addressed with the patient.

A more limited type of cosmetic surgery developed in the 1980s is a form of local fat removal, lipectomy, commonly called liposuction. Lipectomy removes fat deposits under the skin in places of cosmetic concern, such as the hips and thighs. A thin tube is inserted through a small incision in the skin, and the desired amount of fat is suctioned away. This procedure can be quite painful, however, and carries risks such as infection, large disfiguring skin depressions, or blood clots that can lead to dangerous circulatory problems or even kidney failure. Any surgical procedure carries risk and may cause other problems and side effects.

SOUND WEIGHT MANAGEMENT PROGRAM

Essential Characteristics

No shortcuts to successful weight control exist. Weight loss requires hard work and strong individual motivation. Weight management must be a personalized program that focuses on changing food and exercise behaviors and stress and relaxation habits. This program must build a healthy mental and physical lifestyle with ample positive social support.

Behavior Modification

Basic Principles

Food behavior is rooted in many human experiences and associations. Addictive forms of eating responses and conditioning are common within many subgroups of the population. Behavior-oriented therapies are designed to help change patterns that contribute to excessive weight, such as excess caloric intake and physical inactivity. By understanding behaviors and changing associations with undesirable habits, individuals can plan constructive ac-

---

chronic dieting syndrome the cyclic pattern of weight loss by dieting to achieve an unnatural but culturally ideal body thinness, then regaining weight by compulsive food binges in response to stress, anxiety, and hunger. This abnormal psychophysiologic food pattern becomes chronic, changing a person's natural body metabolism and relative body composition to the abnormal state of a metabolically obese person of normal weight.

negative energy balance more total energy is expended than consumed.

lipectomy surgical removal of subcutaneous fat by suction through a tube inserted into a surface incision or by the removal of larger amounts of subcutaneous fat by major surgical incision.

TABLE 15-3

DIET SUMMARIES

DIET	PHILOSOPHY	FOODS TO EAT	FOODS TO AVOID	DIET COMPOSITION (AVERAGE FOR 3 DAYS)	RECOMMENDED SUPPLEMENTS	HEALTH CLAIMS SCIENTIFICALLY PROVEN?	PRACTICALITY	LOSE AND MAINTAIN WEIGHT?
Atkins*	Eating too many carbohydrates causes obesity and other health problems; ketosis leads to decreased hunger	Meat, fish, poultry, eggs, cheese, low-carbohydrate vegetables, butter, oil; no alcohol	Carbohydrates, specifically bread, pasta, most fruits and vegetables, milk	Protein: 27% Carbohydrates: 5% Fat: 68% (saturated: 26%)	Atkins supplement that includes chromium picolinate, carnitine, coenzyme Q10	No long-term validated studies published	Limited food choices; difficult to eat in restaurants because only plain protein sources and limited vegetables/salads allowed	Yes, but initial weight loss is mostly water; does not promote a positive attitude toward food groups; difficult to maintain long term because diet restricts food choices
Eat Right 4 Your Type†	Blood type determines the way your body absorbs nutrients and dictates the diet and exercise plan that will suit you best	Type O: meat, seafood, fruits, vegetables Type A: fruits, vegetables, beans, most seafood Type B: meat, beans, fruits, vegetables, seafood Type AB: seafood, dairy, fruits, vegetables	Type O: wheat, beans Type A: meat, dairy, wheat Type B: chicken, wheat Type AB: meat	Not applicable (diet varies according to blood type, ancestry, etc.)	Depends on your blood type and overall health, including questions on immunity, skin, digestive, bone, joint, circulation, mental, and hormonal health, as well as current medications	No; theories and long-term results not validated	Not applicable (diet varies according to blood type, ancestry, etc.)	Possibly if caloric intake is less than energy output
Protein Power‡	Eating carbohydrates releases insulin in large quantities, which contributes to obesity and other health problems	Meat, fish, poultry, eggs, cheese, low-carbohydrate vegetables, butter, oil, salad dressings, alcohol in moderation	Carbohydrates	Protein: 26% Carbohydrates: 16% Fat: 54% (saturated: 18%) Alcohol: 4%	Multivitamin and mineral supplement	No long-term validated studies published	Not practical for long term; rigid rules	Yes, by caloric restriction; limited food choices not practical for long term

Diet	Theory	Foods Allowed	Foods Avoided	Composition	Supplements	Scientific Evidence	Comments	Weight Loss
The South Beach Diet§	Switching to the "right" carbohydrates stops insulin resistance, reduces cravings, and causes weight loss	Seafood, chicken breast, lean meat, low-fat cheese, nuts oils, most vegetables; (later) whole grains, most grains, low-fat milk or yogurt, beans	Fatty meats, full-fat cheese, refined grains, sweets, juice, potatoes	*Phase 1:* Protein: 34% Carbohydrates:14.8% Fat: 50%	Multivitamins and omega-3 fatty acids; Metamucil recommended during phase 1	Evidence does exist linking the avoidance of saturated fats and reduced risk of heart disease	First phase is more difficult, similar to Atkins diet; later phases are mostly healthy foods and practical	Yes, although initial weight loss is mostly water; sustained weight loss through reduced calorie intake
Sugar Busters‖	Sugar is toxic to body and causes release of insulin, which promotes fat storage	Protein and fat; low glycemic index foods; olive oil, canola oil, and alcohol in moderation	Potatoes, white rice, corn, carrots, beets, white bread, all refined white flour products	Protein: 27% Carbohydrates: 52% Fat: 21% (saturated: 4%)	None	No long-term validated studies published	Eliminates many carbohydrate foods; discourages eating fruit with meals	Yes, by caloric restriction; limited food choices not practical for long term
Stillman¶	High-protein foods burn body fat; if carbohydrates are consumed, body stores fat instead of burning it	Lean meats, skinless poultry, lean fish and seafood, eggs, cottage cheese, skim milk cheeses; no alcohol	All carbohydrates: bread, pasta, fruit, vegetables, fats, oils, dairy products	Protein: 64% Carbohydrates: 3% Fat: 33% (saturated: 13%)	Multivitamin and mineral supplement	No long-term validated studies published	Extreme limitations in food choices; very little variety	Yes, but loss is mostly water; maintenance based on strict calorie counting; very limited food choices not practical for long term
Zone#	Eating right combination of foods leads to metabolic state at which body functions at peak performance, leading to decreased hunger, increased weight loss, and increased energy	Protein, fat, carbohydrates in exact portions only (40/30/30), low glycemic index foods, alcohol in moderation	Carbohydrates, specifically bread, pasta, fruit (some types), saturated fats	Protein: 34% Carbohydrates: 36% Fat: 29% (saturated: 9%) Alcohol: 1%	200 IU vitamin E	No; theories and long-term results not validated	Food must be eaten in required proportions of protein, fat, carbohydrates; menus plain and unappealing; vegetable portions very large; difficult to calculate portions	Yes, by caloric restriction; could result in weight maintenance if carefully followed; diet rigid and difficult to maintain

Modified from Jeor ST and others: Dietary protein and weight reduction: a statement for healthcare professionals from the Nutrition Committee of the Council on Nutrition, Physical Activity, and Metabolism of the American Heart Association, *Circulation* 104(15):1869, 2001.

* Atkins C: *Dr. Atkins' new diet revolution*, New York, 1999, Avon Books.
† D'Adamo PJ, Whitney C: *Eat right 4 your type*, New York, 2002, Riverhead Books.
‡ Eades MR, Eades MD: *Protein power*, New York, 1996, Bantam Books.
§ Agatston A: *The South Beach diet*, Emmaus, NJ, 2003, Rodale Inc.
‖ Steward HL ard others: *Sugar busters*, New York, 1998, Ballantine Books.
¶ Stillman IM, Baker SS: *The doctor's quick weight loss diet*, New York, 1967, Dell.
# Sears B: *The zone*, New York, 1995, HarperCollins.

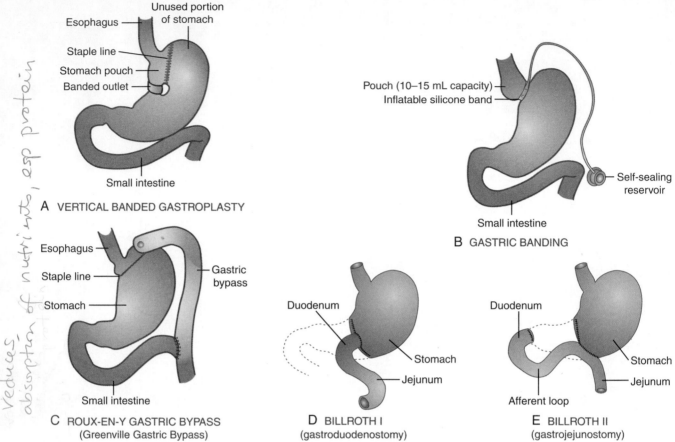

reduces absorption of nutrients, esp protein

Figure 15–7 Surgical procedures for the treatment of clinically severe obesity. (Reprinted from Mahan LK, Escott-Stump S: *Krause's food & nutrition therapy*, ed 12, Philadelphia, 2008, Saunders.)

tions to meet personal health goals. This behavioral approach must begin with a detailed examination of the following three basic aspects of each undesirable eating behavior:

1. *Cues or antecedents.* What stimulates the behavior?
2. *Response.* What happens during the eating or sedentary behavior after the cue?
3. *Consequences.* What happens after the response to the eating or sedentary behavior that reinforces it?

Basic Strategies and Actions

A program of personal behavior modification for weight management is directed toward the following: (1) control of eating behavior (e.g., a food diary: the when, why, where, how, and how much); (2) promotion of physical activity to increase energy output; and (3) emotional, social, and psychological health. Three progressive actions follow in planning individual strategies.

Defining Problem Behavior. *Specifically* define the problem behavior and the desired behavior outcome.

This process clearly establishes goals and contributing objectives.

Recording and Analyzing Baseline Behavior. Record eating and exercise behavior and carefully analyze it in terms of physical setting and persons involved. What types of patterns emerge? How often do these patterns occur? What conditions seem to trigger the behavior? What consequent events seem to maintain the habits (e.g., time and pace, place, persons, social responses, hunger before and after, emotional mood, other factors)?

Planning a Behavior Management Strategy. Set up controls of the external environment involving the situational forces related to each of the three behavior areas involved: (1) what goes before the behavior, (2) the response to the behavior, and (3) the results of the behavior. Then break these identified links to old, undesirable behaviors and recondition them to the desired new eating and exercise behaviors. The Clinical Applications box, "Breaking Old Links: Strategies for Changing Food Behavior," provides a few examples of recondition-

CLINICAL APPLICATIONS

BREAKING OLD LINKS: STRATEGIES FOR CHANGING FOOD BEHAVIOR

Old habits die hard. They are never easy to change, but the effort is worthwhile in the case of undesirable eating behaviors that contribute to excess body fat and are harmful to health. Following are some behavioral suggestions.

1. Deal with Behavioral Cues

Minimize as many cues for the problem behavior as possible. Minimize situations and contacts associated with problem foods, put temptation out of reach, and make the problem behavior as difficult as possible to do. Freeze leftovers, remove problem food items from the kitchen or store them in hard-to-get places, and take a route home other than by the familiar bakery or candy shop.

Suppress the cues that cannot be entirely eliminated. Control social situations that maintain the behavior, reward the alternate desired behavior, have a trusted person monitor eating patterns, reduce stress, minimize contact with excessive food, use smaller plates to make smaller food portions appear larger, and make use of positive nonfood "treat" activities such as physical activity.

Strengthen cues for desirable behaviors. Follow the MyPyramid guidelines and the *U.S. Dietary Guidelines for Americans* for appropriate food choices and amounts. Use food behavior aids (e.g., records, a diary, or a journal). Distribute appropriate foods among meal and snack patterns. Make desirable food behavior as attractive and as enjoyable as possible.

2. Deal with Actual Food Behavior in Response to Cues

Slow the pace of eating. Take one bite at a time and place the utensil on the plate between bites. Chew each bite slowly.

Sip a beverage. Consciously plan conversation with meal companions for between bites. Visualize eating in slow motion. Enhance the social aspect of eating.

Savor the food. Eat slowly, sensing the taste, smell, and texture of the food. Develop and practice these sensory feelings to the extent that they can be described and brought to mind afterward. Look for food seasonings and combinations that will enhance this process and bring to mind positive feelings about the food experience.

3. Deal with the Follow-up Behavior that Results

Decelerate the problem behavior. Slow down its frequency and respond neutrally when it occurs rather than with negative talk or thoughts. Give social reinforcement to the decreasing number of times the problem behavior occurs. Acknowledge the ultimate consequences of the undesirable behavior in health problems.

Accelerate the desired behavior. Update the progress records or personal journal daily. Respond positively to all desired behavior; provide material reinforcement for positive behavior. Provide social reinforcement by enlisting the help of close friends or family for constructive efforts to modify behavior.

Such a program requires effort, motivation, and work. Continuously evaluate progress toward desired behavior while maintaining a realistic goal. Then plan individual or group maintenance and support activities during an extended follow-up period.

---

ing personal food and exercise habits to more positive behaviors.

Dietary Principles

The central dietary approach in a weight management program that could achieve a degree of *lasting* success must be based on the following five characteristics:

1. *Realistic goals:* Goals must be realistic in terms of overall weight loss and rate of loss, averaging ½ to 1 lb/week (no more than 1 to 2 lb/week for clinically severe obese patients).
2. *Energy (kilocalories) reduced according to need:* The diet must have sufficient energy intake in relation to individual energy output to produce gradual weight loss.
3. *Nutritional adequacy:* The diet must be nutritionally adequate. Consuming less food requires conscious choices of nutrient-dense foods and may require vitamin and mineral supplements. In addition, the ratio of macronutrients (carbohydrate, fat, and protein)

should have an appropriate balance based on a wide variety of food sources.
4. *Cultural appeal:* The food plan must be similar enough to an individual's cultural eating patterns to form the basis for a *permanent* alteration of eating habits. It must be a quality, personal lifetime plan.
5. *Energy (kilocalorie) readjustment to maintain weight:* When the desired weight level is reached, the energy level is adjusted according to maintenance needs.

Basic Energy Balance Components

The two sides of energy balance are energy *intake*, in the form of food, and energy *output*, in the form of metabolic work and physical activity. For successful weight reduction, both basic components must be addressed.

Energy Input: Food Behaviors

The energy value of food intake may need to be reduced. Arbitrary serving sizes and number of servings should not be assigned without knowledge of the patient's actual eating patterns. Food diaries are helpful in establishing what the patient's normal food choices are, the amounts typically eaten, and distribution of meals throughout the day. From this baseline information, clinicians can help identify minor changes to start with, such as eating smaller portions, replacing soda with water, and encouraging patients to eat *slowly* to savor the taste and texture. Whole primary foods should be emphasized and processed foods minimized. Ideally, meals should be evenly distributed throughout the day. The use of fat, sugar, salt, and fiber should be quantified and modified if necessary to meet the *Dietary Guidelines for Americans, 2005*. Table 15-4 provides suggested servings of the food groups and subgroups to meet recommended nutrient intakes. These guides can serve as a focal point for sound nutrition education. Some additional practical suggestions are provided in the Clinical Applications box, "Practical Suggestions for Changing Food Behaviors."

Energy Output: Exercise Behaviors

Energy output in physical activity must be increased relative to normal activity. For someone who has no planned physical activity, a regular daily exercise schedule, starting with simple walking for approximately a half hour each day and building to a brisk pace, is a great start. Some form of aerobic exercise (e.g., swimming or running) or resistance exercises should be added (see the For Further Focus box, "Benefits of Aerobic Exercise in Weight Management"). An exercise class may be helpful to maintain motivation (Figure 15-8). Encourage patients to experiment with various activities until they find one they enjoy and can maintain long term. Following are current recommendations by the *Dietary Guidelines for Americans, 2005* regarding exercise and weight maintenance or weight loss[8]:

- *To help manage body weight and prevent gradual, unhealthy body weight gain in adulthood:* Engage in approximately 60 minutes of moderate-intensity to vigorous activity on most days of the week while not exceeding caloric intake requirements.
- *To sustain weight loss in adulthood:* Participate in at least 60 to 90 minutes of daily moderate-intensity physical activity while not exceeding caloric intake requirements. Some people may need to consult a health care provider before participating in this level of activity.

CLINICAL APPLICATIONS

PRACTICAL SUGGESTIONS FOR CHANGING FOOD BEHAVIORS

Goals
Be realistic. Do not set your goals too high. Adapt your rate of loss to ½ lb to 1 lb per week. If visible tools are helpful motivation techniques, use them.

Kilocalories
Do not be an obsessive calorie counter. Simply become familiar with food exchanges in your diet list and learn the general values of some of your home dishes, then modify recipes or make occasional substitutes.

Plateaus
Anticipate plateaus; they happen to everyone. As the body adjusts to a new energy balance, lean:fat body mass ratio, and metabolic rate, weight loss rates can slow down. Increase exercise during these periods to help get started again.

Binges
Do not be discouraged if you have a binge. Individuals who have previously struggled with binge eating behavior may have an occasional setback. Try to keep them infrequent and, when possible, plan ahead for special occasions. Adjust the following day's diet or the remainder of the same day accordingly. Changing binge eating behavior is not easy. The assistance of a psychological and nutritional expert may be helpful.

Special Diet Foods
Purchasing special low-calorie foods is not necessary. Learn to read labels carefully. Most special diet foods are expensive foods that are not much lower in kilocalories than regular foods. All foods can fit with moderation. The amount of kilocalories and fat should be chosen within the context of the overall diet.

Home Meals
Try to avoid making a separate menu for yourself. Adapt your needs to the family meal, adjusting the seasonings or method of preparation to lower kilocalories, especially by reducing or omitting fat.

Eating Away from Home
Watch portions. When you are a guest, limit extras such as sauces and dressings and trim meat well. In restaurants, select singly prepared items rather than combination dishes. Avoid items with heavy sauces or fat seasonings and fried foods. Select fruit or sherbet for dessert rather than pastries.

Appetite Control
Avoid dependence on appetite-depressant medications, which typically are only crutches. Try nibbling on food items from the free food list or save other meal items, such as fruit or bread exchanges, for use between meals.

Meal Pattern
Eat three or more meals a day. If snacks between meals help you, then plan part of your day's allowance to account for them. The point is to spread your daily energy allowance throughout the day. Avoid the common pattern of no breakfast, little or no lunch, and a huge dinner.

FOR FURTHER FOCUS

BENEFITS OF AEROBIC EXERCISE IN WEIGHT MANAGEMENT

The goal of weight management is to reduce excess body fat and, in most cases, build lean body mass. However, both tissues are lost when a person tries to reach a weight goal merely by reducing food intake.

Optimal body composition can be achieved by combining food restriction with aerobic exercise. Aerobic exercise consists of activities sustained long enough to draw on the body's fat reserve for fuel while oxygen intake is increased (thus the term *aerobic*). Lean body tissue burns fats in the presence of oxygen. Therefore aerobic activity is best suited for achieving the ideal balance of high lean body mass and low fatty tissue in the body.

The benefits of aerobic exercise to an overweight person in a weight management program include the following:

- Suppressed appetite
- Reduced total body fat
- Higher BMR
- Increased circulatory and respiratory function
- Increased energy expenditure
- Retention of tissue protein and building of lean body mass levels

Some individuals complain about the slow rate of weight loss, difficulty in controlling appetite, and consistent "flabbiness" despite continuing diet management. These individuals may welcome the suggestion of aerobic activity to help manage weight loss. Suggestions include a brisk daily walk, jumping rope, swimming, bicycling, jogging, running, aerobic or spinning classes, or another activity that increases the heart rate enough to have an aerobic effect and can be maintained for 20 to 30 minutes. Carefully note the physical stress this activity may place on individuals who have not exercised for some time or who have medical problems related to exertion. These individuals should have a medical checkup before beginning such a program on their own or joining a local gym or other community fitness center.

Principles of a Sound Food Plan

A careful diet history (see Chapter 17) can be the basis for a sound personalized food plan and should involve each of the following principles of nutritional balance.

Energy Balance

As previously mentioned, no shortcuts to weight loss exist. Under normal circumstances, when energy expenditure is greater than energy intake, weight loss occurs. Because 1 lb of fat is equal to approximately 3500 kcal, an energy deficit of 500 kcal/day results in a weight loss of approximately 1 lb/week; a deficit of 250 kcal equals a half-pound weight loss per week (see Box 15-1). All persons pursuing weight loss should determine their current total energy needs as a basis for diet planning (Table 15-5). Adjustments to the diet (energy intake) and physical activity (energy output) can then be balanced to produce a negative energy balance. As discussed throughout this text, individual energy needs and intake vary greatly. Therefore assuming all persons on a weight loss program should limit caloric intake to 1400 kcal/day (or any other prefabricated amount) is not appropriate. For a person who normally consumes 2000 kcal/day, the ideal scenario is a deficit of approximately 500 kcal/day. The total of those 500 kcal should not all come from diet. Reducing calorie intake by 25% (2000 × 25% = 500 kcal) would undoubtedly leave a person hungry and constantly thinking about food. Instead, the weight loss program could include a 250-kcal reduction in energy intake and a 250-kcal increase in energy expenditure for a total deficit of 500 kcal (see the Clinical Applications box, "Case Study: John's Energy Balance and Weight Management Plan.")

Nutrient Balance

Basic energy nutrients are outlined in the diet to achieve the following nutrient balance:

- *Carbohydrate:* Approximately 45% to 65% of the total kilocalories, with emphasis on complex forms such as starch with fiber, and a limit on simple sugars
- *Protein:* Approximately 10% to 35% of the total kilocalories, with emphasis on lean food and small portions
- *Fat:* 25% or less of the total kilocalories, with emphasis on little animal fat, scant total use, and alternate non-fat seasonings

The food plan should meet the recommendations of the *Dietary Guidelines for Americans, 2005* (see Figure 1-2).

Figure 15–8 An exercise class provides regular support for an effective weight management plan. (Copyright Photo-Disc.)

TABLE 15-4

RECOMMENDED DAILY AND/OR WEEKLY AMOUNT OF FOOD FROM EACH GROUP*†

FOOD GROUP	CALORIE LEVEL (KILOCALORIES)											
	1000	1200	1400	1600	1800	2000	2200	2400	2600	2800	3000	3200
Fruits (cups [no. servings])	1 (2)	1 (2)	1.5 (3)	1.5 (3)	1.5 (3)	2 (4)	2 (4)	2 (4)	2 (4)	2.5 (5)	2.5 (5)	2.5 (5)
Vegetables (cups [no. servings])	1 (2)	1.5 (3)	1.5 (3)	2 (4)	2.5 (5)	2.5 (5)	3 (6)	3 (6)	3.5 (7)	3.5 (7)	4 (8)	4 (8)
Dark green vegetables (cups/week)	1	1.5	1.5	2	3	3	3	3	3	3	3	3
Orange vegetables (cups/week)	0.5	1	1	1.5	2	2	2	2	2.5	2.5	2.5	2.5
Legumes (cups/week)	0.5	1	1	1.5	2	2	2	2	3.5	3.5	3.5	3.5
Starchy vegetables (cups/week)	1.5	2.5	2.5	2.5	3	3	6	6	7	7	9	9
Other vegetables (cups/week)	4	4.5	4.5	5.5	6.5	6.5	7	7	8.5	8.5	10	10
Grains (ounce equivalents)	3	4	5	5	6	6	7	8	9	10	10	10
Whole grains	1.5	2	2.5	3	3	3	3.5	4	4.6	5	5	5
Other grains	1.5	2	2.5	2	3	3	3.5	4	4.5	5	5	5

Lean meat and beans (ounce equivalents)	2	3	4	5	5	5.5	6	6.5	6.5	7	7
Milk (cups)	2	2	2	3	3	3	3	3	3	3	3
Oils (grams)	15	17	17	22	24	27	29	31	34	36	44
Discretionary calorie allowance (kilocalories)‡	165	171	171	132	195	267	290	362	410	426	512

*Food groups include the following: *Fruits:* All fresh, frozen, canned, and dried fruits and fruit juices, such as oranges and orange juice, apples and apple juice, bananas, grapes, melons, berries, and raisins. Only fruits and juices with no added sugars or fats were used. *Vegetables:* Only vegetables with no added sugars or fats were used. *Dark green vegetables:* All fresh, frozen, and canned dark green vegetables, cooked or raw, such as broccoli; spinach; romaine lettuce; and collard, turnip, and mustard greens. *Orange vegetables:* All fresh, frozen, and canned orange and deep-yellow vegetables, cooked or raw, such as carrots, sweet potatoes, winter squash, and pumpkin. *Legumes:* All cooked dry beans and peas and soybean products, such as pinto beans, kidney beans, lentils, chickpeas, and tofu. Dry beans and peas and soybean products are considered part of this group as well as the lean meat and beans group but should be counted in one group only. *Starchy vegetables:* Vegetables such as white potatoes, corn, and green peas. *Other vegetables:* Vegetables such as artichokes, asparagus, bean sprouts, Brussels sprouts, cabbage, cauliflower, celery, cucumbers, eggplant, green beans, green or red peppers, iceberg (head) lettuce, mushrooms, okra, onions, parsnips, tomatoes, tomato juice, vegetable juice, turnips, wax beans, and zucchini. *Grains:* Only grains in low-fat and low-sugar forms were used. *Whole grains:* All whole-grain products and whole grain products and refined grains used as ingredients, such as whole-wheat and rye breads, enriched grain cereals and crackers, oatmeal, and brown rice. *Other grains:* All refined grain products and refined grains used as ingredients, such as white breads, enriched grain cereals and crackers, enriched pasta, and white rice. *Lean meat and beans:* Meat, poultry, fish, dry beans, eggs, and nuts; dry beans and peas and soybean products are considered part of this group as well as the vegetable group but should be counted in one group only. *Milk:* All milks, yogurts, frozen yogurts, dairy desserts, and cheeses (except cream cheese), including lactose-free and lactose-reduced products. Only fat-free milk was used. Most choices should be fat free or low fat. Calcium-fortified soy beverages are a nondairy calcium source. For all food groups, products with added sugars or fats must be considered under discretionary calories.

†Quantity equivalents for food groups: *Grains:* The following each count as 1 oz equivalent (1 serving) of grains: ½ cup cooked rice, pasta, or cooked cereal; 1 oz dry pasta or rice; 1 slice bread; 1 small muffin (1 oz); 1 cup ready-to-eat cereal flakes. *Fruits and vegetables:* The following each count as 1 cup (2 servings) of fruits or vegetables: 1 cup cut-up raw or cooked fruit or vegetable, 1 cup fruit or vegetable juice, 2 cups leafy salad greens. *Lean meat and beans:* The following each count as 1 oz equivalent: 1 oz lean meat, poultry, or fish; 1 egg; ¼ cup cooked dry beans or tofu; 1 Tbsp peanut butter; ½ oz nuts or seeds. *Milk:* The following each count as 1 cup (1 serving) of milk: 1 cup milk or yogurt, 1½ oz natural cheese such as cheddar cheese, or 2 oz processed cheese. Discretionary calories must be counted for all choices except fat-free milk.

‡The discretionary calorie allowance is the remaining amount of calories in each food pattern after selecting the specified number of nutrient-dense forms of foods in each food group. The number of discretionary calories assumes that food items in each food group are selected in nutrient-dense forms (i.e., forms that are fat free or low fat and that contain no added sugars). Solid fat and sugar calories must always be counted as discretionary calories, as in the following examples: (1) The fat in low-fat, reduced-fat, or whole milk or milk products or cheese and the sugar and fat in chocolate milk, ice cream, pudding, etc. (2) The fat in higher fat meats (e.g., ground beef with more than 5% fat by weight, poultry with skin, higher fat luncheon meats, sausages). (3) The sugars added to fruits and fruit juices with added sugars or fruits canned in syrup. (4) The added fat and/or sugars in vegetables prepared with added fat or sugars. (5) The added fats and/or sugars in grain products containing higher levels of fats and/or sugars (e.g., sweetened cereals; higher fat crackers, pies and pastries, cakes, cookies). Total discretionary calories should be limited to the amounts shown in the table at each calorie level. The number of discretionary calories is lower in the 1600-calorie pattern than in the 1000-, 1200-, and 1400-calorie patterns. These lower calorie patterns are designed to meet the nutrient needs of children 2 to 8 years old. The nutrient goals for the 1600-calorie pattern are set to meet the needs of adult women, which are higher and require that more calories be used in selections from the basic food groups.

Modified from U.S. Department of Health and Human Services: *Dietary guidelines for Americans, 2005,* Washington, DC, 2005, U.S. Government Printing Office.

CLINICAL APPLICATIONS

CASE STUDY: JOHN'S ENERGY BALANCE AND WEIGHT MANAGEMENT PLAN

John is a college student leading a more or less sedentary life because of classes and study. He is interested in wrestling, however, and wants to make the school team. To do so, he must lose some excess weight.

John begins to look carefully at his energy balance picture. He weighs 180 lb and is 5 feet 8 inches tall. John's average food intake is approximately 3000 kcal/day. He wants to lose weight by reversing his energy balance.

Questions for Analysis

1. What are John's present daily total energy (kilocalories) needs (based on weight and activity level)?

2. How does this total energy need compare with his food energy intake?

3. To lose approximately 1 lb/week, how much should he reduce the caloric value of his daily diet?

4. Besides reducing his diet kilocalories, what else could John do to help reverse his energy balance and improve his body condition?

TABLE 15-5

GENERAL APPROXIMATIONS FOR DAILY ADULT BASAL AND ACTIVITY ENERGY NEEDS

DAILY ENERGY NEEDS (BASIS FOR CALCULATIONS)	ACTIVITY ENERGY NEEDS ABOVE BASAL (%)	MALE (70 KG) (KCAL)	FEMALE (58 KG) (KCAL)
Basal Energy Needs 1 kcal/kg per hour		70 kg × 24 hours = 1680	58 kg × 24 hours = 1392
Activity Energy Needs			
Sedentary	+20% basal	1680 + + 336 = 2016	1392 + + 278 = 1670
Very light	+30% basal	1680 + + 504 = 2484	1392 + + 418 = 1810
Moderate	+40% basal	1680 + + 672 = 2352	1392 + + 557 = 1949
Heavy	+50% basal	1680 + + 840 = 2520	1392 + + 696 = 2088

Distribution Balance

Spreading food fairly evenly throughout the day helps meet energy needs. Hunger usually peaks every 4 to 5 hours. If an individual has certain "problem times" of the day, planning simple snacks for those periods helps maintain balance. Long periods without refueling can result in low blood sugar and subsequent periods of overeating, usually whatever can be found at the time, such as high-fat or high-sugar foods in vending machines. Balanced meals require the foresight of planning and preparation.

Food Guide

The 2003 food exchange lists (Appendix E) follow the general *Dietary Guidelines for Americans*. This basic food exchange system is a good general reference guide for comparative food values and portions, variety in food choices, and basic meal planning. Table 15-4 provides examples of food plans that meet nutrient needs at 12 different calorie levels. A simple plan also can be outlined by using the food groups of the MyPyramid guidelines (see Figure 1-1).

Preventive Approach

The most positive work with weight management is aimed at *prevention*. Current studies indicate that the U.S. population of children and adolescents continues to gain excess weight, and these overweight children are becoming obese adults. A major culprit in this health epidemic is physical inactivity. Support for young parents and children before obesity develops can help prevent many problems later in adulthood. This support and guidance should include early nutrition counseling and education, helping to build positive health habits, especially in positive eating behaviors and increased exercise through active play and physical activities for the *entire family*. Many programs for young children, such as Head Start, school lunch programs, and the WIC program (see Chapter 13), address obesity issues through education and prevention for both parents and children.

FOOD MISINFORMATION AND FADS

A fad is any popular fashion or pursuit embraced with fervor. Food fads are scientifically unsubstantiated beliefs about certain foods that may persist for a short time in a given community or society. The word *fallacy* means "a deceptive, misleading, or false notion or belief." Food fallacies are false or misleading beliefs that underlie food fads. The jargon term *quack* is a shortened form of *quicksalver,* a term invented centuries ago by the Dutch to describe the pseudophysician or pseudoprofessor who sold worthless salves, magic elixirs, and cure-all tonics. He proclaimed his wares in a patter that skeptical people compared to the quacking of a duck. In medicine, nutrition, and allied health fields, a quack is a fraudulent pretender who claims to have skill, knowledge, or qualifications that he or she does not possess. The motive for such quackery usually is money, and the quack uses a cruel hoax to feed on the physical and emotional needs of his or her victims. The food quack exists because food faddists exist.

Unscientific statements about food often mislead consumers and contribute to poor food habits. False information may come from folklore or fraud. Food choices should be based on sound scientific knowledge from responsible authorities; misinformation should be recognized as such.

Food Fads

Types of Claims

Food faddists make exaggerated claims for certain types of food. These claims fall into the following four basic groups:

1. *Food cures:* Certain foods cure specific conditions.
2. *Harmful foods:* Certain foods are harmful and should be omitted from the diet.
3. *Food combinations:* Special food combinations restore health and are effective in reducing weight.
4. *Natural foods:* Only "natural" foods can meet body needs and prevent disease. The term *natural* may be used on unprocessed or minimally processed products that contain no artificial ingredients, coloring ingredients, or chemical preservatives. Some people consider all processed foods unhealthy, including those that are enriched or fortified.

Erroneous Claims

Claims that simply are erroneous require careful examination. On the surface they seem to be simple statements about food and health. However, further observation reveals that they focus on a food *itself,* not on the specific *nutrients* in food, which are the actual physiologic agents of life and health. Some individuals may be allergic to specific foods and obviously should avoid them. Also, certain foods may supply relatively large amounts of individual nutrients and therefore are good sources of those nutrients. However, the nutrients, not the whole foods, have specific functions in the body. Each nutrient is found in a wide variety of different foods. Remember, persons require specific nutrients, not necessarily specific foods.

Dangers

Why should health care workers be concerned about food fads and their effect on food habits? What harm do food fads cause? Food fads generally involve four possible negative effects.

Danger to Health. Responsibility for one's health is fundamental. Self-diagnosis and self-treatment can be dangerous, however, especially when such action follows questionable sources. By following such a course, persons with real illness may fail to seek appropriate medical care. Many ill and anxious people have been misled by fraudulent claims of cures and have postponed effective therapy.

Cost. Some foods and supplements used by faddists are harmless, but many are expensive. Money spent for useless items is wasted. When dollars are scarce, a family may neglect to buy foods that fill basic needs and instead purchase a "guaranteed cure."

Lack of Sound Knowledge. Misinformation hinders the development of individuals and society and ignores scientific progress. The perpetuation of certain superstitions can counteract sound teaching about health.

Distrust of the Food Market. America's food environment is changing. People should be watchful, but a blanket rejection of *all* modern food production is unwarranted. People must develop intelligent concerns and rational approaches to meet their nutrition needs. A wise course is to select a variety of primary foods "closer to the source" or those that have minimal processing and then add a few carefully selected processed items for specific uses if desired.

Vulnerable Groups

Food fads appeal to certain groups of people with particular needs and concerns.

The Elderly. Fear of the changes associated with aging may lead many middle-aged and older adults to grasp at exaggerated claims that some products restore vigor. Persons in pain living with chronic illness reach out for the "special supplement" that promises a cure. Desperately ill and lonely persons are easy prey for cruel hoaxes.

Young Persons. Figure-conscious girls and muscle-minded boys may respond to crash programs and claims offering the perfect body. Many who are lonely or have exaggerated ideas of glamour hope to achieve peer group acceptance by these means.

Obese Persons. Obesity is one of the most disturbing personal concerns and frustrating health problems in America today. Obese persons face a constant barrage of propaganda that pushes diets, pills, candies, wafers, formulas, and devices. Many are susceptible to fad diets.

Athletes and Coaches. Individuals involved in athletics are a prime target for those who push miracle supplements. Always looking for the competitive edge, athletes tend to fall prey to nutrition myths and hoaxes. One substance used by well-known athletes who influence many young players is anabolic steroids. Abuse of steroids is harmful and potentially lethal in the long run. Athletes in competition who are found guilty of steroid use are banned from competition.

Entertainers. Persons in the public eye often are taken in by false claims that certain foods, drugs, or dietary combinations will maintain the physical appearance and strength on which their careers depend.

Others. The vulnerability of the groups mentioned above is obvious, but many other people in the general population are susceptible to the appeal of various food fads. Misinformation hinders the efforts of health professionals and concerned consumers to raise community nutrition standards.

What Is the Answer?

What can be done to counter food habits associated with food fads, misinformation, or even outright deception? Helpful instruction is based on personal conviction, practice, and enthusiasm. The following approaches to positive teaching can then be used.

Using Reliable Sources

Sound background knowledge is essential, as follows:

1. Know the product being pushed and the people or company behind it.
2. Know how human physiology and biochemistry really work.
3. Know the scientific method of problem solving (e.g., collect the facts, identify the real problem, determine a reasonable solution or action, carry it out, and evaluate the results).

Sound community resources include the following:

- Extension educators work in the community through state and county Extension Service offices and direct highly successful community nutrition activities, such

as their Expanded Food and Nutrition Education Program. These specialists develop many food and nutrition guides, especially for those with limited education or little skill with English as a second language. Information about the program can be found at *www.csrees. usda.gov/nea/food/efnep/efnep.html.*
- The FDA and USDA produce many educational materials related to food and nutrition (see Chapter 13). Requests for these mostly free materials can be directed to FDA and USDA agency offices.
- Access the *Cultural and Ethnic Food and Nutrition Education Materials: A Resource List for Educators* at *www.nal.usda.gov/fnic/pubs/bibs/gen/ethnic.html.*
- Public health nutritionists located in county and state public health offices and special programs, such as WIC, can provide information. WIC state agencies are listed at *www.fns.usda.gov/wic/Contacts/statealpha.htm.*
- Registered dietitians in local medical care centers and those serving hospitalized patients, outpatient clinics, and others in private practice also are valuable resources. The ADA's nationwide nutrition network can be accessed at *www.eatright.org.*
- In addition, state dietetic associations maintain lists of registered dietitians within the state.

Recognizing Human Needs

Consider the emotional needs that food and food rituals help fulfill. These needs are part of life. Use these needs in a positive way in nutrition teaching. Even if a person is using food as an emotional crutch, the emotional need is still real. Never take away crutches without offering a bet-

On Test

BOX 15-2

THE FOOD AND NUTRITION SCIENCE ALLIANCE'S 10 RED FLAGS OF JUNK SCIENCE

1. Recommendations that promise a quick fix
2. Dire warnings of danger from a single product or regimen
3. Claims that sound too good to be true
4. Simplistic conclusions drawn from a complex study
5. Recommendations based on a single study
6. Dramatic statements that are refuted by reputable scientific organizations
7. Lists of "good" and "bad" foods
8. Recommendations made to help sell a product
9. Recommendations based on studies published without peer review
10. Recommendations from studies that ignore differences among individuals or groups

Reprinted from Food and Nutrition Science Alliance (FANSA): *10 red flags of junk science*, Chicago, 1995, Food and Nutrition Science Alliance.

ter and wiser form of support. Food, and all the associations with it, is a basic enjoyment of life. Maintaining a balance between food as entertainment and food as fuel is the challenge of identifying what human needs are being met by certain foods. Establishing a healthy diet must consider all such human needs and may involve specialized help such as psychotherapy.

Remaining Alert to Teaching Opportunities

Use any opportunity that arises to present sound nutrition and health information, formally or informally. Learn about the available resources described above. Develop communication skills, avoid monotony, and use a well-disciplined imagination.

Thinking Scientifically

Even very young children can be taught to use the problem-solving approach to everyday situations. Children are naturally curious. With their eternal "why?" they often seek evidence to support statements they hear. Three basic questions help evaluate claims in any situation: (1) "What do you mean?" (2) "How do you know?" and (3) "What is your evidence?"

The Food and Nutrition Science Alliance is a partnership of four professional societies: the ADA, American Society for Nutritional Sciences, American Society for Clinical Nutrition, and Institute of Food Technologists. This organization issued a list of 10 red flags to help guide consumers in making educated decisions about nutrition and health issues (Box 15-2). This list is an excellent guide when evaluating reports and claims about various diets, supplements, and other nutrition-related fads.

Knowing Responsible Authorities

The FDA is legally responsible for controlling the quality and safety of food and drug products marketed in the United States. However, this is a tremendous task and requires public help. Other government, professional, and private organizations can provide additional resources (see the "Further Reading and Resources" list at the end of the chapter).

UNDERWEIGHT
General Causes and Treatment

Extremes in underweight, just as in overweight, can bring serious health problems. Although general malnutrition and excessive thinness is a less-common problem in the U.S. population than is overweight, it does occur and usually is associated with poor living conditions or long-term disease. A person who is more than 10% below

the average weight for height and age is considered underweight; being at least 20% below the average is cause for concern. Physiologic and psychological effects may occur, especially in young children. Their resistance to infection is lowered, general health is poor, and strength is reduced.

Causes

Underweight is associated with conditions that cause general malnutrition, including the following:
- *Wasting disease:* long-term disease with chronic infection and fever that raise the BMR
- *Poor food intake:* diminished food intake resulting from (1) psychological factors that cause a person to refuse to eat, (2) loss of appetite, or (3) personal poverty and limited available food supply
- *Malabsorption:* poor nutrient absorption resulting from (1) chronic diarrhea, (2) a diseased GI tract, (3) excessive use of laxatives, or (4) drug-nutrient interactions
- *Hormonal imbalance:* hyperthyroidism, or a variety of other hormonal imbalances, increasing the caloric needs of the body
- *Energy imbalance:* resulting from greatly increased physical activity without a corresponding increase in food or a lack of available food supply
- *Poor living situation:* an unhealthy home environment resulting in irregular and inadequate meals and where eating is considered unimportant and an indifferent attitude toward food exists

Dietary Treatment

Underweight persons require special nutrition care to rebuild body tissues and regain health. Food plans should be adapted to each person's unique situation, whether it involves personal needs, living situation, economic needs, or any underlying disease. The dietary goal, according to each person's tolerance, is to increase energy and nutrient intake, with adherence to the following needs:
- *High-caloric diet:* above the standard requirement for that individual
- *High protein:* to rebuild tissues
- *High carbohydrate:* to provide the primary energy source in an easily digested form
- *Moderate fat:* to provide essential fatty acids and add energy without exceeding tolerance limits
- *Good sources of vitamins and minerals:* including supplements when individual deficiencies require them

A variety of foods, attractively served, help revive the appetite and increase the desire to eat more. Nourishing meals and snacks should be spread throughout the day and often include favorite foods. A basic aim is to help

CLINICAL APPLICATIONS   *On Test*

PROBLEMS OF WEIGHT LOSS AMONG OLDER ADULTS IN LONG-TERM CARE FACILITIES

The American population of adults aged 65 years and older is rapidly increasing. The most rapid population increase over the next decade will be among those older than 85 years. Many of these elderly persons will require long-term care in nursing homes.

One of the problems encountered in elderly residents is low body weight and rapid unintentional weight loss. These can become serious health problems and are a sensitive indicator of malnutrition, contributing to illness and death. Because weight loss is such a strong predictor of morbidity and mortality in clinical settings, early and continuing observation to assess needs is important, especially in relation to factors that contribute to weight loss.

In general, the weight loss can be caused by the physical effects of metabolic changes of aging or disease or by factors that alter the amount and type of food eaten. Physical disease such as cancer can cause extreme weight loss from metabolic abnormalities, taste changes, loss of appetite, nausea, and vomiting. Other diseases underlying weight include GI problems; uncontrolled diabetes; and cardiovascular disorders such as congestive heart failure; pulmonary disease; infection; and alcoholism. Psychological factors or psychiatric disorders also may contribute to malnutrition and weight loss from depression, memory loss, disorientation, apathy, and appetite disturbance. Some altered mental states may be caused by nutritional deficiencies, such as low levels of folate and B-complex vitamins, as well as by protein calorie malnutrition. These conditions can be corrected with specific nutritional support.

The following additional physiologic, psychological, and social factors may influence food intake and body weight and contribute to malnutrition in elderly persons:

■ *Body composition changes*. Height and body weight gradually decline as people age. Body weight usually peaks between the ages of 34 and 54 years in men and 55 and 75 years in women, decreasing thereafter. Body fat losses generally are not significant. The greatest cause of weight loss is a decline in body water, caused in part by weakening of the normal thirst mechanism. Therefore a feeling of thirst cannot be relied on to secure adequate water intake, so water must frequently be offered and encouraged. More constant attention to fluid intake also helps the common problem of xerostomia (dry mouth) in older adults. Xerostomia results from inadequate salivary secretions, which makes eating difficult, thus contributing to malnutrition. Lean body mass also declines with age, resulting in a lower BMR and decreased physical activity and energy requirements. Thus any possible increase in physical activity and use of nutrient-dense foods is encouraged.

■ *Taste changes*. Regeneration of taste cells slows with age, but the extent and effect on food intake vary widely. The sense of smell also declines with age and may affect taste.

Increased use of appropriate seasoning and flavoring in food preparation is needed.

■ *Dentition*. Nearly 50% of all Americans have lost their teeth by the age of 65 years. Many have dentures, but chewing problems often are present. Approximately half of the nursing home population reports chewing, biting, and swallowing problems that interfere with eating and adequate food intake. Assessment of specific needs and dental care solutions helps correct eating problems.

■ *GI problems*. Delayed gastric emptying may contribute to distention and lack of appetite. A decrease in gastric secretions, including hydrochloric acid, may hinder absorption of vitamin B_{12}, folate, and iron, thus contributing to anemia and loss of appetite. Constipation is a common complaint, often leading to laxative abuse and resulting in interference with nutrient absorption. An increase in dietary fiber and liquids can help provide a more natural approach to establishing normal bowel movement.

■ *Drug-nutrient interactions*. Elderly persons often take a number of prescribed and over-the-counter drugs, some of which are the direct cause of anorexia, nausea, and vomiting. Other drugs are indirect causes by inducing nutrient malabsorption, leading to deficiencies that in turn bring anorexia and weight loss. Drug therapy for elderly patients should have constant medical, nutrition, and nursing attention to ensure appropriate use.

■ *Functional disabilities*. Eating problems can prevent or alter the capacity of elderly persons to take in sufficient food. These problems may vary from more difficult functional disabilities that interfere with putting food into the mouth and swallowing (e.g., problems that often require a trained therapist) to dependence on feeding assistance that can be provided by sensitive nursing care.

■ *Social problems*. Socioeconomic problems often are involved with care of the elderly. A specially trained geriatric social worker can help secure possible sources of financial assistance. A sense of social isolation also can lead to decreased food intake. Family support is necessary, as is sensitive contact with nursing home staff and residents and as much involvement as possible in group activities.

Health workers in geriatric settings need continuing education and sensitization to the potential dangers of low body weight and weight loss. Aged persons with acute and chronic illnesses and functional disabilities are at the greatest risk for nutrition-related problems. These persons need continual nutrition assessment and monitoring of body weight. Some of the restrictions of "special diets" should be relaxed or discontinued when the risk of malnutrition is evident, with the goal of increasing nutrient intake and making eating as enjoyable as possible.

DRUG-NUTRIENT INTERACTION

DEPRESSION AND MEDICATIONS IN THE ELDERLY

According to the National Mental Health Association, depression occurs in approximately 15% of community-dwelling older people and up to 25% of those living in nursing homes. The effects can be seen in part by the increased suicide rates among the elderly population, with men far outnumbering women.*

Fluoxetine (Prozac) is a commonly prescribed antidepressant for geriatric patients.† It is a selective serotonin reuptake inhibitor that works by raising levels of serotonin in the brain. Side effects can include nausea and loss of appetite.

These side effects can be intensified by another common problem in the elderly: polypharmacy. Taking many medications at one time can alter the taste of foods and lead to anorexia. Extra care should be taken when working with the elderly to ensure adequate nutrition and weight maintenance.

Sara Oldroyd

*He W and others: *U.S. Census Bureau, Current population reports, 65+ in the United States: 2005*, Washington, DC, 2005, U.S. Government Printing Office.
†Ferguson JM, Hill H: Pharmacokinetics of fluoxetine in elderly men and women, *Gerontology* 52(1):45, 2006.

---

build good food habits so that improved nutritional status and weight can be maintained once they are regained. Residents in long-term care facilities are especially vulnerable to weight loss problems and have special needs (see the Clinical Applications box, "Problems of Weight Loss among Older Adults in Long-Term Care Facilities"). In addition, several medications often prescribed to elderly individuals may result in anorexia or weight loss (see the Drug-Nutrient Interaction box, "Depression and Medications in the Elderly"). This rehabilitation process requires creative counseling for the patient and family along with practical guides and support. In some cases tube feeding or intravenous feeding (e.g., total parenteral nutrition) may be necessary (see Chapter 22).

Ideal weight gain includes both lean and fat tissue. To gain muscle, physical exercise must be part of the treatment. Resistance training increases lean tissue and, in turn, boosts appetite. A variety of weight lifting and strength training programs can be designed depending on the desires of the individual and should be encouraged as an important part of healthy weight gain.

Disordered Eating

A subset of the population has difficulty maintaining "normal" eating behaviors. Normal eating is when an individual is capable of the following:

- Eats when he or she is hungry and stops when full
- Demonstrates moderate restraint in food selection
- Recognizes that overeating and undereating are sometimes acceptable and trusts his or her body to establish a balance
- Can be flexible with his or her eating schedule

Disordered eating is defined as any eating pattern that is not normal and can include a variety of subclinical problems. Disordered eating can range from an insur-

mountable fear of eating fat to an inability to eat in public. Family and personal tensions, as well as social pressures for thinness, sometimes result in serious body image disturbances and eating problems that may become psychiatric disorders. No matter what they weigh, these individuals always see themselves as fat and develop a deep-seated fear of food and fatness. The most recent position paper from the ADA on eating disorders stated that the prevalence occurs less frequently in males than females but the effects are similar, and homosexual males are at higher risk than their heterosexual counterparts.[33]

The three most common eating disorders are anorexia nervosa, bulimia nervosa, and binge eating disorder (Box 15-3). An estimated 5 to 10 million Americans currently battle an eating disorder. Eating disorders are secretive in nature; therefore, establishing a true estimate in the population is difficult.

anorexia nervosa extreme psychophysiologic aversion to food resulting in life-threatening weight loss; a psychiatric eating disorder resulting from a morbid fear of fatness in which a person's distorted body image is reflected as fat when the body is malnourished and extremely thin from self-starvation.

bulimia nervosa a psychiatric eating disorder related to a person's fear of fatness in which cycles of gorging on large quantities of food are followed by compensatory mechanisms, such as self-induced vomiting and use of diuretics and laxatives, to maintain a "normal" body weight.

binge-eating disorder a psychiatric eating disorder characterized by the occurrence of binge eating episodes at least twice a week for a 6-month period.

5-10 million Americans have eating disorders

BOX 15-3

AMERICAN PSYCHIATRIC ASSOCIATION DIAGNOSTIC CRITERIA

Anorexia Nervosa

A. Refusal to maintain body weight at or above a minimally normal weight for age and height (e.g., weight loss leading to maintenance of body weight less than 85% of that expected or failure to make expected weight gain during period of growth, leading to body weight less than 85% of that expected).

B. Intense fear of gaining weight or becoming fat even though underweight.

C. Disturbance in the way in which one's body weight or shape is experienced; undue influence of body weight or shape on self-evaluation; or denial of the seriousness of the current low body weight.

D. In postmenarcheal women, amenorrhea (i.e., the absence of at least three consecutive menstrual cycles).

   1. *Restricting type*: During the current episode of anorexia nervosa, the person has not regularly engaged in binge eating or purging behavior.

   2. *Binge eating/purging type*: During the current episode of anorexia nervosa, the person has regularly engaged in binge eating and purging behavior.

Bulimia Nervosa

A. Recurrent episodes of binge eating, characterized by both of the following:

   1. Eating, in a discrete period of time (e.g., within any 2-hour period), an amount of food that is larger than most people would eat during a similar period of time and under similar circumstances.

   2. A sense of a lack of control regarding eating during the episode (e.g., a feeling that one cannot stop eating or control what or how much one is eating).

B. Recurrent inappropriate compensatory behavior to prevent weight gain, such as self-induced vomiting; misuse of laxatives, diuretics, enemas, or other medications; fasting; or excessive exercise.

C. The binge eating and inappropriate compensatory behaviors both occur, on average, at least twice a week for 3 months.

D. Self-evaluation is unduly influenced by body shape and weight.

E. The disturbance does not occur exclusively during episodes of anorexia nervosa.

   1. *Purging type:* During the current episode of bulimia nervosa, the person has regularly engaged in self-induced vomiting or the misuse of laxatives, diuretics, or enemas.

   2. *Nonpurging type:* During the current episode of bulimia nervosa, the person has used other inappropriate compensatory behaviors such as fasting or excessive exercise but has not regularly engaged in self-induced vomiting or the misuse of laxatives, diuretics, or enemas.

Eating Disorder not Otherwise Specified

This category is for disorders of eating that do not meet criteria for any specific eating disorder. For example:

   1. For females, all the criteria for anorexia nervosa are met except that the individual has regular menses.

   2. All the criteria for anorexia nervosa are met except that, despite significant weight loss, the individual's current weight is in the normal range.

   3. All the criteria for bulimia nervosa are met except that the binge eating and inappropriate compensatory mechanisms occur at a frequency of less than twice a week or for a duration of less than 3 months.

   4. The regular use of inappropriate compensatory behavior by an individual of normal body weight after eating small amounts of food.

   5. Repeatedly chewing and spitting out, but not swallowing, large amounts of food.

Binge Eating Disorder

A. Recurrent episodes of binge eating in the absence of the regular use of inappropriate compensatory behaviors characteristic of bulimia nervosa.

B. Binge episodes must occur at least 2 days per week for a period of 6 months.

Modified from American Psychiatric Association: *Diagnostic and statistical manual of mental disorders, DSM-IV-TR,* ed 4 (text revision), Washington, DC, 2000, APA Press.

Anorexia Nervosa

This complex psychological disorder results in self-imposed starvation. Patients with anorexia nervosa generally are characterized as high achievers who constantly push themselves toward perfection. They see food and their bodies as things that can be controlled. Their distorted body image (seeing themselves as fat even when they are emaciated; Figure 15-9) keeps them in a state of near panic. These patients may plan their days around ways to avoid food, which becomes a full-time obsession. Patients generally grow more depressed, irritable, and anxious as the disease progresses.

The American Psychological Association's *Diagnostic and Statistical Manual of Mental Disorders, Fourth Edition* sets the criteria for anorexia nervosa as a weight that is less than 85% expected for height.[34] Individuals with anorexia nervosa often are preoccupied with food, calories, and weight. Warning signs include dramatic weight loss, avoidance of food-related events, mood swings, excessive exercise, and other obsessive-compulsive behaviors.

Bulimia Nervosa

Individuals with bulimia nervosa also have similar obsessions about their body and food. Bulimia is an eating

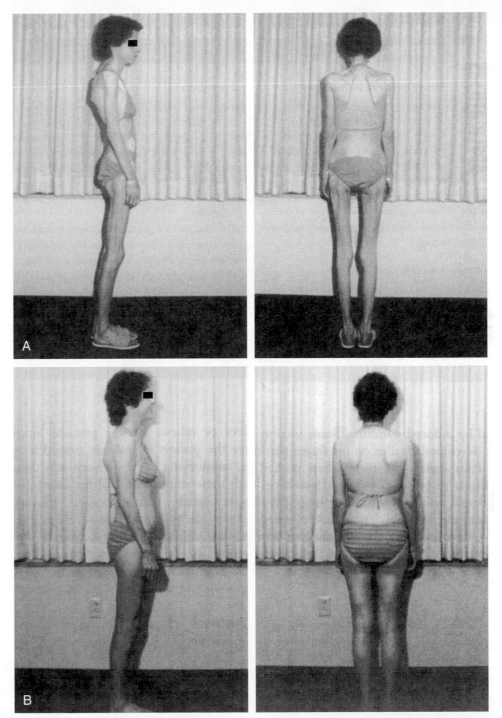

Figure 15–9 **A,** Woman with anorexia nervosa before treatment. **B,** Same patient after gradual refeeding, nutrition management, and psychological therapy.   (Courtesy Sycamore Hospital, a division of Kettering Medical Center, Dayton, Ohio.)

disorder involving repeated episodes of binge eating followed by one or more compensatory mechanisms to rid the body of excess calories. By definition, this behavior occurs at least twice per week for 3 months. Compensatory mechanisms include self-induced vomiting, laxa-

tive abuse, strict dieting or fasting, and excessive exercise. A binge will vary among patients but generally involves the consumption of excessive quantities of food in a short period. Some individuals consume several thousand kilocalories within 20 to 30 minutes. Oral and dental problems from the purging behavior may involve oral mucosal irritation, decreased salivary secretions and dry mouth (xerostomia), and irreversible tooth enamel erosion.

Individuals with bulimia nervosa often go unnoticed and undiagnosed for much longer than individuals with anorexia nervosa. Body weight generally is within a normal range but may fluctuate. Warning signs include excessive concern about weight, cycles of strict dieting and binge eating, self-criticism and low self-esteem, depression, and absences after meals.

Binge Eating Disorder

This eating disorder includes binging episodes without compensatory behaviors. This reactive type of eating often follows some stress or anxiety as an emotional eating pattern to soothe or relieve painful feelings. The binges may be triggered by psychological factors involving the self and body image. Dietary restriction and failure to achieve satiety or relieve hunger precede binges and relentlessly drive individuals toward a continuous, unsatisfying cycle. Persons who attempt to reach unrealistic, and for them unnatural, weight goals are forever dieting (chronic dieting syndrome). After each weight loss rebound eating occurs, followed by more attempts to lose weight. Thus the weight cycling, with its psychologic and physiological effects, continues.

Treatment

These psychological disorders require therapy from a team of skilled professionals, including physicians, psychologists, and dietitians. Even with the best of care, recovery is slow and the word *cure* often is not used. Approximately two thirds of patients with eating disorders have persistent food and weight preoccupations throughout life. Patients with eating disorders often have neurologic disturbances. These chemical disturbances were first thought of as the cause for disordered eating behavior. However, researchers have found that once a normal weight and eating pattern are reestablished in the patient, the neurologic chemistry returns to normal. Therefore one of the first issues to address in treatment of an eating disorder is establishing a healthy weight in the patient. Psychological therapy is more successful once neurologic disturbances are reduced. Next the team of professionals must work together to restore eating habits and attitudes toward food, optimize physical and mental health, and restore intrapersonal and interpersonal problems. Continuing support groups, including friends, family, and health care professionals, are critical for long-term treatment.

SUMMARY

In the traditional medical model, obesity has been viewed as an illness and a health hazard, which is true in cases of clinically severe obesity. Newer approaches view moderate overweight differently, however, in terms of the important aspect of fatness and leanness or body composition and propose a more person-centered positive health model.

Planning a weight management program, either for an overweight or underweight person, must involve the metabolic and energy needs of the individual. Personal food choices and habits, as well as fatty tissue needs during different stages of the life cycle, must be considered. Important aspects of such a weight reduction program include changing food behaviors, and increasing physical activity. A sound program is based on reduced energy intake for gradual weight loss and nutrient balance to meet the health standards of the U.S. dietary goals, with meals distributed throughout the day for energy needs. The ideal plan begins with prevention, stressing the formation of positive food habits in early childhood to prevent major problems later in life.

Food fads and misinformation are increasingly popular within all facets of American society. Identifying harmful practices and providing accurate information are basic functions of the health care provider.

The American obsession with thinness has created extreme weight management problems such as eating disorders that result in self-starvation. These psychological disorders require professional team therapy, including medical, psychological, and nutrition care.

CRITICAL THINKING QUESTIONS

1. Why is the term *ideal weight* difficult to define? Explain some of the problems in determining this measure. What role does it play in weight management?

2. What does *set point* mean in relation to individual weight? How does it relate to diet and exercise in a personal weight management program?

3. Describe the components of a positive health model for weight management. What are the basic principles of a sound food plan for such a program?

4. Describe two major eating disorders associated with a growing obsession with thinness. What are the contributing social and psychological factors? What is the treatment? How does chronic dieting syndrome relate and contribute to the prevalence of disordered eating?

CHAPTER CHALLENGE QUESTIONS

True-False

Write the correct statement for each statement that is false.

1. *True or False:* Development of childhood obesity results exclusively from genetic inheritance.

2. *True or False:* Increasing the energy expended in physical activity is a means of weight reduction.

3. *True or False:* A certain percentage of stored fat in the body is necessary for life.

4. *True or False:* A reasonable weight reduction diet for an adult has an energy value of approximately 1200 to 1800 kcal, depending on individual size and need.

5. *True or False:* A weight reduction diet should not use between-meal snacks.

6. *True or False:* Food fads usually are long lasting and seldom change.

Multiple Choice

1. Overweight is a direct risk factor in which of the following conditions? *(Circle all that apply.)*
   a. Surgery
   b. Type 2 diabetes mellitus
   c. Liver disease
   d. Hypertension

2. A 500-kcal deficit in the daily energy expenditure of an obese person enables him or her to lose weight at which of the following rates?
   a. 1 lb/week
   b. 2 lb/week
   c. 3 lb/week
   d. 4 lb/week

3. An individual who has repeated binge-purge episodes, expresses severe self-criticism, and often is depressed may have which of the following?
   a. Anorexia nervosa
   b. Bulimia nervosa
   c. Compulsive overeating
   d. None of the above

evolve Please refer to the Students' Resource section of this text's Evolve Web site for additional study resources.

REFERENCES

1. National Center for Health Statistics: *Health, United States, 2006, with chartbook on trends in the health of Americans,* Hyattsville, MD, 2006, U.S. Government Printing Office.

2. Nader PR and others: Identifying risk for obesity in early childhood, *Pediatrics* 118(3):e594, 2006.

3. Demura S and others: Percentage of total body fat as estimated by three automatic bioelectrical impedance analyzers, *J Physiol Anthropol Appl Human Sci* 23(3):93, 2004.

4. Ittenback RF and others: Statistical validation of air-displacement plethysmography for body composition assessment in children, *Ann Hum Biol* 33(2):187, 2006.

5. Bosy-Westphal A and others: Validation of air-displacement plethysmography for estimation of body fat mass in healthy elderly subjects, *Eur J Nutr* 42(4):207, 2003.

6. Silva AM and others: Body fat measurement in adolescent athletes: multicompartment molecular model comparison, *Eur J Clin Nutr* 60(8):955, 2006.

7. Ginde SR and others: Air displacement plethysmography: validation in overweight and obese subjects, *Obes Res* 13(7):1232, 2005.

8. U.S. Department of Health and Human Services: *Dietary guidelines for Americans, 2005,* Washington, DC, 2005, U.S. Government Printing Office.

9. Inoue K and others: Body mass index as a predictor of mortality in community-dwelling seniors, *Aging Clin Exp Res* 18(3):205, 2006.

10. Lawlor DA and others: Reverse causality and confounding and the associations of overweight and obesity with mortality, *Obesity* 14(12):2294, 2006.

11. Miller KK and others: Preservation of neuroendocrine control of reproductive function despite severe undernutrition, *J Clin Endocrinol Metab* 89(9):4434, 2004.

12. Wannamethee SG and others: Overweight and obesity and weight change in middle aged men: impact on cardiovascular disease and diabetes, *J Epidemiol Community Health* 59(2):134, 2005.

13. Centers for Disease Control and Prevention: *Overweight and obesity*, www.cdc.gov/nccdphp/dnpa/obesity, accessed January 2007.

14. Tejada T and others: Nonpharmacologic therapy for hypertension: does it really work? *Curr Cardiol Rep* 8(6):418, 2006.

15. Shapiro JR and others: "Structure-size me": weight and health changes in a four week residential program, *Eat Behav* 7(3):229, 2006.

16. Schneider PL and others: Effects of a 10,000 steps per day goal in overweight adults, *Am J Health Promot* 21(2):85, 2006.

17. Zhang Y and others: Positional cloning of the mouse obese gene and the human homologue, *Nature* 372(6505):425, 1994.

18. Eikelis N, Esler M: The neurobiology of human obesity, *Exp Physiol* 90:673, 2005.

19. Eikelis N and others: Extra adipocyte leptin release in human obesity and its relation to sympathoadrenal function, *Am J Physiol Endocrinol Metab* 286:E744, 2004.

20. Farooqi IS and others: Clinical and molecular genetic spectrum of congenital deficiency of the leptin receptor, *N Engl J Med* 356(3):237, 2007.

21. Kalra SP and others: Stimulation of appetite by ghrelin is regulated by leptin restraint: peripheral and central sites of action, *J Nutr* 135:1331, 2005.

22. Popovic V, Duntas LH: Brain somatic cross-talk: ghrelin, leptin and ultimate challengers of obesity, *Nutr Neurosci* 8(1):1, 2005.

23. Walley AJ and others: Genetics of obesity and the prediction of risk for health, *Hum Mol Genet* 15:R124, 2006.

24. Dong C and others: Interacting genetic loci on chromosomes 20 and 10 influence extreme human obesity, *Am J Hum Genet* 72:115, 2003.

25. Speakman JR: Obesity: the integrated roles of environment and genetics, *J Nutr* 134(8 suppl):2090s, 2004.

26. Salsberry PJ, Reagan PB: Dynamics of early childhood overweight, *Pediatrics* 116:1329, 2005.

27. American Dietetic Association: Position of the American Dietetic Association: individual-, family-, school-, and community-based interventions for pediatric overweight, *J Am Diet Assoc* 106:925, 2006.

28. Sachdev M and others: Effect of fenfluramine-derivative diet pills on cardiac valves: a meta-analysis of observational studies, *Am Heart J* 144(6):1065, 2002.

29. Ioannides-Demos LL and others: Pharmacotherapy for obesity, *Drugs* 65(10):1391, 2005.

30. Schnee DM and others: An update on the pharmacological treatment of obesity, *Curr Med Res Opin* 22(8):1463, 2006.

31. Christou NV and others: Surgery decreases long-term mortality, morbidity, and health care use in morbidly obese patients, *Ann Surg* 240:416, 2004.

32. Kelly J and others: Best practice recommendations for surgical care in weight loss surgery, *Obes Res* 13:227, 2005.

33. American Dietetic Association: Position of the American Dietetic Association: nutrition intervention in the treatment of anorexia nervosa, bulimia nervosa, and other eating disorders, *J Am Diet Assoc* 106:2073, 2006.

34. American Psychiatric Association: *Diagnostic and statistical manual of mental disorders, SSM-IV-TR*, ed 4 (test revision), Washington, DC, 2000, APA Press.

FURTHER READING AND RESOURCES

Speakman JR: Obesity: the integrated roles of environment and genetics, *J Nutr* 134(8 suppl):2090S, 2004.

Colmers WF: What makes people fat? View from the chair, *Obesity (Silver Spring)* 14(5):190S, 2006.
> *The first article explores the various facets of genes and environment that contribute to obesity and specifically discusses the "lipostatic model" and the role of evolution within this context. The second article summarizes four papers discussing theories regarding the etiology of obesity.*

Pawlak L: *Stop gaining weight*, ed 2, Emeryville, CA, 2005, Jeblar, Inc.
> *The author establishes three steps to stopping weight gain with insightful tips in an easy-to-read textbook.*

Soliah L: The psychological appeal of fad diets, *Today's Dietitian* 5(4):22, 2003.
> *The author takes a fascinating look into the psychological appeal and complications of fad diets.*

CHAPTER 16

Nutrition and Physical Fitness

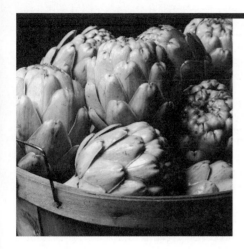

KEY CONCEPTS

- Regular physical activity is an important part of a healthy lifestyle.
- Healthy muscle structure and function depend on appropriate energy fuels and tissue-building material as well as oxygen and water.
- Different levels of physical activity and athletic performance draw on different body fuel sources.
- A sedentary lifestyle contributes to health problems.
- A healthy personal exercise program combines both strengthening and aerobic activities.

Public interest in physical fitness has continued to grow over the past few decades, as encouraged by preventive medicine and health promotion. This approach has been stimulated by an effort to prevent various chronic diseases in America's aging population and extend the number of healthy years of life.

This chapter demonstrates that nutrition and physical fitness are essential interrelated parts of a healthy lifestyle. Both reduce risks associated with chronic diseases, and both are important therapies in the treatment of chronic conditions. Health care workers should provide their patients with sound guidelines for nutrition and physical fitness and also set good examples.

PHYSICAL ACTIVITY RECOMMENDATIONS AND BENEFITS

Guidelines and Recommendations

Technology is rapidly reducing the requirement for physical activity in everyday life. Of course, these are considered technological advances, such as moving sidewalks, yet the overall health of some people suffers from the consequences of too much convenience. Approximately 40% of American adults do not engage in any form of leisure-time physical activity, and only 30% of adults participate in 30 minutes of moderate physical activity five or more times per week.[1]

Increased participation in regular physical activity is a national health goal. The USDHHS has set nutrition and physical fitness goals for Americans, among many other health-related goals, in their *Healthy People 2010: Understanding and Improving Health* report. The 2010 target for participation in regular moderate to vigorous physical activity is 30% of adults and 85% of adolescents.[2] In addition to the goals of *Healthy People 2010*, the *Dietary*

Guidelines for Americans, the MyPyramid guidelines, and the DRIs address the need to participate in physical activity on a daily basis. The most recent publication from the Institute of Medicine increases its recommendations from 30 minutes of moderate exercise on most days of the week to 60 minutes of moderate exercise every day. The increased recommendations were made because the former were not enough to maintain a body weight within the recommended BMI range (18.5 to 25 kg/m^2).[3]

Physical activity differs from exercise according to the following definition[3]:

- *Physical activity:* bodily movement produced by the contraction of muscles that substantially increases energy expenditure
- *Exercise:* planned, structured, and repetitive bodily movement performed to promote or maintain one or more components of physical fitness

The Food and Nutrition Board identifies moderate activity as walking (3 to 4 mph), leisurely swimming and cycling, and playing golf. The recommendations state that to achieve health benefits from physical activity, the 60 minutes of moderate activity should be in addition to activities of daily living (house cleaning, walking to the bus stop, light gardening, etc.). Figure 16-1 suggests guidelines on how to incorporate the recommended activity into daily life.

Health Benefits

The health benefits of physical activity are not reserved only for athletes. In a personalized program designed to meet individual needs, any person can develop a healthy lifestyle. The longer people follow some form of regular exercise, the more committed they become.[4] Water aerobics, walking, and other low-impact workouts are becoming more and more popular in health clubs and have enabled more people to participate (e.g., those who cannot lift heavy weights or participate in "go for the burn" aerobics). Several of these new gym members are older adults who have health problems that may improve with moderate exercise. Regular exercise helps manage health and reduces the risk of chronic disease, promotes independence, and increases quality of life.

For most people physical activity should not pose any problem or hazard. The Physical Activity Readiness Questionnaire (PAR-Q) has been designed to identify the small number of adults for whom physical activity might be inappropriate or those who should have medical advice concerning the type of activity most suitable for them (Figure 16-2). All practitioners in the health care field should be well informed of their scope of practice regarding exercise recommendations and prescriptions. This chapter discusses general recommendations. Much like dietetics, in which the registered dietitian is recognized as the nutrition expert, exercise scientists, physiologists, and certified personal trainers are the experts in exercise.

The sense of fitness that exercise creates helps people feel good physically, emotionally, and psychologically. However, in addition to this general sense of well-being, exercise (especially aerobic exercise) has special benefits for persons with certain health problems.[5]

Coronary Heart Disease

Exercise reduces risks for heart disease in several ways, including improved heart function, blood cholesterol levels, and oxygen transport.

Heart Muscle Function. The heart is a four-chambered organ of muscle that is approximately the size of an adult fist. Exercise, especially aerobic conditioning, strengthens the heart, thereby enabling it to pump more blood per beat (stroke volume). A heart strengthened by exercise has an increased aerobic capacity; that is, the heart can pump more blood per minute without an undue increase in the heart rate. Therefore exercises relying primarily on the aerobic oxygen system for energy, such as walking, jogging, and light cardiovascular machines, improve heart function.

Blood Cholesterol Levels. Exercise raises blood levels of HDL, referred to as good cholesterol because it carries surplus cholesterol from the tissues to the liver for breakdown and removal from the body (see Chapter 19). Exercise also lowers blood levels of LDL, referred to as bad cholesterol because it carries at least two thirds of the total blood cholesterol to body tissues, raising the potential of cholesterol deposits in major arteries of the heart. Both exercise effects (improved heart function and cholesterol profile) lower the risks for diseased arteries.

Oxygen-Carrying Capacity. Exercise also enhances the circulatory system by increasing the oxygen-carrying capacity of the blood. As training continues, a person's VO$_2$max will improve, thus increasing the efficiency of oxygen use and uptake.

Hypertension

The risk for cardiovascular complications increases along with increasing levels of blood pressure. According to the CDC, approximately one in four adults in the United States has hypertension.[1] Persons with stage 1 hypertension (systolic 140 to 159 mm Hg or diasystolic 90 to 104 mm Hg) represent the overwhelming majority of hypertensive individuals in the general population, and exercise has become one of the most effective nondrug treatments. Even for people with higher levels of blood pressure, exercise has proved to be an important adjunct to drug therapy, offsetting adverse drug effects and lowering medication dosage.

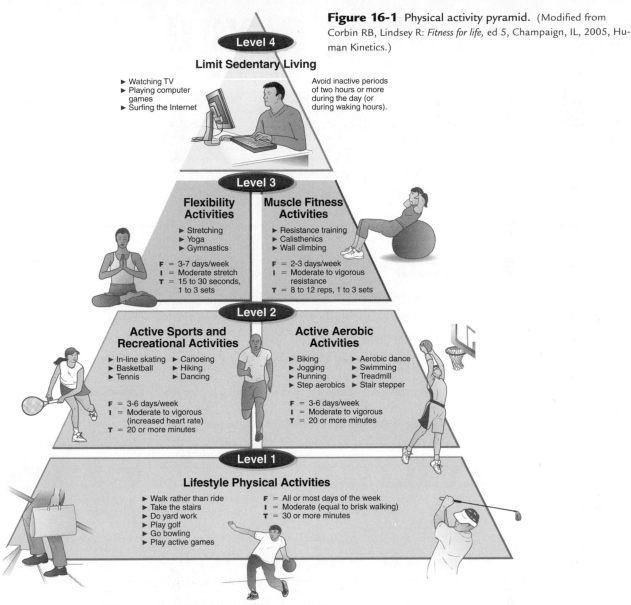

Figure 16-1 Physical activity pyramid. (Modified from Corbin RB, Lindsey R: *Fitness for life,* ed 5, Champaign, IL, 2005, Human Kinetics.)

Level 4

Limit Sedentary Living

▶ Watching TV
▶ Playing computer games
▶ Surfing the Internet

Avoid inactive periods of two hours or more during the day (or during waking hours).

Level 3

Flexibility Activities

▶ Stretching
▶ Yoga
▶ Gymnastics

F = 3-7 days/week
I = Moderate stretch
T = 15 to 30 seconds, 1 to 3 sets

Muscle Fitness Activities

▶ Resistance training
▶ Calisthenics
▶ Wall climbing

F = 2-3 days/week
I = Moderate to vigorous resistance
T = 8 to 12 reps, 1 to 3 sets

Level 2

Active Sports and Recreational Activities

▶ In-line skating ▶ Canoeing
▶ Basketball ▶ Hiking
▶ Tennis ▶ Dancing

F = 3-6 days/week
I = Moderate to vigorous (increased heart rate)
T = 20 or more minutes

Active Aerobic Activities

▶ Biking ▶ Aerobic dance
▶ Jogging ▶ Swimming
▶ Running ▶ Treadmill
▶ Step aerobics ▶ Stair stepper

F = 3-6 days/week
I = Moderate to vigorous
T = 20 or more minutes

Level 1

Lifestyle Physical Activities

▶ Walk rather than ride
▶ Take the stairs
▶ Do yard work
▶ Play golf
▶ Go bowling
▶ Play active games

F = All or most days of the week
I = Moderate (equal to brisk walking)
T = 30 or more minutes

Accumulate moderate activity from the pyramid on all or most days of the week, and vigorous activity at least three days a week.

Eating well helps you stay active and fit.

Normal rises in blood pressure occur during both aerobic and resistance-type exercises. Both forms of exercise are beneficial for individuals with hypertension. However, exercisers with diagnosed hypertension should avoid excess exertion to prevent severe stress on the cardiovascular system. An example would be holding your breath during the exertion phase of the exercise, as with heavy weight lifting.

VO$_2$max maximal uptake volume of oxygen during exercise; used to measure the intensity and duration of exercise a person can perform.

hypertension chronically elevated blood pressure in which systolic blood pressure is consistently 140 mm Hg or greater and/or diastolic blood pressure is consistently 90 mm Hg or greater.

Physical Activity Readiness
Questionnaire - PAR-Q
(revised 2002)

PAR-Q & YOU

(A Questionnaire for People Aged 15 to 69)

Regular physical activity is fun and healthy, and increasingly more people are starting to become more active every day. Being more active is very safe for most people. However, some people should check with their doctor before they start becoming much more physically active.

If you are planning to become much more physically active than you are now, start by answering the seven questions in the box below. If you are between the ages of 15 and 69, the PAR-Q will tell you if you should check with your doctor before you start. If you are over 69 years of age, and you are not used to being very active, check with your doctor.

Common sense is your best guide when you answer these questions. Please read the questions carefully and answer each one honestly: check YES or NO.

YES	NO	
☐	☐	**1. Has your doctor ever said that you have a heart condition <u>and</u> that you should only do physical activity recommended by a doctor?**
☐	☐	**2. Do you feel pain in your chest when you do physical activity?**
☐	☐	**3. In the past month, have you had chest pain when you were not doing physical activity?**
☐	☐	**4. Do you lose your balance because of dizziness or do you ever lose consciousness?**
☐	☐	**5. Do you have a bone or joint problem (for example, back, knee or hip) that could be made worse by a change in your physical activity?**
☐	☐	**6. Is your doctor currently prescribing drugs (for example, water pills) for your blood pressure or heart condition?**
☐	☐	**7. Do you know of <u>any other reason</u> why you should not do physical activity?**

If you answered

YES to one or more questions

Talk with your doctor by phone or in person BEFORE you start becoming much more physically active or BEFORE you have a fitness appraisal. Tell your doctor about the PAR-Q and which questions you answered YES.

• You may be able to do any activity you want — as long as you start slowly and build up gradually. Or, you may need to restrict your activities to those which are safe for you. Talk with your doctor about the kinds of activities you wish to participate in and follow his/her advice.

• Find out which community programs are safe and helpful for you.

NO to all questions

If you answered NO honestly to <u>all</u> PAR-Q questions, you can be reasonably sure that you can:

• start becoming much more physically active – begin slowly and build up gradually. This is the safest and easiest way to go.

• take part in a fitness appraisal – this is an excellent way to determine your basic fitness so that you can plan the best way for you to live actively. It is also highly recommended that you have your blood pressure evaluated. If your reading is over 144/94, talk with your doctor before you start becoming much more physically active.

DELAY BECOMING MUCH MORE ACTIVE:

• if you are not feeling well because of a temporary illness such as a cold or a fever – wait until you feel better; or

• if you are or may be pregnant – talk to your doctor before you start becoming more active.

PLEASE NOTE: If your health changes so that you then answer YES to any of the above questions, tell your fitness or health professional. Ask whether you should change your physical activity plan.

<u>Informed Use of the PAR-Q</u>: The Canadian Society for Exercise Physiology, Health Canada, and their agents assume no liability for persons who undertake physical activity, and if in doubt after completing this questionnaire, consult your doctor prior to physical activity.

Figure 16-2 Physical Activity Readiness Questionnaire. (Courtesy Canadian Society for Exercise Physiology, copyright 2002.)

Diabetes

Regular, moderate-intensity exercise programs help individuals with type 2 diabetes control blood glucose levels and reduce the risk of chronic complications associated with diabetes.[6] Exercise increases glucose uptake in skeletal muscle despite insulin resistance. In managing type 1 diabetes mellitus, the type of exercise and when it is performed must be balanced with food and insulin to prevent reactions caused by drops in blood glucose (see Chapter 20 for a more detailed discussion of diabetes).

Weight Management

Exercise is extremely beneficial to weight management in the following ways: (1) it helps regulate appetite, (2) it increases BMR, and (3) it reduces the genetic fat deposit set point level. Together with a well-planned diet, physical exercise corrects the energy balance in favor of increased energy output (see Chapter 15). Fat is used efficiently as the primary fuel source during lower intensity (30% to 60% VO_2max) aerobic exercise such as walking, jogging, swimming, and light cycling (Table 16-1).

Bone Disease

Weight-bearing exercises, such as walking and running, help strengthen bones by increasing osteoblast activity. The weight-bearing load increases calcium deposits in bone, thus increasing bone density and reducing the risk for osteoporosis. The benefits of exercise on bone density are most notable during peak bone growth of the adolescent and young adult. However, excessive or extreme forms of training can have a rebound effect in which bone density is lost because of overtraining and/or undernutrition.

Mental Health

Exercise stimulates the production of brain opiates, substances called *endorphins*. These natural chemicals decrease pain and improve mood, which may include an exhilarating type of "high." Mental health benefits from physical activity are persistent throughout life. A recent study evaluating quality of life in older healthy subjects found mental health benefits such as improved vitality and social functioning in those who exercised more than 1 hour per week at moderate intensity.[7]

Types of Physical Activity

A variety of exercises in a person's fitness plan is best. A well-balanced exercise program incorporates resistance training, aerobic activities, flexibility and stretching exercises, and a variety of activities of daily living. A good fitness plan is a combination of different enjoyable activities that most effectively reduce the risk of several chronic diseases.

Activities of Daily Living

Many activities of daily living do not reach aerobic levels (e.g., walking to work or the store, walking the dog, playing catch with children) but are enjoyable and should be incorporated into daily life. If the activity of choice is not enjoyable and appreciated, it will likely be discontinued—along with any potential benefit. Many people question whether exercise is most beneficial in the morning or at night. Again, the bottom line is it is best whenever one can commit to doing it. No significant differences occur in the overall outcome as long as exercise is incorporated into a daily routine and consistently maintained.

Resistance Training

Resistance training creates and maintains muscle and bone strength, a physical trait necessary for health and enhanced quality of life. Two position statements by the American College of Sports Medicine established guidelines for a beginning resistance training program and for progressive models of advanced training for healthy adults.[8,9] An ideal resistance program should include 8 to 10 separate exercises (with 8 to 12 repetitions of each), focusing on all major muscle groups and performed 2 to 3 days per week.[8] A more progressive model incorporates gradual load increases to stimulate muscle overload, more muscle specificity and variation, and a training regimen of 4 to 5 days per week.[9]

Aerobic Exercise

Forms of exercise that can be sustained at a necessary level of intensity to provide aerobic benefits include activities such as swimming, running, jogging, bicycling, and aerobic dancing routines and similar workouts (Table 16-2).

TABLE 16-1

SOURCE OF ENERGY FOR VARYING EXERCISE INTENSITY

EXERCISE INTENSITY	FUEL USED BY MUSCLE
<30% VO_2max (easy walking)	Mainly muscle fat stores
40%-60% VO_2max (jogging, brisk walking)	Fat and carbohydrate used evenly
75% VO_2max (running)	Mainly carbohydrate
>80% VO_2max (sprinting)	Nearly 100% carbohydrate

osteoblast cells responsible for mineralization and formation of bone.

TABLE 16-2

AEROBIC EXERCISES FOR PHYSICAL FITNESS

TYPE OF EXERCISE	AEROBIC FORMS
Ball playing	Handball
	Racquetball
	Squash
Bicycling	Stationary
	Touring
Dancing	Aerobic routines
	Ballet
	Disco
Jumping rope	Brisk pace
Running, jogging	Brisk pace
Skating	Ice skating
	Roller skating
Skiing	Cross-country
Swimming	Steady pace
Walking	Brisk pace

Maintained at aerobic level for at least 30 minutes.

TABLE 16-3

APPROXIMATE ENERGY EXPENDITURE PER HOUR DURING VARIOUS ACTIVITIES

ACTIVITY	KILOCALORIES PER HOUR
Sleeping	63
Lying or sitting, awake	70
Standing, relaxed	84
Rapid typing, sitting	105
Dressing and undressing	140
Walking slowly (24 min/mile)	210
Water aerobics	280
High-impact aerobics	490
Football, flag or touch	560
Walking quickly (12 min/mile)	560
Stair, treadmill	630
Swimming, vigorous effort	700
Running (8 min/mile)	875

For an adult weighing 70 kg (154 lb).

Perhaps the simplest and most popular form of stimulating exercise is *walking*. Figure 16-3 illustrates that aerobic walking can fit into almost anyone's lifestyle. If the pace is fast enough to elevate pulse rate and is maintained for at least the required 30 minutes, walking can be an excellent form of aerobic exercise. It is convenient and requires no equipment other than good walking shoes. Table 16-3 provides information on energy expenditure per pound of body weight per hour for various activities.

Meeting Personal Needs

Health Status and Personal Gains

In planning a personal exercise program, first assess an individual's health status, present level of fitness, personal needs, and resources necessary for equipment or cost. The exercise chosen should be something that is both enjoyable and of aerobic value. Also, start slowly and

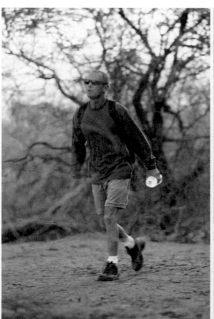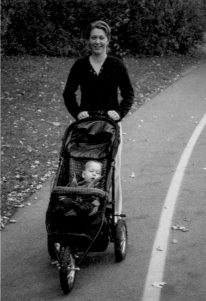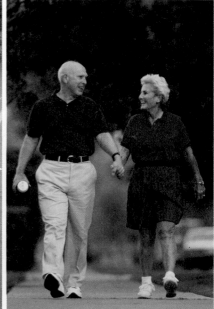

Figure 16-3 Aerobic walking is an exercise that can fit into almost anyone's lifestyle. (*Left and center,* Copyright JupiterImages Corporation; *right,* copyright PhotoDisc.)

build gradually to avoid burnout and injury. Moderation and regularity are the chief guides.

Achieving Aerobic Benefits

To build aerobic capacity, the level of exercise must raise the pulse rate to within 60% to 90% of an individual's maximal *heart rate*. An acceptable way to estimate maximal heart rate is to subtract the person's age from 220. Approximately 70% of this figure is the *target zone rate*, the level to which the pulse hopefully will be raised during exercise (Table 16-4). Check the pulse before the exercise period, then again during and immediately after exercising.

The *Dietary Guidelines for Americans* recommend the following for physical activity[10]:

- To reduce the risk of chronic disease in adulthood, engage in at least 30 minutes of moderate-intensity physical activity, above usual activity at work or home, on most days of the week.
- For most people, greater health benefits can be obtained by engaging in physical activity of more vigorous intensity or longer duration.
- To help manage body weight and prevent gradual, unhealthy weight gain in adulthood, engage in approximately 60 minutes of moderate-intensity to vigorous activity on most days of the week while not exceeding caloric intake requirements.
- To sustain weight loss in adulthood, participate in at least 60 to 90 minutes of daily moderate-intensity physical activity while not exceeding caloric intake requirements. Some people may need to consult a health care provider before participating in this level of activity.

Exercise Preparation and Care

Whatever the choice of exercise, preparation and continuing care are important. Before beginning, a person should warm up his or her muscles to prevent stress or injury and take time to cool down afterward. Do not go beyond tolerance limits; instead, listen to the body. Rest when tired. Stop when hurting. When more challenge is desired, gradually increase the exercise level by number of repetitions, weight intensity, or endurance.

DIETARY NEEDS DURING EXERCISE

Muscle Action and Fuel

Structure and Function

Millions of special cells and fibers make up skeletal muscle mass. These coordinated structures make all physical activity possible. A finely coordinated series of small bundles within the muscle fibers triggered by nerve endings produce a smooth symphony of action through simultaneous and alternating contraction and relaxation

Fuel Sources

Muscle action requires fuel to burn for energy. These fuel sources are the basic energy nutrients (primarily carbohydrate and some fat). Their metabolic products—

TABLE 16-4

TARGET ZONE HEART RATE ACCORDING TO AGE TO ACHIEVE AEROBIC PHYSICAL EFFECT OF EXERCISE

AGE (YEARS)	MAXIMAL ATTAINABLE HEART RATE (PULSE = 220 − AGE)	TARGET ZONE	
		70% MAXIMAL RATE	85% MAXIMAL RATE
20	200	140	170
25	195	136	166
30	190	133	161
35	185	129	157
40	180	126	153
45	175	122	149
50	170	119	144
55	165	115	140
60	160	112	136
65	155	108	132
70	150	105	127
75	145	101	124

glucose, glycogen, and fatty acids—provide ready fuels for immediate, short-, and long-term energy needs. A good diet to meet these needs is essential, whatever the level of physical activity.

Oxygen

The constant supply of oxygen necessary for life becomes even more important during exercise. A person's ability to deliver this vital oxygen to the tissues for energy production determines how much exercise can be done. Aerobic capacity depends on two basic factors: (1) the fitness of the lungs, heart, and blood vessels; and (2) body composition.

Body Fitness. Physical fitness may be defined in terms of aerobic capacity, which is the body's ability to deliver and use oxygen in sufficient quantities to meet the demands of increasing levels of exercise, as measured in terms of VO_2max. The lungs, heart, and blood vessels deliver oxygen to the cells, so their health is essential to overall fitness. Aerobic capacity is measured by the amount of oxygen consumed per kilogram of body weight per minute. To measure VO_2max, an individual must either run on a treadmill or ride a stationary bike to exhaustion while oxygen consumption is measured. As aerobic fitness improves, so does VO_2max.

Body Composition. Body tissues that use more oxygen make up the *lean body mass* (muscle tissue). These tissues are the active metabolic tissues of the body. A person's aerobic capacity depends, in part, on the percentage of body fat and lean body mass. Body composition is determined by the relative amounts of these two components of body weight (see Chapter 15).

Fluid and Energy Needs

Fluid

Dehydration can be a serious problem for athletes and may greatly limit exercise capacity, especially in endurance events.[11,12] Its extent depends on the intensity and duration of the exercise, the surrounding temperature, the level of fitness, and the preexercise or pregame state of hydration. With continued exercise, the body temperature rises because of the release of heat as part of the energy produced. To control this temperature rise, the body sends as much heat as possible to the skin, where it is released in sweat. Over time, and especially in hot weather, this excessive sweating can lead to *dehydration*. To prevent dehydration, water must be frequently replaced. If dehydration continues, athletes may experience problems such as cramps, delirium, vomiting, hypothermia, or hyperthermia. With careful planning for athletic events and providing fluid replacement through-

out, many of these problems can be prevented. Regular fluid intake should be planned for all types of athletes, not just runners. Athletes who are engaged in longer and more demanding endurance events, especially in a warm environment, however, may choose one of the many mild saline and glucose (4% to 8% solution) sports drinks that have rapid gastric emptying and intestinal absorption times (see the For Further Focus box, "Sorting out Sports Drinks").[13]

Energy and Nutrient Stores

Physical activity requires energy in the form of kilocalories. See Table 16-3 for some examples of the amount of kilocalories expended in general activities. Exercise raises the kilocalorie need and helps regulate the appetite to meet this need. For athletes, as well as any active person, proper diet choices are essential for daily energy needs, nutrient reserves, and winning performances. With prolonged exercise, nutrient levels fall too low to sustain the body's continued demands. Fatigue follows, and exhaustion may result. Carbohydrate and fat are the fuels used to maintain these energy reserves; very little energy is drawn from protein (see Table 16-1).

Macronutrient and Micronutrient Recommendations

Nutrient Ratios

Highly active people and some athletes have slightly increased protein requirements when compared with inactive persons, but recommendations for fat intake do not vary from standard guidelines. Carbohydrate is the preferred fuel and is the critical energy source for an active person both before an exercise period and during the recovery period. The complex carbohydrate forms (e.g., starches) sustain energy needs and supply added fiber, vitamins, and minerals. Thus the recommended ratio of energy nutrients to support physical activity is summarized as follows:

- *Carbohydrate:* 45% to 70% of total kilocalories
- *Fat:* 15% to 25% of total kilocalories
- *Protein:* 10% to 35% of total kilocalories

Carbohydrate

The major nutrient used for energy support during exercise is carbohydrate. The carbohydrate energy reserve comes from circulating *blood glucose* and *glycogen* stored in muscle cells and the liver. Athletes competing in prolonged endurance events should increase their energy from carbohydrates to 60% to 70% of their daily total (6 to 10 g/kg body weight).[13] Complex carbohydrates, or starches, are preferable to simple sugars. On the whole, complex starches break down more slowly and help maintain blood sugar

FOR FURTHER FOCUS

SORTING OUT SPORTS DRINKS

Sports drinks developed from the belief that water alone does not meet hydration needs during exercise. Current knowledge, however, states that the ideal fluid to prevent dehydration depends on how demanding the exercise is and how long it lasts.

For nonendurance exercise, physically fit athletes can maintain hydration with plain water. However, long-term endurance athletes need both water and fuel (i.e., carbohydrate), especially in hot weather. For example, without carbohydrate replacement, a long-distance marathon runner would soon run out of muscle glycogen and the ability to use stored fat for energy and "hit the wall" or "bonk." Also, in a demanding run, when the body can sweat as much as 6% of its weight, it cannot keep cool enough and the overall system overheats, leading to heatstroke and collapse. Simply adding table sugar to water causes the water to remain in the stomach longer, where it does nothing for the immediate needs of the body tissues.

The first group of sports drinks began with a solution called *Gatorade*, named by its developers for their university's football team (the University of Florida Gators). They reasoned that if they analyzed their players' sweat, they could appropriately replace lost minerals and water, thus better meeting the needs of athletes than plain water would. The manufacturers also added some flavoring, coloring, and sugars to make it more palatable. Although Gatorade was highly profitable for the university and the manufacturer, subsequent studies have shown that regular nonendurance athletes do not need it. Plain water serves their needs well, and they obtain minerals in their diet.

A second category of sports drinks has been developed to meet both the water and energy needs of athletes in longer lasting endurance events. More dilute 8% sugar solutions, using glucose or glucose polymers (i.e., short chains of approximately five glucose molecules) that are not sweet are being used. In the more dilute solutions, energy-sustaining sugars quickly leave the stomach and provide a continuing fuel and water source for the endurance athlete.

Other products entering the sports drink market have been Gatorade "clones" that claim to add no sugar but supply ample amounts of fructose and glucose in their fruit juice base. Fructose does not leave the stomach rapidly and is absorbed more slowly from the intestine than is glucose, often causing bloating or diarrhea. Still other products add multiple vitamins (yielding substantially more than the RDA in a single 10-oz bottle) to their fruit juice base but contain no minerals. These vitamins do not help performance, and on a hot day a sweating athlete can easily down a megadose in four or five bottles.

Be sure to sort out the claims of sports drinks; they are not for everyone. Furthermore, several functional foods (food components with physiologic actions) are marketed specifically to athletes as performance enhancers. Examples include the addition of citric acid, branched-chain amino acids, creatine, caffeine, carnitine, antioxidants, glutamine, and arginine to drinks or foods. Scientific evidence exists for beneficial physiologic function for some of these components, but most do not yet have evidence indicating efficacy.* In the long run, sports drinks meet the needs of athletes in endurance events. For nonendurance activities, however, most persons do not need them. After all, water is the best solution for regular needs and costs far less.

*Wataru A and others: Exercise and functional foods, *Nutr J* 5:15, 2006.

---

levels more evenly, avoiding high and low blood sugar spikes. Starches also are more readily converted to glycogen to maintain this store of constant primary fuel.

Simple sugars, on the other hand, are less efficient at maintaining the body's glycogen stores and are more easily converted to fat for storage. Simple sugars also trigger a sharper insulin response, contributing to the dangers of rebound hypoglycemia. However, simple carbohydrates can supply immediate energy sources for athletes engaging in endurance events for which a continued dietary source of glucose is needed.

Recent studies have shown that low-carbohydrate diets hinder exercise performance.[14] This is due to reduced glucose deposit in skeletal muscle when following a low-carbohydrate diet.[15] Over time, a low-carbohydrate diet decreases the body's capacity for work. Conversely, a high-carbohydrate diet restores glycogen concentrations to their regular levels. Athletes on a low-carbohydrate diet

are susceptible to fatigue, ketoacidosis, dehydration, and hypoglycemia. However, athletes given carbohydrate feedings before and during exercise maintain glucose concentrations and rates of glucose oxidation necessary to exercise strenuously and thus are able to delay fatigue.[16]

Fat

In the presence of oxygen, *fatty acids* serve as a fuel source from stored fat tissue. No evidence supports improved physical performance with dietary fat intake greater than

---

aerobic capacity requiring oxygen to proceed; milliliters of oxygen consumed per kilogram of body weight per minute, as influenced by body composition.

hypoglycemia an abnormally low blood sugar level that may lead to muscle tremors, cold sweat, headache, and confusion.

30% of the total daily energy intake. The essential fatty acids, *linoleic acid* and *linolenic acid*, are important for regulating the inflammatory process evoked by heavy exertion during exercise.

The relative use of stored fat for energy during exercise depends on the level of fitness of the person and the exercise intensity. Trained endurance athletes are more efficient at using fat for energy than are their untrained counterparts. However, the use of fat for energy declines as the exercise intensity increases above approximately 70% VO_2max, at which point the body becomes more reliant on glucose utilization for immediate energy (see Table 16-1).[17] Mild- or moderate-intensity exercise, at 25% to 65% VO_2max, increases fatty acid oxidation by fivefold to tenfold more than resting oxidation levels.

Protein

Dietary protein has only a small role as a fuel substrate in energy production during exercise. Although a number of amino acids can feed into the Kreb's cycle, authorities agree that under normal circumstances protein makes a relatively insignificant contribution to energy during exercise. Therefore no more than the usual adult requirement is needed to meet general protein needs of a healthy, physically active adult. However, evidence shows that endurance and strength-trained athletes, specifically, may require as much as 1.2 to 1.7 g protein per kilogram of body weight.[13]

Protein recommendations, even for athletes, usually can be met through the diet alone. The national average for protein intake is 14.7% of total calories and within the general recommendations.[18] Furthermore, excess consumption from whole protein or amino acid supplements may put a taxing load on the kidneys, which can contribute to dehydration because the excess nitrogen must be excreted.

Vitamins and Minerals

Vitamins and minerals cannot be used as fuel. They are not oxidized or used in the energy production process. They are essential in this process but only as a part of needed coenzymes (see Chapters 7 and 8). Increased physical exertion during exercise or athletic training does not require a greater intake of vitamins and minerals beyond currently recommended intakes. A well-balanced diet supplies adequate amounts of vitamins and minerals, and exercise may improve the body's efficient use of them. Because athletes, for example, have an increased dietary need for energy, a larger kilocalorie intake from nutrient-dense foods would automatically boost their general intake of vitamins and minerals.

Multivitamin and mineral supplementation does not improve physical performance in healthy athletes eating a well-balanced diet, and the potential side effects from megavitamin supplements are well known. However, therapeutic iron supplements may be necessary for some

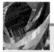

DRUG-NUTRIENT INTERACTION

IRON SUPPLEMENTATION

Body iron stores are determined by testing the following blood indexes:

- *Hemoglobin:* a protein structure that contains iron needed for oxygen transport
- *Hematocrit:* the proportion of RBCs to total blood volume
- *Ferritin:* a protein that stores iron for later use

Improved dietary intake of foods high in iron or iron supplementation is warranted when blood iron indexes are below normal levels. Adolescents and female athletes are at high risk for developing iron deficiency. This can be attributed to iron loss during the menstrual cycle, excessive sweat loss, hemolysis, and inadequate amounts of iron in the diet to meet the needs for growth.

When iron supplements are prescribed, the following precautions should be taken:

- Iron supplements may cause nausea, vomiting, and constipation. Taking the supplement with meals and drinking plenty of fluids can help alleviate side effects.
- Iron and calcium compete for absorption. Avoid taking iron supplements with milk or any other calcium-containing products.

- Iron also competes with other metals, such as zinc and copper, for absorption. These minerals are needed in smaller amounts than calcium but should still be considered. Normal levels of iron found in foods pose an insignificant competition with other metals for absorption. Megadoses can negatively affect absorption, however.
- Ascorbic acid, or vitamin C, aids in iron absorption. This can be useful when eating iron-rich foods (e.g., beef liver, clams, lima beans). Meals high in both ascorbic acid and iron should be encouraged.

Sports anemia, as it has come to be called, can show a false need for iron supplementation. When an athlete begins an exercise program, he or she may have low hemoglobin for a time because of the rapid expansion of blood volume. However, the athlete is not truly anemic, and hemoglobin values will return to normal once the body adjusts to the new lifestyle. Iron supplementation is not necessary and could be harmful in this case.

Sara Oldroyd

athletes who have iron-deficiency anemia (see the Drug-Nutrient Interaction box, "Iron Supplementation"). Also, special assessment of nutrient-energy status is needed for young adolescent amenorrheic female athletes. Chronic negative energy balance is not uncommon in athletes such as gymnasts, ballet dancers, and runners, who also may suffer from eating disorders such as anorexia nervosa. Disordered eating patterns may involve low calcium intake, which can have serious consequences for bone development (see the Clinical Applications box, "The Female Athlete Triad: How Performance and Social Pressure Can Lead to Low Bone Mass").[19]

---

amenorrheic state of having absences or an abnormal cessation of menses.

CLINICAL APPLICATIONS

THE FEMALE ATHLETE TRIAD: HOW PERFORMANCE AND SOCIAL PRESSURE CAN LEAD TO LOW BONE MASS

The female athlete triad consists of three health afflictions faced by women who are extremely physically active: disordered eating, menstrual disturbances and irregularity, and osteopenia (low bone mass) or osteoporosis. Low bone mineral density (BMD) often is the final result of the triad that affects women, and it is the leading cause of stress fractures and injuries throughout the body, some of which may be irreversible. Many women who are in top physical form are ironically the most likely to develop these three linked complications and health problems because social and performance pressure may steer them to extreme eating habits and exercise regimens. The dilemma facing female athletes today is how to maintain optimal physical performance while not tampering with health risks.

Women who participate in competitive sports that require endurance, such as rowing or long-distance running, or who are judged partially on physical appearance, such as in ice skating, diving, or dancing, are more likely to be preoccupied with their weight and have self-image issues. Social and competitive pressure for a woman to be thin can contribute to her sense of imperfection. These demands and pressures can lead some women to develop disordered eating patterns that, in combination with strenuous exercise, result in low energy levels. This drop in energy will be followed by a drop in performance as the athlete loses focus and concentration and is fatigued. Some women develop extreme dietary conditions, such as bulimia nervosa, which is characterized by binge eating followed by forced vomiting, purging, or excessive laxative intake, or anorexia nervosa, which is characterized by the refusal or inability to consume sufficient calories for daily requirements. These more serious disorders can progress to psychological problems (depression or low self-esteem), seizures, cardiac arrhythmia, myocardial infarction, and other health complications. The seriousness of the eating disorder is linked to the amount of stress and concern the woman feels over her body image combined with the amount of emphasis put on weight by trainers, coaches, and instructors. Athletes often believe that leanness enhances performance, and some are willing to take health risks to satisfy perfectionist needs and habits.

Poor caloric intake and disordered eating can cause menstrual irregularity. Amenorrhea is the suppression of menstrual cycles to a level of zero to three menses a year, and primary amenorrhea is the repression of all menstrual cycles until the age of 16 years. This condition is often found in young female gymnasts who, in the most competitive circles, may strive to delay the onset of puberty to maintain small, childlike physiques. Some women may have oligomenorrhea instead, which are sporadic cycles that occur 3 to 9 times a year. The levels of estrogen and progesterone that regulate menses can be affected by metabolism, intensive exercise, dieting, or stress.

Several treatments are available for female athletes: sex steroid replacement, increased caloric intake, decreased exercise, weight gain, and calcium supplements. Evidence suggests that raising estrogen and progesterone levels and increasing calorie intake are the most effective measures. Education and further research are needed to find the optimal course.

Menstrual irregularities are related to low BMD. Bone density reaches its peak before the age of 30 years; young women must strive for dense bones in early adulthood to have healthy bone density later in life. If the density of bones is diminished early, osteopenia occurs and, if severe enough, can be a signal of future osteoporosis. The bone loss in all areas is not permanent, but bone loss in the vertebrae of the spine seems to be irreversible. Although women who were once athletes seem to recover some of their BMD loss, vertebral bone normalization is uncommon. Active young women with tightly regulated diets and menstrual inconsistency can have a BMD as low as that of a 70-year-old woman. These thin bones increase the likelihood of stress fractures and injuries, and women are far more likely to incur such injuries than are men.

Some studies, however, indicate that weight-bearing activities, such as gymnastics, seem to improve BMD, even perhaps in vertebrae, and may help prevent density decreases later in life. Yet the problem facing female athletes who eat improperly is that the rate of decline in BMD intensifies as menstrual cycles continue to be erratic. The longer the menstrual cycles are inconsistent, the sooner BMD is lost. Weight-bearing sports will not overcome the tendency toward low BMD if diet and exercise levels are not carefully monitored.

The best course of action is to have female athletes monitor their diet to include adequate caloric intake and sufficient micronutrient consumption. The prevention of osteoporosis later in life lies in the habits of the individual and the modification of factors that can lead to the triad of eating disturbances, menstrual irregularity, and low BMD. Body weight is individual, depending on height and skeletal

CLINICAL APPLICATIONS

THE FEMALE ATHLETE TRIAD: HOW PERFORMANCE AND SOCIAL PRESSURE CAN LEAD TO LOW BONE MASS—cont'd

structure, and not one specific weight goal should be promoted for all female athletes.

However, the societal and competitive pressures that cause the initial step in this three-step process also must be addressed. Asking female athletes to sacrifice their health for an unrealistic image projected on them and the need for vicarious victory must not dominate the standards of acceptable eating habits. In today's weight-conscious society, the emphasis must not be on a perfect image, size, or body but rather on the perfect balance of health and training. The female athlete's skeletal integrity suffers as she resorts to drastic measures in her aspiration for a perfect lean physical image, but her male athlete counterpart has no such risk because his BMD does not depend on menstrual regularity.

The need now is to educate trainers, athletes, and health professionals about the consequences of neglected nutrition. No single image of the perfect female body should be promoted, and young female athletes must understand that deprivation of life's essential nutrients ultimately does more harm than good.

Meredith Catherine Williams

References

Iacopino L and others: Body composition differences in adolescent female athletes and anorexic patients, *Acta Diabetol* 40(1 suppl):S180, 2003.

Kerstetter JE and others: Dietary protein, calcium metabolism, and skeletal homeostasis revisited, *Am J Clin Nutr* 78(3 suppl):584S, 2003.

Lloyd T and others: Lifestyle factors and the development of bone mass and bone strength in young women, *J Pediatr* 144(6):776, 2004.

Miller KK: Mechanisms by which nutritional disorders cause reduced bone mass in adults, *J Womens Health* 12(2):145, 2003.

Thrash LE, Anderson JJB: The female athlete triad: nutrition, menstrual disturbances, and low bone mass, *Nutr Today* 35(5):168, 2000.

Zeni AI and others: Stress injury to the bone among women athletes, *Phys Med Rehabil Clin N Am* 11(4):929, 2000.

Reprinted from Schlenker ED, Long S: *Williams' essentials of nutrition & diet therapy,* ed 9, St Louis, 2007, Mosby.

ATHLETIC PERFORMANCE

General Training Diet

All individuals who exercise regularly (especially athletes in training) must apply the general principles of exercise and energy previously described. Athletes involved in heavy training are more susceptible to immunosuppression because of the extreme demands placed on the body. A well-balanced diet with plenty of carbohydrates and protein from a variety of foods helps prevent exercise-induced malnutrition and risk for injury and infection.[20]

Carbohydrate

Moderate to high amounts, 5 to 7 g/kg body weight per day of carbohydrate, are needed to support general training. Endurance athletes have higher needs: 7 to 10 g/kg body weight per day. Female endurance athletes are the least likely group to achieve such dietary recommendations despite evidence supporting enhanced performance from high carbohydrate intakes.

Fat

Dietary fat is needed to meet energy needs, supply essential fatty acids, and maintain weight. No performance benefit occurs from consuming a diet less than 15% or greater than 30% fat. Fat delays the emptying of the stomach and does not contribute to the glycogen stores needed during exercise. Therefore a high-fat meal before a workout or competition could hinder performance.

Protein

Protein should make up the remainder of the diet (approximately 10% to 35% total kilocalories or 1.2 to 1.7 g/kg body weight per day for highly active endurance or strength trainers). Similar to fat, protein slows the rate of emptying in the stomach and thus should not be consumed in high quantities immediately before a workout or competition. Muscle recovery is optimal after a strenuous workout, and protein intake during this time is most beneficial.

Total Energy

Athletes need varying amounts of energy, depending on body size and the type of training or competition involved. A small woman may need approximately 1800 kcal/day to sustain body weight and normal daily activities, whereas a larger, muscular man may need 3000 kcal/day. Consider these basic requirements and add the extra energy needed for a given sport. For example, endurance bicycle races in mountainous areas may require an additional 2000 to 3000 kcal/day. Thus some athletes in training may require as many as 5000 to 7000 kcal/day simply to maintain their weight. A well-planned individual program is necessary.

Athletes should consume a variety of foods, such as represented in the My Pyramid guideline (Figure 1-1).

Many choices and portions from the starch and fruit groups replace glycogen losses from the previous day's workouts and provide adequate glycogen stores in the muscles. Box 16-1 gives carbohydrate values for selected foods to use in planning an athlete's low-fat, moderate-protein, and high-carbohydrate diet.

BOX 16-1

GRAMS OF CARBOHYDRATE IN ONE SERVING OF COMMON FOODS

CARBOHYDRATE GROUP

Starches

Bread; cereals and grains; starchy vegetables; crackers and snacks; beans, peas, and lentils; starchy foods prepared with fat. One serving (as follows) contains 15 g carbohydrate:

- ½ cup wheat bran cereal
  ⅓ cup couscous
  1½ cups puffed cereal
  ½ cup grits
- ⅓ cup rice, white or brown
  ½ cup bulgur
  ⅓ cup pasta
- ⅓ cup baked beans
- ½ cup refried beans, canned
- ½ cup beans and peas (black, garbanzo, pinto, kidney, white, lima, navy, split, black-eyed)
  ½ cup lentils (brown, green, yellow)
- ½ cup green peas
- 1 cup winter squash (acorn, butternut)
  ½ cup yam, sweet potato, plain
  1 small (3 oz) potato, boiled
  1 cup (2 oz) French fries (oven baked)
  ¼ (1 oz) bagel
  1 chapatti, 6 inches across
  ½ English muffin
  1 (1 oz) slice bread (white, whole grain, pumpernickel, rye, unfrosted raisin)
  ½ (1 oz) hot dog bun or hamburger bun
- 1 (1½ oz) cube of cornbread
  ¼ naan, 8 inches by 2 inches
- 1 waffle, 4 inches across
  1 pancake, 4 inches across
- 2 taco shells, 5 inches across
  1 tortilla, corn, 6 inches across
  1 tortilla, flour, 6 inches across
- 1 biscuit, 2½ inches across
  ½ pita, 6 inches across

Fruits

One serving (as follows) contains 15 g carbohydrate:
  1 (4 oz) apple, unpeeled, small
- 4 whole (5½ oz) apricots, fresh

  1 (4 oz) banana, extra small
  ½ (4 oz) pear, large, fresh
- 1¼ cup strawberries, whole
  12 (3 oz) cherries, sweet, fresh
  17 (3 oz) grapes, small
  ½ (11 oz) grapefruit, large
  1 (5 oz) nectarine, small
- 1 (6½ oz) orange, small
  1 (4 oz) peach, large, fresh
  1 slice (13½ oz) of 1¼ cup cubes of watermelon
  2 (5 oz) plums, small
  ½ cup apple juice or cider
  ⅓ cup fruit juice blends, 100% juice
  ½ cup orange juice
  ½ cup grapefruit juice

Milk

One serving (as follows) contains 12 g carbohydrate:
  1 cup fat-free, 1%, or 2% milk
  ⅔ cup plain low-fat yogurt

Other Carbohydrates

One serving (as follows) contains 15 g carbohydrate:
  Cake, frosted, 2-inch square
  Cake, unfrosted, 2-inch square
  3 gingersnaps
  5 Vanilla Wafers
  2 small cookies or sandwich cookies with crème filling
  ½ cup light ice cream
  ½ cup sherbet or sorbet
  1 meal replacement bar (1⅓ oz)
  1 granola bar

Vegetables

Carrots, asparagus, beans (green, wax, Italian), beets, broccoli, cauliflower, onions, spinach, summer squash, greens (collard, kale, mustard, turnip), cucumbers, turnips.

One serving (as follows) has 5 g:
  ½ cup cooked vegetables
  1 cup raw vegetables
  ½ cup vegetable juice

Modified from American Dietetic Association, American Diabetes Association: *Choose your foods: exchange lists for diabetes,* Chicago/Alexandria, VA, 2007, American Dietetic Association, American Diabetes Association.

- More than 3 grams of dietary fiber per serving.
- Extra fat, or prepared with added fat. (Add an extra fat choice.)
- 480 milligrams or more of sodium per serving.

Competition

Carbohydrate Loading

To prepare for an athletic event, especially an endurance event, athletes sometimes follow a dietary process called *carbohydrate* or *glycogen loading* (see the For Further Focus box, "Carbohydrate Loading for Endurance"). The current practice, which has been modified from earlier, more stressful plans, takes place the week before the event. The protocol includes a moderate, gradual tapering of exercise while increasing total carbohydrate intake in the diet (Table 16-5).

Pregame Meal

The ideal pregame meal depends on the tolerance of the athlete. It usually is a light meal eaten 3 to 4 hours before the event. This meal should be high in complex carbohydrates (approximately 200 to 300 g carbohydrate) and relatively low in protein, with little fat or fiber.[13] This schedule gives the body time to digest, absorb, and transform the meal into stored glycogen. Good food choices include pasta, bread, bagels, muffins, and cereal with non-fat milk. Box 16-2 outlines a sample pregame meal.

Hydration

Dehydration can be a serious problem for athletes. Fluid needs depend on (1) the intensity and duration of the exercise; (2) the surrounding temperature, altitude, and humidity; (3) fitness level; and (4) the pregame or preexercise state of hydration. The thirst mechanism cannot keep up with the loss of water during exercise; therefore, to prevent dehydration, athletes are advised to drink more water than they think they need (Figure 16-4). In addition to water loss (as much as 1.5 L/hr), sweat also contains a relatively large amount of sodium and small amounts of other minerals (e.g., potassium, iron, and calcium).

Athletes are recommended to drink 6 to 12 oz of fluid every 15 to 20 minutes during athletic events. A number of sports drinks with added sugar, electrolytes, and flavorings have been marketed, but questions have been raised about their use or misuse (see the For Further Focus box, "Sorting out Sports Drinks"). Except for endurance events lasting longer than 1 hour, plain water usually is the rehydration fluid of choice. Electrolytes

FOR FURTHER FOCUS

CARBOHYDRATE LOADING FOR ENDURANCE

Glycogen is the body storage form of carbohydrate designed to provide an immediate source of backup fuel and protect blood glucose levels during the fasting hours of sleep. Glycogen is restored with each day's food intake, but during heavy exercise normal glycogen stores are quickly used and the person reaches the point of exhaustion.

During the 1960s trainers and coaches began to explore ways of avoiding this state of exhaustion in their athletes during endurance events. They reasoned that if the athletes exercised heavily and ate a low-carbohydrate diet for 3 days to use the stored glycogen, and then only exercised lightly and ate a high-carbohydrate diet for the next 3 days, their

glycogen stores would become supersaturated, enabling them to perform at a higher level. When this practice was tested, the increase in glycogen stores in muscle and the athletes' performance was nearly twice their former workload.

This practice has become known as *carbohydrate* or *glycogen loading* and is specifically designed for endurance athletes. Today a less-stressful, modified process of tapered depletion is used to prevent possible injury to muscle tissue. This method can be used more often than the previously used schedule and is more productive in the long run (see Table 16-5).

TABLE 16-5

PRECOMPETITION PROGRAM FOR CARBOHYDRATE LOADING

DAY	EXERCISE	DIET
1	90-min period at 70%-75% VO_2max	Mixed diet, 5 g carbohydrate/kg body weight
2-3	Gradual tapering of time and intensity: ~40-min period	Same as day 1
4-5	Continuation of tapering: ~20-min period	Mixed diet, 10 g carbohydrate/kg body weight
6	Complete rest	Same as days 4-5
7	Day of competition	High-carbohydrate preevent meal

Modified from Coleman EJ: Carbohydrate and exercise. In Dunford M, editor: *Sports nutrition: a practice manual for professionals*, ed 4, Chicago, 2006, The American Dietetic Association.

BOX 16-2

SAMPLE PREGAME MEAL

The following sample pregame meal includes approximately 320 kcal; high complex carbohydrates; and low protein, fat, and fiber:

- ¾ cup spaghetti (150 kcal, 30 g carbohydrate)
- ¼ cup tomato sauce (23 kcal, 4.5 g carbohydrate)
- 1 slice French bread, small (88 kcal, 17 g carbohydrate)
- ½ cup apple juice (58 kcal, 15 g carbohydrate)

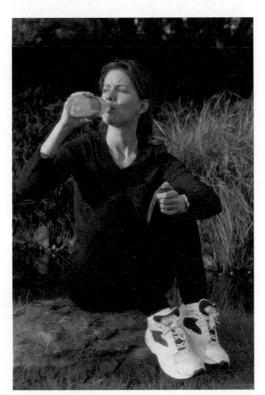

Figure 16-4 Frequent small drinks of cold water during extended exercise prevent dehydration. (Copyright Photo-Disc.)

are replaced during the athlete's next meal. For events lasting longer than 1 hour, beverages containing 4% to 8% glucose concentrations and 0.5 to 0.7 g/L sodium are recommended.[13]

Energy during Exercise

For activities lasting less than 1 hour, most athletes do not need exogenous sources of energy during the exercise period. However, performance is enhanced during longer endurance events with the interval consumption of carbohydrates. The American College of Sports Medicine, the ADA, and the Dietitians of Canada recommend eat-

ing or drinking 0.7 g of carbohydrate per kilogram of body weight per hour (approximately 30 to 60 g/hr) during long events.[13] Consuming equal amounts of the preferred food every 15 to 20 minutes throughout the event is ideal rather than consuming the entire 30 to 60 g at once. Athletes should experiment with various forms of glucose before competition to determine what is best tolerated. A large variety of sports drinks, gels, and other forms of carbohydrates are available for the athlete to choose from. The food of choice should provide carbohydrates primarily from glucose, with little or no fat, protein, or fiber.

Energy after Exercise: Recovery

Proper nutrition is important to the athlete before and during exercise and also plays a major role in recovery after the event. Fluid and carbohydrate replacement beverages consumed immediately after a glycogen-depleting endurance event result in higher glycogen synthesis and muscle recovery than if replacement beverages are delayed for 2 hours or more.[13] Beverages of 6% glucose concentration are adequate during this period, but higher concentrations may be consumed depending on the tolerance of the athlete. For athletes taking only a short break in between events (e.g., triathletes), foods and beverages ingested should primarily be limited to simple carbohydrate-containing substances. However, for athletes recovering for longer periods, a replacement beverage containing 0.8 g of carbohydrate per kilogram body weight results in a greater rate of muscle glycogen recovery.[21]

Ergogenic Aids

Since ancient times athletes have been seeking and experimenting with "magic" substances or treatments to gain the competitive edge. Today these substances are known as ergogenic aids (Table 16-6). Most are worthless fads, but one current practice, the use of steroids, is of great concern because it is dangerous and, in competitive sports, illegal. The use of steroids is widespread among athletes and body builders, sometimes starting as early as high school or even junior high school. Steroids are synthetic sex hormones that have two actions: (1) *anabolic* (tissue growth), and (2) *androgenic* (masculinization). Athletes have been known to take steroids in megadoses—

ergogenic the tendency to increase work output; various substances that increase work or exercise capacity and output.

steroids the group name for lipid-based sterols, including hormones, bile acids, and cholesterol.

TABLE 16-6

ERGOGENIC AIDS IN ATHLETES

PROHIBITED CLASSES OF SUBSTANCES	HOW SUBSTANCE HAS BEEN USED BY ATHLETES (SPORT EXAMPLE)	MECHANISM OF ACTION AND EFFECTS	ADVERSE EFFECTS
Stimulants, amphetamines	CNS stimulant Reduce fatigue Improve reaction times Increase alertness and aggression (endurance sports)	Release: various neurotransmitters Inhibition: uptake of neurotransmitter Direct impact: neurotransmitter receptors Inhibition: monamine oxidase activity	Milder doses: insomnia, irritability, tremor, increase in aggressive behavior, restlessness Higher doses: tachycardia, sweating, arrhythmias, higher blood pressure; can impede ability to reduce body temperature Chronic use: danger of amphetamine psychosis Abuse in endurance sports: contribute to heatstroke
Sympathomimetics (over-the-counter decongestants)	Create vasoconstriction and higher blood pressure (milder), CNS effects (see above) (aid in fat loss, such as ephedrine use by female body builders and in endurance sports)	Activation of α_1 adrenoreceptors in vascular smooth muscle, decrease in mucus secretion Effects on CNS, similar to amphetamines but weaker (see above)	Headache, dizziness, hypertension, irritability, some anxiety tachycardia Higher doses: mania or psychosis, possible cerebral hemorrhage or stroke
Caffeine	Delay of fatigue by enhancing muscle contractility Enhance performance on short, intense periods of exercise Sparing of muscle glycogen levels (various sport activities, endurance sports)	(Milder) CNS effects Antagonist of adenosine receptors Inhibits phosphodiesterase-type enzymes, resulting in activation of cAMP, link between receptor activity and cell response	Mild: insomnia, irritability, GI disturbances More severe: peptic ulcer, seizure, coma, arrhythmias, hallucinations, death
Cocaine	Possible distortion of perception of enhanced performance and reduced strength (ergogenic effects in sport are inconclusive; accumulation more likely from recreational use by athletes)	Includes inhibition of various neurotransmitters, such as dopamine	Note: complex pharmacology Hypertension, seizures, psychosis, negative impact on glycogenolysis, myocardial toxicity/intense exercise (possible ischemia, arrhythmias, sudden death)
Agonists (β_2)	Improve activities that depend on aerobic function Promote muscle growth Reduction in body fat Used as alternative to anabolic steroids (see p. 313) (Endurance sports, sports with an "appearance" aspect, such as weight lifting)	Bronchodilation (also used for asthma) by stimulation of β_2 adrenoreceptors in respiratory tract (smooth muscle) Also anabolic effect (see below) Higher doses: stimulate β_1 adrenoreceptors (with side effects)	β_2 adrenoreceptors: higher doses allow β_1 adrenoreceptor stimulation At higher doses: β_1 adrenoreceptor stimulation: hand tremor, tachycardia, arrhythmias, insomnia, headache, nausea Anabolic effects (related to high dose): example of clenbuterol myalgia, dizziness, nausea, periorbital pain, and/or asthenia (see below)
Narcotics	Pain reliever (Variable use across athletic activities)	Interaction with brain receptors sensitive to endorphin transmitters (also affect emotions)	Absence of pain could exacerbate underlying or mask new condition High doses: coma and stupor, possible lethal from respiratory depression Withdrawal symptoms from dependence: sweating, nausea, insomnia, anxiety, aching muscles More severe: cardiovascular collapse

TABLE 16-6

ERGOGENIC AIDS IN ATHLETES—cont'd

PROHIBITED CLASSES OF SUBSTANCES	HOW SUBSTANCE HAS BEEN USED BY ATHLETES (SPORT EXAMPLE)	MECHANISM OF ACTION AND EFFECTS	ADVERSE EFFECTS
Anabolic androgenic steroids	Improve lean body mass and strength Reduction of body fat Relative to training, enhance recovery time, promote energy and aggressive performance Concomitant drugs (hGH, hCG) have been taken to enhance anabolic effects or to minimize adverse effects (diuretics, opiates, among others) or maximize intensity of training (added stimulant) No solid evidence to support above practices (strength-dependent and endurance sports)	Act on endogenous androgen receptors Increase protein synthesis Antagonist to glucocorticoid hormones/anticatabolic effect Tissue building/anabolic effect Virilizing/androgenic effect	Majority are minor and reversible after cessation Incidence of serious effects are catastrophic but low Long-term effects generally unknown Broad classes: masculinization and gynecomastia (cosmetic effects); liver abnormalities: dysfunction, tumor; infection/injection techniques: hepatitis mycobacterial, HIV/AIDS; cardiovascular: may increase risk of atherosclerosis; reproductive: atrophy of testicles, decreased sperm production; psychiatric/psychological: mood swings, depression and mania/hypomania
Diuretics	No sport-enhancing effects Reduce weight Manage fluid retention Increase urine to dilute other doping agents	Effect on kidney resulting in excessive loss of fluid	Use during exercise produces harmful effects Hypohydration: electrolyte disturbances can compromise the muscles and heart Side effects can worsen if accompanied by fatigue and/or glycogen production
hGH	Increases muscle mass Spares muscle glycogen More intense training may be possible Quicker recovery after training (no support for enhanced performance)	Polypeptide hormone of pituitary gland Activates growth hormone receptors to allow the production of insulinlike growth factor-1 with anabolic effects	Adverse effects in sport are not well evidenced because of short-term substance use, in which effects and features of acromegaly do not occur
Erythropoietin	Increases oxygen capacity of RBCs An alternative to blood doping (endurance sports)	Glycoprotein hormone manufactured mostly in kidney Endogenous production influenced by a decrease in oxygen to the kidney Result: increased number of RBCs produced from bone marrow and increased rate of RBCs into blood circulation	Little published research on substance and athletes In patient use: headaches, flulike symptoms, joint pain (all of which appear to resolve) Abuse risk involves too high a hematocrit; an increase in hematocrit occurs that increases blood viscosity, a state that can be exacerbated by dehydration, possibly viscosity syndrome (hypertension, decreased output, possible heart failure) At a certain level of increased hematocrit, a risk of cerebral or coronary occlusion
Peptide hormones, mimetics, and analogues	Acquire substances that provoke other agents that have ergogenic attributes, such as testosterone with its effects or those that increase muscle tissue (variety of activities)	hCG and luteinizing hormone provoke testosterone release Insulin may ease glucose entry into cells and promote bulking of muscle tissue	Little published research in sports Information becomes constrained to studies of individual agent effects (e.g., hCG may produce symptoms of fatigue, headache, and mood swings) No published reports of adverse effects of insulin use in sports

cAMP, Cyclic adenosine monophosphate; *hGH*, human growth hormone; *hCG*, human chorionic gonadotropin.
Reprinted from Bernstein A, Safirstein J, Rosen JE: Athletic ergogenic aids, *Bull Hosp Jt Dis* 61(3-4):164, 2003.

10 to 30 times their normal body hormonal output—to increase muscle size, strength, and performance. However, the physiologic side effects can be devastating, such as masculinization and gynecomastia; liver abnormalities such as dysfunction, tumor, and hepatitis; increase risk of atherosclerosis; and atrophy of testicles and decreased sperm production. Psychological effects vary from mood swings to depression and mania or hypomania.[22] Many professional athletes confront the hard choice of not using steroids while facing a field of opponents who are using them or of using the drugs and risking the side effects and potential disqualification.

Misinformation

Athletes and their coaches are particularly susceptible to claims and myths about foods and dietary supplements. All athletes, particularly those involved in highly competitive sports, constantly search for the competitive edge. Knowing this, manufacturers sometimes make distorted or false claims regarding their products. In addition, the world of athletics holds numerous superstitions and myths about food and nutrients, including the following:

- Athletes need protein for energy.
- Protein supplements are needed to build bigger and stronger muscles.
- Vitamin supplements are needed to enable athletes to use more energy.
- Vitamins and minerals are burned up in workouts and training sessions.
- Electrolyte solutions are *always* needed during exercise to replace losses from sweat.
- A pregame meal of steak and eggs ensures maximal performance.
- Drinking water during exercise causes cramps.

Health care providers should be familiar with common fads and myths circulating in the community. Understanding these myths is important, as is knowing how to approach them and what to recommend as an effective alternative.

masculinization condition marked by the attainment of male characteristics, such as facial hair, either physiologically as part of male maturation or pathologically by either sex.

gynecomastia excessive development of the male mammary gland; frequently a result of increased estrogen levels.

SUMMARY

Many fine muscle fibers and cells, triggered by nerve endings, work together to make physical activity possible. Carbohydrate, mainly in the form of complex-carbohydrate foods or starches, is the primary fuel for energy to run this system. Carbohydrate metabolism yields circulating blood glucose and stored glycogen in muscles and the liver for fuel. Stored body fat supplies additional fuel as fatty acids while protein provides insignificant energy for exercise. Vitamins and minerals cannot be burned for energy but are important parts of coenzymes for the process of energy production.

Activities of daily living, aerobic exercises, and resistance training have many benefits that increase with practice. Excellent aerobic exercises include sustained fast walking, swimming, jogging, running, and aerobic dancing or similar workouts. Resistance training increases muscle strength, a direct influence on metabolic rate and bone density.

Exercise increases the need for energy and water. Water in small, frequent amounts generally is the best way to avoid dehydration. Electrolytes lost in sweat are replaced in the next meal. The optimal diet for athletes is approximately 60% of the kilocalories from carbohydrate (mainly complex starches), 25% from fat, and 15% from protein. During the week before an athletic event, especially an endurance event, athletes may practice carbohydrate loading to meet the energy demands of competition. However, pregame meals should contain small, mainly complex carbohydrates (starches), with little fat, protein, or fiber.

CRITICAL THINKING QUESTIONS

1. What is the primary role of each energy nutrient (carbohydrates, fats, protein) in terms of fuel for exercise?
2. Outline the nutrition and physical fitness principles you would discuss with a client who is an athlete. Plan a diet for this person that meets nutrient and energy needs.
3. Why is fluid balance vital during exercise periods? How are water and electrolyte balance achieved?
4. Describe the health benefits of exercise for a person with heart disease and a person with hypertension. Also describe the benefits of exercise for an overweight person with type 2 diabetes.
5. Describe several factors to consider when planning a personal exercise program. Define the term aerobic exercise and list its benefits.

CHAPTER CHALLENGE QUESTIONS

True-False

Write the correct statement for each statement that is false.

1. *True or False:* Sports drinks containing electrolytes and sugar are the best way to replace fluids lost during short bouts of exercise, such as a 30-minute jog.
2. *True or False:* Drinking water immediately before and during an athletic event causes cramps.
3. *True or False:* Carbohydrate-containing sports drinks are best absorbed from the stomach when in glucose concentrations of 4% to 8%.
4. *True or False:* Athletes need protein for extra energy.
5. *True or False:* Vitamins and minerals are burned for energy in workouts and training sessions.
6. *True or False:* Protein and fat do not contribute to glycogen stores.
7. *True or False:* Sweating is the main mechanism for dissipating body heat.
8. *True or False:* Aerobic exercise is of limited benefit in controlling heart disease and diabetes.
9. *True or False:* Walking can be an excellent form of aerobic exercise.

Multiple Choice

1. Which of the following activities is most likely to provide aerobic exercise?
   a. Golf
   b. Swimming
   c. Gardening
   d. Baseball
2. To develop aerobic capacity, an exercise should
   a. raise the pulse to 50% of the maximal heart rate.
   b. be maintained for alternating 10-minute periods.
   c. be practiced consistently every day.
   d. be practiced several times a week at an appropriate pulse rate for sustained periods.
3. Characteristics of a healthful exercise program should include which of the following? *(Circle all that apply.)*
   a. Enjoyable activities
   b. Moderation
   c. Regularity
   d. Going beyond tolerance limits
4. Exercise is beneficial in weight management because it serves which of the following purposes? *(Circle all that apply.)*
   a. Helps regulate appetite
   b. Decreases BMR
   c. Reduces stress-related eating
   d. Increases the set point for fat deposit
5. Which of the following meals is the best choice for an athlete's pregame meal?
   a. Large grilled steak, fried potatoes, ice cream
   b. Fried fish, vegetable salad with cream dressing, fresh fruit
   c. Spaghetti with tomato sauce, French bread, fruit
   d. Hamburger, French fries, cola

evolve Please refer to the Students' Resource section of this text's Evolve Web site for additional study resources.

REFERENCES

1. National Center for Health Statistics: *Health, United States, 2006, with chartbook on trends in the health of Americans,* Hyattsville, MD, 2006, U.S. Government Printing Office.

2. U.S. Department of Health and Human Services: *Healthy people 2010: understanding and improving health,* Washington, DC, 2000, U.S. Government Printing Office.

3. Food and Nutrition Board, Institute of Medicine: *Dietary reference intakes for energy, carbohydrate, fiber, fat, fatty acids, cholesterol, protein, and amino acids,* Washington, DC, 2002, National Academies Press.

4. Simonen RL and others: Factors associated with exercise lifestyle—a study of monozygotic twins, *Int J Sports Med* 24(7):499, 2003.

5. Bauman AE: Updating the evidence that physical activity is good for health: an epidemiological review 2000-2003, *J Sci Med Sport* 7(1):6, 2004.

6. Snowling NJ, Hopkins WG: Effects of different modes of exercise training on glucose control and risk factors for complications in type 2 diabetic patients, *Diabetes Care* 29(11):2518, 2006.

7. Acree LS and others: Physical activity is related to quality of life in older adults, *Health Qual Life Outcomes* 4:37, 2006.

8. American College of Sports Medicine: Position stand: the recommended quantity and quality of exercise for developing and maintaining cardiorespiratory and muscular fitness, and flexibility in healthy adults, *Med Sci Sports Exerc* 30:975, 1998.

9. American College of Sports Medicine: Position stand: progressive models in resistance training for healthy adults, *Med Sci Sports Exerc* 34:364, 2002.

10. U.S. Department of Health and Human Services: *Dietary Guidelines for Americans, 2005,* Washington, DC, 2005, U.S. Government Printing Office.

11. Von Duvillard SP and others: Fluids and hydration in prolonged endurance performance, *Nutrition* 20(7-8):651, 2004.

12. Shirreffs SM and others: Fluid and electrolyte needs for preparation and recovery from training and competition, *J Sports Sci* 22(1):57, 2004.

13. American College of Sports Medicine, American Dietetic Association, Dietitians of Canada: Joint position statement: nutrition and athletic performance, *Med Sci Sports Exerc* 32(12):2130, 2000.

14. Havemann L and others: Fat adaptation followed by carbohydrate loading compromises high-intensity sprint performance, *J Appl Physiol* 100(1):194, 2006.

15. Pehleman TL and others: Enzymatic regulation of glucose disposal in human skeletal muscle after a high-fat, low-carbohydrate diet, *J Appl Physiol* 98:100, 2005.

16. Utter AC and others: Carbohydrate supplementation and perceived exertion during prolonged running, *Med Sci Sports Exerc* 36(6):1036, 2004.

17. Horowitz JF, Klein S: Lipid metabolism during endurance exercise, *Am J Clin Nutr* 72(2):558S, 2000.

18. Wright JD and others: *Dietary intake of ten key nutrients for public health, United States: 1999-2000. Advanced data from vital and health statistics; No. 334,* Hyattsville, MD, 2003, National Center for Health Statistics.

19. Kerstetter JE and others: Dietary protein, calcium metabolism, and skeletal homeostasis revisited, *Am J Clin Nutr* 78:584S, 2003.

20. Gleeson M: Can nutrition limit exercise-induced immunodepression? *Nutr Rev* 64(3):119, 2006.

21. Williams MB and others: Effects of recovery beverages on glycogen restoration and endurance exercise performance, *J Strength Cond Res* 17(1):12, 2003.

22. Bernstein A and others: Athletic ergogenic aids, *Bull Hosp Jt Dis* 61(3-4):164, 2003.

FURTHER READING AND RESOURCES

Washington Coalition for Promoting Physical Activity: *www.beactive.org*

National Center for Chronic Disease Prevention and Health Promotion, Centers for Disease Control and Prevention: *Physical activity and health: a report of the surgeon general: www.cdc.gov/nccdphp/sgr/sgr.htm*

American College of Sports Medicine: *www.acsm.org*

National Institutes of Health, Office of Dietary Supplements: *http://dietary-supplements.info.nih.gov*

National Academies Press: *www.nap.edu*
   Review the above Web sites for information, guidelines, research, and suggestions on exercise and physical fitness.

Bauman AE: Updating the evidence that physical activity is good for health: an epidemiological review 2000-2003, *J Sci Med Sport* 7(1):6, 2004.
   This review of current scientific literature discusses benefits of physical activity on several areas of health, including cardiovascular disease, diabetes, stroke, mental health, falls and injuries, and obesity.

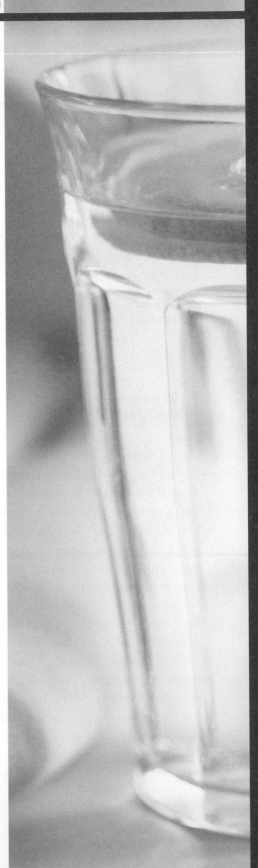

Clinical Nutrition

CHAPTER 17

Nutrition Care

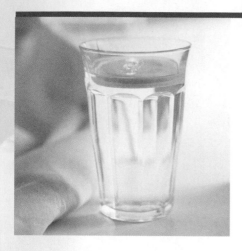

KEY CONCEPTS

- Valid health care is centered on the patient and his or her individual needs.
- Comprehensive health care is best provided by a team of health professionals and support staff.
- A personalized health care plan, evaluation, and follow-up care guide actions to promote healing and health.

People face acute illness or chronic disease and treatment in a variety of settings: the hospital, extended-care facility, clinic, and home. Nutrition support is fundamental in the successful treatment of disease and often is the primary therapy. To meet individual needs, a broad knowledge of nutrition status, requirements, and ways of meeting the identified needs is essential. The clinical dietitian, along with the physician, carries the major responsibility for this care. Each member of the health care team plays an important role in developing and maintaining a person-centered health care plan.

This chapter focuses on the comprehensive care of the patient's nutrition needs as provided by the registered dietitian. Nurses are intimately involved in the care process and often identify nutrition needs within the nursing diagnosis. An effective care plan involves all health care members as well as the patient, family, and support system.

THE THERAPEUTIC PROCESS

Setting and Focus of Care

Health Care Setting

Modern hospitals are a marvel of medical technology, but medical advances sometimes bring confusion to many patients, whose illnesses place them in the midst of a complex system of care. Various members of the medical staff come and go, and sometimes the day's schedule does not proceed as planned. Patients need personal advocates. Primary health care providers such as the nurse and dietitian provide essential support and personalized care.

Person-Centered Care

Nutrition care must be based on individual needs and be *person centered*. Figure 17-1 demonstrates the nutrition care process model, with the person-centered approach defining the relationship between patient and dietetic professional. Needs must constantly be updated with the patient's status. Such personalized care demands great commitment from the health care team. Despite all methods, tools, and technologies described in this text and elsewhere, remember this basic fact: *therapeutic use of self is the most healing tool a person will ever use.* This is a

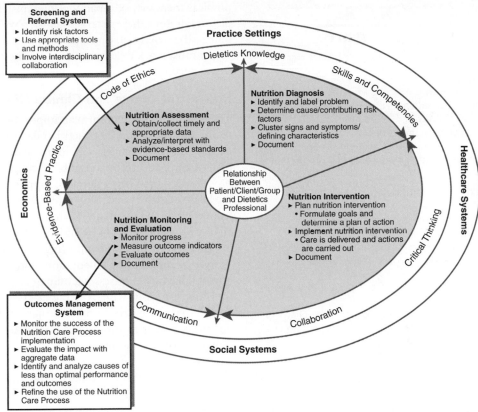

Figure 17–1 The nutrition care process model. (Reprinted from Lacey K, Pritchett E: Nutrition care process and model: ADA adopts road map to quality care and outcomes management, *J Am Diet Assoc* 103(8):1061, 2003.)

simple yet profound truth because the *human* encounter is where health care workers bring themselves and their skills.

Health Care Team

In the area of nutrition care, the registered dietitian (RD) carries the major responsibility of medical nutrition therapy (MNT). Box 17-1 outlines the qualifications of an RD. Working closely with the physician, the dietitian determines individual nutrition therapy needs and plan of care. Team support is essential throughout this process. Nurses are in a unique position to provide additional nutrition support, referring patients to the dietitian when necessary. Of all the health care team members, nurses are in the closest continuous contact with patients and their families. Patients and caretakers with emotional and social support have a more positive experience with hospitalizations and overall medical care, regardless of clinical status.[1,2] Such a relationship is important to ensure the most beneficial health care approach. In developing this

team relationship, all involved parties need each others' expertise for a successful outcome.

Physician and Support Staff

The health care team is headed by the physician and may include several other allied health professionals depending on the need of the patient. The team may include some or all of the following members: nurse, dietitian,

---

nursing diagnosis a statement about the health of a client based on information gathered during the nursing assessment. The North America Nursing Diagnosis Association defines standard diagnoses.

medical nutrition therapy (MNT) is a specific nutrition service and procedure used to treat an illness, injury, or condition. It involves an in-depth nutrition assessment of the patient; nutrition diagnosis; nutrition intervention, which includes diet therapy, counseling, or use of specialized nutrition supplements; and nutrition monitoring and evaluation.

BOX 17-1

QUALIFICATIONS OF A REGISTERED DIETITIAN

WHAT IS AN RD?

An RD is a food and nutrition expert who has met minimal academic and professional requirements to qualify for the credential of registered dietitian. In addition to RD credentialing, many states have regulatory laws for dietitians and nutrition practitioners. State requirements frequently are met through the same education and training required to become an RD.

WHAT ARE EDUCATIONAL AND PROFESSIONAL REQUIREMENTS FOR AN RD?

The following criteria must be met to earn the RD credential:

- Receive a bachelor's degree from an American, regionally accredited university or college and complete coursework approved by the Commission on Accreditation for Dietetics Education of the American Dietetic Association.
- Complete a Commission on Accreditation for Dietetics Education accredited, supervised practice program at a health care facility, community agency, or a food service corporation or in combination with graduate studies. A practice program typically takes 6 to 12 months.
- Pass a national examination administered by the Commission on Dietetic Registration (CDR).
- Complete continuing professional educational requirements to maintain registration.

Some RDs hold additional certifications in specialized areas of practice, such as pediatric or renal nutrition, nutrition support and diabetes education, and sports nutrition. These certifications are awarded through the CDR, the credentialing agency for the ADA and other medical and nutrition organizations, and are recognized within the profession but are not required.

WHAT IS THE DIFFERENCE BETWEEN AN RD OR DIETETIC TECHNICIAN, REGISTERED, AND A NUTRITIONIST?

The credentials RD and DTR (dietetic technician, registered) can only be used by dietetics practitioners who are currently authorized to use the credential by the CDR. These are legally protected titles. Individuals with these credentials have completed specific academic and supervised practice requirements, successfully completed a registration examination, and maintained requirements for recertification.

Some RDs and DTRs call themselves nutritionists. However, the definition and requirements for the term "nutritionist" vary. Some states have licensure laws that define the scope of practice for someone using the designation nutritionist.

Reprinted from American Dietetic Association: *Registered dietitian information sheet,* www.eatright.org/cps/rde/xchg/ada/hs.xsl/home_6658_ENU_HTML.htm, accessed September 2007.

physical therapist, occupational therapist, speech therapist, respiratory therapist, radiologist, physician assistant, kinesiotherapist, pharmacist, and social worker. The group must work together as a unit to best serve the patient's needs.

Role of the Nurse and Clinical Dietitian

The nurse and dietitian form an important team for providing nutrition care. The dietitian determines nutrition needs, plans and manages nutrition therapy, evaluates the plan of care, and records results. Throughout this entire process the nurse helps develop, support, and carry out the plan of care. Successful care depends on the close teamwork of the dietitian and nurse. The nursing process is a specific process by which nurses deliver care to patients and includes the following steps: assessment, diagnosis, planning, implementation, and evaluation. The nursing diagnosis addresses a human response need that the nurse can assist with. Nursing diagnoses may include several that are nutrition related, such as diarrhea, malnutrition, failure to thrive, and fluid volume deficit. Although covering the nursing process is not within the scope of this text, an appreciation of the interconnected work of the nurse and dietitian on the health care team is important.

When necessary, the nurse also may serve as an essential coordinator, advocate, interpreter, teacher, or counselor.

Coordinator and Advocate. Nurses work more closely with patients than do any other practitioners. They are best able to coordinate the patient's special services and treatments and can consult and refer as needed. Unfortunately, malnutrition is common in hospital settings. Many factors are involved in malnutrition (e.g., lack of appetite because of pain, medicine-induced anorexia, surgery, emotional and psychological distress). However, sometimes patients have reduced food intake because of conflict with medical procedures or appointments during meal time. The nurse may be able to help resolve such conflicts by coordinating meal delivery times in consideration of the patient's scheduled procedures.

Interpreter. The nurse can help reduce a patient's anxiety by careful, brief, easily understood explanations about various treatments and plans of care. This may include a basic reinforcement of special diet needs, resulting food choices from menus, and illustrations of needs from foods on the tray. These activities may be difficult with uninterested patients, but efforts to understand such patient behaviors are important. A patient's psychological and emotional status has a strong influence on his or her overall ability to deal with the medical problem at hand. Patients who are discharged without proper interpretation of their prognosis or plan of continued care may experience unnecessary stress and confusion. A group of researchers has developed a useful questionnaire that may help identify gaps in patient understanding and help the health care professional address unresolved issues.[3] The questionnaire is short and focuses on communication, emotions, short-term outcome, barriers, and relations with auxiliary staff (Figure 17-2). Such tools may help identify and address the personal needs of each patient.

Teacher or Counselor. Basic teaching and counseling skills are essential in nursing. Many opportunities exist during daily care for planned conversations about sound nutrition principles, which will reinforce the dietitian's work with the patient. Learning about the patient's nutrition needs should begin with hospital admission or initial contact, carry through the entire period of care, and continue in the home environment, supported by community resources as needed.

PHASES OF THE CARE PROCESS

The ADA has developed a standardized Nutrition Care Process for RDs (see the Student Resources section on the Evolve Web site). The Nutrition Care Process is defined as "a systematic problem-solving method that dietetics professionals use to critically think and make decisions to address nutrition-related problems and provide safe and effective quality nutrition care."[4] It is composed of the following four distinct and interrelated nutrition steps: (a) assessment, (b) diagnosis, (c) intervention, and (d) monitoring and evaluation.

Nutrition Assessment

To assess nutrition status and provide person-centered care, as much information as possible about the patient's situation must be collected. Family and medical history questionnaires are useful methods of gathering pertinent information on admission or during the initial office visit. Appropriate care considers the patient's nutrition status, food habits, and living situation as well as his or her needs, desires, and goals. The patient and family are the primary sources of this information (Figure 17-3). Other sources include the patient's medical chart, oral or written communication with hospital staff, and related research. The ABCD approach to nutrition assessment includes anthropometry, biochemical tests, clinical observations, and dietary evaluations.

Anthropometric Data
Anthropometric data include the following:
- Age

- Gender
- Height
- Weight
- Body frame
- Body composition

Practice taking correct anthropometric measurements to avoid errors. Also maintain proper equipment and careful technique. Three types of measurements are common in clinical practice.

Weight. Weigh hospital patients at consistent times (e.g., in the early morning after the bladder is emptied and before breakfast). Weigh patients without shoes in light indoor clothing or an examination gown. Ask about their usual body weight and compare it with standard BMI tables (see Chapter 15). Ask about any recent weight loss (e.g., how much over what period?). Rapid undesirable weight loss is significantly associated with increased health risks. Patients who have lost more than 5% body weight in 1 month or more than 10% body weight over any amount of time for unknown reasons should be referred to an RD for a thorough evaluation. Ask about any recent weight gain as well. Sometimes asking about general weight history over time is helpful (e.g., peaks and lows at what ages).

Height. Use a fixed measuring stick against the wall if possible. Otherwise, use the moveable measuring rod on the platform clinic scales. Have the person stand as straight as possible, without shoes or cap. Note the growth of children as well as the diminishing height of older adults. BMI is calculated by using both weight and height measurements and is a helpful assessment tool throughout the life cycle.

Children younger than 2 years should be measured while lying down with a stationary headboard and movable footboard (Figure 17-4). Alternative measures for nonambulatory patients provide estimates for persons who are confined to a bed, cannot stand up straight, or have lower body amputations (Box 17-2).

kinesiotherapist a health care professional who treats the effects of disease, injury, and congenital disorders through the application of scientifically based exercise principles adapted to enhance the strength, endurance, and mobility of individuals with functional limitations or those requiring extended physical conditioning.

nursing process how nurses deliver care to patients; includes the steps of assessment, diagnosis, planning, implementation, and evaluation.

anthropometric measurements physical measurements of the human body used for health assessment, including height, weight, skinfold thickness, and circumference (head, hip, waist, wrist, mid-arm muscle).

PEQ
Patient experience questionnaire
2000

In order to provide better service, we ask for your experience in this medical visit, what it felt like for you and what you think it will mean to you and your health situation

(Please answer all questions, even if you saw your doctor without any specific ailment or problem in mind)

Outcome of this specific visit

1. Do you know what to do to reduce your health problem(s)? (Or how to prevent problems?)
   - Much more ☐5
   - Some more ☐4
   - A bit more ☐3
   - Not much more ☐2
   - No more ☐1

2. Do you know what to expect from now on?
   - Much more ☐5
   - Some more ☐4
   - A bit more ☐3
   - Not much more ☐2
   - No more ☐1

3. Will you be able to handle your health problems differently?
   - No, no at all ☐5
   - Not much ☐4
   - A bit ☐3
   - Some ☐2
   - A lot ☐1

4. Will it lead to fewer health problem(s)? (Or help prevent problems?)
   - No, no at all ☐5
   - Not much ☐4
   - A bit ☐3
   - Some ☐2
   - A lot ☐1

Communication experiences

5. We had a good talk
   - Agree completely ☐5
   - Agree ☐4
   - So-so ☐3
   - Disagree ☐2
   - Disagree completely ☐1

6. I felt reassured
   - Agree completely ☐5
   - Agree ☐4
   - So-so ☐3
   - Disagree ☐2
   - Disagree completely ☐1

7. The doctor understood what was on my mind
   - Agree completely ☐5
   - Agree ☐4
   - So-so ☐3
   - Disagree ☐2
   - Disagree completely ☐1

8. I felt I was taken care of
   - Agree completely ☐5
   - Agree ☐4
   - So-so ☐3
   - Disagree ☐2
   - Disagree completely ☐1

Communication barriers

9. It was a bit difficult to connect with the doctor
   - Agree completely ☐5
   - Agree ☐4
   - So-so ☐3
   - Disagree ☐2
   - Disagree completely ☐1

10. Too much time was spent on small talk
    - Agree completely ☐5
    - Agree ☐4
    - So-so ☐3
    - Disagree ☐2
    - Disagree completely ☐1

11. It was a bit difficult to ask questions
    - Agree completely ☐5
    - Agree ☐4
    - So-so ☐3
    - Disagree ☐2
    - Disagree completely ☐1

12. Important decisions were made over my head
    - Agree completely ☐5
    - Agree ☐4
    - So-so ☐3
    - Disagree ☐2
    - Disagree completely ☐1

Experience with the auxiliary staff

13. I sensed that other patients could listen in when I was talking to the staff
    - Agree completely ☐5
    - Agree ☐4
    - So-so ☐3
    - Disagree ☐2
    - Disagree completely ☐1

14. I felt like one of the crowd
    - Agree completely ☐5
    - Agree ☐4
    - So-so ☐3
    - Disagree ☐2
    - Disagree completely ☐1

Emotions immediately after the visit

After this visit I felt:

(Please circle one number for each line)

Relieved	7	6	5	4	3	2	1	Worried
Sad	1	2	3	4	5	6	7	Cheerful
Strengthened	7	6	5	4	3	2	1	Worn out
Relaxed	1	2	3	4	5	6	7	Tense

Thank you for your time and collaboration!

Figure 17–2 Patient Experience Questionnaire (PEQ). Steine S and others: A new, brief questionnaire (PEQ) developed in primary health care for measuring patients' experience of interaction, emotion and consultation outcome, *Fam Pract* 18:410, 2001.

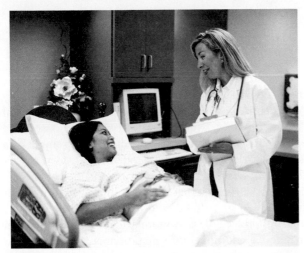

Figure 17–3 Interviewing a patient to plan personal care. (Copyright JupiterImages Corporation.)

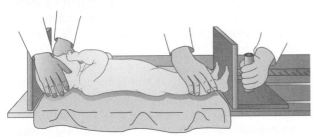

Figure 17–4 Measuring height in an infant. (Reprinted from Mahan LK, Escott-Stump S: *Krause's food & nutrition therapy*, ed 12, Philadelphia, 2008, Saunders.)

BOX 17-2

ALTERNATIVE MEASURES FOR NONAMBULATORY PATIENTS

TOTAL ARM SPAN
- With a flexible metric tape, measure the patient's full arm span from fingertip to fingertip across the front of the clavicles.
- For patients with limited movement in one arm, measure from fingertip to the midpoint of the sternum and then double the measurement.

KNEE HEIGHT
- With the client's knees bent at a 90-degree angle, measure knee-to-floor height from the outside bony point just under the kneecap (fibular head) down to the floor surface.
- Use the following equations to calculate total body height from knee height (KH):
  - Height for women: $([1.833 \times KH] - [0.24 \times Age]) + 84.88$
  - Height for men: $([2.02 \times KH] - [0.04 \times Age]) + 64.19$

Body Frame. Height (in centimeters) divided by wrist circumference (in centimeters) provides an estimate to body frame size. For an accurate measurement, the patient's arm should be flexed at the elbow with palm facing up and hand relaxed. With a flexible measuring tape, measure the wrist circumference at the joint distal (toward hand) to the styloid process (bony wrist protrusion). The following example indicates the standards for body frame size, which are useful for interpreting ideal body weight:

Example: Height: 5 ft, 4 in = 64 in ×
2.54cm/in = 162.56 cm

Wrist circumference = 15.4 cm

162.56/15.4 = 10.56 = Medium frame

FRAME SIZE	MALE RATIO	FEMALE RATIO
Small	>10.4	>10.9
Medium	10.4-9.6	10.9-9.9
Large	<9.6	<9.9

Body Composition. The dietitian usually measures various aspects of body size and composition to determine relative levels of fat versus muscle. Several methods used to measure body composition are covered in Chapter 15. Some methods include skinfold thickness measurement with calipers, hydrostatic weighing, bioelectrical impedance analysis, dual-energy x-ray absorptiometry, and the BOD POD body composition tracking system (Life Measurement, Inc., Concord, Calif.).

Biochemical Tests

Biochemical tests include the following:
- Plasma proteins (serum albumin and prealbumin)
- Liver enzymes (evaluate liver function)
- Blood urea nitrogen, serum electrolytes (evaluate renal function)
- Urinary urea nitrogen excretion
- Creatinine height index (evaluate protein tissue breakdown)
- Complete blood count (evaluate for anemia)
- Fasting glucose (evaluate for high or low blood glucose levels)
- Total lymphocyte count (evaluate immune function)

Laboratory and radiographic tests aid in nutrition status assessment. Such reports generally are available in the patient's chart. Several of the most frequently used tests are listed above. Additional details for some biochemical tests are described below.

Plasma Protein. Basic measures are serum albumin, prealbumin, and hemoglobin. Additional tests may include serum transferrin or total iron-binding capacity and ferritin. These tests help detect protein and iron deficiencies.

Protein Metabolism. Basic 24-hour urine tests measure the byproducts of protein metabolism (e.g., urinary creatinine and urea nitrogen). Elevated levels may indicate excess breakdown of body tissue.

Immune System Integrity. Lymphocyte count is the ratio of special white cells to the total white blood cell count. Skin testing also may be done to check for sensitivity to common antigens and, hence, the strength of the general immune system.

Skeletal System Integrity. Several tests may be used, especially with older patients, to determine the status of bone integrity and possible osteoporosis. Some tests commonly used are x-ray, dual-energy x-ray absorptiometry, and full-body bone scan.

Gastrointestinal Function. X-rays also are useful to evaluate GI function and problems, such as peptic ulcer disease and malfunctions along the GI tract.

The medical tests used for nutrition assessment generally are reliable in persons of any age, but some conditions may interfere with test results and should be considered when evaluating laboratory values. For example, laboratory values are affected by hydration status, presence of chronic diseases, changes in organ function, and certain medications.

Clinical Observations

Clinical observations include the following:
- Clinical signs of nutrition status
- Physical examination

Observation. Careful observation of various areas of the patient's body may reveal signs of poor nutrition. Table 17-1 lists some clinical signs of nutrition status that should be kept in mind when providing general patient care.

Physical Examination. Other members of the health care team, such as the physician, nurse, or physical therapist, may perform physical examinations that are useful for evaluating nutrition status. Such evaluations include inspection of skin for the presence of edema and skin turgor, evaluation of nail integrity, and assessment of body organ sounds in the intestine and lungs.

Diet Evaluations

Evaluation of the diet includes the following assessments:
- Usual intake, current intake, restrictions, modifications (use 24-hour recall and food diaries)
- Support system (caregivers to help with nutrition care plan)

- Nutrition supplements, vitamin or mineral supplements
- Food allergies, intolerances
- Activity level (average energy expended per day)

In most cases, the RD is responsible for evaluating the diet. Knowledge of the patient's basic eating habits may help identify possible nutrition deficiencies. The Clinical Applications box, "Nutrition History: Activity-Associated Food Pattern of a Typical Day," shows an example of a general guide for gathering a nutrition history. Sometimes a more specific food history is obtained by using a 3-day food record; that is, recording everything consumed, food items used, and amounts and methods of preparation for 3 days. A more extended view of the diet may reveal additional information about food habits or problems as they relate to the individual's socioeconomic status, family and/or living situation, and general support system.

Clinicians should be aware that underreporting energy intake is quite common and may affect dietary assessment and recommendations.[5-7] A recent study of elderly individuals reported that 25% of the participants underreported usual intake.[8] A variety of methods are used to collect dietary intake, all of which have strengths and weaknesses (Table 17-2). Specific questioning on various supplements (vitamins, minerals, multivitamin/mineral combinations, and herbs) is more likely to yield accurate answers and give insight to overall consumption. Patients often do not report supplement intake (see the Drug-Nutrient Interaction box, "The Safety of Supplements"). Allergies and intolerances should be noted so that alternative recommendations meet nutrition needs without causing negative reactions.

Physical activity logs are similar to dietary intake logs in that all activity is recorded throughout the day to access energy expenditure. Also similar to diet logs, physical activity reporting tends to be inaccurate relative to fitness in a portion of the population. A recent study found that 10% of men overreported their physical activity and fitness level on a standard questionnaire—another important consideration when providing recommendations.[9]

Nutrition Diagnosis

A nutrition diagnosis is "identification and labeling an actual occurrence, risk of, or potential for developing a nutrition problem that dietetics professionals are responsible for treating independently."[4] A careful study of all information gathered reveals basic patient needs. Other needs develop and guide the care plan as the hospitalization or consultation continues. The nutrition diagnosis

TABLE 17-1

CLINICAL SIGNS OF NUTRITION STATUS

BODY AREA	SIGNS OF GOOD NUTRITION	SIGNS OF POOR NUTRITION
General appearance	Alert, responsive	Listless, apathetic, cachectic
Weight	Normal for height, age, and body type	Overweight or underweight (special concern for underweight)
Posture	Erect, straight arms and legs	Sagging shoulders, sunken chest, humped back
Muscles	Well developed, firm, good tone; some fat under skin	Flaccid, poor tone; underdeveloped; tender, "wasted" appearance; inability to walk properly
Nervous control	Good attention span, not irritable or restless, normal reflexes, psychologic stability	Inattentive, irritable, confused; burning and tingling of hands and feet (paresthesia); loss of position and vibratory sense; weakness and tenderness of muscles (may result in inability to walk); decrease or loss of ankle and knee reflexes
GI function	Good appetite and digestion; normal, regular elimination; no palpable (perceptible to touch) organs or masses	Anorexia, indigestion, constipation or diarrhea, liver or spleen enlargement
Cardiovascular function	Normal heart rate and rhythm, no murmurs, normal blood pressure for age	Rapid heart rate (>100 beats/min, tachycardia), enlarged heart, abnormal rhythm, elevated blood pressure
General vitality	Good endurance, energetic, sleeps well, vigorous	Easily fatigued, no energy, falls asleep easily, looks tired or apathetic
Hair	Shiny, lustrous, firm, not easily plucked, healthy scalp	Stringy, dull, brittle, dry, thin, sparse; depigmented; can be easily plucked
Skin (general)	Smooth, slightly moist, good color	Rough, dry, scaly, pale, pigmented, irritated; bruised; petechiae
Face and neck	Skin color uniform; smooth, pink, healthy appearance; not swollen	Greasy, discolored, scaly, swollen; skin dark over cheeks and under eyes; lumpiness or flakiness of skin around nose and mouth
Lips	Smooth, good color; moist, not chapped or swollen	Dry, scaly, swollen; redness and swelling (cheilosis) or angular lesions at corners of the mouth or fissures or scars (stomatitis)
Mouth, oral membranes	Good pink color, healthy, no swelling or bleeding	Swelling, scarlet and raw, magenta color, beefy (glossitis), hyperemic and hypertrophic papillae, atrophic papillae
Teeth	No cavities, no pain, bright, straight, no crowding, well-shaped jaw, clean, no discoloration	Unfilled caries, absent teeth, worn surfaces, mottled (fluorosis), malpositioned
Eyes	Bright, clear, shiny; no sores at corners of eyelids; membranes moist and healthy pink color; no prominent blood vessels or amount of tissue or sclera; no fatigue circles beneath	Eye membranes pale (pale conjunctiva), redness of membrane (conjunctival infection), dryness, signs of infection, Bitot's spots, redness and fissuring of eyelid corners (angular palpebritis), dryness of eye membrane (conjunctival xerosis), dull appearance of cornea (corneal xerosis), soft cornea (keratomalacia)
Neck (glands)	No enlargement	Thyroid enlarged
Nails	Firm, pink	Spoon shaped (koilonychia), brittle, ridged
Legs, feet	No tenderness, weakness, or swelling; good color	Edema, tender calf, tingling, weakness
Skeleton	No malformations	Bowlegs, knock-knees, deformity at diaphragm, beaded ribs, prominent scapulas

Reprinted from Williams SR: Nutritional assessment and guidance in prenatal care. In Worthington-Roberts BS, Williams SR: *Nutrition in pregnancy and lactation*, ed 5, New York, 1993, McGraw-Hill.

CLINICAL APPLICATIONS

NUTRITION HISTORY: ACTIVITY-ASSOCIATED FOOD PATTERN OF A TYPICAL DAY

Name _____ Date_____

Height _____ Weight (lb) _____ (kg) _____ Ideal weight _____ Usual weight _____

Referral:

Diagnosis:

Diet order:

Occupation:

Recreation, physical activity:

Present food intake:

Time/location	Food (and method of preparation)	Serving size	Tolerance/comments
Breakfast:			
Snack:			
Lunch:			
Snack:			
Dinner:			
Snack:			

Summary: Total servings of foods in each category:

Breads/grains:_____ Vegetables:_____ Fruits:_____ Dairy:_____ Meat:_____ Fat/sugar:_____

Dietary supplements and herbs:

Name of Supplement	Dose per Day

TABLE 17-2

STRENGTHS AND LIMITATIONS OF TECHNIQUES USED TO MEASURE DIETARY INTAKE

TECHNIQUE	BRIEF DESCRIPTION	STRENGTHS	LIMITATIONS
24-Hour food record	Trained interviewer asks respondent to recall, in detail, all food and drink consumed during a period in the recent past	Requires <20 min to administer Inexpensive Easy to administer Can provide detailed information on types of foods consumed Low respondent burden More objective than dietary history Does not alter usual diet Useful in clinical settings	One recall rarely illustrates typical intake Underreporting and overreporting occur Depends on memory Omissions of sauces, dressings, and beverages can lead to low estimates of energy intake Data entry can be labor intensive
1- to 7-day food record or diary	Respondent records, at time of consumption, identity and amounts of all foods and beverages consumed for a period, usually ranging from 1 to 7 days	Does not rely on memory Can provide detailed intake data Can provide information about eating habits Multiple-day data more representative of usual intake Reasonably valid up to 5 days	Requires high degree of cooperation Subject must be literate Takes more time to obtain data Act of recording may alter usual intake
Food frequency questionnaires	Respondents indicate how many times a day, week, month, or year they usually consume foods by using a questionnaire consisting of a list of approximately 150 foods or food groups important to the intake of energy and nutrients	Can be self-administered Machine readable Modest demand on respondents Relatively inexpensive May be more representative of usual intake than a few days of diet records	May not represent usual food or portion sizes chosen by respondent Intake data can be compromised when multiple foods are grouped within single listings Depends on ability of respondent to describe diet
Diet history	Respondents are interviewed by a trained interviewer about number of meals eaten per day; appetite; food dislikes; presence or absence of nausea and vomiting; use of nutritional supplements and herbal products; cigarette smoking; habits related to sleep, rest, work and exercise	Assess usual nutrient intake Can detect seasonal changes Data on all nutrients can be obtained Can correlate well with biochemical measures	Lengthy interview process Requires highly trained interviewers May overestimate nutrient intake Requires cooperation of respondent with ability to recall usual diet

Modified from Lee RD, Neiman DC. *Nutrition assessment,* ed 3, New York, 2003, McGraw-Hill.

will change as the patient's nutrition needs change. An example of a nutrition diagnosis statement is:

Excessive caloric intake (problem) related to frequent consumption of large portions of high-fat meals (etiology) as evidenced by average daily intake of calories exceeding recommended amount by 500 kcal and 12-pound weight gain during the past 18 months (signs).[4]

Problem

After careful assessment of nutrition indexes, data are analyzed and a nutrition diagnostic category is assigned. The nutrition diagnostic statement helps identify nutri-

tion problems, which may include nutrient deficiencies (e.g., evidence of iron-deficiency anemia) or underlying disease requiring a special modified diet (e.g., diabetes or liver disease). The diagnosis(es) also "provides a link to setting realistic and measurable expected outcomes, selecting appropriate interventions, and tracking progress in attaining those expected outcomes."[4]

Etiology

The cause or contributing risk factors are identifiable factors directly leading to the stated problem. The ADA defines etiology as the "factors contributing to the existence of, or maintenance of pathophysiological, psychosocial,

DRUG-NUTRIENT INTERACTION

THE SAFETY OF SUPPLEMENTS

The Dietary Supplement Health and Education Act was passed by Congress in 1994 and opened the door to what could be called the supplement boom. Since that time some companies have attached claims to supplements that may not have reliable scientific backing. Indeed, many of these claims are based on studies that may not have a control group (placebo), or the study may not be double blinded. The same rigorous testing that must be completed before a pharmaceutical goes on the market is not required for supplements.

Many people do not report supplement intake when asked about current prescriptions simply because they do not consider supplements potentially dangerous. However, side effects and interactions with other medications are a possibility. The following are red flags to look for when determining the efficacy and validity of a supplement claim:

- If it sounds too good to be true, it probably is.
- If it claims to be a cure-all, be on your guard. The human body is complex, and one supplement will probably not relieve a variety of pains or deficiencies.

- If it promises greater weight loss than 2 lb/week, the weight loss will probably not be sustainable and may be harmful.
- If the claim made by using an "inferiority" approach (i.e., claims stating that without supplement X a person will not be as beautiful, intelligent, or active as he or she could be), understand it may be playing on emotion, not logic.

When speaking with clients or patients about supplements, take an objective role. Ask why they use the supplement and discuss reasons why they may or may not need it. If the supplement may be harmful, let the patient know without being confrontational. The decision of starting or ending supplement use is personal and should be respected even if different from what is advised. Always encourage patients to speak with their physicians and pharmacists about possible drug-nutrient interactions.

Sara Oldroyd

situational, developmental, cultural, and/or environmental problems."[4] Correctly identifying the cause is the only way to design an intervention plan adequately.

Signs and Symptoms

Signs and symptoms of nutrition problems are an accumulation of subjective and objective changes in the patient's health status that indicate a nutrition problem and are results of the identified etiology. Signs of general malnutrition requiring rebuilding of body tissue and nutrient stores may be evidenced.

Nutrition Intervention

Objectives of the health care plan are designed to meet identified needs of the patient. This written care plan gives attention to personal needs and goals as well as the identified requirements of medical care. Suitable and realistic actions then carry out the personal care plan. For example, nutrition care and teaching include an appropriate food plan with examples of food choices, food buying, and food preparation. Such activities ideally include family members as well.

Psychological and emotional problems can weigh heavily on the overall outcome of a patient's prognosis and well-being. For example, geriatric patients in long-term health care facilities often suffer from depression and weight loss, a confounding problem when individuals are already in poor health. The most important link to this type of malnutrition is decreased food intake. Researchers

have found everyday emotions to have a significant influence on food intake in the elderly population.[10] Thus, by addressing emotional tribulations, energy needs may be better met and complications associated with malnutrition avoided. Unfortunately, such problems often are not discussed with the physician. By inquiring about a patient's psychological well-being, perhaps some of the confounding factors can be alleviated. Likewise, economic needs are paramount for many persons in high-risk populations. By considering the patient's personal goals and needs, the health care team and patient can help establish priorities for immediate and long-term care.

Disease Modifications

The primary principle of diet therapy is that it is based on a patient's normal nutrition requirements and is only modified as an individual's specific condition requires. Nutrition components of the normal diet may be modified in the following three ways:

1. *Energy:* The total energy value of the diet, expressed in kilocalories, may be increased or decreased.
2. *Nutrients:* One or more of the essential nutrients (protein, carbohydrate, fat, mineral, vitamin, and water) may be modified in amount or form.
3. *Texture:* The texture or seasoning of the diet may be modified (e.g., liquid or low-residue diets).

Personal Adaptation

Successful nutrition therapy can occur only when the diet is *personalized* (i.e., adapted to meet individual needs).

This can be done only by planning *with the patient or family*. Four areas must be explored together, as follows:

1. *Personal needs:* What personal desires, concerns, goals, or life situation needs must be met?
2. *Disease:* How does the patient's disease or condition affect the body and its normal metabolic functions?
3. *Nutrition therapy:* How and why must the diet be changed to meet needs created by the patient's particular disease or condition?
4. *Food plan:* How do these necessary nutritional modifications affect daily food choices? How can these needs be met?

Mode of Feeding

The method of feeding used in the nutrition care plan depends on the patient's condition. The dietitian and nurse work together to manage the diet by using oral, enteral, or parenteral feeding.

Routine House Diets. A schedule of routine "house" diets, based on a cycle menu, is typically followed in most hospitals. The basic modification is in texture, ranging from clear liquid (no milk) to full liquid (including milk) and soft food to a full regular diet. *Mechanically altered soft diets* are designed for patients with chewing or swallowing problems. Small amounts of liquid may be added to regular foods to achieve an appropriate consistency when pureed. These diets may be further modified depending on the patient's needs. For example, low-sodium, low-fat, or high-protein requirements can still be met with mechanically altered diets. *Therapeutic soft diets* are used to transition between liquid and regular diets. Whole foods low in fiber and limited seasoning are included as tolerated. Table 17-3 summarizes details of routine hospital diets.

Oral Feeding. For as long as possible, regular oral feedings are the preferred method of feeding. If needed, nutrient supplements may be added.

Assisted Oral Feeding. According to the patient's condition, the nurse or assistant may need to help the patient eat. Patients usually like to maintain independence as much as possible and should be encouraged to do so with whatever degree of assistance necessary. Plate guards or special utensils to facilitate independence usually are welcomed by both patient and staff. Try to learn each patient's needs and limitations so that little things (e.g., having the meat cut up or the bread buttered before bringing the tray to the bedside) can be done without making a patient feel inadequate. When complete assistance is needed, the following guidelines may help with the feeding experience:

- Have the tray securely placed within the patient's sight.
- Sit down beside the bed if this is more comfortable and make simple conversation or remain silent as the patient's condition indicates.
- Offer small amounts and do not rush the feeding.
- Give ample time for a patient to chew and swallow or rest between mouthfuls.
- Offer liquids between the solids, with a drinking straw if necessary.
- Wipe the patient's mouth with a napkin during and after each meal.
- Let the patient hold the bread if desired and able to do so.
- When feeding a patient who is blind or has eye dressings, describe the food on the tray so that a mental image helps create a desire to eat. Sometimes the analogy of the face of a clock allows a patient to visualize the position of certain foods on the plate (indicate that the meat is at 12 o'clock, the potatoes are at 3 o'clock, etc.).
- Warn the patient that the soup feels particularly hot when taken through a straw and identify each food being served beforehand.

Assisted feeding times can provide a special opportunity for nutrition counseling and support. Important observations can be made during this time. The nurse can closely observe the patient's physical appearance and responses to the foods served, appetite and tolerance for certain foods, and the meaning of food to the person. These observations can help the nurse adapt the patient's diet to meet any particular individual needs. Helping patients learn more about their diets and nutrition needs is an important part of personal care. Persons who understand the role of good food in health (e.g., that it helps them regain strength and recover from illness) are more likely to accept the diet. Patients also feel more encouraged to maintain sound eating habits after discharge from the hospital as well as improve their eating habits in general. Health care providers who are cognizant of personal, cultural, and ethnic needs of their patients will be more effective when helping a patient plan for immediate and long-term nutrition needs (see the Cultural Considerations box, "Cultural Differences in Advanced Care Planning").

Enteral Feeding. When a patient cannot eat, but the remaining portions of the GI tract can be used, an alternate form of **enteral** feeding by tube provides nutrition support. The saying, "if you don't use it, you lose it" also applies to gut function. Therefore any time the pa-

enteral a mode of feeding that uses the GI tract through oral or tube feeding.

TABLE 17-3

ROUTINE HOSPITAL DIETS

FOOD	CLEAR LIQUID	FULL LIQUID	MECHANICAL SOFT	REGULAR HOUSE DIET
Soup	Clear, fat-free broth, bouillon	Same as clear, plus strained or blended cream soups	Same as clear and full, plus all cream soups	All
Cereal	Not included	Cooked refined cereal	Cooked cereal, corn flakes, rice, noodles, macaroni, spaghetti	All
Bread	Not included	Not included	White bread, crackers, melba toast, Zwieback	All
Protein foods	Not included	Milk, cream, milk drinks, yogurt	Same as full, plus eggs (not fried), mild cheese, cottage and cream cheeses, fowl, fish, tender beef, veal, lamb, liver, bacon	All
Vegetables	Not included	Vegetable juices or pureed vegetables	Potatoes: baked, mashed, creamed, steamed, scalloped; tender cooked whole, bland vegetables; fresh lettuce, tomatoes	All
Fruit and fruit juices	Strained fruit juices (as tolerated), flavored fruit drinks	Fruit juices	Same as clear and full, plus cooked fruit: peaches, pears, applesauce, peeled apricots, white cherries; ripe peaches, pears, bananas, orange and grapefruit sections without membrane	All
Desserts and gelatin	Fruit-flavored gelatin, fruit ices and popsicles	Same as clear, plus sherbet, ice cream, puddings, custard, frozen yogurt	Same as clear and full, plus plain sponge cakes, plain cookies, plain cake, puddings, pie made with allowed foods	All
Miscellaneous	Soft drinks (as tolerated), coffee and tea, decaffeinated coffee and tea, cereal beverages such as Postum, sugar, honey, salt, hard candy, Polycose (Abbott Nutrition, Columbus, OH), residue-free supplements	Same as clear, plus margarine, pepper, all supplements	Same as clear and full, plus mild salad dressings	All

tient can tolerate feedings through the gut, it is the feeding method of choice. A small tube is placed through the patient's nasal cavity, running down the back of the throat into either the stomach or small intestine (nasogastric or nasojejunal tube, respectively) to administer an appropriate source of nutrients and energy. For long-term enteral feedings, the tubes may be placed surgically into the stomach or small intestine through the abdominal wall. Various commercial formulas are available and usually are preferred over locally mixed ones. A blended formula from table food may be calculated and prepared but carries a greater risk for contamination during preparation and storage. Enteral feedings, along with diagrams, are covered in greater detail in Chapter 22.

Parenteral Nutrition. If a patient cannot tolerate food or formula through the GI tract, intravenous feeding is necessary. Compared with tube feeding, parenteral feedings are more invasive and expensive and introduce more risk. However, for patients in whom part or all of the GI tract or accessory organs (liver, pancreas, etc.) are not functioning, it is necessary. Parenteral nutrition comes in two forms: (1) peripheral vein feeding and (2) central vein feeding. Both forms of parenteral nutrition are covered in detail in Chapter 22, but a brief description follows:

- *Peripheral vein feeding:* Various solutions of dextrose, amino acids, vitamins, minerals, and lipids can be directly administered into peripheral veins. The nutrient

CULTURAL CONSIDERATIONS

CULTURAL DIFFERENCES IN ADVANCED CARE PLANNING

Advanced care planning is the process in which future treatment of a patient is determined before it is needed. *Advanced directives* and *living wills* are examples of documents recognized in the United States by all health care institutions. The Patient Self Determination Act of 1991 was intended to promote the use of advanced care procedures and strengthen the rights of patients during end-of-life medical procedures. Such documents are the only way treatment preferences of the patient can be ensured during times of unconsciousness or otherwise inability to communicate.

MNT, such as enteral and parenteral nutrition, may be considered a life-sustaining intervention by some people. Several recent studies have compared the cultural discrepancy in attitudes about advanced care planning.[*†‡] Researchers suggest significant differences exist between various racial and ethnic patients and their caregivers about advanced care planning and end-of-life decisions. Kwak and Haley[‡] summarized the findings of 33 published studies

addressing these issues and found trends within certain ethnic groups: (1) Caucasians exhibited more knowledge and support of advanced directives than did other ethnic groups, and (2) Hispanics and Asians prefer family-centered decision making.[‡] Researchers have also found African-American patients to be more likely than Caucasians to request life-supportive treatments.[†‡]

By recognizing such cultural differences in desired treatment and knowing the likelihood of patients having advanced care planning, health care professionals can assist the patient with greater awareness and sensitivity. Educate patients about advanced directives and living wills and explain all methods of life support that may be available. Even if the patient has verbally expressed his or her wishes to the family, sometimes family members find making these decisions to be too difficult. Advanced care planning can alleviate the burden on the family and ensure that the patient's wishes are granted.

* Shrank WH and others: Focus group findings about the influence of culture on communication preferences in end-of-life care, *J Gen Intern Med* 20(8):703, 2005.
†Phipps E and others: Approaching the end of life: attitudes, preferences, and behaviors of African-American and white patients and their family caregivers, *J Clin Oncol* 21(3):549, 2003.
‡Kwak J, Haley WE: Current research findings on end-of-life decision making among racially or ethnically diverse groups, *Gerontologist* 45(5):634, 2005.

and energy intake is limited in this method of feeding, however, so peripheral vein feeding is used only when the need for nutrition support is not extensive or long term. Patients should be told that this is still a method of "feeding."

■ *Central vein feeding:* When a patient's nutrition need is great (e.g., for massive injury or debilitating disease) and parenteral nutrition may be necessary for a longer time, a larger central vein is required. Total parenteral nutrition (TPN) through a central line involves a surgical procedure in which a catheter is inserted into the large subclavian vein for easy access. This mode of parenteral feeding allows for higher volumes of nutrients and can be used long term. A team of specialists (physicians, dietitians, pharmacists, and nurses) works closely together in the administration of TPN nutrition. Throughout this procedure, the patient needs special care and support, including instruction for continued TPN use at home as needed (see Chapter 22).

Nutrition Monitoring and Evaluation

The nutrition care plan is evaluated in terms of nutrition diagnosis and treatment objectives. Efficacy of the care plan is evaluated and changes are made if necessary. This evaluation continues through the period of care and terminates

at the point of discharge or the end of the care period. The questions listed in the following sections are important.

Nutrition Goals. What is the effect of the diet or feeding method on the illness or the patient's situation? Did the diet plan adequately address nutritional concerns?

Required Changes. Should any of the nutrition care plan components be changed? Are any changes in the nutrients, energy, meal/snack patterns, or feeding methods necessary? Should the type of food or feeding equipment, environment for meals, counseling procedures, or types of learning activities for nutrition education be changed?

Ability to Follow Diet. Does any hindrance or disability prevent the patient from following the treatment plan? What is the effect of the diet on the patient, family, and staff?

More Information or Resources. Was all the necessary nutrition information gathered? Do the patient and family understand all the self-care instructions provided? Are needed community resources available and convenient? Have necessary food-assistance programs been sufficient for the patient's care, if needed?

---

parenteral a mode of feeding that does not use the GI tract but instead provides nutrition support by intravenous delivery of nutrient solutions.

DRUG INTERACTIONS

Gathering information about all drug use is essential to the care process—including over-the-counter self-medications and prescribed drugs as well as alcohol and street drugs. The nurse should be particularly familiar with drug-food interactions because he or she is most commonly administering both items to patients. Research each drug to determine any possible problems from the interaction of drugs with foods or nutrients (Figure 17-5). Pocket guides, such as "Food-Medication Interactions" (Food-Medication Interactions, PO Box 204, Birchrunville, PA 19421-0204, phone: 800-746-2324), are helpful for on-site references. Many negative reactions can occur with multiple drug use, especially in elderly patients with chronic diseases. A total of 45.3% of the U.S. population takes at least one prescription drug, and 17.7% take three or more prescription drugs at any given time.[11] Patients may respond quite differently from one another depending on normal dietary habits, specific disease, compliance, and other medications or supplements currently taken.

Drug-Food Interactions

Interactions in which food increases or decreases the effect of a drug can adversely influence the health of a patient. Certain foods may affect the absorption, distribu-

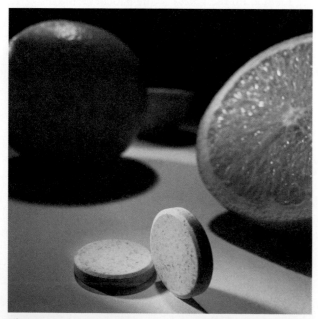

Figure 17–5 Many drugs, foods, and nutrients interact and cause medical problems. (Copyright JupiterImages Corporation.)

tion, metabolism, or elimination of a drug, thus altering the intended dose response (Table 17-4). Timing, size, and composition of meals relative to medication administration are all common causes of drug-food interactions. For example, a high-fat meal increases the absorption of some drugs that are lipophilic ("fat loving"), whereas a high-fiber meal may bind other drugs and reduce their absorption. The interaction of grapefruit juice and several drugs has been under critical evaluation in recent years. Researchers have found that a substance called furanocoumarin in grapefruit juice can dramatically alter the bioavailability of certain drugs to a dangerous level.[12,13] The anticoagulation medication warfarin is a commonly prescribed drug for patients with heart disease and also is one of the most highly interactive medications with certain foods, specifically those high in vitamin K.[14]

Drug-Nutrient Interactions

Drug-nutrient interactions primarily refer to reactions that occur when medications are taken in combination with over-the-counter vitamin and mineral supplements (see the Clinical Applications box, "Case Study: Drug-Nutrient Interaction"). Unfortunately, the use of vitamin and mineral supplements is seldom reported to physicians or pharmacists by patients. A recent study published in the *Journal of the American Dietetic Association* reported that 73% of noninstitutionalized adults in the United States use a dietary supplement.[15] Patients must be asked what other medications they are taking, specifically questioning supplement use. Drug-nutrient interactions may result in a depletion of a nutrient (e.g., corticosteroids deplete vitamin C, antibiotics destroy the gut flora and thus microbial production of vitamin K), or the vitamin may induce a change in the rate of metabolism of the drug (e.g., vitamin B_6 reduces the effectiveness of the anticonvulsant medication phenytoin but improves the effectiveness of certain tricyclic antidepressants).[14]

Drug-Herb Interactions

Interactions involving prescription drugs and herbs are the least well-defined drug interactions. St. John's wort *(Hypericum perforatum),* one of the most commonly taken herbs (as an antidepressant), has been extensively studied for drug interactions. The exact mechanism by which St. John's wort interacts with medications is not clear because it is not the same with all drugs. Some researchers have found the herb decreased the activity of key enzymes involved in the metabolism of drugs, whereas others have found the herb increased the enzymatic activ-

TABLE 17-4

FOODS AND NUTRIENTS AFFECTING MEDICATIONS

DRUG CLASS	EXAMPLES	USE	FOOD/NUTRIENT	ACTION	HOW TO AVOID
Alcohol, particularly excessive use	Beer, wine, spirits	Lowers inhibitions, CNS depressant	Food	Slowed absorption	Consume alcohol with food or meals
Analgesics and non-steroidal antiin-flammatory drugs	Salicylates (aspirin), Ibuprofen (Motrin, Advil), naproxen (Anaprox, Aleve, Naprosyn), Acetaminophen (Tylenol)	Pain and fever	Alcohol	Alcohol ingestion increases hepatotoxicity, liver damage, and stomach bleeding	Limit alcohol intake to 2 drinks/day for men, 1 drink/day for women
Antibiotics	Ciprofloxacin (Cipro)	Infection	Dairy products	Decreased absorption	Avoid dairy products
Anticoagulant	Warfarin (Coumadin)	Blood clots	Vitamins K and E (supplements) may reduce efficacy, alcohol and garlic may increase anticoagulation	Reduced efficacy, increased anticoagulation	Limit foods high in vitamin K, e.g, broccoli, spinach, kale, turnip greens, cauliflower, Brussels sprouts; avoid high doses of vitamin E (400 IU)
Anticonvulsants	Phenobarbital	Seizures, epilepsy	Alcohol	Increased sedation	Avoid alcohol
Antidepressants (monoamine oxidase inhibitors)	Phenelzine (Nardil), tranylcypromine (Parnate)	Depression, anxiety	Foods or alcoholic beverages containing tyramine	Rapid, potentially fatal increase in blood pressure	Avoid beer; red wine; American processed, cheddar, bleu, brie, mozzarella, and parmesan cheeses; yogurt and sour cream; beef and chicken liver; cured meats such as sausage and salami; game meats; caviar and dried fish; avocados, bananas, raisins, broad (fava) beans; sauerkraut; yeast extracts; soy sauce and miso soup; ginseng; caffeine-containing products (colas, chocolate, coffee, tea)
Antiemetics	Amitriptyline (Elavil), chlorpromazine (Thorazine)	Antidepressant, antipsychotic/antiemetic	Alcohol	Increased sedation	Avoid alcohol
Antihistamines	Fexofenadine (Allegra), loratadine (Claritin), cetirizine (Zyrtec), astemizole (Hismanal)	Allergies	Alcohol	Increased drowsiness and slowed mental and motor performance	Use caution when operating machinery or driving
Antihyperlipidemics (HMG-CoA reductase inhibitors) or statins	Atorvastatin (Lipitor), lovastatin (Mevacor), pravastatin (Pravachol), simvastatin (Zocor)	High serum LDL cholesterol	Food and meals, alcohol	Enhanced absorption, increased risk of liver damage	Lovastatin should be taken with evening meal to enhance absorption, avoid large amounts of alcohol

Continued

TABLE 17-4

FOODS AND NUTRIENTS AFFECTING MEDICATIONS—cont'd

DRUG CLASS	EXAMPLES	USE	FOOD/NUTRIENT	ACTION	HOW TO AVOID
Antihypertensives	Angiotensin-converting enzyme inhibitors, angiotensin II receptor antagonists, beta-blockers, verapamil	Hypertension	Natural licorice (*Glycyrrhiza glabra*) and tyramine-rich foods	Reduced effectiveness	Avoid tyramine-containing foods (see list under Antidepressants)
Antineoplastic drugs	Methotrexate	Cancer	Alcohol	Increased hepatotoxicity with chronic alcohol use	Avoid alcohol
Antiparkinson agents	Levodopa (Dopar, Larodopa)	Parkinson's disease	High-protein foods (eggs, meat, protein supplements), vitamin B_6	Decreased absorption	Spread protein intake equally in three to six meals/day to minimize reaction; avoid vitamin B_6 supplements or multivitamin supplement in doses >10 mg
Antituberculotics	Isoniazid (INH)	Tuberculosis	Alcohol	Reduced absorption with foods, increased hepatotoxicity and reduced isoniazid levels with alcohol	Take on empty stomach, avoid alcohol
Antiulcer agents (histamine blockers)	Cimetidine (Tagamet)	Ulcers	Alcohol, caffeine-containing foods and beverages	Increased blood alcohol levels, reduced caffeine clearance	Limit caffeine intake; limit alcohol intake to ≤2 drinks/day for men, ≤1 drink/day for women
Bronchodilators	Theophylline (Slo-Bid, Theo-Dur)	Asthma, chronic bronchitis, emphysema	Caffeine, alcohol	Increased stimulation of CNS; alcohol can increase nausea, vomiting, headache, and irritability	Avoid caffeine-containing foods and beverages (chocolate, colas, teas coffee); avoid alcohol if taking theophylline medications
Corticosteroids	Prednisone (Pediapred, Preline, Solu-Medrol), hydrocortisone	Inflammation and itching	Food	Stomach irritation	Take with food or milk to decrease stomach upset
Hypoglycemic agents	Sulfonylurea (Diabinese), metformin (Glucophage)	Diabetes	Alcohol	Severe nausea and vomiting	Avoid alcohol

HMG-CoA, 3-hydroxy-3-methylglutaryl coenzyme A.
Data from Anderson J, Hart H: *Nutrient-drug interactions and food*, Fort Collins, CO, 2004, Colorado State University Cooperative Extension. Available at *www.ext.colostate.edu/pubs/foodnut/09361.html*; Bland SE: Drug-food interactions, *J Pharm Soc Wisc* Nov/Dec:28, 1998; Bobroff LB and others: *Food/drug and drug/nutrient interactions: what you should know about your medications*, Gainesville, FL, 1994, University of Florida Cooperative Extension Service, Institute of Food and Agricultural Science. Available at *edis.ifas.ufl.edu*; Brown CH: Overview of drug interactions, *US Pharmacist* 25(5), 2000. Available at *www.uspharmacist.com/index.asp?show=archive&issue=5_2000*; Kuhn MA: Drug interactions with medications and food [online course], Hoffman Estates, IL, 2005, Nursing Spectrum Online. Available at *nsweb.nursingspectrum.com/ce/ce174.htm*; and Food and Drug Administration/National Consumers League: *Food & drug interactions* [brochure], Washington, DC, Food and Drug Administration. Available at *www.nclnet.org/Food%20%26%20Drug.pdf*.

CLINICAL APPLICATIONS

CASE STUDY: DRUG-NUTRIENT INTERACTION

Linda, a 32-year-old woman, reported to her doctor with symptoms including fatigue; headaches; muscle, joint, and bone pain; dry, flaking skin; amenorrhea; nausea and vomiting; and weight loss. After a physical examination and laboratory work, Linda was determined to have liver damage. The only prescription medication Linda takes is isotretinoin (Accutane) for acne. She also reported taking several dietary supplements, including a multivitamin, a fat-soluble vitamin mixture with 500% of the RDA for all fat-soluble vitamins, an antioxidant liquid mix, and an occasional multimineral.

1. Could her dietary supplement use have anything to do with her liver problems? Why?
2. What foods and/or nutrients should be avoided when taking isotretinoin?
3. What would you counsel Linda on regarding to her supplement and medication use?

Linda also mentions that she is trying to become pregnant. Would you recommend she change anything with her supplement or medication use?

ity.[14] Other common herbs involved in drug interactions include papaya extract *(Carica papaya)*, devil's claw *(Harpagophytum procumbens)*, *Ginkgo biloba*, evening primrose *(Oenothera biennis)*, valerian *(Valeriana officinale)*, kelp *(Fucus vesiculosus)*, ginseng *(Panax ginseng)*, and ginger *(Zingiber officinale)*.[14] Many herbs also have clinically documented medicinal properties and should be evaluated on an individual basis to determine appropriateness with the patient's current dietary habits and prescribed medications.

SUMMARY

The basis for effective nutrition care begins with the patient's nutrition needs and must involve the patient and family. Such person-centered care requires initial assessment and planning by the dietitian and continuous close teamwork among all team members providing primary care. Careful assessment of factors influencing nutrition status requires a broad foundation of pertinent information (e.g., physiologic, psychosocial, medical, and personal). The patient's medical record is a basic means of communication among health care team members.

Nutrition therapy is based on the personal and physical needs of the patient. Successful therapy requires a close working relationship among dietetics, medical, and nursing staff in the health care facility. The nurse is in a unique position to reinforce nutrition principles of the diet with the patient and family.

Drug interactions with nutrients, foods, or other medications can present complications with patient care. Careful questioning to determine all prescription and over-the-counter supplements and medications taken will help guide education needs for the patient.

CRITICAL THINKING QUESTIONS

1. Identify and discuss the possible effects of various psychosocial factors on the outcome of nutrition therapy.
2. Describe commonly used measures for determining nutrition status in an outpatient setting and a long-term care facility. Include the following measurement tools: (1) anthropometric measures, (2) biochemical tests, (3) clinical observations, and (4) diet evaluation.
3. Describe the roles of the dietitian and nurse in the nutrition care plan. What part of the care plan are nurses closely involved in? In what situation would a nurse refer a patient to the dietitian?
4. When questioning a patient about diet history after bypass surgery, you determine the patient is fond of spinach, kale, and broccoli. The patient reports eating at least two servings of the above foods almost every day. Knowing that most patients undergoing bypass take an anticoagulant medication after surgery, what would you counsel the patient on?

CHAPTER CHALLENGE QUESTIONS

True-False

Write the correct statement for each statement that is false.

1. *True or False:* Nutrition care is based on the needs of individual patients.

2. *True or False:* Patients' housing situations have little relation to their illnesses or continuing care.

3. *True or False:* History taking is an important skill in planning nutrition care.

4. *True or False:* Once a diet treatment plan has been established, it should be continuously followed without change.

6. *True or False:* The involvement of the patient's family in the diet therapy and teaching usually creates problems and is best avoided.

7. *True or False:* Patients' personal goals do not relate to their diet therapy and instruction.

8. *True or False:* Drug-nutrient interactions only create complications when the patient is taking dietary supplements; they do not occur with whole foods.

Multiple Choice

1. Which of the following personal details help determine a patient's nutrition needs? *(Circle all that apply.)*

    a. GI function
    b. Blood protein level
    c. Skinfold thickness
    d. Symptoms of illness

2. A nutrition history should include which of the following items of nutrition information? *(Circle all that apply.)*

    a. General food habits
    b. Food buying practices
    c. Cooking methods
    d. Food likes and dislikes

3. Knowledge of which of the following items is necessary for carrying out valid nutrition therapy for a hospitalized patient? *(Circle all that apply.)*

    a. The specific diet and its relation to the patient's disease

    b. Foods affected by the diet modification
    c. The mode of the hospital's food service and the patient's need for any eating assistance devices
    d. The patient's response to the diet

4. Which of the following actions would be helpful to a disabled patient who needs assistance in eating? *(Circle all that apply.)*

    a. Learning the extent of the disability and encouraging her to do as much of the feeding as she can herself
    b. Feeding the patient completely, regardless of the problem, because it saves her time and energy
    c. Hurrying the feeding to get in as much food as possible before the patient's appetite wanes
    d. Sitting comfortably by the patient's bed, offering mouthfuls of food, with ample time for chewing, swallowing, and rest as needed

evolve **Please refer to the Students' Resource section of this text's Evolve Web site for additional study resources.**

REFERENCES

1. Okkonen E, Vanhanen H: Family support, living alone, and subjective health of a patient in connection with a coronary artery bypass surgery, *Heart Lung* 35(4):234, 2006.
2. Raina P and others: The health and well-being of caregivers of children with cerebral palsy, *Pediatrics* 115(6):e626, 2005.
3. Steine S and others: A new, brief questionnaire (PEQ) developed in primary health care for measuring patients' experience of interaction, emotion and consultation outcome, *Fam Pract* 18(4):410, 2001.
4. Lacey K, Pritchett E: Nutrition care process and model: ADA adopts road map to quality care and outcomes management, *J Am Diet Assoc* 103(8):1061, 2003.
5. Scagliusi FB and others: Underreporting of energy intake in developing nations, *Nutr Rev* 64(7):319, 2006.
6. Scagliusi FB and others: Selective underreporting of energy intake in women: magnitude, determinants, and effect of training, *J Am Diet Assoc* 103(10):1306, 2003.
7. Harnack L and others: Accuracy of estimation of large food portions, *J Am Diet Assoc* 104(5):804, 2004.
8. Bailey RL and others: Assessing the effects of underreporting energy intake on dietary patterns and weight status, *J Am Diet Assoc* 107(1):64, 2007.
9. Fogelholm M and others: International Physical Activity Questionnaire: validity against fitness, *Med Sci Sports Exerc* 38(4):753, 2006.
10. Paquet C and others: Direct and indirect effects of everyday emotions on food intake of elderly patients in institutions, *J Gerontol A Biol Sci Med Sci* 58(2):153, 2003.
11. National Center for Health Statistics: *Health, United States, 2006, with chartbook on trends in the health of Americans*, Hyattsville, MD, 2006, U.S. Government Printing Office.
12. Mertens-Talcott SU and others: Grapefruit-drug interactions: can interactions with drugs be avoided? *J Clin Pharmacol* 46(12):1390, 2006.

13. Paine MF and others: A furanocoumarin-free grapefruit juice establishes furanocoumarins as the mediators of the grapefruit juice-felodipine interaction, *Am J Clin Nutr* 83(5):1097, 2006.
14. Sorensen JM: Herb-drug, food-drug, nutrient-drug, and drug-drug interactions: mechanisms involved and their medical implications, *J Altern Complement Med* 8(3):293, 2002.
15. Timbo BB and others: Dietary supplements in a national survey: prevalence of use and reports of adverse events, *J Am Diet Assoc* 106(12):1966, 2006.

FURTHER READING AND RESOURCES

National Policy and Resource Center on Nutrition and Aging, Nutrition Screening and Assessment: Nutrition Screening Initiative and Mini Nutritional Assessment: *www.fiu.edu/~nutreldr/SubjectList/N/Nutrition_Screening_Assessment.htm*

This site provides research, reports, resources, and additional Web links for nutrition assessment tools.

American Society for Parenteral and Enteral Nutrition: *www.clinnutr.org*

This association provides education, publications, conferences, and resources on clinical nutrition therapy for health care professionals. The association is made up of physicians, dietitians, nurses, pharmacists, scientists, and other allied health care professionals.

Lacey K, Pritchett E: Nutrition care process and model: ADA adopts road map to quality care and outcomes management, *J Am Diet Assoc* 103(8):1061, 2003.

The authors discuss the development, purpose, model, and future implications for standardized nutrition.

Sorensen JM: Herb-drug, food-drug, nutrient-drug, and drug-drug interactions: mechanisms involved and their medical implications, *J Altern Complement Med* 8(3):293, 2002.

Sorensen presents a thorough review of adverse interactions between drugs and herbs, food, nutrients, and other drugs. Internet resources for additional information on drug interactions are provided.

CHAPTER 18

Gastrointestinal and Accessory Organ Problems

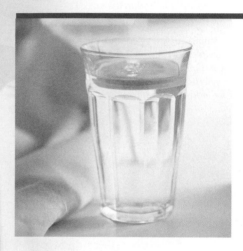

KEY CONCEPTS

- Diseases of the GI tract and its accessory organs interrupt the body's normal cycle of digestion, absorption, and metabolism.
- Food allergies result from sensitivity to certain proteins.
- Underlying genetic diseases may cause metabolic defects that block the body's ability to handle specific foods.

The body's highly organized and intricate system for handling food often is taken for granted. However, when something goes wrong with the system the whole being is affected. The GI tract is a sensitive mirror, both directly and indirectly, of the individual human condition.

This chapter looks at the sensitive system that handles food and its nutrients to provide energy and maintain body tissues. The digestive process requires a series of cascading events throughout the GI tract and the accessory organs—the pancreas, liver, and gallbladder. Nutrition therapy must be based on the functioning of this finely integrated network and on the person whose life it affects.

THE UPPER GASTROINTESTINAL TRACT

Major diseases affecting the GI tract are not limited to the small or large intestine. The most affected areas are discussed in this chapter under the sections where their primary problems exist.

Problems of the Mouth

Dental Problems

Although the incidence of dental caries has declined somewhat in recent years, tooth decay still plagues children and adults. Some of the decline is associated with increased use of fluoridated public water and toothpaste as well as better dental hygiene. Researchers concluded in a thorough review of the literature over the past half century that the benefits of fluoride toothpastes are clearly effective in preventing dental caries in children and adolescents.[1] In elderly persons, loss of teeth or ill-fitting dentures may cause problems with eating, swallowing, and overall nutrition. According to the CDC, tooth decay is more common in individuals from a lower socioeconomic background. More than 40% of poor adults have at least one untreated decayed tooth.[2] Sometimes a mechanical soft diet is helpful for individuals lacking teeth. In such a diet, all foods are soft cooked and meats are ground and mixed with sauces or gravies so that less chewing is necessary.

Surgical Procedures

A fractured jaw or other mouth or neck surgery poses obvious eating problems. Healing nutrients must be supplied, usually in the form of high-protein, high-caloric liquids. Table 18-1 provides an example of a simple milkshake. Other commercial formulas also are available (see Chapter 22). As healing progresses, soft foods requiring little chewing effort can be added, building to a full diet according to individual tolerance.

Oral Tissue Inflammation

The tissues of the mouth often reflect a person's general nutrition status. Malnutrition, especially severe states, causes deterioration of oral tissues, resulting in local infection or injury that brings pain and difficulty eating. The following conditions of malnutrition in the oral cavity affect all its parts:

- *Gingivitis:* Inflammation of the gums involving the mucous membrane and its supporting fibrous tissue circling the base of the teeth (Figure 18-1, *A*).
- *Stomatitis:* Inflammation of the oral mucous lining of the mouth (Figure 18-1, *B*).
- *Glossitis:* Inflammation of the tongue (Figure 18-1, *C*).
- *Cheilosis:* A dry, scaling process at the corners of the mouth affecting the lips and corner angles, making opening the mouth quite painful (Figure 18-1, *D*).

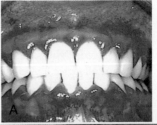
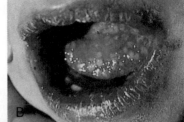
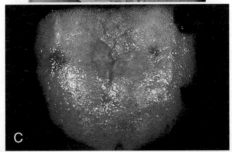
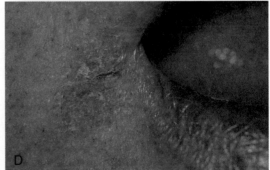

Figure 18–1 Tissue inflammation of the mouth. **A,** Gingivitis. **B,** Stomatitis. **C,** Glossitis. **D,** Cheilosis. (**A** reprinted from Murray PR and others: *Medical microbiology,* ed 2, St Louis, 1994, Mosby. **B** reprinted from Doughty DB, Broadwell-Jackson D: *Gastrointestinal disorders,* St Louis, 1993, Mosby. **C** reprinted from Hoffbrand AV, Pettit JE (eds): *Sandoz atlas of clinical hematology,* London, 1988, Gower Medical. **D** reprinted from Lemmi FO, Lemmi CAE: *Physical assessment findings* [CD-ROM], Philadelphia, 2000, Saunders.)

TABLE 18-1

HIGH-PROTEIN, HIGH-KILOCALORIE FORMULA FOR LIQUID FEEDINGS

INGREDIENT	AMOUNT
Milk	1 cup
Egg substitute	Equivalent of 2 eggs
Skim milk powder or enteral nutrition formula	6-8 Tbsp
Sugar	2 Tbsp
Ice cream	2.5-cm (1-inch) slice or 1 scoop
Cocoa or other flavoring	2 Tbsp
Vanilla	Few drops, as desired

Approximate food value: 40 g protein, 30 g fat, 70 g carbohydrate, 710 kcal.
Prepackaged supplemental feedings generally are used instead of homemade liquid feedings.

Mouth ulcers may develop from three infectious sources: (1) the herpes simplex virus, which causes mouth sores on the inside mucous lining of the cheeks and lips or on the external portion of the lips, where they are commonly called cold sores or fever blisters; (2) *Candida albicans,* a fungus causing similar sores on the oral mucosa, a condition called candidiasis or thrush; and (3) hemolytic *Streptococcus,* a bacteria causing mucosal ulcers commonly called canker sores. Mouth ulcers usually are self-limiting and short lived. Other causes include simple toothbrush abrasions or allergies. Patients with an underlying illness such as cancer or HIV, both of which lower the body's immune system, often have mouth ulcers. Chemotherapy and radiation treatment to the mouth destroy the fast-replicating cells and can result in mouth sores.

In these situations eating is painful; adequate nutrition should be considered in severe cases. Progressing from nutritionally dense liquids, high in protein and calories, to soft foods (e.g., usually nonacidic and bland to avoid irritation) is well tolerated. Extremes in temperature are avoided if they cause pain. Room temperature soft or liquid foods usually are better accepted. In severe disease, such as in cancer and its treatments, a mouthwash containing a mild topical local anesthetic before meals helps relieve the pain of eating.

Salivary Gland Problems

Disorders of the salivary glands in the mouth also affect eating and related nutrition status. Problems may arise from infection, such as the mumps virus that attacks the parotid gland (Figure 18-2). Other problems arise from excess salivation. This is seen in numerous disorders affecting the nervous system, local mouth infections, injury, and drug reactions. Conversely, a dry mouth from lack of salivation may be temporary and caused by fear, infection, or drug reaction. Chronic dry mouth, called xerostomia, sometimes occurs in middle-aged and elderly adults and often is associated with rheumatoid arthritis,

radiation therapy, or as a side effect from many drugs taken on a long-term basis. Xerostomia causes difficulty in swallowing and speaking, taste interference, and tooth decay. More liquid food items such as beverages, soups, stews, juicy fruits, and gravies or sauces may facilitate the eating process. Extreme mouth dryness may be partially relieved by spraying an artificial saliva solution inside the mouth.

Swallowing Disorders

Swallowing is not as simple an act as it may seem. It involves highly integrated actions of the mouth, pharynx, and esophagus and, once started, is beyond voluntary control. Swallowing difficulty is a fairly common problem with a variety of causes. It may be only temporary (e.g., a piece of food lodged in the back of the throat), and the Heimlich maneuver may be appropriate first aid. However, dysphagia is a more chronic problem in some patients and may be associated with insufficient production of saliva, dry mouth, abnormal peristaltic motility of the esophagus, complications of medication, or neurologic disorders. To treat dysphagia effectively, the problem must be identified as either a mechanical obstruction or a neuromuscular disorder and usually is diagnosed by a speech-language pathologist. Such dysfunctional swallowing may cause aspiration of food particles, which may be evident in coughing or choking episodes. Swallowing disorders are particularly common in cases of head trauma or brain tumor, stroke, advanced Alzheimer's disease, and Parkinson's disease.[3]

Dysphagia has been estimated to affect 35% to 60% of nursing home residents.[4] Subtle symptoms include an unexplained drop in food intake or repeated episodes of

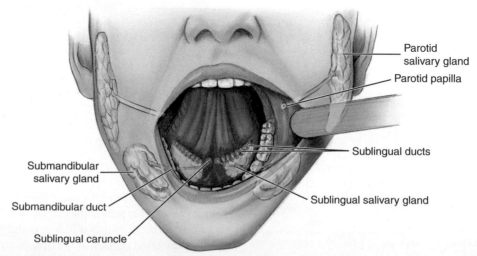

Figure 18–2 Location of the salivary glands. (Reprinted from Fehrenbach MJ, Herring SW: *Illustrated anatomy of the head and neck,* ed 3, 2007, Saunders.)

pneumonia, possibly related to aspiration of food particles. Watch for warning signs of dysphagia and report them immediately. These signs may include reluctance to eat certain food consistencies or any food at all, very slow chewing or eating, fatigue from eating, frequent throat clearing, complaints of food "sticking" in the throat, pockets of food held in the cheeks, painful swallowing, regurgitation, and coughing or choking during attempts to eat.

The problem usually is referred to a team of specialists that includes a physician, nurse, dietitian, and speech-language pathologist, who is especially important for both the evaluation and treatment of swallowing problems. Thin liquids are the most difficult food form to swallow. Thus the diet is adapted to individual needs, in stages of added thickened liquids and pureed foods. Pureed foods generally are the consistency of mashed potatoes or pudding. Regular table food can be pureed in a food processor to achieve the desired consistency. Several manufacturers produce pureed foods or food molds shaped like various meats or vegetables. Placing pureed foods in a food mold to take the shape of the original food (e.g., corn on the cob or chicken breast) enhances the appeal and appetite of patients faced with swallowing disorders and has been shown to improve overall nutrition intake.[4]

Problems of the Esophagus

Central Tube Problems

The esophagus is a long muscular tube extending from the throat to the stomach. It is bound on both ends by circular muscles, or sphincters, that act as valves to control food passage. The upper sphincter muscle remains closed except during swallowing, preventing airflow into the esophagus and stomach. On swallowing, the sphincter automatically opens and then closes immediately afterward. Various disorders along the tube may disrupt normal swallowing, including (1) muscle spasms or uncoordinated contractions, and (2) stricture or narrowing of the tube caused by a scar from a previous injury, ingestion of caustic chemicals, a tumor, or esophagitis (inflammation of the esophagus). These problems hinder eating and require medical attention through stretching procedures or surgery to widen the tube and drug therapy to heal the inflammation. The diet during such problems is liquid to soft in texture, depending on the extent of the problem and individual tolerance.

Lower Esophageal Sphincter Problems

Defects in the function of the lower esophageal sphincter (LES) may come from changes in the smooth muscle itself or from the nerve-muscle hormone control of peri-

stalsis (see Chapter 5). Spasms occur when the LES muscles maintain an excessively high muscle tone, even while resting, thus failing to open normally when the person swallows. This condition is medically termed achalasia, from its tense muscle state, but commonly is called cardiospasm because of its proximity of the heart, although the condition does not relate to the heart at all. Symptoms include swallowing problems, frequent vomiting, a feeling of fullness in the chest, weight loss from eating difficulty, serious malnutrition, and pulmonary complications and infection caused by aspiration of food particles, especially during sleep. Surgical treatment involves dilating the LES or cutting the muscle, a procedure called an esophagomyotomy. Both procedures can improve relaxation of the LES, but neither affects the lack of peristalsis. The postoperative course starts with oral liquids and progresses to a regular diet within a few days, depending on tolerance. Patients should avoid very hot or cold foods, citrus juices, and highly spiced foods to prevent irritation. Patients also should eat frequent small meals as tolerated and eat slowly in small bites.

---

parotid glands the largest of three pairs of salivary glands situated near the ear. The parotid glands lie, one on each side, above the angle of the jaw, below and in front of the ear. They continually secrete saliva, which passes along the duct of the gland and into the mouth through an opening in the inner cheek, level with the second upper molar tooth. Normal saliva flow facilitates the chewing and swallowing of food and prevents dry mouth problems.

xerostomia dryness of the mouth from lack of normal secretions.

pharynx the muscular membranous passage between the mouth and the posterior nasal passages and the larynx and esophagus.

Heimlich maneuver a first-aid maneuver to relieve a person who is choking from blockage of the breathing passageway by a swallowed foreign object or food particle. Standing behind the person, clasp the victim around the waist, placing one fist just under the sternum (breastbone) and grasping the fist with the other hand. Then make a quick, hard, thrusting movement inward and upward to dislodge the object.

dysphagia difficulty swallowing.

speech-language pathologist a specialist in the assessment, diagnosis, treatment, and prevention of speech, language, cognitive communication, voice, swallowing, fluency, and other related disorders.

Gastroesophageal Reflux Disease

Ongoing LES problems and esophageal motor impairment contribute to chronic gastroesophageal reflux disease (GERD).[5] Constant regurgitation of acidic gastric contents into the lower part of the esophagus creates tissue irritation and inflammation, called esophagitis (Figure 18-3). GERD is a serious and difficult problem that has been described as "acid setting up shop in the esophagus." The problem is likely more widespread than the number of cases reported because only a few chronic sufferers seek medical help. In addition, acid reflux may be attributed to pregnancy, obesity, pernicious vomiting, or nasogastric tubes. Gastric acid and pepsin from the stomach cause tissue erosion, resulting in the most common symptom of frequent, severe heartburn that occurs 30 to 60 minutes after eating. The pain sometimes moves into the neck or jaw or down the arms. The most common complications are (1) stenosis, a narrowing or stricture of the esophagus, and (2) esophageal ulcer.

Treatment for GERD and its relentless esophagitis includes weight management because obesity often is a causative factor.[6,7] Other conservative measures include acid control and a low-fat diet. High-fat diets make closure of the esophageal sphincter less effective. Patients must avoid lying down after eating and must sleep with the head of the bed elevated. Frequent use of antacids helps control the symptoms. The goals and actions of dietary care are outlined in Table 18-2.

Hiatal Hernia

The lower end of the esophagus normally enters the chest cavity through an opening in the diaphragm membrane called the hiatus. A hiatal hernia occurs when a portion of the upper stomach also protrudes through this opening, as shown in Figure 18-4. Hiatal hernias are not uncom-

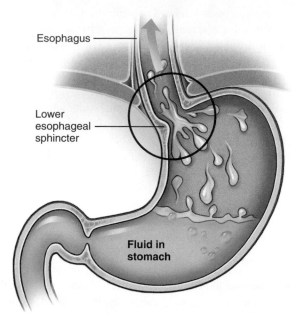

Figure 18-3 Reflux of gastric acid up into the esophagus through the LES in GERD. (Reprinted from Thibodeau GA, Patton KT: *Anatomy and physiology*, ed 6, St Louis, 2007, Mosby.)

mon, especially in obese adults, for whom weight reduction is essential. Patients with a hiatal hernia are advised to eat small amounts of food at a time, avoid lying down after meals, and sleep with the head of the bed elevated to prevent reflux of acidic stomach contents. Frequent use of antacids helps control the symptoms of heartburn, which is caused by the acid-enzyme-food mixture irritating the lower esophagus and the upper herniated area of the stomach. A meta-analysis of the literature found the risk for GERD symptoms and erosive esophagitis increased with overweight or obesity compared with normal BMI, indicating that patients may respond well to

TABLE 18-2

DIETARY CARE OF GERD

GOAL	ACTION
Decrease esophageal irritation	Avoid common irritants such as coffee, carbonated beverages, tomato and citrus juices, and spicy foods
Increase LES pressure	Increase lean protein foods
	Decrease fat to approximately 45 g/day or less; use nonfat milk
	Avoid strong tea, coffee, and chocolate if poorly tolerated
	Avoid peppermint and spearmint
Decrease reflux frequency and volume	Eat small, frequent meals
	Sip only a small amount of liquid with meal; drink mostly between meals
	Avoid constipation; straining increases abdominal pressure reflux
Clear food materials from the esophagus	Sit upright at the table and elevate the head of the bed
	Do not recline for 2 hours or more after eating

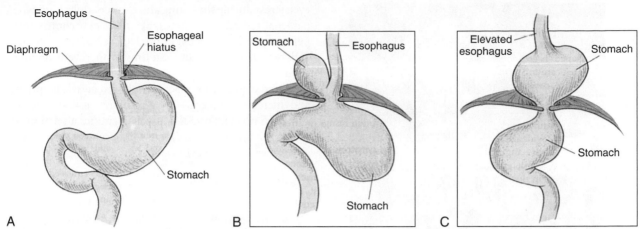

Figure 18–4 Hiatal hernia compared with normal stomach placement. **A,** Normal stomach. **B,** Paraesophageal hernia (esophagus in normal position). **C,** Esophageal hiatal hernia (elevated esophagus). (Courtesy Bill Ober.)

weight reduction and other conservative measures.[8] Large hiatal hernias or smaller sliding hernias, however, usually require surgical repair.

Problems of the Stomach and Duodenum: Peptic Ulcer Disease

An ulcer is a craterlike lesion in the wall of the stomach or duodenum that erodes the mucosal layers (Figure 18-5, *A*).

Incidence

Throughout the United States, lifetime prevalence of peptic ulcer disease (PUD) is approximately 10%, with similar occurrences in men and women. PUD affects 4.5 million people annually, with an estimated death rate of 1 per 100,000 cases.[9] It can occur at any age but is mostly seen in middle-aged and older adults.

Causes

The underlying cause of PUD in most cases has been identified as *Helicobacter pylori* infection (Figure 18-5, *B*).[10] *H. pylori,* responsible for up to 85% of gastric and duodenal ulcers, are common spiraling, rod-shaped bacteria inhabiting the GI area around the pyloric valve. This muscular valve connects the lower part of the stomach to the head of the small intestine, the duodenal bulb. Infection by *H. pylori* is a major determinant of chronic active gastritis and also is a necessary ingredient, along with gastric acid and pepsin, in the ulcerative process. Although approximately half of the world's population is infected with *H. pylori,* not all persons develop ulcers (see the Cultural Considerations box, "Risk for Gastric Ulcer Disease: Environmental or Genetic?"). However, persons

with chronic *H. pylori* infections are at a much greater risk for developing gastric cancer.[10] Tobacco smoking also was found to be highly correlated to PUD in a recent large-scale study in Denmark, confirming it as a major risk factor. The same study noted a negative association with physical activity.[11] Thus increased physical activity may lessen the occurrence of PUD in some individuals.

Long-term use of nonsteroidal antiinflammatory drugs (NSAIDs) also may contribute to PUD development.[12] These widely used drugs, including ibuprofen (Advil, Motrin) and aspirin (acetylsalicylic acid), irritate the gastric mucosa and cause bleeding, erosion, and ulceration, especially with prolonged or excessive use. The NSAIDs, including at least a dozen antiinflammatory drugs, are so named to distinguish them from steroid drugs, which are synthetic variants of natural adrenal hormones. However, both physical and psychological factors are involved in PUD development.

Physical Factors. The general term peptic ulcer refers to an eroded mucosal lesion in the central portion of the GI tract. This lesion can occur in the lower esophagus, stomach, or first portion of the duodenum, the duodenal bulb. Most ulcers occur in the duodenal bulb because the gastric contents emptying there are most concentrated. The lesion results from an imbalance among the following three factors: (1) the amount of gastric acid and pepsin secretions (a powerful gastric enzyme for digestion of protein), (2) extent of the *H. pylori* infection, and (3) the degree of tissue resistance to these secretions and the infection. The more acidic the environment, the more favorable the conditions for *H. pylori* colonization.

Psychological Factors. The influence of psychological factors in the development of peptic ulcer varies. No distinct personality type is free from the disease. How-

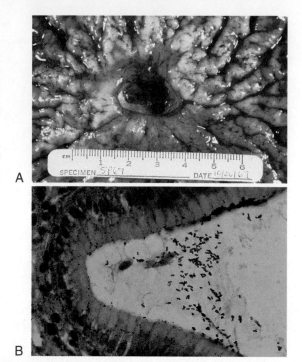

A

B

Figure 18–5 **A,** Gastric ulcer. **B,** *H. pylori (black particles)* infecting the stomach mucosa. (Reprinted from Thibodeau GA, Patton KT: *Anatomy and physiology,* ed 6, St Louis, 2007, Mosby Elsevier.)

ever, stress during the young and middle adult years, when personal and career striving is at a peak, may contribute to peptic ulcer development in predisposed individuals. Several neurologic changes resulting from severe or long-term stress have specific effects on the GI tract, such as increased colonic motor activity, slowed gastric emptying, and increased susceptibility to colonic inflammation.[13] Although no evidence definitively identifies a relation between psychological stress and the development of PUD, an association likely exists and is under investigation.[14]

Clinical Symptoms

General symptoms of PUD include increased gastric muscle tone and painful contractions when the stomach is empty. With duodenal ulcers, the amount and concentration of hydrochloric acid secretions are increased; with gastric ulcers, the secretions may be normal. Hemorrhage may be one of the first signs. Low plasma protein levels, anemia, and weight loss reveal nutrition deficiencies. Diagnosis is confirmed by radiographs and visualization by gastroscopy.

Medical Management

In treating patients with PUD, physicians have four basic goals: (1) alleviate the symptoms, (2) promote healing, (3) prevent recurrences by eliminating the cause, and (4)

CULTURAL CONSIDERATIONS

RISK FOR GASTRIC ULCER DISEASE: ENVIRONMENTAL OR GENETIC?

Before the bacteria *Helicobacter pylori* was shown in 1982 to be the causative organism of PUD, the disease was thought to be the result of excess stress, acid, and spicy foods. Although these factors may still contribute to the disease, infection with *H. pylori* is now known to cause 80% to 90% of duodenal and gastric ulcers. Long-term use of NSAIDs is responsible for the majority of the other cases.

INFECTION WITH *H. PYLORI*

H. pylori infection is more common in certain ethnic and age groups. In the United States older adults, African Americans, and Hispanics have the highest prevalence of infection. Also, individuals of a lower socioeconomic status have a higher risk of *H. pylori* infection than do individuals of a higher socioeconomic status. The mechanism by which *H. pylori* infection is transmitted is not yet known; however, it is believed to be spread through the fecal-oral or oral-oral routes. This may be one of the reasons that *H. pylori* infection is higher in developing countries than in developed countries. Remember that not all carriers of the bacteria develop a peptic ulcer, however.

ACTIVE *H. PYLORI* ULCERS

H. pylori ulcers are more common in men than women in the United States. In other countries such as Japan, where PUD is quite common, men are reported to have twice the prevalence of peptic ulcers than women. The risks for developing an ulcer are not easily defined by genetics, gender, ethnicity, or environment. A combination of all these factors seems to lead to ulceration. Researchers believe that genetics are less important than environment in determining risk of ulceration, but both physiologic and psychological factors are involved in the overall environmental risk.

Physiologic trauma and emotional stress can lead to excess acid secretions in the stomach. For individuals already infected with *H. pylori* bacteria, that may be the missing link for creating a perfect environment for rapid growth and inflammation, ultimately resulting in an ulcer. Therefore treatment for peptic ulcers must focus on eliminating the cause (bacteria or drugs) and focus on the environmental cues involved in promoting excessive acidic secretions.

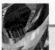

DRUG-NUTRIENT INTERACTION

TETRACYCLINE AND MINERAL ABSORPTION

Tetracycline is a broad-spectrum antibiotic used to treat conditions such as respiratory tract infections, acne, infections of the skin, and stomach ulcers. Minerals with a 2+ charge, including magnesium, calcium, and iron, bond with tetracycline to form a new compound that the body can no longer absorb.* Thus tetracycline is less effective and mineral absorption is poor.

To ensure optimal absorption, avoid the following foods or medications 1 hour before and/or 2 hours after taking tetracycline:

- Foods containing high amounts of calcium, such as milk
- Calcium supplements
- Antacids
- Laxatives containing magnesium
- Iron supplements should be taken at least 2 hours before or 3 hours after tetracycline.†

Sara Oldroyd

*Merck Manual's Online Medical Library: *Tetracyclines, www.merck.com/mmpe/sec14/ch170/ch170o.html,* accessed April 2007.
†MedlinePlus: *Tetracycline, www.nlm.nih.gov/medlineplus/druginfo/medmaster/a682098.html,* accessed April 2007.

---

prevent complications. In addition to general traditional measures, the recently expanded knowledge base about the cause of PUD and the development of a number of new drugs have increased the physician's available management tools.

Rest. Adequate rest, relaxation, and sleep have long been the foundation of general care to enhance the body's natural healing process. Incorporating positive coping and relaxation skills into daily life may help patients deal with personal psychosocial stress factors. Encouraging patients to talk about anxieties, anger, and frustrations may help them work through issues. Appropriate physical activity helps some patients work out tension. Habits that contribute to ulcer development, such as smoking and alcohol use, should be eliminated. Irritating drugs (e.g., aspirin, NSAIDs) should be avoided. Sometimes sedatives are prescribed to aid rest.

Drug Therapy. Advances in knowledge and therapy have provided physicians with the following four basic types of drugs for managing PUD:

- Histamine H_2-receptor antagonists (H_2-blockers) control hydrochloric acid production and secretion (e.g., cimetidine [Tagamet], ranitidine [Zantac], famotidine [Pepcid], and nizatidine [Axid]).
- Proton pump inhibitors also reduce hydrochloric acid production by inhibiting hydrogen ion secretion needed to produce hydrochloric acid (e.g., lansoprazole [Prevacid], omeprazole [Prilosec], esomeprazole [Nexium], pantoprazole [Protonix], and rabeprazole [Aciphex]).
- Mucosal protectors inactivate pepsin and produce a gel-like substance to cover the ulcer and protect it from acid and pepsin while it heals itself (e.g., sucralfate [Carafate]).
- Antibiotics address the *H. pylori* infection (e.g., amoxicillin, clarithromycin, tetracycline, and metronida-

zole). See the Drug-Nutrient Interaction box, "Tetracycline and Mineral Absorption," regarding potential interactions with tetracycline and other nutrients.

- Antacids counteract or neutralize the acid. Magnesium-aluminum compounds (e.g., Mylanta II, Maalox TC) are typical antacids of choice in treating PUD.

Maintenance drug therapy is imperative to stabilize the growth rate of bacteria. A continuous low-dose drug therapy follows initial treatment, with intermittent full-dose treatment or symptomatic self-care with the same agents used to heal the initial ulcer infection. Success rates depend on the relative strengths of the risk factors that influence recurrence (Box 18-1).

Dietary Management

In the past, a highly restrictive, bland diet was used in the care of patients with PUD. A bland diet has long since proved to be ineffective and lacking in adequate nutrition support for the healing process. Such a restrictive diet is unnecessary today because newer and better drugs are available to control acid secretions and assist healing. Thus current diet therapy is based on a liberal individual approach, guided by individual responses to food. In this positive nutrition support for medical management, two basic goals guide food habits.

Eating a Well-Balanced, Healthy Diet. Supply a well-balanced, regular healthy diet to aid tissue healing and maintenance. Nutrient energy needs are outlined in the current RDAs and DRIs (see inside front cover) and

---

gastroscopy examination of the upper intestinal tract with a flexible tube with a small camera on the end. The tube is approximately 9 mm in diameter and takes color pictures as well as biopsy samples, if necessary.

RISK FACTORS FOR RECURRING PEPTIC ULCER

HIGH RISK

Medical/Physical
- Hypersecretion of gastric acid
- Previous recurrences of peptic ulcer with complications
- *H. pylori* infection

Emotional
- Continuous, unrelieved emotional stress
- Denial of emotional problems

Behavioral
- Poor dietary habits
- Failure to maintain prescribed diet and drug therapy
- Cigarette smoking (10 or more/day)

MODERATE RISK

Medical/Physical
- Family history of PUD among close relatives
- Recurring discomfort after eating

Emotional
- Emotionally stressful environment
- Recognition of emotional problems

Behavioral
- Frequent use of aspirin and other NSAIDs
- Distilled alcohol consumption
- Irregular meals

expressed in simple food choices in the MyPyramid guideline (see Figure 1-1). Further focus is provided by the goals of the *Dietary Guidelines for Americans* (see Figure 1-2).

Avoiding Acid Stimulation. Avoid stimulating excess gastric acid secretion, which irritates gastric mucosa. Only a few food-related habits have been shown to affect acid secretion, as follows:

- *Food quantity:* To avoid stomach distension, do not eat large quantities at meals. Avoid eating right before going to bed; food intake stimulates acid output.
- *Milk intake:* Avoid drinking high-fat milk because it stimulates significant acid secretion, has only a transient buffering effect, and its animal fat content is undesirable.
- *Seasonings:* Individual tolerance is the rule, but hot chili peppers, black pepper, and chili powder have shown variable results and perhaps should be limited.
- *Dietary fiber:* No evidence exists for restricting dietary fiber. Some fibers, especially soluble forms, are beneficial.
- *Coffee:* Avoid regular and decaffeinated coffee, including drinks made with coffee. Coffee stimulates acid secretion and may cause indigestion. The comparative effect

of regular tea and colas may be milder to some persons, but these beverages also stimulate acid secretion.

- *Citric acid juices:* These juices may cause discomfort in persons with existing esophagitis.
- *Alcohol:* Avoid alcohol in concentrated forms, such as 40% (80 proof) alcohol. Other less-concentrated forms of wine, taken with food in moderation, are tolerated well by some patients. Avoid beer; it has been shown to be a potent stimulant of gastric acid. For those who find completely avoiding alcohol and coffee to be difficult, an occasional small glass of dinner wine or a small cup (demitasse) of coffee at the close of a meal may minimize the acid secretion.
- *Smoking:* Complete smoking cessation is best because smoking hinders ulcer healing. It affects gastric acid secretion and hinders the effectiveness of drug therapy.
- *Food environment:* Finally, consider the food environment. Eat slowly and savor the food in a calm environment. Respect individual responses or tolerances to specific foods. Remember that the same food may bring different responses at different times depending on stress factors.

In the long run, a wide range of foods that are attractive to the eye and taste and regular, relaxed eating habits provide the best course of action.

LOWER GASTROINTESTINAL TRACT

Small Intestine Diseases

Malabsorption

Malabsorption syndromes are characterized by a defect in the absorption of fats, proteins, carbohydrates, vitamins, minerals, and/or water. Malabsorption results from a disturbance in the normal digestive process, and the defect may include any of the following processes:

- *Digestion of macronutrients:* Carbohydrates, proteins, and fat are broken down into their basic building blocks (monosaccharides and disaccharides, amino acids, and fatty acids and glycerol, respectively) with the aid of salivary and pancreatic enzymes and bile acid.
- *Terminal digestion at the brush border mucosa:* Disaccharides and peptides are hydrolyzed by disaccharidases and peptidases for the final step of digestion.
- *Transport:* The final products of macronutrient digestion, micronutrients (vitamins, minerals, electrolytes) and water, are absorbed across the epithelium of the small intestine into the general or lymphatic circulation. Several organ systems and functions are affected by malabsorption disorders. Chronic deficiencies of vita-

TABLE 18-3

MAJOR MALABSORPTION SYNDROMES

SYMPTOMS	CAUSE
Defective Intraluminal Digestion	
Defective digestion of fats and proteins	Pancreatic insufficiency from pancreatitis or CF
	Zollinger-Ellison syndrome,* with inactivation of pancreatic enzymes by excess gastric acid secretion
Solubilization of fat as a result of defective bile secretion	Ileal dysfunction or resection with decreased bile salt uptake
	Cessation of bile flow from obstruction, hepatic dysfunction
Nutrient preabsorption or modification	Bacterial overgrowth
Primary Mucosal Cell Abnormalities	
Defective terminal digestion	Disaccharidase deficiency (lactose intolerance)
	Bacterial overgrowth with brush border damage
Defective epithelial transport	Abetalipoproteinemia (inherited disorder of fat metabolism from the inability to synthesize beta lipoproteins)
	Primary bile acid malabsorption resulting from mutations in the ileal bile acid transporter
Reduced Small Intestinal Surface Area	Gluten-sensitive enteropathy (CD)
	Crohn's disease
Lymphatic Obstruction	Lymphoma
	Tuberculosis and tuberculous lymphadenitis
Infection	Acute infectious enteritis
	Parasitic infestation
	Whipple disease (bacterial infection)
General malabsorption resulting from surgery	Subtotal or total gastrectomy
	Short-gut syndrome after extensive surgical resection
	Distal ileal resection or bypass

*Rare disorder that causes tumors in the pancreas and duodenum and ulcers in the stomach and duodenum. The tumors secrete a hormone called gastrin that causes the stomach to produce too much hydrochloric acid, which in turn causes stomach and duodenal ulcers. The symptoms include signs of a peptic ulcer: gnawing, burning pain in the abdomen; diarrhea; nausea; vomiting; fatigue; weakness; weight loss; and bleeding. (National Digestive Disease Information Clearinghouse: *Zollinger-Ellison Syndrome*, http://digestive.niddk.nih.gov/ddiseases/pubs/Zollinger, accessed June 2008.)

mins, minerals, and macronutrients can lead to several forms of anemia (iron, pyridoxine, folate, vitamin B_{12}); osteopenia and tetany (from calcium, vitamin D, and magnesium deficiency); and other musculoskeletal, endocrine, and nervous system abnormalities. The most common symptom of malabsorption disorders is chronic diarrhea and/or steatorrhea.

Three of these malabsorption conditions—cystic fibrosis, inflammatory bowel disease, and celiac sprue—are reviewed in this chapter. Other malabsorption syndromes are listed in Table 18-3. Diarrhea and steatorrhea usually are symptoms of a disease or disorder rather than diseases themselves. However, they are discussed in this section because they pertain to most malabsorption disorders.

Cystic Fibrosis

Disease Process. Cystic fibrosis (CF) is the most common fatal genetic disease in North America and occurs in approximately 1 in 3300 live Caucasian births and 1 in

15,300 African-American births.[15] Although the disease is characterized as a pulmonary disease, it is a multisystem disorder with a profound GI tract impact. Because pulmonary diseases are outside the scope of this text, only the nutrition implications of CF are discussed.

CF is a generalized genetic disease of childhood inherited as an autosomal recessive trait that can include multiple defects. In past years, children with CF generally lived to approximately age 10 years, dying from complications such as damaged airways and lung infections as well as a fibrous pancreas and lack of essential pancreatic enzymes to digest nutrients. However, recent discovery of the CF gene and the underlying metabolic defect has improved management of the disease and helped push the life expectancy into adulthood. Nevertheless, mortality

steatorrhea fatty diarrhea; excessive amounts of fat in the feces often caused by malabsorption diseases.

rates from CF have a strong correlation with poverty status. A recent study reported individuals in the lowest socioeconomic category as having a 44% increased risk of death compared with patients in the highest income category.[16] Identifying and addressing differences between socioeconomic classes in terms of treatment factors, environment, and overall care are important to improve the life of all patients with CF.

The metabolic defect of CF inhibits the normal movement of chloride (Cl−) and sodium (Na+) ions in body tissue fluids (see Chapter 9). These ions become trapped in cells, causing thick mucus to form that clogs ducts and passageways. Involved organ tissues are damaged so that they no longer function normally. The classic CF symptoms include the following:

- Thick mucus in the lungs, which leads to damaged airways, more difficult breathing, and pulmonary infections such as bronchitis and pneumonia
- Pancreatic insufficiency, which leads to lack of normal pancreatic enzymes (see Chapter 5) to digest the macronutrients and progressive loss of insulin-producing beta cells and eventual diabetes mellitus in approximately 15% of adult patients (see Chapter 20)
- Malabsorption of undigested food nutrients, with consequential malnutrition and stunted growth
- Liver disease from progressive degeneration of functional liver tissue, initiated by clogged bile ducts
- Inflammatory complications, including arthritis, finger clubbing, and/or vasculitis
- Increased salt concentration (formed from Na+ and Cl−) in body perspiration, leading to salt depletion

Nutrition Management. Nutrition therapy is a critical component of the treatment regimen and can have a significant impact on normal growth. Treatment is based on (1) increased knowledge of the disease process, (2) early newborn screening and diagnosis, and (3) improved pancreatic enzyme replacement products. These products, such as pancrelipase (Pancrease), contain the normal pancreatic enzymes for each energy nutrient (lipase for fat digestion; amylase for starch digestion; and the protein enzymes trypsin, chymotrypsin, and carboxypeptidase [see Chapter 5]). These enzymes are processed into very small enteric-coated beads encased in capsules designed not to open or dissolve until they reach the alkaline medium of the intestine. Generous doses of these enzyme-replacement capsules, varying with a child's age, weight, and symptoms, are divided among three meals and usually are taken just before eating. Adequate enzyme replacement is the foundation that makes aggressive diet therapy a possibility for meeting growth needs.

Children with CF require 105% to 150% of the recommended nutrients for their age, depending on the severity of the disease. A low-fat diet is no longer used. Instead, a nutritionally adequate diet is recommended and provides 15% to 20% of the kilocalories as protein, 35% to 40% as fat (as tolerated), and the remaining as carbohydrate. Routine care is based on regular nutrition assessment, diet counseling, food plans, enzyme replacement, vitamin supplements (especially fat-soluble vitamins A, D, E, and K), nutrition education, and exploration of individual problems, as outlined in Table 18-4. Try applying these principles of care in the Clinical Applications box, "Case Study: Paul's Adaptation to CF." This specialized care is administered by the medical genetics division of hospitals with a team of CF specialists.

Inflammatory Bowel Disease

The term inflammatory bowel disease applies to both Crohn's disease and ulcerative colitis. The related condition of short-bowel syndrome results from repeated surgical removal of parts of the small intestine as the disease progresses. Crohn's disease and ulcerative colitis are considered idiopathic diseases because their etiology is unknown. These diseases share many symptoms and management but differ in clinical manifestations. Both diseases result from chronic inflammation and inappropriate mucosal immune activation by normal gut flora for unknown reasons. As a result, portions of the GI tract develop lesions and malabsorption.

Crohn's Disease. Crohn's disease may affect any portion of the GI tract from mouth to anus but is most commonly localized to the ileum and colon. In the United States approximately three per 100,000 individuals are affected by Crohn's disease, with certain subgroups of the population demonstrating higher rates (females slightly more than males, Caucasians more than other ethnic groups). Inflammation may skip sections of the GI tract and affect more than one section at a time (Figure 18-6).

Ulcerative Colitis. UC is an inflammatory disease limited to the colon and occurs in approximately four to 12 per 100,000 individuals in the United States. Symptoms include diarrhea with blood and mucus, abdominal pain, and cramping. The inflammation does not skip sections of the bowel but is progressive from the anus (see Figure 18-6).

All inflammatory bowel conditions can have severe, often devastating, nutrition results as more and more of the absorbing surface area becomes involved. Restoring positive nutrition is a basic requirement for tissue healing and health. Elemental formulas of amino acids, glucose, fat, minerals, and vitamins are more easily absorbed and support initial healing in response to antibacterial and antiinflammatory medications. The diet is gradually advanced to restore optimal nutrient intake. The princi-

TABLE 18-4

LEVELS OF NUTRITION CARE FOR MANAGEMENT OF CF

LEVEL OF CARE	PATIENT GROUPS	NUTRITION ACTIONS
Level I: routine care	All	Diet counseling, food plans, enzyme replacement, vitamin supplements, nutrition education, exploration of problems
Level II: anticipatory guidance	Above 90% ideal weight/height index but at risk for energy imbalance, severe pancreatic insufficiency, frequent pulmonary infections, normal periods of rapid growth	Increased monitoring of dietary intake, complete energy nutrient analysis, increased kilocalorie density as needed, assessment of behavioral needs, counseling and nutrition education
Level III: supportive intervention	85% to 90% ideal weight/height index, decreased weight/growth velocity	Reinforcement of all the above actions, addition of energy nutrient–dense oral supplements
Level IV: rehabilitative care	Consistently below 85% ideal weight/height index, nutrition and growth failure	All the above plus enteral nutrition support by nasoenteric or enterostomy tube feeding (see Chapter 22)
Level V: resuscitative or palliative care	Below 75% ideal weight/height index, progressive nutrition failure	All the above plus continuous enteral tube feedings or TPN (see Chapter 22)

Modified from Ramsey B and others: Nutrition assessment and management in cystic fibrosis: a consensus report, *Am J Clin Nutr* 55:108, 1992. Copyright the American Society for Clinical Nutrition.

CLINICAL APPLICATIONS

CASE STUDY: PAUL'S ADAPTATION TO CF

Paul is a 12-year-old boy with CF. He is hospitalized with pneumonia and has difficulty breathing. Paul is a thin child with little muscle development who tires easily, although he has a large appetite. His stools are large and frequent and contain undigested food material.

Questions for Analysis
1. What is CF? Account for the clinical effects of the disease as evidenced by Paul's appearance and symptoms.
2. What are the basic goals of treatment in CF? Why is vigorous nutrition therapy a main part of treatment?

Describe the current role of enzyme replacement therapy in this aggressive nutrition support.
3. Outline a day's food plan for Paul. Check the amount of protein and kilocalories by calculating the total food values in your food plan to ensure the extra amount he needs is provided.
4. Why does Paul require therapeutic doses of multivitamins, including B-complex vitamins? Why does he need to have these in water-soluble form?

ples of continuing dietary management include the following[17]:
1. During periods of inflammation:
   - Use enteral or parental nutrition feedings if necessary
   - Progress to high-protein, high-calorie, low-residue foods in small, frequent meals
   - Increase vitamins and minerals, usually with supplements
2. During periods of remission:
   - Meet energy and protein needs specific for weight and activity level
   - Avoid suspected intolerable foods
   - Increase probiotic foods or supplements

vasculitis inflammation of the walls of blood vessels.

idiopathic of unknown cause.

etiology the cause or origin of a disease.

elemental formula a nutrition support formula composed of simple elemental nutrient components that require no further digestive breakdown and are thus readily absorbed; formulas with the protein as free amino acids and the carbohydrate as the simple sugar glucose.

probiotic food that contains live microbials thought to benefit the consumer by improving intestinal microbial balance (e.g., lactobacilli in yogurt).

CROHN'S DISEASE   ULCERATIVE COLITIS

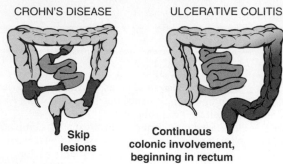

Skip   Continuous
lesions   colonic involvement,
                    beginning in rectum

Figure 18–6 Comparison of the distribution pattern of CD and ulcerative colitis. (Reprinted from Kumar V and others: *Robbins and Cotran pathologic basis of disease,* ed 7, Philadelphia, 2005, Saunders.)

- Increase antioxidant and essential fatty acids intake

Current study and clinical practice indicate the benefit of a regular nourishing diet, respecting individual tolerances and disease status. A close working relationship among the physician, dietitian, and nurse is essential. Appetite often is poor, but adequate nutrition intake is imperative. A range of feeding modes, including enteral and parenteral nutrition support as needed, are explored in individual cases to achieve the vigorous nutrition care necessary. However, whatever the mode of feeding, it always must be provided with personal support, warmth, and encouragement.

Diarrhea

Diarrhea typically is not a disease of the small intestine, but rather a symptom or result of another underlying cause. In some cases diarrhea may result from intolerance to specific foods or nutrients, such as in lactose intolerance (see Chapter 2) or acute food poisoning from a specific food-borne organism or toxin (see Chapter 13). A variety of parasites *(Giardia lamblia, Cryptosporidium parvum, Cyclospora cayetanensis, Entamoeba histolytica),* bacteria *(Campylobacter, Clostridium difficile, Escherichia coli, Listeria monocytogenes, Salmonella enteritidis, Shigella),* and viral infections (HIV, rotavirus, Norwalk agent) are known causes of diarrhea. Traveler's diarrhea, often attributed to irregular meals, unfamiliar foods, and travel tensions, also is a well-known GI disturbance, and infection with *E. coli* is the most common cause.[18]

Chronic diarrhea (diarrhea lasting more than 2 weeks) can be a life-threatening illness, especially for young children or individuals with a weak immune system. Diarrhea in infants is a more serious problem that can quickly lead to dehydration and nutrient losses, especially if prolonged. Acute infectious diarrhea is the second most common form of death in children in developing countries.[19] Intravenous fluid and electrolyte replacement may be necessary, or an oral solution of water, glucose, and electrolytes (e.g., Polycose [Abbott Nutrition, Columbus, Ohio]) may be used. As soon as it is tolerated, a regular refeeding schedule is needed to avoid malnutrition.

In severely malnourished patients, resumption of nutrient intake should be carefully monitored. Refeeding syndrome is a potentially fatal metabolic disturbance with fluid and electrolyte imbalances that can result in cardiac failure. When malnourished patients are started on a feeding schedule that is too aggressive, sudden shifts in electrolytes leave low serum phosphate, potassium, magnesium, glucose, and thiamine. Malnourished patients need slow reintroduction to nutrients; supplemental phosphate, potassium, and magnesium; and close monitoring.

Large Intestine Diseases

Diverticular Disease

Diverticulosis is a lower intestinal condition characterized by the formation of many small pouches, or pockets, along the muscular mucosal lining, usually in the colon (Figure 18-7). These little pouches are called diverticula. They most often occur in older persons and develop at

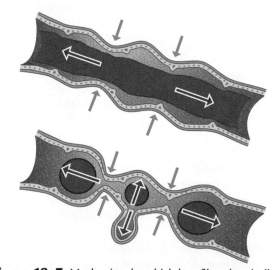

Figure 18–7 Mechanism by which low-fiber, low-bulk diets might generate diverticula. Where the colon contents are bulky *(top),* muscular contractions exert pressure longitudinally. If the lumen is small in diameter *(bottom),* contractions can produce occlusions and exert pressure against the colon wall, which may produce a diverticular "blowout." (Reprinted from Mahan LK, Escott-Stump S: *Krause's food & nutrition therapy,* ed 12, Philadelphia, 2008, Saunders Elsevier.)

points of weakened muscles in the bowel wall. The direct cause is a progressive increase in pressure within the bowel from segmental circular muscle contractions that normally move the remaining food mass along and form the feces for elimination. When pressures become sufficiently high in one of these segments and insufficient fiber is present to maintain the necessary bulk for preventing high internal pressures within the colon, small diverticula develop. As the pockets become infected, a condition called diverticulitis, the affected area becomes painful. Epidemiologic studies estimate that 60% of people in western societies will develop diverticulosis.[20,21] One conclusion about the development of diverticulosis is that "fiber deficiency results in diverticular formation and a chronic inflammation that may progress to acute or chronic diverticulitis that can be treated medically but may require surgical intervention."[20] Such conclusions speak to the seriousness and preventability of the disease.

The commonly used collective term covering diverticulosis and diverticulitis is diverticular disease. As the inflammatory process advances, increased pain and tenderness are localized in the lower left side of the abdomen and are accompanied by nausea, vomiting, distention, diarrhea, intestinal spasm, and fever. Perforation sometimes occurs, and surgery is indicated. Underlying malnutrition also may be present. Aggressive nutrition therapy hastens recovery from an attack, shortens the hospital stay, and reduces costs. Current studies and clinical practice have demonstrated better management of chronic diverticular disease with an increased amount of dietary fiber (25 to 30 g/day).[20] Avoiding certain foods, such as nuts and seeds that can accumulate in the small diverticula pouches, is recommended but little evidence suggests this is truly protective against inflammation.

Irritable Bowel Syndrome

As much as 20% of the general U.S. population has problems consistent with the condition called irritable bowel syndrome (IBS), yet a large majority do not seek medical attention. Although IBS is one of the most common GI disorders, its precise nature and cause continue to puzzle practitioners (Figure 18-8).

Accumulating evidence indicates, however, that IBS is a multicomponent disorder of physiologic, emotional, environmental, and psychologic function. Medical guidelines define IBS as a benign functional, nonorganic disorder displaying three major types of symptoms: (1) chronic and recurrent pain in any area of the abdomen; (2) small-volume bowel dysfunction, varying from constipation or diarrhea to a combination of both; and (3) excess gas formation with increased distention and bloating, ac-

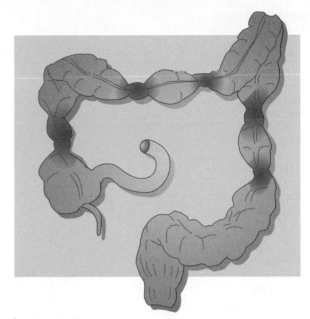

Figure 18–8 Irritable bowel syndrome. (Reprinted from Mahan LK, Escott-Stump S: *Krause's food, nutrition, & diet therapy,* ed 10, Philadelphia, 2000, Saunders.)

companied by rumbling abdominal sounds, belching, and passing of gas. Patients appear tense and anxious, and stress is a major triggering factor.[22] No permanent damage to the intestinal wall occurs after episodes, and no immunologic involvement occurs. A highly individual and personal approach to nutrition care is essential, based on careful nutrition assessment (see Chapter 17). Guided by this personal food and symptom pattern, a reasonable food plan can be devised with the patient. In general, the food plan should give attention to the following basic principles:

- *Increase dietary fiber:* A regular diet with optimal energy-nutrient composition and dietary fiber food sources (e.g., whole grains, legumes, fruits, and vegetables) provides basic therapy (Table 18-5).

---

refeeding syndrome a potentially lethal condition occurring when severely malnourished individuals are fed high-carbohydrate diets too aggressively. A sudden shift in electrolytes, fluid retention, and drastic drop in serum phosphorus levels cause a series of complications involving several organs.

diverticulitis inflammation of pockets of tissue (diverticula) in the lining of the mucous membrane of the colon.

TABLE 18-5

DIETARY FIBER AND KILOCALORIE VALUES FOR SELECTED FOODS

FOODS	SERVING SIZE	KILOCALORIES	DIETARY FIBER (G)
Breads and Cereals			
Fiber One	½ cup	59	14.4
All Bran	½ cup	70	8.5
Bran (100%)	½ cup	75	8.4
Bran Buds	⅓ cup	75	7.9
Barley, whole grain	½ cup	135	6.8
Corn bran	⅔ cup	100	5.4
40% Bran	¾ cup	119	5.2
Whole-wheat bagel	1 small	145	5.1
Bran Chex	⅔ cup	90	4.6
Whole-wheat English muffin	1	134	4.4
Cracklin' Oat Bran	½ cup	110	4.3
Bran flakes	¾ cup	90	4.0
Wheat germ	¼ cup	108	3.6
Bran muffin	1	172	3.5
Whole-wheat matzo	2	100	3.4
Wheaties	1 cup	107	3.0
Shredded Wheat	1 oz	101	2.8
Bulgur	½ cup	50	2.7
Air-popped popcorn	1 cup	25	2.5
Oatmeal	1 cup	144	2.2
Wheat Chex	⅔ cup	69	2.2
Whole-wheat roll	1	75	2.1
Whole-wheat pita	1 small	75	2.1
Legumes, Cooked			
Cooked dried peas	½ cup	116	8.1
Cooked lentils	½ cup	115	7.8
Cooked dry black beans	½ cup	114	7.5
Cooked dry pinto beans	½ cup	117	7.4
Kidney beans	½ cup	110	7.3
Cooked dry northern beans	½ cup	104	6.2
Cooked dry navy beans	½ cup	129	5.8
Lima beans	½ cup	130	4.5
Vegetables, Cooked			
Green peas	½ cup	55	3.6
Corn	½ cup	70	2.9
Parsnips	½ cup	50	2.7
Potato, with skin	1 medium	95	2.5
Brussels sprouts	½ cup	30	2.3
Carrots	½ cup	25	2.3
Broccoli	½ cup	20	2.2
Spinach	½ cup	21	2.2
Fruits			
Raspberries	½ cup	30	4.2
Apple	1 medium	80	3.5
Raisins	¼ cup	110	3.1
Prunes, dried	3	60	3.0
Strawberries	1 cup	45	3.0
Orange	1 medium	60	2.6
Pear	½ large	62	2.5
Banana	1 medium	105	2.4
Blueberries	½ cup	40	2.0

■ *Recognize gas formers:* Some foods are recognized gas formers because of known constituents (e.g., indigestible short chains of glucose [oligosaccharides] in the case of legumes). Others may cause gaseous discomfort on an individual basis.

■ *Eliminate food intolerances:* Lactose intolerance, for example, in people who lack the digestive enzyme lactase is well known (see Chapter 2).

■ *Reduce total fat content:* Excess fat delays gastric emptying and contributes to malabsorption problems.

■ *Avoid large meals:* Large amounts of food in one meal create discomfort from gastric distention and gas. Smaller, more frequent meals usually reduce these symptoms.

■ *Decrease air-swallowing habits:* These habits include eating rapidly and in large amounts, excessive fluid intake, especially of carbonated beverages, and gum chewing.

Patients are highly individualized regarding the symptoms they most often experience. For example, the predominant symptom may be diarrhea, constipation, abdominal pain, gas, or bloating, but not necessarily all of them. Therefore the dietary recommendations are equally as individualized. Experienced practitioners have learned that in helping patients manage IBS, an honest and creative relationship is essential. Lifestyle and diet are highly personal, and wise nutrition management involves realistic counseling toward a healthier life.

Constipation

The general complaint of constipation is common. Americans spend a quarter of a billion dollars each year on laxatives to treat their regularity problems. "Normal" intestinal elimination is ill defined and can vary greatly. However, a daily bowel movement is not necessary for good health. This common short-term problem usually results from various sources of nervous tension and worry, neurologic or neuromuscular problems, changes in routines, frequent laxative use, low-fiber diets, and lack of exercise. Improved diet, exercise, and bowel habits usually remedy the situation. Any regular laxative or enema routine should be avoided. The diet should include increased fiber, naturally laxative fruits (e.g., dried prunes and figs), and adequate fluid intake, based on the assessment of current fiber and fluid intake, as well as any diuretic medication use. Constipation occurs at all ages but is almost epidemic among elderly persons. In all cases a personalized approach to management is fundamental.

FOOD ALLERGIES AND INTOLERANCES

Food Allergies

The Problem

Several conditions may cause certain food allergies or intolerances. Intolerances, unlike true allergies, are not life threatening and are nonimmunologic in etiology. The underlying problem of an allergic reaction is the body's immune system reacting to a protein as if it were a threatening foreign object and launching a powerful attack against it. The word allergy comes from two Greek words meaning altered reactivity and refers to the abnormal reactions of the immune system to a number of substances in the environment. A particular allergic condition results from a disorder of the immune system.

Common Food Allergens

The most common food allergens include proteins in cow's milk, eggs, peanuts, wheat, soy, fish, shellfish, and tree nuts. Early foods of infancy and childhood often are offenders in sensitive individuals, especially if introduced to the child before the GI tract is fully capable of sophisticated digestion. In a child's diet, solid foods should be added one at a time, with common offenders excluded in early feedings. If a child shows signs of allergic reaction, a process of food elimination is sometimes used to identify disagreeable foods. A core of less-often offending foods is used at first; other single foods are then gradually added to test the response. If a given food causes an allergic reaction, the food is identified as an allergen and eliminated from the diet. The food may be tried again later to see if it still causes the same reaction, validating the initial response. Individuals commonly outgrow allergies to milk, soy, and eggs. However, peanuts, tree nuts, and shellfish tend to elicit an allergic response, sometimes fatally, throughout life. Peanut allergy elicits the most severe form of food allergy and carries a high risk of anaphylaxis. Much effort has been devoted to understanding the

---

allergy a state of hypersensitivity to particular substances in the environment that works on body tissues to produce problems in functions of affected tissues; the agent involved (allergen) may be a certain food eaten or a substance (e.g., pollen) inhaled.

anaphylaxis severe allergic, sometimes fatal, reaction resulting from exposure to a protein the body perceives as foreign and eliciting a systemic response that includes multiple organs.

immunologic response to peanuts and developing effective methods for avoiding such severe reactions.[23,24]

Recognizing signs and symptoms of allergic reactions may save a life. Anaphylactic shock is the most severe form of allergic reaction and can result in death relatively quickly. The person's throat, lips, and tongue swell to the point of blocking the airway, ultimately suffocating the individual. The most common symptoms of food allergies are hives, nausea, diarrhea, and abdominal pain. Individuals in anaphylactic shock have swelling of the face and throat, difficulty breathing, anxiety, increased heart rate and, if not treated, decreased blood pressure and loss of consciousness.

Referring any person with food allergies to a dietitian to provide family support, education, and counseling may be helpful. Guidance regarding food substitutions or special food products and modified recipes to maintain nutrition needs for growth is necessary. Children tend to become less allergic as they grow older, but family education on deciphering the labels of food products and cooking guides are essential from the beginning. Furthermore, if anaphylaxis is a known risk, patients should be under the care of a physician for provision of self- and/or family-administered emergency medications if anaphylaxis occurs.

Celiac Disease

Disease Process. The childhood disorder celiac disease and the adult disease nontropical sprue are now known to be a single disease, both of which are referred to as celiac disease (CD). In all cases, the cause is hypersensitivity to proteins found in wheat, barley, and rye. The CD-activating proteins have all come to be known as gluten. However, gluten protein is found only in wheat products. The proteins causing an adverse reaction in barley and rye are hordein and secalin, respectively. For simplicity, all dietary proteins involved in disease pathogenesis are referred to as gluten in this text in keeping with the general public's understanding. Oat products are not problematic for all individuals with CD. However, oats often are processed in facilities that process wheat products, which can result in cross-contamination.

In reaction to ingestion of a CD-activating protein, the eroded mucosal surface leaves villi that are malformed and deficient in number, with few microvilli (Figure 18-9). This damaged mucosa effectively reduces the surface area for micronutrient and macronutrient absorption. In addition, decreased release of peptide hormones, bile, and pancreatic secretions attenuates malabsorption. The underlying cause is unknown, but the pathogenesis involves environmental, genetic, and immunologic factors and is estimated to affect 1% of the U.S. popula-

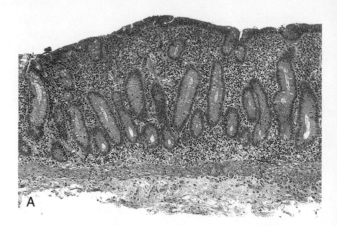
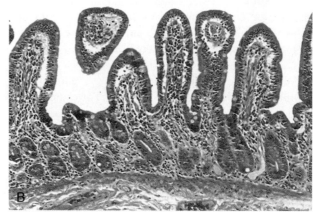

Figure 18–9 CD (gluten-sensitive enteropathy). **A,** Peroral jejunal biopsy specimen of diseased mucosa shows severe atrophy and blunting of villi, with a chronic inflammatory infiltrate of the lamina propria. **B,** Normal mucosal biopsy. (Reprinted from Kumar V and others: *Robbins and Cotran pathologic basis of disease,* ed 7, Philadelphia, 2005, Saunders.)

tion.[25] The major symptom of steatorrhea (large amounts of ingested fat in stool) and progressive malnutrition are secondary effects to the gluten reaction.

Nutrition Management. The goal of nutrition management is to control the dietary gluten intake and prevent malnutrition. Thus wheat, rye, and barley are eliminated from the diet and corn, potato, and rice are used as substitutes. Some individuals with CD are sensitive to oats and also must eliminate this grain. Careful label reading is important for parents and children because many commercial products use gluten-containing grains as thickeners or fillers. Some commercial products have a gluten-free symbol on their labels to assist in the identification of acceptable foods (Figure 18-10). With the increasing number of processed foods and ethnic dishes available in the marketplace, detecting all food sources of gluten is difficult. Home test kits for gluten are available and may be beneficial for individuals consum-

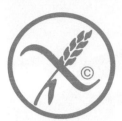

Figure 18–10 Gluten-free symbol. (Copyright Coeliac UK, Bucks, United Kingdom, 2004.)

ing foods without standard ingredient lists. Adhering to a gluten-free diet is the only effective treatment in maintaining a healthy mucosa and must be followed for life (Table 18-6). Because of the nature of the malabsorption disorder, patients with CD must be monitored for potential vitamin and mineral deficiencies and partake in supplementation as necessary.

PROBLEMS OF THE GASTROINTESTINAL ACCESSORY ORGANS

Three major accessory organs—the liver, gallbladder, and pancreas—produce important digestive agents that enter the intestine and aid in the handling of food substances (Figure 18-11). Diseases of these organs easily affect normal GI function and cause problems with the handling of specific types of food. The normal structure of the liver's functional units, the lobule and its cells, is shown in Figure 18-12.

Liver Disease

The liver has several critical roles in basic metabolism and regulation of body functions. Some essential functions include bile production for fat digestion; synthesis of proteins and blood clotting factors; metabolism of hormones, medications, macronutrients, and micronutri-

TABLE 18-6

GLUTEN-FREE DIET FOR INDIVIDUALS WITH CD

FOOD GROUPS	FOODS INCLUDED	FOODS EXCLUDED
Milk	Milk (plain or flavored with chocolate or cocoa), buttermilk, yogurt, ice cream, cottage cheese, cream cheese	Malted milk; preparations such as Cocomalt, Hemo, Postum, Nestle's chocolate
Meat or substitute	Lean meat, trimmed well of fat Eggs Poultry, fish Creamy peanut butter (if tolerated)	Luncheon meats, corned beef, frankfurters, all common prepared meat products with any possible wheat filler (stuffed turkey) Fish canned in broth Meat prepared with bread, crackers, or flour
Fruits and juices	All cooked and canned fruits and juices Frozen or fresh fruits as tolerated, with no skins and seeds	Prunes, plums (unless tolerated)
Vegetables	All cooked, frozen, canned as tolerated (prepared without wheat, rye, oat, or barley products); raw as tolerated	All prepared with wheat, rye, oat, or barley products (batter dipped)
Breads, flours, cereal products	Hot or cold cereals made with amaranth, corn, quinoa, or rice products Breads, pancakes, or waffles made with suggested flours (cornmeal, cornstarch, rice, soybean, lima bean, potato, buckwheat) Pasta made from beans, corn, pea, potato, quinoa, rice, soy or rice flours	All bread or cereal products made with gluten; wheat, rye, oat, barley, macaroni, noodles, spaghetti; any sauces, soups, or gravies prepared with gluten flour, wheat, rye, oat, or barley
Soups	Broth, bouillon (no thickening with wheat, rye, oat, or barley products); soups and sauces may be thickened with cornstarch	All soups containing wheat, rye, oat, or barley products

Dietary principles: (1) High kilocalories, usually approximately 20% above normal requirement to compensate for fecal loss. (2) High protein as tolerated to promote growth in children and maintenance in adults. (3) Low fat, but not fat free because of impaired absorption. (4) Simple carbohydrates, including easily digested sugars (fruits, vegetables) to provide approximately half the kilocalories. (5) Small, frequent feedings during ill periods; afternoon snack for older children. (6) Smooth, soft texture, initially avoiding irritating roughage; use of strained foods longer than usual for age, adding whole foods as tolerated and according to age of child. (7) Supplements of B vitamins, vitamins A and E in water-miscible forms, and vitamin C. (8) Iron supplements if anemia is present.

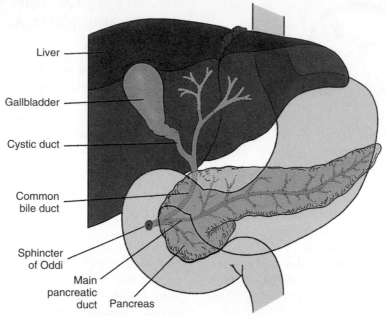

Figure 18–11 Biliary system organs.

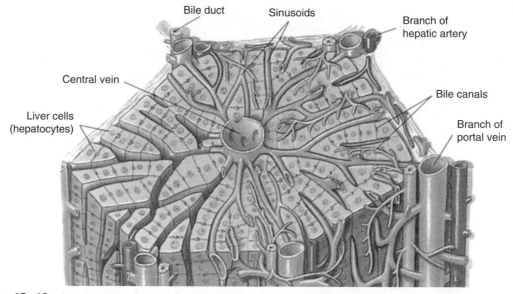

Figure 18–12 Liver structure showing hepatic lobule and hepatic cell. (Copyright Medical and Scientific Illustration.)

ents; the regulation of blood glucose levels; and urea production to remove waste products of normal metabolism. Diseases of the liver are among the leading causes of death in the United States for individuals of Hispanic, Native-American, and Alaskan-Native ancestry.[26]

Steatohepatitis

Inflammation and fat accumulation in the liver is known as the silent liver disease—steatohepatitis. Some patients have no known risk factors and have normal cholesterol and triglyceride levels but still have elevated liver enzymes. The exact cause of steatohepatitis is unknown, and few patients have physical symptoms such as pain or nausea. It most often is associated with alcohol abuse. However, steatohepatitis also affects an estimated 2% to 5% of Americans who drink little or no alcohol. When the cause is not linked to alcohol, the condition is called nonalcoholic steatohepatitis. Incidence of this form of the disease is higher for individuals with diabetes and/or obesity.

If left untreated, steatohepatitis can advance to cirrhosis, a condition from which the liver cannot recover. Patients typically have fatigue and weight loss. A balanced diet, the avoidance of alcohol (if indicated), increased physical activity, and tight blood glucose control are the main focus of treatment.

Hepatitis

Acute hepatitis is an inflammatory condition caused by viruses, alcohol, drugs, or toxins. The viral agent causing infection often is transmitted by the oral-fecal route (hepatitis A), which is common in many epidemic diseases. The carrier usually is contaminated food or water. In other cases the virus may be transmitted by transfusions of infected blood or contaminated syringes or needles (hepatitis B). Symptoms include anorexia and jaundice with underlying malnutrition. Treatment centers on bed rest and nutrition therapy to support healing of the liver tissue. The following requirements govern the principles of the diet therapy and relate to the liver's function in metabolizing each nutrient:

- *Adequate protein:* Protein is essential for building new liver cells and tissues. It also combines with fats (lipoproteins) to remove them, preventing damage from fatty infiltration in liver tissue. The diet should supply 1.0 to 1.2 g/kg of high-quality protein daily if no complications are present. If the individual has complications and a positive nitrogen balance is desirable, 1.2 to 1.3 g/kg of protein is warranted (Box 18-2).

BOX 18-2

HIGH-PROTEIN, HIGH-CARBOHYDRATE, MODERATE-FAT DAILY DIET

- 1 L (1 qt) low-fat milk
- ¼ cup egg substitute (e.g., Egg Beaters)
- 8 oz lean meat, fish, poultry
- 4 servings vegetables:
  - 2 servings potato or substitute
  - 1 serving green leafy or yellow vegetable
  - 1 to 2 servings other vegetables, including 1 raw
- 3 to 4 servings fruit (including juices):
  - 1 to 2 citrus fruits (or other good source of ascorbic acid)
  - 2 servings other fruit
- 6 to 8 servings bread and cereal (whole grain or enriched):
  - 1 serving cereal
  - 5 to 6 slices bread, crackers
- 2 to 4 Tbsp butter or fortified margarine
- Additional jam, jelly, honey, and other carbohydrate foods as patient desires and is tolerated
- Sweetened fruit juices to increase both carbohydrates and fluid

- *High carbohydrate:* Available glucose restores protective glycogen reserves in the liver. It also helps meet the energy demands of the disease process and prevents the breakdown of protein for energy, thus ensuring its use for the vital tissue building necessary for healing. The diet should supply 50% to 55% total kilocalories as carbohydrates. Glucose intolerance and hypoglycemia are sometimes problematic with liver disease. Therefore the amount of carbohydrates in the diet depends on individual needs and condition.
- *Low fat:* Some fat helps season food to encourage eating despite a poor appetite. A moderate amount of easily used fat, from milk products and vegetable oil, is beneficial. The diet should incorporate a maximum of 30% of total kilocalories from fat. Energy supply depends more on fat as the disease progresses.
- *High energy:* From 2500 to 3000 kcal (approximately 120% of basal energy expenditure) is needed daily to meet energy demands. This increased amount is necessary to support the healing process, make up losses from fever and general debilitation, and renew strength for recuperating from the disease.
- *Meals and feedings:* At first, liquid feedings (e.g., milkshakes high in protein and kilocalories [see Table 18-1] or special formula products) may be necessary. As a patient's appetite and food tolerance improve, a full diet is needed while observing likes and dislikes and planning ways to encourage optimal food intake. Nutrition is the basic therapy during acute hepatitis (see the Clinical Applications box, "Case Study: Bill's Bout with Infectious Hepatitis").

Cirrhosis

Liver disease may advance to a chronic state of cirrhosis (Figure 18-13). The most common problem is fatty cirrhosis associated with malnutrition and alcoholism. Malnutrition leads to multiple nutrition deficiencies as alcohol increasingly replaces balanced meals. Alcohol and its metabolic byproducts also may cause direct damage to liver cells. Although alcohol is a major cause of cirrhosis, other causes include chronic hepatitis types B and C; autoimmune hepatitis; inherited diseases such as Wilson's disease and galactosemia; nonalcoholic steatohepatitis; blocked bile ducts; and drugs, toxins, and infections.

Wilson's disease an autosomal recessive genetic disorder in which copper accumulates in tissue and causes damage to organs.

galactosemia an autosomal recessive genetic disorder in which the liver does not produce the enzyme needed to metabolize galactose.

CLINICAL APPLICATIONS

CASE STUDY: BILL'S BOUT WITH INFECTIOUS HEPATITIS

Bill is a college student who spent part of his summer vacation in Mexico. Shortly after he returned home, he began to feel ill. He had little energy, no appetite, and severe headaches. Nothing he ate seemed to agree with him. He felt nauseated, began to have diarrhea, and soon developed a fever. He began to show evidence of jaundice.

Bill was hospitalized for diagnosis and treatment, and his tests indicated impaired liver function. His liver and spleen were enlarged and tender. The physician's diagnosis was infectious hepatitis. Bill's hospital diet was high in proteins, carbohydrates, and kilocalories and moderately low in fats, but Bill had difficulty eating. He had no appetite, and food seemed to nauseate him even more.

Questions for Analysis

1. What are the normal functions of the liver in relation to the metabolism of carbohydrates, proteins, and fats? What other metabolic functions does the liver have?
2. What is the relation of normal liver functions to the effects or clinical symptoms that Bill had during his illness?
3. Why does vigorous nutrition therapy in liver disease (e.g., hepatitis) present a problem in planning a diet?
4. Outline a day's food plan for Bill. Calculate the amount of kilocalories and protein to ensure that he is getting the necessary amount. Bill is 5'10" and 168 lbs.
5. What vitamins and minerals would be significant aspects of Bill's nutrition therapy? Why?

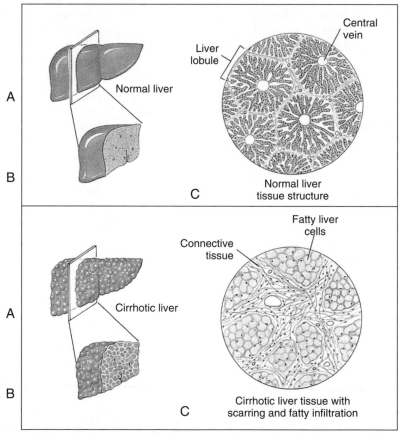

Figure 18–13 Comparison of normal liver and liver with cirrhotic tissue changes. **A,** Anterior view of organ. **B,** Cross-section. **C,** Tissue structure. (Copyright Medical and Scientific Illustration.)

During steatohepatitis the accompanying fatty infiltration kills liver cells, leaving only nonfunctioning fibrous scar tissue. Low plasma protein levels eventually lead to ascites, which is abdominal fluid accumulation. Scar tissue impairs blood circulation in the liver, resulting in elevated venous blood pressure and esophageal varices. The rupture of these enlarged veins with massive hemorrhage often is the cause of death. Treatment is difficult when alcoholism is the underlying problem. Nutrition therapy focuses on as much healing support as possible, as follows:

- *Energy:* 30 to 35 kcal/kg of actual body weight. Practitioners must carefully distinguish body weight from fluid weight.
- *Protein:* 1 to 2 g/kg body weight in the absence of impending hepatic encephalopathy. Sufficient protein is needed to correct severe malnutrition, heal liver tissue, and restore plasma proteins. If signs of encephalopathy begin, the protein must be reduced according to individual tolerance.
- *Low sodium:* Sodium is restricted to 2000 mg/day to help reduce fluid retention (ascites).
- *Soft texture:* If esophageal varices develop, soft foods help prevent the danger of rupture and hemorrhage.
- *Fluids:* Water intake is encouraged unless ascites or edema is present.
- *Optimal general nutrition:* The remaining diet principles outlined for hepatitis are continued for cirrhosis for the same reasons. Kilocalories, carbohydrates, and vitamins, especially B-complex vitamins such as thiamine and folate, are important. Moderate fat is used. Alcohol is prohibited.

Hepatic Encephalopathy

One of the main functions of the liver is to remove ammonia, and hence nitrogen (see Chapter 4), from the blood by converting it to urea for urinary excretion. When cirrhosis continues and fibrous scar tissue replaces more and more functional liver tissue, the blood can no longer circulate normally through the liver. Therefore other vessels develop around this scar tissue, bypassing the liver. The blood, carrying its ammonia load, cannot get to the liver for its normal removal of ammonia and nitrogen. Instead it must follow the bypass and proceed to the brain, producing ammonia intoxication. The resulting hepatic encephalopathy results in apathy, confusion, inappropriate behavior, drowsiness, and eventually coma. Treatment focuses on removing the sources of excess ammonia. Because ammonia is a nitrogen compound and its main source is protein, the chief dietary goal is to reduce protein intake. High biologic value protein equaling 0.5 g/kg body weight is the standard; however, individual tolerance should guide intake. Box 18-3 provides a menu for reducing protein to 30 g/day, with additional increases to tolerance.

Gallbladder Disease

The basic function of the gallbladder is to concentrate and store bile and then release the concentrated bile into the small intestine when fat is present there. In the intestine, bile emulsifies fat, preparing it for initial digestion, and then carries it into the cells of the intestinal wall for its continued metabolism.

BOX 18-3

LOW-PROTEIN DIETS

The following diets are used when dietary protein is to be restricted. The patterns limit foods containing large percentages of protein (e.g., milk, eggs, cheese, meat, fish, fowl, and legumes). Meat extractives, soups, broth, bouillon, gravies, and gelatin desserts also should be limited.

30 g PROTEIN
Breakfast
- ½ cup fruit or fruit juice
- ½ cup cereal
- ½ cup milk
- 1 slice toast
- Butter
- Jelly
- Sugar
- 2 Tbsp cream
- Coffee

Lunch
- ½ cup pasta
- ¼ cup pasta sauce
- ½ cup vegetable
- Tossed green salad
- 1 slice bread
- Butter
- 1 serving fruit
- Sugar
- Coffee or tea

Dinner
- 1 small potato
- 2 oz chicken breast
- ½ cup vegetable
- Tossed green salad
- 1 slice bread
- Butter
- 1 serving fruit
- Sugar
- Coffee or tea

40 g PROTEIN
- Add 1 cup milk, 2½ oz meat, or 1 egg and 1½ oz meat*

50 g PROTEIN
- Add 1 cup milk, 4 oz meat, or 2 eggs and 2 oz meat†

---

*For example, 2½ oz meat = 1 ground beef patty (e.g., 5 patties made from 1 lb beef), 1 slice roast.
†For example, 4 oz meat = 2 lamb chops or 1 small steak.

---

varices pathological dialation of the blood vessels within the wall of the esophagus due to liver cirrhosis. These vessels can continue to expand to the point of rupturing.

Cholecystitis and Cholelithiasis

Inflammation of the gallbladder, or cholecystitis, usually results from a low-grade chronic infection. Cholesterol in bile, which is not soluble in water, is normally kept in solution. When chronic infection alters the solubility of bile ingredients, however, cholesterol separates out and forms gallstones. This condition is called cholelithiasis. When infection, stones, or both are present the normal contraction of the gallbladder, triggered by fat entering the intestine, causes pain. Thus high-fat meals usually are avoided. The treatment is surgical removal of the gallbladder, a cholecystectomy. If a patient is obese, some weight loss before surgery may be indicated. In any case, diet therapy centers on controlling fat intake. Table 18-7 outlines a general low-fat diet guide, but the degree of its application depends on individual need.

Pancreatic Disease

The pancreas is a key organ in normal digestion and metabolism, acting as both an exocrine and endocrine gland. Digestive enzymes and bicarbonate, necessary for the breakdown of carbohydrates, proteins, and fats, are excreted by the pancreas under hormonal control during digestion. The endocrine functions of the pancreas are primarily related to blood glucose regulation by glucagon and insulin.

Pancreatitis

Acute inflammation of the pancreas, or pancreatitis, results when the enzymes the organ produces (principally trypsin [see Chapter 4]) digest the organ tissue. Obstruction of the common duct through which the inactive enzymes normally enter the intestine causes the enzymes

TABLE 18-7

LOW-FAT AND FAT-FREE DIETS

FOODS	FOODS ALLOWED	FOODS NOT ALLOWED
Beverages	Skim milk, coffee, tea, carbonated beverages, fruit juices	Whole milk, cream, evaporated and condensed milk
Bread and cereals	Most all	Rich rolls or breads, waffles, pancakes
Desserts	Gelatin, sherbet, water ices, fruit whips made without cream, angel food cake, rice and tapioca puddings made with skim milk	Pastries, pies, rich cakes and cookies, ice cream
Fruits	All fruits as tolerated	Avocado
Eggs	3 allowed per week, cooked any way except fried	Fried eggs
Fats	3 tsp butter or margarine daily	Salad and cooking oils, mayonnaise
Meats	Lean meat such as beef, veal, lamb, liver, lean fish, and fowl baked, broiled, or roasted without added fat	Fried meats, bacon, ham, pork, goose, duck, fatty fish, fish canned in oil, cold cuts
Cheese	Dry or fat-free cottage cheese	All other cheese
Potato or substitute	Potatoes, rice, macaroni, noodles, and spaghetti prepared without added fat	Fried potatoes, potato chips
Soups	Bouillon or broth without fat, soups made with skim milk	Cream soups
Sweets	Jam, jelly, sugar candies without nuts or chocolate	Chocolate, nuts, peanut butter
Vegetables	All vegetables as tolerated	Omit if causing distress: broccoli, cauliflower, corn, cucumber, green pepper, radishes, turnips, onions, dried peas, and beans
Miscellaneous	Salt in moderation	Pepper, spices, highly spiced foods, olives, pickles, cream sauces, gravies

Foods are prepared without the addition of fat. Fatty meats, gravies, oils, cream, lard, avocados, and desserts containing eggs, butter, cream, and nuts are avoided.
Suggested food patterns for a low-fat diet: *Breakfast:* fruit, cereal, toast, jelly, 1 tsp butter or margarine, egg (three times per week), 1 cup skim milk, coffee, sugar. *Lunch and dinner:* broiled or baked meat, potato, vegetable, salad with fat-free dressing, bread, jelly, 1 tsp butter or margarine, fruit or dessert (as allowed), 1 cup skim milk, coffee, sugar. This pattern contains approximately 85 g protein, 50 g fat, 220 g carbohydrates, and 1670 kcal.
A relatively fat-free diet omits meat, eggs, and butter or margarine; a substitute for meat at the noon and evening meals is 3 oz fat-free cottage cheese.

and bile to back up into the pancreas. This mixing of digestive materials activates the powerful enzymes within the gland. In this active form they begin to digest the pancreatic tissue itself, causing severe pain. Mild or moderate episodes may completely subside, but the condition tends to recur, leading to chronic pancreatitis. Excessive alcohol consumption and gallstones are the major culprits leading to pancreatitis in the United States. Other causes of chronic pancreatitis include a blocked or narrowed pancreatic duct, heredity, and other unknown causes. Initial care includes the following measures for acute disease involving shock: complete intravenous feeding to allow GI rest, replacement of fluid and electrolytes, blood transfusion, antibiotics, pain medications, and gastric suction. As healing progresses, oral feedings are resumed. A low-fat, moderate-protein diet is used to reduce stimulation of pancreatic secretions. Alcohol and excess coffee also should be avoided to decrease pancreatic stimulation.

SUMMARY

Nutrition management of GI diseases is based on the degree of interference in the normal process of ingestion, digestion, absorption, and metabolism that the diseases cause. Problems in the upper GI tract relate to conditions that hinder chewing, swallowing, or transporting the food mass down the esophagus into the stomach. Esophageal problems such as muscle constriction, acid reflux causing esophagitis, or a hiatal hernia at the entry of the esophagus into the chest cavity interfere with passage of food into the stomach. These problems cause general tissue irritation and discomfort after eating. PUD, a common GI problem, is acidic erosion of the mucosal lining of the stomach or the duodenal bulb. The ulcerated tissue causes nutrition problems such as anemia and weight loss. Medical management consists of drug therapy and rest. Diet therapy is liberal and individual, with the goal of correcting malnutrition and supporting the healing process.

Problems of the lower GI tract include common functional disorders such as malabsorption and diarrhea, for which symptomatic and personalized treatment is indicated. Diseases such as CD, which is caused by sensitivity to gluten in certain grains and results in malabsorption problems, and the genetic disease CF, require individualized nutrition support. The inflammatory bowel diseases

(e.g., Crohn's disease and ulcerative colitis) involve extensive tissue damage that often requires surgical resection and results in short-bowel syndrome from the decreased absorbing surface area. Large intestine problems (e.g., diverticular disease, IBS, and constipation) often involve anxiety and stress and thus are more difficult to resolve. Nutrition therapy requires modification of the diet's protein and energy content and food texture, increased vitamins and minerals, and replacement of fluids and electrolytes. Continuous adjustment of the diet is made according to individual need.

Diseases of the GI accessory organs also contribute to nutrition problems. Common liver disorders include hepatitis and cirrhosis. Uncontrolled cirrhosis leads to hepatic encephalopathy and eventual liver failure and death. Nutrient and energy levels of the necessary diet therapy vary with the progression of the disease process. Gallbladder disease, infection, and stones involve some limit to fat tolerance, which is modified according to individual need. The treatment for gallstones is surgical removal of the gallbladder followed by moderate use of dietary fat. Pancreatic disease (pancreatitis) is a serious condition requiring immediate measures to counter the symptoms of shock followed by restorative nutrition support.

CRITICAL THINKING QUESTIONS

1. What general nutrition guidance would you give to a person with esophageal reflux? What would be the basic goal of your suggestions?
2. What are the basic principles of diet planning for patients with PUD? How do these principles differ from the traditional therapy of the past? What other elements may be involved in the treatment process besides nutrition therapy?
3. Describe the causes, clinical signs, and treatment for diverticular disease, CD, and IBS.

4. Considering the nutrients digested and absorbed in the small intestine, what long-term deficiencies would you expect to encounter in a patient with chronically inflamed Crohn's disease affecting more than 40% of the gut? Explain why this may happen and what alternative method of feeding would be beneficial.
5. What is the rationale for treatment in the progressive course of liver disease (e.g., hepatitis, cirrhosis, and hepatic encephalopathy)?

CHAPTER CHALLENGE QUESTIONS

True-False
Write the correct statement for each statement that is false.

1. *True or False:* A high-fiber diet rich in raw vegetables is appropriate for a person with dental problems.

2. *True or False:* Remaining upright after eating helps prevent discomfort in a person with esophageal reflux.

3. *True or False:* The fundamental cause of PUD is a bacteria.

4. *True or False:* Peptic ulcer pain is eliminated by consuming decaffeinated coffee and colas instead of the fully caffeinated forms of these beverages.

5. *True or False:* A low-fiber diet (no more than 12 g/day) is encouraged in the treatment of diverticulosis.

6. *True or False:* All food sources of wheat must be eliminated in the gluten-free diet for treatment of CD.

7. *True or False:* The nutrition objective in CF is to meet growth needs and help compensate for nutrient losses along with enzyme replacement therapy.

Multiple Choice

1. In a gluten-free diet for CD, which of the following foods is eliminated?
   a. Eggs
   b. Milk
   c. Rice
   d. Whole-wheat crackers

2. The symptoms of anemia in malabsorption diseases are caused by poor absorption of which of the following nutrients?
   a. Vitamins B_2 and C
   b. Iron and folic acid
   c. Calcium and phosphorus
   d. Fats and protein

3. Treatment for hepatic encephalopathy includes
   a. increased protein to aid healing of liver cells.
   b. decreased protein to reduce ammonia levels in blood.
   c. increased kilocalories to reduce the metabolic load.
   d. increased fluid intake to stimulate output.

4. Which of the following is a swallowing disorder?
   a. Dysphagia
   b. Xerostomia
   c. CD
   d. CF

5. Crohn's disease differs from ulcerative colitis in that
   a. Crohn's disease is progressive from the rectum up.
   b. Crohn's disease is temporary and easily treated with medication.
   c. Crohn's disease skips lesions throughout the small and large intestine.
   d. Crohn's disease only affects the small intestine.

evolve Please refer to the Students' Resource section of this text's Evolve Web site for additional study resources.

REFERENCES
1. Marinho VC and others: Fluoride toothpastes for preventing dental caries in children and adolescents, *Cochrane Database Syst Rev* (1):CD002278, 2003.
2. Centers for Disease Control and Prevention: *Fact sheet: oral health for adults, www.cdc.gov/oralhealth/publications/factsheets/adult.htm,* accessed March 2008.
3. Morris H: Dysphagia in the elderly: a management challenge for nurses, *Br J Nurs* 15(10):558, 2006.
4. Germain I and others: A novel dysphagia diet improves the nutrient intake of institutionalized elders, *J Am Diet Assoc* 106(10):1614, 2006.
5. Chrysos E and others: Factors affecting esophageal motility in gastroesophageal reflux disease, *Arch Surg* 138:241, 2003.
6. Nilsson M, Lagergren J: The relationship between body mass and gastro-oesophageal reflux, *Best Pract Res Clin Gastroenterol* 18(6):1117, 2004.
7. Nocon M and others: Lifestyle factors and symptoms of gastro-oesophageal reflux: a population-based study, *Aliment Pharmacol Ther* 23(1):169, 2006.
8. Hampel H and others: Meta-analysis: obesity and the risk for gastroesophageal reflux disease and its complications, *Ann Intern Med* 143(3):199, 2005.
9. Le TH, Fantry GT: *Peptic ulcer disease, www.emedicine.com/med/topic1776.htm,* accessed March 2007.
10. Beswick EJ and others: *H pylori* and host interactions that influence pathogenesis, *World J Gastroenterol* 12(35):5599, 2006.
11. Rosenstock S and others: Risk factors for peptic ulcer disease: a population based prospective cohort study comprising 2416 Danish adults, *Gut* 52:186, 2003.
12. Ji KY, Hu FL: Interaction or relationship between *Helicobacter pylori* and non-steroidal anti-inflammatory drugs in upper gastrointestinal diseases, *World J Gastroenterol* 12(24):3789, 2006.

13. Bhatia V, Tandon RK: Stress and the gastrointestinal tract, *J Gastroenterol Hepatol* 20(3):332, 2005.

14. Jones MP: The role of psychosocial factors in peptic ulcer disease: beyond *Helicobacter pylori* and NSAIDs, *J Psychosom Res* 60(4):407, 2006.

15. Merck, Inc.: *Cystic fibrosis (CF)*, www.merck.com/mmhe/au/sec04/ch053/ch053a.html, accessed March 2007.

16. O'Connor GT and others: Median household income and mortality rate in cystic fibrosis, *Pediatrics* 111(4):333, 2003.

17. American Dietetic Association: *ADA nutrition care manual*, Chicago, 2005, American Dietetic Association.

18. Qadri F and others: Enterotoxigenic *Escherichia coli* in developing countries: epidemiology, microbiology, clinical features, treatment, and prevention, *Clin Microbiol Rev* 18(3):465, 2005.

19. King CK, and others: Managing acute gastroenteritis among children: oral rehydration, maintenance, and nutritional therapy, *MMWR Recomm Rep* 52:1, 2003.

20. Floch MH, Bina I: The natural history of diverticulitis: fact and theory, *J Clin Gastroenterol* 38(5 Suppl):S2, 2004.

21. Kang JY and others: Epidemiology and management of diverticular disease of the colon, *Drugs Aging* 21(4):211, 2004.

22. Spence MJ, Moss-Morris R: The cognitive behavioral model of irritable bowel syndrome: a prospective investigation of gastroenteritis patients, *Gut* 56(8):1066, 2007.

23. Palmer K, Burks W: Current developments in peanut allergy, *Curr Opin Allergy Clin Immunol* 6(3):202, 2006.

24. Li XM: Beyond allergen avoidance: update on developing therapies for peanut allergy, *Curr Opin Allergy Clin Immunol* 5(3):287, 2005.

25. Kagnoff MF: Celiac disease: pathogenesis of a model immunogenetic disease, *J Clin Invest* 117(1):41, 2007.

26. National Center for Health Statistics: *Health, United States, 2006, with chartbook on trends in the health of Americans*, Hyattsville, MD, 2006, U.S. Government Printing Office.

FURTHER READING AND RESOURCES

Dysphagia Resource Center: *www.dysphagia.com*

Cystic Fibrosis Foundation: *www.cff.org*

Cystic Fibrosis.com: *www.cysticfibrosis.com*

Celiac Sprue Association: *www.csaceliacs.org*

Crohn's and Colitis Foundation of America: *www.ccfa.org*

International Foundation for Functional Gastrointestinal Disorders: *www.iffgd.org*

National Digestive Diseases Information Clearinghouse, Irritable Bowel Syndrome: *http://digestive.niddk.nih.gov/ddiseases/pubs/ibs/*

American Academy of Allergy, Asthma, & Immunology: *www.aaaai.org*

Asthma and Allergy Foundation of America: *www.aafa.org*
  These organizations provide support for individuals affected by disorders of the GI tract. Health care providers should be familiar with these organizations, as well as their Web sites, to refer patients to organizations that can continue to give them support, understanding, and up-to-date information about their disease.

Case S: *Gluten-free diet: a comprehensive resource guide*, Regina, Canada, 2002, Case Nutrition Consulting.
  An excellent guide for individuals with CD. The author provides up-to-date information for a gluten-free diet.

Spanier JA and others: A systematic review of alternative therapies in the irritable bowel syndrome, *Arch Intern Med* 163:265, 2003.
  IBS is a frustrating disorder of the GI tract. A variety of medical and psychological factors contribute to the disorder, which is more prevalent in women than men, and a variety of treatment modalities have been explored. This article reviews the wide array of alternative and complementary treatment methods proposed for IBS.

CHAPTER 19

Coronary Heart Disease and Hypertension

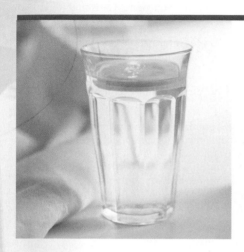

KEY CONCEPTS

- Cardiovascular disease is a leading cause of death in the United States.
- Several risk factors contribute to the development of cardiovascular disease and hypertension, many of which are preventable by improved food habits and lifestyle behaviors.
- Other risk factors are nonmodifiable, such as age, gender, family history, and race.
- Hypertension, or chronically elevated blood pressure, may be classified as essential (primary) or secondary hypertension.
- Hypertension damages the endothelium of blood vessels.
- Early education is critical for the prevention of cardiovascular disease.

Cardiovascular disease (CVD) is a leading cause of death in the United States, accounting for more than 650,000 deaths each year.[1] A similar situation exists in most other developed Western societies. Every day thousands of people have heart attacks and strokes, and more than 1 million others continue to live with various forms of rheumatic and congestive heart disease.

This chapter discusses the primary underlying disease processes of atherosclerosis and hypertension, as well as the various risk factors involved, and explores ways to use nutrition approaches to reduce risk factors and help prevent disease.

CORONARY HEART DISEASE

Atherosclerosis

Disease Process

The major cause of CVD and the underlying pathologic process in coronary heart disease is atherosclerosis. Ongoing studies have strengthened the earlier association of key risk factors (including diet) and the progressive development of the atherosclerotic process.[2-4] This process is characterized by fatty fibrous plaques that may begin in childhood and develop into fatty streaks, largely composed of cholesterol, on the inside lining of major blood vessels. When tissue is examined, cholesterol can be seen with the unaided eye in the debris of advanced lesions. This fatty fibrous plaque gradually thickens over time, narrowing the interior part of the blood vessel. The thickening of the vessel or a blood clot may eventually cut off blood flow (Figure 19-1).

Cells die when deprived of their normal blood supply. The local area of dying or dead tissue is called an infarct. If the affected blood vessel is a major artery supplying

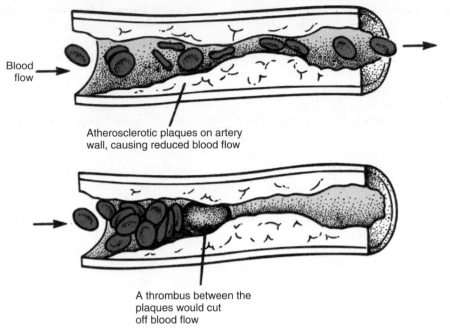

Blood flow →

Atherosclerotic plaques on artery wall, causing reduced blood flow

A thrombus between the plaques would cut off blood flow

Figure 19–1 Atherosclerotic plaque in artery.

vital blood nutrients and oxygen to the heart muscle, the myocardium, the event is called a myocardial infarction (MI), or heart attack. If the affected vessel is a major artery going to the brain, the event is called a cerebrovascular accident, or stroke. The major arteries and their many branches serving the heart are called coronary arteries because they lie across the brow of the heart muscle and resemble a crown. Thus the overall disease process is identified as coronary heart disease. A common symptom of its presence is angina pectoris, or chest pain, usually radiating down the left arm and sometimes brought on by excitement or physical effort.

Relation to Fat Metabolism

Elevated blood lipids are associated with CVD. Lipid is the class name for all fats and fat-related compounds. Lipid substances involved in the disease process are described in more detail in Chapter 3. Three of these substances are detailed in this chapter.

Triglycerides. The chemical name for fat, describing its basic structure, is triglyceride. All simple fats, whether in the body or in food, are triglycerides (see Chapter 3). The blood test for total triglycerides measures the level circulating in the blood. Studies assessing the effect of dietary fat on blood lipid profiles show adverse results from diets high in saturated fat. Conversely, diets low in overall

atherosclerosis the underlying pathology of coronary heart disease; a common form of arteriosclerosis characterized by the formation of yellow, cheeselike, fatty streaks containing cholesterol that develop into hardened plaques in the inner lining of major blood vessels such as the coronary arteries.

myocardial infarction (MI) a heart attack; caused by failure of the heart muscle to maintain normal blood circulation because of blockage of coronary arteries with fatty cholesterol plaques that cut off delivery of oxygen to the affected part of the heart muscle.

cerebrovascular accident a stroke; caused by arteriosclerosis within blood vessels of the brain that cuts off oxygen supply to the affected portion of brain tissue, thus paralyzing body muscle actions controlled by the affected brain area.

coronary heart disease the overall medical problem resulting from the underlying disease of atherosclerosis in the coronary arteries, which serve the heart muscle with blood, oxygen, and nutrients.

angina pectoris spasmodic, choking chest pain caused by lack of oxygen to the heart muscle; symptom of a heart attack; also may be caused by severe effort or excitement.

lipids the chemical group name for fats and fat-related compounds such as cholesterol and lipoproteins.

fat and that replace saturated fat with monounsaturated fats and polyunsaturated fats produce more desirable profiles.[5,6] Body fat distribution, using measurement methods such as waist circumference, dual-energy x-ray absorptiometry, and ultrasonography, help identify persons more likely to have elevated triglyceride levels.[7]

Cholesterol. Cholesterol is a fat-related compound produced in the liver and is an important part of normal cell functioning. Cholesterol is found in foods of animal origin (e.g., meat, dairy, and butter); it is not found in plant foods. Although it is an essential compound in the body, excess dietary cholesterol has been shown to raise total blood cholesterol levels and increase the risk of heart disease in predisposed individuals.[8] Blood cholesterol levels above that needed by the body increase the risk for deposition of cholesterol, fats, fibrous tissue, and macrophages in arteries throughout the body, which is the beginning of atherosclerosis. The CDC reports that 16.5% of American adults (20 to 74 years of age) have high blood cholesterol.[1] Many patients with hypercholesterolemia have the related problems of obesity and hypertension, requiring medical advice and intervention with diet as the primary treatment. A total blood cholesterol level of less than 200 mg/dl is considered desirable by the NIH.[9]

Lipoproteins. Because fat is not soluble in water, it is carried in the bloodstream in small packages wrapped with protein called lipoproteins. These compounds are produced in the intestinal mucosal cells after a meal containing fat and in the liver as part of the ongoing process of fat metabolism. Lipoproteins carry fat and cholesterol to tissues for cell metabolism and then back to the liver for breakdown and excretion as needed. Lipoproteins are grouped and named according to their protein, fat, and cholesterol content (their density) (Figure 19-2). Those with the highest protein content have the highest density and vice versa. Five lipoproteins are significant in relation to heart disease risk, as follows:

- *Chylomicrons:* made predominantly (85%) from dietary triglycerides that accumulate in the portal vein after absorption from the GI tract. Chylomicrons are exogenous lipoprotein particles that transport dietary triglycerides to plasma and tissues (Figure 19-2, A).
- *Very low-density lipoproteins (VLDLs):* formed in the liver from endogenous fat. These VLDLs carry a rela-

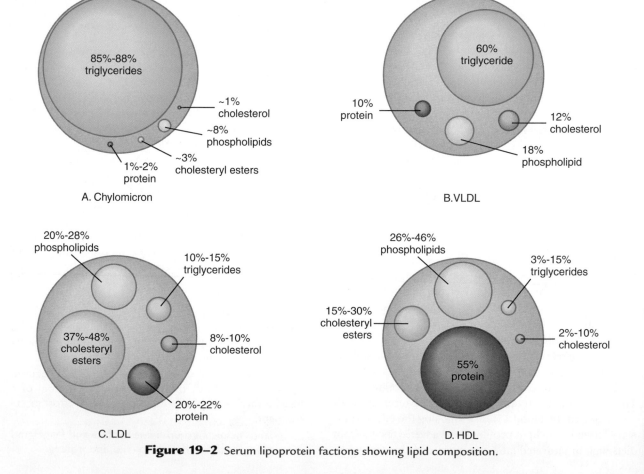

Figure 19–2 Serum lipoprotein factions showing lipid composition.

tively large load of triglycerides to cells but also contain approximately 12% cholesterol (Figure 19-2, B).

- *Intermediate-density lipoproteins:* continue delivering endogenous triglycerides to cells and tissue.
- *LDLs:* carry, in addition to other lipids, at least two thirds of the total plasma cholesterol to body tissues. LDLs are formed endogenously in the liver and in serum from catabolism of VLDLs. Because LDLs constantly send cholesterol to tissues, they have been called the source of bad cholesterol. In blood lipid tests, total LDL is the major lipoprotein of concern (Figure 19-2, C).
- *HDLs:* carry less total fat and more protein. HDLs transport cholesterol from the tissues to the liver for catabolism and elimination from the body. HDL is not found in food; rather, it is endogenously produced in the liver. When compared with LDL, HDL often is called good cholesterol, and higher serum levels are considered protective against CVD. Values less than 40 mg/dl imply increased risk for CVD, and a value of 60 mg/dl or greater contributes protection and decreased risk. Unlike other lipoproteins, HDL cholesterol is more closely associated with regular exercise than diet, which is one of the reasons the Expert Panel on Detection, Evaluation, and Treatment of High Blood Cholesterol in Adults recommends regular physical activity (Figure 19-2, D).[9]

Table 19-1 outlines the recommended blood levels of each lipid component.

Risk Factors

The underlying disease process of atherosclerosis is caused by multiple risk factors (Box 19-1). Note the modifiable risk factors which people have control compared with those they cannot control (nonmodifiable), as follows:

- *Gender:* CVD occurs more often in men than women until women reach menopause, at which time the relative risks are the same for both genders. Researchers have not concluded whether the increased risk for women is solely due to menopause because separating risks associated with age from menopause is difficult.[10]
- *Age:* General risk for CVD increases with the aging process (men older than 45 years, women older than 55 years).
- *Family history:* A positive family history is defined as a history of premature (before age 55 years in father or before 65 years in mother) CVD or high blood cholesterol above 240 mg/dl in a parent or first-degree relative. Early screening for children and adolescents with a high risk resulting from family history is important so that appropriate therapy may be started when the fatty streaks in coronary arteries are just beginning.

TABLE 19-1

CHOLESTEROL AND LIPOPROTEIN PROFILE CLASSIFICATION

CHOLESTEROL READING	CLASSIFICATION
Total Cholesterol (mg/dl)	
<200	Desirable
200-239	Borderline high risk
≥240	High risk
LDL Cholesterol (mg/dl)	
<100	Optimal
100-129	Near optimal
130-159	Borderline high risk
160-189	High risk
≥190	Very high risk
HDL Cholesterol (mg/dl)	
≥60	Optimal
<40	Low
Triglycerides (mg/dl)	
<150	Normal
150-199	Borderline high risk
200-499	High risk
≥500	Very high risk

Data from National Cholesterol Education Program: *Third report of the NCEP Expert Panel on Detection, Evaluation, and Treatment of High Blood Cholesterol in Adults (Adult Treatment Panel III)*, Washington, DC, 2002, National Institutes of Health.

- *Heredity:* Certain ethnic groups (African Americans, Hispanics, Native Americans, Native Hawaiians, and some Asian Americans) have a higher incidence of risk factors and CVD. Genetic defects that result in abnormally high serum lipids include familial hypercholes-

waist circumference measurement of the waist at its narrowest point width-wise, just above the navel. Waist circumference is a rough measurement of abdominal fat and a predictor of risk factors for CVD. This risk increases with a waist measurement of more than 40 inches in men and more than 35 inches in women.

dual-energy x-ray absorptiometry radiography using two beams (dual) that measure bone density and body composition.

ultrasonography ultrasound-based diagnostic imaging technique used to visualize muscles and internal organs; also referred to as sonography.

hypercholesterolemia condition of elevated blood cholesterol levels.

familial hypercholesterolemia genetic disorder resulting in elevated blood cholesterol levels despite lifestyle modifications; caused by absent or nonfunctional LDL receptors and requires drug therapy.

BOX 19-1

RISK FACTORS IN CVD

Lipid Risk Factors
- LDL cholesterol >130 mg/dl
- HDL cholesterol <40 mg/dl
- Total cholesterol >200 mg/dl
- Triglycerides >150 mg/dl
- Atherogenic dyslipidemia*

Nonlipid Risk Factors
Nonmodifiable
- Male gender
- Age (men >45 years, women >55 years)
- Heredity (including race)
- Family history of premature CVD (MI or sudden death <55 years in father or other male first-degree relative or <65 years in mother or other female first-degree relative)

Modifiable
- Cigarette smoking
- Hypertension (>140/90 mm Hg or on antihypertensive medication)
- Physical inactivity
- Obesity (BMI >30 kg/m²) and overweight (BMI 25 to 29.9 kg/m²)
- Diabetes mellitus
- Atherogenic diet (high intake of saturated fats and cholesterol)

Emerging Risk Factors
Emerging Lipid Risk Factors
- Elevated lipoprotein remnants
- Elevated lipoprotein(a)
- Small LDL particles
- Elevated apolipoprotein B
- Low apolipoprotein A-I
- High total cholesterol/HDL cholesterol ratio

Emerging Nonlipid Risk Factors
- Hyperhomocysteinemia
- Thrombogenic or hemostatic factors
- Inflammatory markers such as C-reactive protein
- Impaired fasting glucose level

*Atherogenic dyslipidemia is a disorder with four components: borderline high-risk LDL cholesterol (130 to 159 mg/dL), moderately raised (often high normal) triglycerides, small LDL particles, and low HDL cholesterol.
Modified from National Cholesterol Education Program: *Third report of the NCEP Expert Panel on Detection, Evaluation, and Treatment of High Blood cholesterol in Adults (Adult Treatment Panel III)*, Washington, DC, 2002, National Institutes of Health.

terolemia and familial hypertriglyceridemia. Both conditions require diet and drug therapy beginning in the second or third decade of life.

Elevated serum cholesterol is one of the major risk factors for the disease process, which is worsened by obesity, physical inactivity, diets high in saturated fat and cholesterol, stress, and smoking. The National Choles-terol Education Program recommends cholesterol screening every 5 years for adults without existing risk factors and more often for those with higher risks.

Compounding diseases such as diabetes, hypertension, and metabolic syndrome (Table 19-2) increase the risk for developing CVD.[11,12]

Dietary fat can affect serum cholesterol. Thus diets aimed at lowering cholesterol and overall fat intake, especially saturated fat and trans fat, are an important part of the treatment for CVD.

Dietary Recommendations for Reduced Risk

Dietary Guidelines. Because control of dietary fat and cholesterol is important in reducing risks for heart disease, the *Dietary Guidelines for Americans* (see Chapter 1)

TABLE 19-2

DIAGNOSTIC CRITERIA FOR METABOLIC SYNDROME

MEASURE*	CATEGORIC CUT POINTS
Increased waist circumference†‡	≥102 cm (≥40 in) in men ≥88 cm (≥35 in) in women
Elevated triglycerides	≥150 mg/dl (1.7 mmol/L) or drug treatment for elevated triglycerides§
Reduced HDL cholesterol	<40 mg/dl (1.03 mmol/L) in men <50 mg/dl (1.3 mmol/L) in women or drug treatment for reduced HDL cholesterol§
Elevated blood pressure	≥130 mm Hg systolic or ≥85 mm Hg diastolic or drug treatment for hypertension
Elevated fasting glucose	≥100 mg/dl or drug treatment for elevated glucose

Reprinted from Grundy SM and others: Diagnosis and management of metabolic syndrome: an American Heart Association/National Heart, Lung, and Blood Institute Scientific Statement, *Circulation* 112:2735, 2005.
*Any three of these five criteria constitute a diagnosis of metabolic syndrome.
†To measure waist circumference, locate the top of the right iliac crest. Place a measuring tape in a horizontal plane around the abdomen at the level of the iliac crest. Before reading the tape measure, ensure that the tape is snug but does not compress the skin and is parallel to the floor. The measurement is made at the end of a normal expiration.
‡Some U.S. adults of non-Asian origin (e.g., Caucasian, African American, Hispanic) with marginally increased waist circumference (e.g., 94 to 101 cm [37 to 39 in] in men and 80 to 87 cm [31 to 34 in] in women) may have a strong genetic contribution to insulin resistance and should benefit from changes in lifestyle habits, similar to men with categoric increases in waist circumference. A lower waist circumference cut point (e.g., 90 cm [35 in] in men and 80 cm [31 in] in women) appears to be appropriate for Asian Americans.
§Fibrates and nicotinic acid are the most commonly used drugs for elevated triglycerides and reduced HDL cholesterol. Patients taking one of these drugs are presumed to have high triglycerides and low HDL.

and the American Heart Association (Box 19-2) recommend dietary restriction in both nutrients.

National Cholesterol Education Program Adult Treatment Panel III Guidelines. The National Heart, Lung, and Blood Association's National Cholesterol Education Program (NCEP) began a campaign against high blood cholesterol in 1988 with the release of its Report of the Expert Panel on Detection, Evaluation, and Treatment of High Blood Cholesterol in Adults, Adult Treatment Panel (ATP). The NCEP designed the Step I and Step II diets, also endorsed by the American Heart Association, to lessen the risk of CVD by reducing high blood cholesterol levels. Since the inception of the Step I and Step II diets, the NCEP has released two follow-up reports. In the most recent (ATP III) the organization moved toward an intensive life habit intervention focused on appropriate weight, diet, physical activity, and other controllable risk factors.[9] This comprehensive approach is referred to as the Therapeutic Lifestyle Changes (TLC). Although the Step I and Step II diets are no longer used, historic information can be found at *www.americanheart. org/presenter.jhtml?identifier=4764.* Table 19-3 outlines the recommendations for the TLC diet. Essential components of the approach are as follows:

- Total energy intake should reflect energy expenditure to maintain desirable body weight and prevent weight gain.
- Total fat intake should not exceed 25% to 35% of total kilocalories, with saturated fat contributing no more

TABLE 19-3

AMERICAN HEART ASSOCIATION AND NCEP RECOMMENDATIONS FOR LOWERING CHOLESTEROL

NUTRIENT*	RECOMMENDED INTAKE AS PERCENT OF TOTAL CALORIES
Total fat	25%-35%
Saturated	<7%
Polyunsaturated	≤10%
Monounsaturated	≤20%
Carbohydrate	50%-60%
Protein	~15%
Cholesterol	<200 mg/day
Fiber	20-30 g
Total calories	Balance energy intake and expenditure to maintain desirable body weight and prevent weight gain

Modified from Krauss RM and others: AHA dietary guidelines (revision 2000): a statement for healthcare professionals from the Nutrition Committee of the American Heart Association, *Circulation* 102(18):2284, 2000; and National Cholesterol Education Program: *Third report of the NCEP Expert Panel on Detection, Evaluation, and Treatment of High Blood cholesterol in Adults (Adult Treatment Panel III)*, Washington, DC, 2002, National Institutes of Health.
*Calories from alcohol not included.

than 7%, polyunsaturated fat up to 10%, and monounsaturated fats up to 20%. Individuals with metabolic syndrome or diabetes can increase their intake of mono- and polyunsaturated fats in place of carbohydrates.

- Avoid trans fatty acids.
- Carbohydrates, mainly from complex carbohydrates such as whole grains, fruits, and vegetables, should make up 50% to 60% of the total energy intake per day. The diet should allow for 10 to 25 g of soluble fiber and 2 g of plant-derived sterols or stanols per day.
- Total protein intake should account for approximately 15% of the total energy intake. Soy protein is encouraged as a low-fat alternative to other animal products

BOX 19-2

AMERICAN HEART ASSOCIATION DIETARY GUIDELINES

- Burn at least as many calories as you take in.
- Aim for at least 30 minutes of physical activity on most, if not all, days. To lose weight, do enough activity to burn more calories than you eat every day.
- Eat a diet rich in vegetables and fruits.
- Choose whole-grain, high-fiber foods.
- Eat fish at least twice a week.
- Limit how much saturated fat, trans fat, and cholesterol you eat.
- Select fat-free, 1% fat, and low-fat diary products.
- Cut back on foods containing partially hydrogenated vegetable oils to reduce trans fat in your diet.
- Cut back on beverages and foods high in calories and low in nutrition, such as soft drinks and foods with added sugar.
- Choose and prepare foods with little or no salt.
- If you drink alcohol, drink in moderation.

Reprinted from American Heart Association: *Dietary guidelines, www. americanheart.org/presenter.jhtml?identifier=1330*, accessed September 2007.

familial hypertriglyceridemia genetic disorder resulting in elevated blood triglyceride levels despite lifestyle modifications; requires drug therapy.

metabolic syndrome a combination of disorders that, when occurring together, increases the risk of CVD and diabetes. Also known as syndrome X and insulin resistance syndrome.

Therapeutic Lifestyle Changes an intensive lifestyle intervention focused on appropriate weight, diet, physical activity, and other controllable risk factors to reduce cholesterol and prevent other heart disease complications.

(see the For Further Focus box, "Soy Protein and Heart Disease").

- Total cholesterol intake should be less than 200 mg/day.
- Include enough exercise to expend at least 200 kcal/day.

A diet rich in vegetables, fruits, and whole grains and low in saturated and trans fatty acids, with moderate use of polyunsaturated and monounsaturated food fats (e.g., mostly from olive oil or corn oil and other vegetable oils and products), is the basic guideline. Low-fat and fat-free dairy products and lean meat, fish, and poultry are used instead of their high-fat alternatives.

When the risk factor of obesity is present, the overall excess energy value of the diet (kilocalories) also is reduced accordingly, and increased physical activity is encouraged (see Chapter 15). A treadmill exercise tolerance test is ideal to determine the exercise limit for individuals who are older, obese, or have a history of CVD or hypertension before starting an exercise program (Figure 19-3).

Drug Therapy

In the event that LDL cholesterol is above goal range, the NCEP ATP III guidelines recommend cut points for the TLC diet and drug therapy depending on the level of risk (Table 19-4). As the number and severity of risk factors increase, the point at which TLC and drug therapy should begin declines. For example, a person with little or no risk factors associated with CVD may wait to initiate drug therapy until LDL levels exceed 190 mg/dL, whereas an individual with significant risk for CVD would consider drug therapy when LDL levels rise above 100 mg/dL.

FOR FURTHER FOCUS

SOY PROTEIN AND HEART DISEASE

In recent years soy protein has been linked to a reduced risk for coronary heart disease. Ingestion of soy protein has lead to a reduction in LDL cholesterol, an increase in HDL cholesterol, and a reduction in triglycerides. The findings are so significant that the FDA has approved an official health claim linking soy protein consumption and a reduced risk of coronary heart disease.*

One of the main focuses of research in this area is to narrow the recommendations for the amount and type of phytosterols and phytostanols needed on a daily basis to receive the most beneficial results. Phytosterols and phytostanols are the molecules found in plant foods that have the cholesterol-lowering effect. One way in which they work is by preventing the absorption of cholesterol in the digestive tract. Previous research had found a huge range (18 to 124 g/day) in the amount of soy protein needed to achieve the desired results. One reason for this large difference is the low water solubility of the compounds. Because the compound requires fat as a carrier, consuming that amount of soy protein could drastically increase total fat consumption. (Even if it is the heart-healthy fat, it still carries the potential for increasing weight gain.) The FDA recommends consuming four servings per day of soy protein, with each serving containing a minimum of 6.25 g, for a total of 25 g/day.

Researchers are exploring alternative methods for introducing the protein without drastically changing diet or fat intake. One study found that a soy protein supplement of soybean beta-conglycinin (a component of soy protein isolate) in the form of candy produced a significant reduction in triglyceride concentrations and may be an effective alternative, or addition, to soy protein foods.† A similar study combined soy protein with small amounts of lecithin, dried it, and added it to otherwise fat-free foods as an alternative source of phytosterols and phytostanols.‡ b-Sitosterol and lecithin increased the water solubility of the compound and allowed better absorption without the fat. In both cases the beneficial effects of soy protein were seen in the form of lowered cholesterol and improved lipid profiles.

Incorporating soy protein into a low-fat, high-fiber diet with plenty of fruits and vegetables is a sound start to reducing the risk for coronary heart disease.§ Soy protein can be found in the following foods:

- Soy-based meat alternatives
- Miso
- Nondairy frozen desserts
- Okara
- Soy beverages
- Soy cheese
- Soy nut butter
- Soy yogurt
- Soybeans
- Soybean oil
- Soy milk
- Soy nuts
- Tempeh
- Textured vegetable protein
- Tofu

*U.S. Food and Drug Administration: *Health claim: soy protein and coronary heart disease (CHD)*, www.cfsan.fda.gov/~lrd/cf101-82.html, accessed March 2007.
†Kohno M and others: Decreases in serum triacylglycerol and visceral fat mediated by dietary soybean beta-conglycinin, *J Atherscler Thromb* 13(5):247, 2006.
‡Spilburg CA and others: Fat-free foods supplement with soy stanol-lecithin powder reduce cholesterol absorption and LDL cholesterol, *J Am Diet Assoc* 103(5):577, 2003.
§Sacks FM and others: Soy protein, isoflavones, and cardiovascular health: an American Heart Association Science Advisory for professionals from the Nutrition Committee, *Circulation* 113(7):1034, 2006.

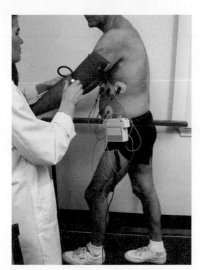

Figure 19–3 A patient with a history of cardiac disease is evaluated for exercise tolerance with a treadmill test. (Copyright PhotoDisc.)

Acute Cardiovascular Disease

When CVD progresses to the point of cutting off the blood supply to major coronary arteries, a critical vascular event (i.e., MI) may occur (see the Clinical Applications box, "Case Study: The Patient with an MI"). In the initial, acute phase of the attack, additional diet modifications are necessary for healing.

Objective: Cardiac Rest

The term *infarction* means tissue death from a lack of oxygen. Blood tests reveal enzymes and proteins released from the damaged heart muscle after infarction. These cardiac markers are one of the tests used for diagnosis. During the care immediately after an MI, patients are given analgesics (e.g., Morphine), supplemental Oxygen, intravenous Nitroglycerine, and Aspirin (the MONA protocol). All care, including diet, is directed toward ensuring cardiac rest so that the damaged heart may be restored to normal functioning.

TABLE 19-4

ATP III LDL CHOLESTEROL GOALS AND CUT POINTS FOR TLC AND DRUG THERAPY

RISK CATEGORY	LDL GOAL	LDL LEVEL AT WHICH TO INITIATE TLC	LDL LEVEL AT WHICH TO CONSIDER DRUG THERAPY*
High risk: CHD† or CHD risk equivalents‡ (10-year risk >20%)	<100 mg/dl (optional goal: <70 mg/dl)§	≥100 mg/dl¶	≥100 mg/dl#(<100 mg/dl: consider drug options)*
Moderately high risk: 2+ risk factors** (10-year risk 10% to 20%)††	<130 mg/dl‡‡	≥130 mg/dl¶	≥130 mg/dl (100-129 mg/dl; consider drug options)§§
Moderate risk: 2+ risk factors** (10-year risk <10%)††	<130 mg/dl	≥130 mg/dl	≥160 mg/dl
Lower risk: 0-1 risk factor¶¶	<160 mg/dl	≥160 mg/dl	≥190 mg/dl (160-189 mg/dl: LDL-lowering drug optional)

CHD, Chronic heart disease.

Reprinted from Grundy S and others: Implications of recent clinical trials for the NCEP-ATP III Guidelines, *Circulation* 110:227, 2004.

*When LDL-lowering drug therapy is used, intensity of therapy should be sufficient to achieve at least a 30% to 40% reduction in LDL cholesterol levels.

†CHD includes history of myocardial infarction, unstable angina, stable angina, coronary artery procedures (angioplasty or bypass surgery), or evidence of clinically significant myocardial ischemia.

‡CHD risk equivalents include clinical manifestations of noncoronary forms of atherosclerotic disease (peripheral arterial disease, abdominal aortic aneurysm, and carotid artery disease [transient ischemic attacks or stroke of carotid origin or >50% obstruction of a carotid artery]), diabetes, and 2+ risk factors with 10-year risk for hard CHD >20%.

§Very high risk favors the optional LDL cholesterol goal of <70 mg/dl and, in patients with high triglycerides, non-HDL cholesterol <100 mg/dl.

¶Any person at high risk or moderately high risk who has lifestyle-related risk factors (e.g., obesity, physical inactivity, elevated triglycerides, low HDL cholesterol, or metabolic syndrome) is a candidate for therapeutic lifestyle changes to modify these risk factors regardless of LDL cholesterol level.

#If baseline LDL cholesterol is <100 mg/dl, institution of an LDL-lowering drug is a therapeutic option on the basis of available clinical trial results. If a high-risk person has high triglycerides or low HDL cholesterol, combining a fibrate or nicotinic acid with an LDL-lowering drug can be considered.

**Risk factors include cigarette smoking, hypertension (blood pressure 140/90 mm Hg or on antihypertensive medication), low HDL cholesterol (<40 mg/dl), family history of premature CHD (CHD in male first-degree relative <55 years old; CHD in female first-degree relative <65 years old), and age (men, 45 years; women, 55 years).

††Electronic 10-year risk calculators are available at *www.nhlbi.nih.gov/guidelines/cholesterol*.

‡‡Optional LDL cholesterol goal <100 mg/dl.

§§For moderately high-risk persons, when LDL cholesterol level is 100 to 129 mg/dl, at baseline or on lifestyle therapy, initiation of an LDL-lowering drug to achieve an LDL cholesterol level <100 mg/dl is a therapeutic option on the basis of available clinical trial results.

¶¶Almost all people with zero or 1 risk factor have a 10-year risk <10%; 10-year risk assessment in people with zero or 1 risk factor is thus not necessary.

CLINICAL APPLICATIONS

CASE STUDY: THE PATIENT WITH AN MI

Charles Carter is a successful young businessman who works long hours and carries the major responsibility of his struggling small business. At his last physical checkup, the physician cautioned him about his pace because he was already showing mild hypertension. His blood cholesterol was elevated, and he was overweight (BMI of 28). In his desk job he got little exercise and found himself smoking more and eating irregularly under the stress of his increasing financial pressures.

One day while commuting in the heavy freeway traffic, he felt a pain in his chest and became increasingly apprehensive. When he arrived home, the pain persisted and increased. He broke out into a cold sweat and felt nauseated. When he became more ill after trying to eat dinner, his wife called their physician and Mr. Carter was admitted to the hospital.

After emergency care and tests, the physician placed Mr. Carter in the coronary care unit at the hospital. His test results showed elevated total cholesterol, triglycerides, and lipoproteins, especially LDL, but low HDL. The electrocardiogram revealed an infarction of the posterior myocardium wall.

When Mr. Carter was first able to take oral nourishment, he could only consume a liquid diet. As his condition stabilized, his diet was increased to 1200 kcal (soft diet) with low cholesterol and low fat. By the end of the first week, his diet was increased to 1600 kcal (full diet) with low cholesterol and only 25% of the total kilocalories from fat and a polyunsaturated/saturated ratio of 1:1.

Mr. Carter gradually improved over the next few days and was able to go home. The physician, nurse, and dietitian discussed with Mr. Carter and his wife the need for care at home during a period of convalescence. They explained that he had an underlying lipid disorder and needed to continue his weight loss and follow a TLC diet.

Questions for Analysis

1. Identify factors in Mr. Carter's personal and medical history that place him at high risk for coronary heart disease. Give reasons why each factor contributes to heart disease.
2. Identify as many laboratory tests as you can that the physician may have ordered. Relate these tests to Mr. Carter's condition.
3. Why did Mr. Carter receive only a liquid diet at first? What is the reason for each modification in his first diet of solid food?
4. What occurs in the underlying disease process that causes a heart attack? What relation do fat and cholesterol have to this underlying process?
5. Outline a day's menu for Mr. Carter on his 1600-kcal TLC diet.
6. What needs might Mr. Carter have when he goes home? How would you help him prepare to go home? Name some community resources you might use to help him understand his illness and plan self-care.

Principles of Medical Nutrition Therapy

The diet is modified in energy value and texture as well as in fat and sodium content.

Energy. A brief period of reduced energy intake during the first day after the heart attack reduces the metabolic workload on the damaged heart. The metabolic demands for digestion, absorption, and metabolism of food require a generous cardiac output. Thus, to decrease the level of metabolic activity that the weakened heart can handle, small feedings are spread over the day when an oral diet is started. The patient progresses to eating more as healing occurs. During the recovery period, caloric intake is adjusted to meet energy needs of the person's ideal body weight.

Texture. Early feedings may include foods that are relatively soft in texture or easily digested to avoid excess effort in eating or the discomfort of gas formation. Some patients benefit from assistance in the feeding process for a short period, especially those with poor appetite or weakness or who become short of breath from the exertion of feeding. Smaller, more frequent meals may give needed nourishment without undue strain or pressure.

Depending on the patient's condition, gas-forming foods, caffeine-containing beverages, and hot or cold temperature extremes in foods (both solids and liquids) should be avoided.

Fat. The TLC diet controls the amount and types of fat and cholesterol (see Table 19-3). Table 19-5 outlines the maximal amount of fat allowed in a TLC diet. Research supports the adoption of a Mediterranean-type diet (see Chapter 14) for patients who have had an MI. The Mediterranean diet replaces saturated fats with omega-3 fats.[13]

Sodium. General attention to reduced sodium content in food selection is important as well. A mild sodium restriction to approximately 2 to 4 g/day typically is sufficient (Box 19-3). This restriction can be achieved by using little or no salt in cooking, adding no salt when eating, and avoiding salty processed foods. Appendixes C and D provide the sodium values of select foods and a salt-free seasoning guide. Food labels on canned and other processed foods, as mandated by Congress and administered by the FDA, provide specific information about the item's sodium content (see Chapter 13).

TABLE 19-5

MAXIMAL AMOUNTS OF FAT ALLOWED PER DAY ON A TLC DIET

TOTAL CALORIES	TOTAL FAT (g)	SATURATED FAT (g)
1200	33-47	9
1400	39-54	11
1600	44-62	12
1800	50-70	14
2000	56-78	16
2200	61-86	17
2400	67-93	19
2600	72-101	20
2800	78-109	22
3000	83-117	23

Modified from Krauss RM and others: AHA dietary guidelines: revision 2000: a statement for healthcare professionals from the Nutrition Committee of the American Heart Association, *Circulation* 102:(18):2284, 2000; and National Cholesterol Education Program: *Third report of the NCEP Expert Panel on Detection, Evaluation, and Treatment of High Blood cholesterol in Adults (Adult Treatment Panel III)*, Washington, DC, 2002, National Institutes of Health.

BOX 19-3

SODIUM-RESTRICTED DIET RECOMMENDATIONS

- No salt served with meals.
- Avoid salt-preserved foods such as salted or smoked meat (e.g., bacon and bacon fat, bologna, dried or chipped beef, corned beef, frankfurters, ham, kosher meats, luncheon meats, salt pork, sausage, smoked tongue), salted or smoked fish (e.g., anchovies, caviar, salted and dried cod, herring, sardines), sauerkraut, and olives.
- Avoid highly salted foods such as crackers, pretzels, potato chips, corn chips, salted nuts, and salted popcorn.
- Limit spices and condiments such as bouillon cubes, catsup, chili sauce, celery salt, garlic salt, onion salt, monosodium glutamate, meat sauces, meat tenderizers, pickles, prepared mustard, relishes, Worcestershire sauce, and soy sauce.*
- Limit processed foods such as cheese and peanut butter.*

Restrictions for mild low-sodium diet (2 to 4 g/day).
*Low-sodium brands may be used.

Chronic Heart Disease

Congestive heart failure, a form of chronic heart disease, may develop over time. The progressively weakened heart muscle is unable to maintain an adequate cardiac output to sustain normal blood circulation. The resulting fluid imbalances cause edema, especially pulmonary edema. This condition makes breathing difficult and places more stress on the laboring heart. Worldwide, more than 7 million people die each year from chronic heart disease.[14]

Objective: Control of Pulmonary Edema

The basic objective of diet therapy in congestive heart failure is to control the fluid imbalance that results in pulmonary edema. The primary causes of fluid accumulation are (1) altered fluid shift mechanisms and (2) inappropriate hormonal responses.

Fluid Shift Mechanism. With decreased heart function, blood accumulates in the vascular system. This buildup offsets the delicate balance of filtration pressures and causes fluid to collect within intracellular spaces instead of flowing between fluid compartments.

Hormonal Alterations. Kidney nephrons sense decreased renal blood flow, normally an indication of dehydration, and respond by triggering the vasopressin and renin-angiotensin-aldosterone systems to increase blood pressure (see Chapter 9). Unlike dehydration, reduced blood flow is caused by inadequate pumping of the heart instead of low blood volume. Vasopressin, also known as antidiuretic hormone, from the pituitary gland stimulates resorption of water in the kidneys. Additionally, aldosterone, secreted by the adrenal glands, causes resorption of sodium in the kidneys and the water that follows. Thus edema is exacerbated.

Principles of Medical Nutrition Therapy

Because of sodium's role in tissue fluid balance, the diet used to treat pulmonary edema restricts sodium intake. The main source of dietary sodium is common table salt, or sodium chloride.

The taste for salt is acquired. Some people heavily salt food by habit without even tasting it first, thus habituating their taste to high salt levels. Others acquire a taste for less salt by gradually using smaller and smaller amounts. Daily adult intakes of sodium range widely in the typical American diet, with an average intake for adults of 3.4 g/day.[15] Other than the salt used in cooking or added at the table, a large amount is used in food processing. Remaining sources of sodium include that found as a naturally occurring mineral in certain foods. Nutrition therapy includes the following:

- *Sodium restriction (2 to 3 g):* No salt is served with meals. Fresh foods are encouraged with sodium-free flavorings such as herbs. Salty processed foods are

congestive heart failure chronic condition of gradually weakening heart muscle unable to pump normal blood through the heart-lung circulation, resulting in congestion of fluids in the lungs.

pulmonary edema accumulation of fluid in lung tissues.

avoided (e.g., pickles, olives, bacon, ham, corn chips, potato chips). Some processed foods with low sodium are available in food markets.

- *Fluid restriction:* Limited to 1500 ml/day when indicated.
- *Texture:* Patients may tolerate soft foods better if eating is laborious or uncomfortable.
- *Small meals:* Frequent small meals (5 to 6 per day) are better suited than large meals.
- *Alcohol:* Intake is limited or avoided if it contributes to heart disease.

ESSENTIAL HYPERTENSION

The Problem of Hypertension

Incidence and Nature

Hypertension, or high blood pressure, is one of the most common vascular diseases. The CDC reports 29.7% of American adults (older than 20 years) have hypertension, with an additional 19% of the population at risk with elevated blood pressure. The incidence is highest among African-American women (44.7%).[1] When speaking of the chronic disease of elevated blood pressure, the term *hypertension* is more appropriate than *high blood pressure* because blood pressure occasionally may be elevated in situations such as overexertion or stress. With **essential (or primary) hypertension** the specific cause is unknown, although injury to the inner lining of the blood vessel wall appears to be an underlying link. More than 90% of cases are considered essential hypertension. **Secondary hypertension** is the result of a known cause and is a symptom or side effect of another primary condition. For example, individuals with kidney disease often have secondary hypertension.

Hypertension has been called the silent killer because no signs indicate its presence. It can have serious effects if not detected, treated, and controlled. Hypertension is a highly inherited disorder; children of hypertensive parents may develop the condition at an early age, often in their adolescent years. Obesity worsens the condition by forcing the heart to work harder to circulate blood through the excess tissue, thus maintaining higher pressure. Smoking also increases blood pressure because nicotine constricts the small blood vessels. Other risk factors include physical inactivity, chronic stress, alcohol abuse, certain drugs (e.g., birth control pills), and sodium intake.

Hypertensive Blood Pressure Levels

Common blood pressure measurements indicate the pressure of the blood surge in the arteries of the upper arm with each heartbeat. The power of each surge is mea-sured in millimeters of mercury (mm Hg). Two forces are counted and represented by separate numbers. The numerator of the fraction (top value) measures the force of the blood surge when the heart contracts, known as the systolic pressure. The denominator of the fraction (bottom value) measures the pressure remaining in the arteries when the heart relaxes between beats, known as the diastolic pressure. Adult blood pressure usually is considered normal if it is less than 120/80 mm Hg. Current hypertension screening and treatment programs identify persons with hypertension according to degree of severity of these pressures (Table 19-6). Specific care is then outlined depending on the severity.

Prehypertension. The initial focus of hypertension treatment is on lifestyle modifications. Lifestyle choices encouraged include (1) reduced salt and increased potassium intake, (2) increased fruit and vegetable consumption, (3) reduced saturated fat and cholesterol intake, (4) moderation of alcohol use, (5) weight loss if indicated, and (6) physical fitness. Such lifestyle changes are able to reduce the risk of chronic disease and improve blood pressure (Table 19-7).[16,17]

Stage 1 Hypertension. In addition to the diet therapy for prehypertension, drugs are used according to need and usually include a diuretic. Continuous use of some, although not all, diuretic drugs causes loss of potassium along with the increased loss of water from the body. Because potassium is necessary for maintaining normal heart muscle action, depletion could become dangerous. Potassium replacement is necessary. Dietary replacement by increased use of potassium-rich foods (e.g., fruits, especially bananas and orange juice, vegetables, legumes, nuts, and whole grains) is an important part of therapy. Appendix C provides the sodium and potassium values of various foods.

Stage 2 Hypertension. In addition to the diet for stage 1 hypertension, vigorous drug therapy is necessary for stage 2 hypertension. (See the Drug-Nutrient Interaction box, "The Grapefruit Conundrum," regarding potential interactions with medications often used for hypertension.) Nutrition therapy is important for all types of hypertension, along with other nondrug therapies such as physical activity and stress reduction.

Principles of Medical Nutrition Therapy

Weight Management

According to individual need, weight management requires losing excess weight and maintaining a healthy weight for height. A sound approach to managing weight loss is given in Chapter 15, and guidance for increasing

TABLE 19-6

CLASSIFICATION OF BLOOD PRESSURE FOR ADULTS

BP CLASSIFICATION	SBP (mm Hg)	DBP (mm Hg)	LIFESTYLE MODIFICATION	INITIAL DRUG THERAPY	
				WITHOUT COMPELLING INDICATION	WITH COMPELLING INDICATION
Normal	<120	and <80	Encourage		
Prehypertension	120-139	or 80-89	Yes	No antihypertensive drug indicated	Drug(s) for compelling indications*
Stage 1 hypertension	140-159	or 90-99	Yes	Thiazide-type diuretics for most; may consider ACEI, ARB, BB, CCB, or combination	Drug(s) for compelling indications,* other antihypertensive drugs as needed (diuretics, ACEI, ARB, BB, CCB)
Stage 2 hypertension	≥160	or ≥100	Yes	Two-drug combination for most† (usually thiazide-type diuretic and ACEI, ARB, BB, or CCB)	

Adults aged 18 years and older. Treatment determined by highest blood pressure category.
BP, Blood pressure; *SBP,* systolic blood pressure; *DBP,* diastolic blood pressure; *ACEI,* angiotensin-converting enzyme inhibitor; *ARB,* angiotensin receptor blocker; *BB,* β-blocker; *CCB,* calcium channel blocker.
Reprinted from National Heart, Lung, and Blood Institute, National Institutes of Health: *Seventh report of the Joint National Committee on Prevention, Detection, Evaluation, and Treatment of High Blood Pressure (JNC 7) express,* NIH publication #03-5233, Bethesda, MD, 2003, National Institutes of Health.
*Patients with chronic kidney disease or diabetes should be treated with a blood pressure goal of <130/80 mm Hg.
†Initial combined therapy should be used cautiously in individuals at risk for orthostatic hypotension.

physical activity is given in Chapter 16. Because excess weight has been closely associated with hypertension risk factors, a wisely planned personal program of weight reduction and physical activity is a cornerstone of therapy.

Sodium Control

In sodium-sensitive persons, additional attention is given to restricting sodium in the diet.[18] Substantial evidence exist to support a direct correlation with decreasing sodium intake and decreasing blood pressure. However, in light of the current food supply (rich in processed foods), achieving a palatably diet with sodium restrictions set below 2 g/day is difficult. Therefore the current recommendation of 2.3 g/day as a maximal intake generally is sufficient.[17] A value of 2.4 g of sodium is equivalent to approximately 6 g sodium chloride (i.e., table salt). See Box 19-3 for ideas on ways to limit sodium intake.

Other Minerals

In addition to sodium control, other minerals have been discussed in relation to hypertension. Evidence suggests that increased calcium, potassium, and magnesium intake is beneficial for everyone, especially those with hypertension. High potassium intake has an independent and inverse relation with blood pressure.[17] The *Dietary Guidelines for Americans* and American Heart Association encourage a diet with a wide variety of fruits, vegetables, and low-fat dairy products specifically to ensure adequate intake of these minerals.

The DASH Diet

The DASH diet is the result of the successful Dietary Approaches to Stop Hypertension landmark study, which was able to lower blood pressure significantly by diet alone within a short period (14 days).[19] The diet recommends eating four to six servings of fruits, four to six servings of vegetables, and two to three servings of low-fat dairy foods per day in addition to lean meats and high-fiber grains. Studies have found that individuals following the diet have an average decrease in systolic blood pressure of 6 to 11 mm Hg.[19] When combining the DASH diet with a low-sodium diet, the blood pressure–lowering effects are even greater.[20] More recent studies have found that the DASH diet also can

essential (or primary) hypertension an inherent form of high blood pressure with no specific discoverable cause; considered to be familial; also called primary hypertension.

secondary hypertension elevated blood pressure for which the cause can be identified and is a symptom or side effect of another primary condition.

TABLE 19-7

LIFESTYLE MODIFICATIONS TO PREVENT AND MANAGE HYPERTENSION

MODIFICATION	RECOMMENDATION	APPROXIMATE SBP REDUCTION (RANGE)*
Weight reduction	Maintain healthy body weight (BMI 18.5-24.9)	5-20 mm Hg/10 kg
Adopt DASH eating plan	Consume a diet rich in fruits, vegetables, and low-fat dairy products with a reduced content of saturated and total fat	8-14 mm Hg
Dietary sodium reduction	Reduce dietary sodium intake to no more than 100 mmol per day (2.4 g of sodium or 6 g of sodium chloride)	2-8 mm Hg
Physical activity	Engage in regular aerobic physical activity such as brisk walking (at least 30 min/day most days of the week)	4-9 mm Hg
Moderation of alcohol consumption	Limit consumption to no more than 2 drinks/day (e.g., 24 oz beer, 10 oz wine, or 3 oz 80-proof whiskey) in most men and no more than 1 drink/day in women and lighter weight persons	2-4 mm Hg

For overall cardiovascular risk reduction, stop smoking.
SBP, systolic blood pressure.
Reprinted from National Institutes of Health, National Heart, Lung, and Blood Institute National High Blood Pressure Education Program: *The seventh report of the Joint National Committee on Prevention, Detection, Evaluation, and Treatment of High Blood Pressure,* NIH Publication No. 04-5230, Bethesda, MD, 2004, National Institutes of Health.
*The effects of implementing these modifications are dose and time dependent and could be greater for some individuals.

DRUG-NUTRIENT INTERACTION

THE GRAPEFRUIT CONUNDRUM

Calcium channel blockers (antihypertensives) and 3-hydroxy-3methylglutaryl coenzyme A (HMG-CoA) reductase inhibitors (statin drugs used for lowering cholesterol) are both lipid soluble and easily absorbed. Water solubility leads to urinary excretion. This is important in understanding the grapefruit conundrum.

The body detects all medications as toxins. Through a mechanism specifically designed for detoxification called CYP3A-mediated drug metabolism, the polarity of a drug is changed to become more water soluble and available for excretion through urine. As more of the drug is changed, more of the drug is excreted. This system is anticipated, and standardized dosages for medications consider that only a percentage of the original active ingredients will make it to the general circulation.

Grapefruit juice puts a kink in this reaction. A substance called furanocoumarin, found in grapefruit juice, blocks enzymes responsible for making the drug more polar. As a result less drug is excreted, which can lead to adverse side effects and even toxicity.

Eight ounces of grapefruit juice, or 1 cup, can cause increased drug absorption up to 72 hours after consumption. Normal side effects of calcium channel blockers and HMG-CoA reductase inhibitors are listed below. Excess absorption of the medication can exacerbate these side effects to a potentially lethal degree.

Grapefruit juice is not served in hospitals and should be avoided in the home by individuals taking either of these medications or any others that follow the same mechanism.

Calcium Channel Blockers	HMG-CoA Reductase Inhibitors
GI symptoms such as constipation and nausea	GI complaints such as stomach pain, heartburn, nausea, constipation, diarrhea, gas
Headache	Headache
Flushing	Muscle pain
Bradycardia or reflex tachycardia	Increased risk of myopathy
Skin rash	Skin rash

produce a significant reduction in total and LDL cholesterol, an added benefit for preventing heart disease.[21]

The DASH diet is recommended for individuals with high blood pressure, blood pressure in the prehypertension range, and a family history of high blood pressure or for those who are trying to eliminate the use of blood pressure medications. The first step in following the DASH diet is to determine the appropriate energy (kilocalories) level based on desired weight and activity level (see Chapter 6). The appropriate number of servings per day of each food group should then be based on the total energy need. Table 19-8 outlines the DASH diet and serv-

TABLE 19-8

DASH EATING PLAN

CALORIC INTAKE	GRAINS*	VEGETABLES	FRUITS	FAT-FREE OR LOW-FAT MILK AND MILK PRODUCTS	LEAN MEATS, POULTRY, AND FISH	NUTS, SEEDS, AND LEGUMES	FATS AND OILS†	SWEETS AND ADDED SUGARS
1600	6	3-4	4	2-3	3-6	3 per week	2	0
2000	6-8	4-5	4-5	2-3	6	4-5 per week	2-3	5 or less per week
2600	10-11	5-6	5-6	3	6	1	3	2
3100	12-13	6	6	3-4	6-9	1	4	2
Serving sizes	1 slice bread; 1 oz dry cereal‡; ½ cup cooked rice, pasta, or cereal	1 cup raw leafy vegetable, ½ cup cut-up raw or cooked vegetable, ½ cup vegetable juice	1 medium fruit; ¼ cup dried fruit; ½ cup fresh, frozen, or canned fruit; ½ cup fruit juice	1 cup milk or yogurt, 1½ oz cheese	1 oz cooked meats, poultry, or fish; 1 egg§	⅓ cup or 1½ oz nuts, 2 Tbsp peanut butter, 2 Tbsp or ½ oz seeds, ½ cup cooked legumes (dry beans and peas)	1 tsp soft margarine, 1 tsp vegetable oil, 1 Tbsp mayonnaise, 2 Tbsp salad dressing	1 Tbsp sugar, 1 Tbsp jelly or jam, ½ cup sorbet, gelatin; 1 cup lemonade

Modified from National Institutes of Health, National Heart, Lung, and Blood Institute: *Your guide to lowering your blood pressure with DASH*, NIH Publication No. 06-4082, Washington, DC, 2006, US Department of Health and Human Services.

*Whole grains are recommended for most grain servings as a good source of fiber and nutrients.

†Fat content changes serving amount for fats and oils. For example, 1 Tbsp of a low-fat dressing equals one-half serving; 1 Tbsp of a fat-free dressing equals zero servings.

‡Serving sizes vary between ½ cup and 1¼ cups depending on cereal type. Check the product's Nutrition Facts label.

§Because eggs are high in cholesterol, limit egg yolk intake to no more than four per week; two egg whites have the same protein content as 1 oz meat.

ing sizes; Box 19-4 provides a 1-day sample menu based on a 2000-calorie diet.

Additional Lifestyle Factors

The National High Blood Pressure Education Program recommends limiting alcohol intake to 1 oz/day ethanol for men and 0.5 oz/day for most women and smaller men. One ounce of ethanol is equal to 24 oz regular beer, 10 oz wine, or 2-oz 100-proof whiskey. Additional recommendations to prevent or treat hypertension include stopping smoking, limiting saturated fat and cholesterol intake, and increasing aerobic physical activity to a minimum of 30 to 45 minutes per day on most days of the week.[22]

BOX 19-4

SAMPLE 1-DAY MENU ON THE DASH DIET (2000 CALORIES)

BREAKFAST
- ¾ cup bran flakes cereal
  - 1 medium banana
  - 1 cup low-fat milk
- 1 slice whole-wheat bread
  - 1 tsp soft (tub) margarine
  - 1 cup orange juice

LUNCH
- ¾ cup chicken salad
  - 2 slices whole-wheat bread
  - 1 Tbsp Dijon mustard
- Salad with:
  - ½ cup fresh cucumber slices
  - ½ cup tomato wedges
  - 1 Tbsp sunflower seeds
  - 1 tsp Italian dressing, low calorie
- ½ cup fruit cocktail, juice pack

DINNER
- 3 oz beef, eye of round
  - 2 Tbsp beef gravy, fat free
- 1 cup green beans, sautéed with ½ tsp canola oil
- 1 small baked potato
  - 1 Tbsp sour cream, fat free
  - 1 Tbsp grated natural cheddar cheese, reduced fat
  - 1 Tbsp chopped scallions
- 1 small whole-wheat roll
  - 1 tsp soft (tub) margarine
- 1 small apple
- 1 cup low-fat milk

SNACKS
- ⅓ cup almonds, unsalted
- ¼ cup raisins
- ½ cup fruit yogurt, fat free, no sugar added

Modified from National Institutes of Health, National Heart, Lung, and Blood Institute: *Your guide to lowering your blood pressure with DASH,* NIH Publication No. 06-4082, Washington, DC, 2006, U.S. Department of Health and Human Services.

EDUCATION AND PREVENTION

Practical Food Guides

Food Planning and Purchasing

The *Dietary Guidelines for Americans, 2005* (see Chapter 1) provide a basic outline to guide sound food habits. The food exchange list, described in Chapter 20 and listed in Appendix E, provides the food groups with the fat and sodium modifications discussed in this chapter. These lists also provide a guide for controlling energy intake to help plan weight management.

An important part of purchasing food is carefully reading labels. The Nutrition Facts labels provide basic nutrition information in a standard format that is easily recognized and clearly expressed (see Chapter 13). All food products that make health claims must follow the strict guidelines provided by the FDA. A good general guide is to use primarily fresh foods with informed selection of processed foods as necessary. Refer to Chapter 13 for background material about food supply and health.

Food Preparation

The public is more aware of the need to prepare foods with less fat and salt than ever before. Consequently, the cookbook industry has responded by providing an abundance of guides and recipes for various age groups and customs. Many seasonings (e.g., herbs, spices, lemon, wine, onion, garlic, nonfat milk and yogurt, and fat-free broth) can help train the taste for less salt and fat (see Appendix D). Less meat in leaner and smaller portions can be combined with more complex carbohydrate foods (e.g., starches such as potato, pasta, rice, bulgur, and beans) to make more healthful main dishes. Whole-grain breads and cereals provide needed fiber, and more use of fish can add healthier forms of fat in smaller quantities. A variety of vegetables may be used (e.g., in salads or steamed and lightly seasoned), and fruits add interest, taste appeal, and nourishment to meals. The American Heart Association publishes several cookbooks that are excellent guides to newer, lighter, tasteful, and healthier food preparation (*www.american-heart.org*).

Special Needs

Individual adaptation of diet principles is important in all nutrition teaching and counseling. Special attention must be given to personal desires, ethnic diets, individual situations, and food habits (see Chapter 14). Successful diet planning must meet both personal and health needs.

Education Principles

Starting Early

Prevention of hypertension and heart disease begins in childhood, especially with children in high-risk families. Preventive measures in family food habits relate to healthy weight maintenance and limited use of foods high in salt and fat. For adults with heart disease and hypertension, learning should be an integral part of all therapy. If a heart attack occurs, education should begin early in convalescence, not at hospital discharge, to give patients and their families clear and practical knowledge of positive needs.

Focusing on High-Risk Groups

Education about heart disease and hypertension should be particularly directed to individuals and families with one or more high-risk factors (see Box 19-1). For example, hypertension has been closely associated with certain high-risk groups, including African Americans, persons with strong family history of the disease, and obese individuals (see the Cultural Considerations box, "Influence of Ancestors on a Person's Risk for Heart Disease").

Using a Variety of Resources

As researchers learn more about heart disease and hypertension, the American Heart Association and other health agencies are providing many excellent resources. The ADA provides a series of pamphlets that are helpful in client education, several of which are applicable to heart disease (available at *www.eatright.org/cps/rde/xchg/ada/hs.xsl/nutrition.html*). As professionals and the public have become more aware of health needs and disease prevention, an increasing number of resources and programs are available in most communities. These include various weight management programs, RDs in private practice or in health care centers who provide nutrition

CULTURAL CONSIDERATIONS

INFLUENCE OF ANCESTORS ON A PERSON'S RISK FOR HEART DISEASE

Although the mortality rate from heart disease has declined since the 1960s, it is still the leading cause of death in the United States. The mortality rate for CVD in the Americas (North, South, and Central) ranges from 141 to 526 deaths per 100,000 persons (see the figure at right). Relative to other countries within the Americas, the United States has a reasonably low rate (188/100,000). Unlike weight and dietary habits, family history is a nonmodifiable risk factor for CVD. Therefore distinguishing between environmental factors and the genetics associated with a culture is important to identify the specifics regarding cause of disease. Only when those factors have been recognized can prevention and treatment programs be directed on an individual basis.

Interestingly, the major conditions of heart disease (hypertension and high blood cholesterol) are more prevalent in certain ethnic and age groups than others within the United States. The prevalence of both hypertension and high blood cholesterol increases with age. However, hypertension is most prevalent in the African-American population, whereas hypercholesterolemia (high blood cholesterol) is most common in Caucasian and non-Hispanic women and least common in African-American men.* As a health care provider, you should be aware of the risk associated with CVD among various ethnic groups. By acknowledging the risk associated with ethnicity, warning signs may be detected earlier than they would otherwise.

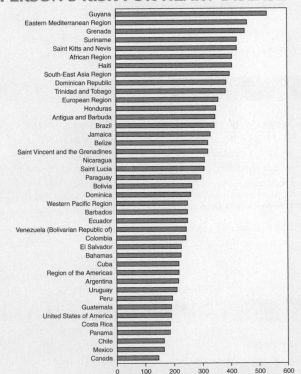

Age-standardized mortality rate for CVD in the Americas (per 100,000 population). (Modified from World Health Organization: *World Health Statistics 2006, www.who.int/whosis/database/core/core_select_process.cfm#.*)

*National Center for Health Statistics: *Health, United States, 2006, with chartbook on trends in the health of Americans,* Hyattsville, MD, 2006, U.S. Government Printing Office.

counseling, and practical food preparation materials found in a number of "light cuisine" cooking classes and cookbooks. Bookstores and public libraries, as well as health education libraries in health centers and clinics, provide an abundance of materials on health promotion and self-care. For example, local health care centers teach people with hypertension and their families how to take their own blood pressure so they can assume more control in managing their health needs and provide other resources for such self-care.

SUMMARY

Coronary heart disease is the leading cause of death in the United States. Its underlying blood vessel disease is atherosclerosis, which involves buildup of the fatty substance containing cholesterol on the interior surfaces of blood vessels, interfering with blood flow and damaging blood vessels. If this fatty buildup becomes severe, it cuts off the supply of oxygen and nutrients to tissue cells, which in turn die. When this occurs in a major coronary artery, the result is an MI, or heart attack.

The risk for atherosclerosis increases with the amount and type of blood lipids (fats), or lipoproteins, available. Elevated serum cholesterol is a primary risk factor for development of atherosclerosis.

Current recommendations to help prevent coronary heart disease involve a low-fat and balanced diet, weight management, and increased physical activity. Such a diet limits fats to 25% to 30% of total energy intake, sodium intake to 2 to 3 g/day, and cholesterol intake to 200 mg/day. Dietary recommendations for acute CVD include measures to ensure cardiac rest (e.g., energy restriction and small meals modified in fat, cholesterol, and sodium). Persons with chronic heart disease involving congestive heart failure benefit from a low-sodium diet to control pulmonary edema.

Persons with hypertension may improve their condition with weight control, exercise, sodium restriction, and adequate calcium and potassium intake.

CRITICAL THINKING QUESTIONS

1. Why are fat and cholesterol primary factors in heart disease? How are they carried in the bloodstream? Which of these lipoproteins carry so-called good cholesterol and which carry bad cholesterol, the cholesterol of concern?
2. How can people influence the relative amounts of fat and cholesterol in the blood? Describe the food changes involved.
3. Identify the risk factors for heart disease. What control do people have over these risk factors?
4. Identify four dietary recommendations for a patient who has had a heart attack. Describe how each recommendation facilitates recovery.
5. Discuss the three levels of hypertension and the treatment options for each.
6. What does essential hypertension mean? Why would weight control and sodium restriction contribute to its control? What other nutrient factors may be involved in hypertension?

CHAPTER CHALLENGE QUESTIONS

True-False
Write the correct statement for each statement that is false.

1. *True or False:* In the disease process underlying heart disease (atherosclerosis), the fatty deposits in blood vessel linings are made up mainly of cholesterol.
2. *True or False:* Hypertension occurs more frequently in Caucasians than in African Americans.
3. *True or False:* The problem of CVD could be solved if cholesterol could be removed entirely from the body.
4. *True or False:* Cholesterol is a dietary essential because people depend entirely on food sources for their supply.
5. *True or False:* Lipoproteins are the major transport form of lipids in the blood.
6. *True or False:* One of the basic clinical objectives in treating acute a heart attack is cardiac rest.

7. *True or False:* In chronic congestive heart disease, the heart eventually may fail because its weakened muscle must work at a faster rate to pump the body's necessary blood supply.

8. *True or False:* The taste for salt is instinctive to ensure a sufficient supply.

9. *True or False:* High sodium intake is an effective therapy for congestive heart failure and hypertension.

10. *True or False:* Essential hypertension can be cured by drugs and diet.

Multiple Choice

1. A low-cholesterol diet restricts which of the following foods? *(Circle all that apply.)*

   a. Fish
   b. Liver
   c. Butter
   d. Nonfat milk

2. Helpful seasonings to use in a sodium-restricted diet include which of the following? *(Circle all that apply.)*

   a. Lemon juice
   b. Soy sauce
   c. Herbs and spices
   d. Seasoned salt

3. Prehypertension is defined as a blood pressure of _____ (systolic) / _____(diastolic) mm Hg.

   a. Less than 120 and less than 80
   b. 120 to 139 and 80 to 89
   c. 140 to 159 and 90 to 99
   d. More than 160 and more than 100

4. Which of the following foods may be used freely on a low-sodium diet?

   a. Fruits
   b. Milk
   c. Meat
   d. Spinach and carrots

---

evolve **Please refer to the Students' Resource section of this text's Evolve Web site for additional study resources.**

REFERENCES

1. National Center for Health Statistics: *Health, United States, 2006, with chartbook on trends in the health of Americans,* Hyattsville, MD, 2006, U.S. Government Printing Office.
2. De Caterina R and others: Nutritional mechanisms that influence cardiovascular disease, *Am J Clin Nutr* 83:421S, 2006.
3. Krauss RM: Dietary and genetic probes of atherogenic dyslipidemia, *Arterioscler Thromb Vasc Biol* 25:2265, 2005.
4. Sies H and others: Nutritional, dietary, and postprandial oxidative stress, *J Nutr* 135:969, 2005.
5. Montoya MT and others: Fatty acid saturation of the diet and plasma lipid concentrations, lipoprotein particle concentrations, and cholesterol efflux capacity, *Am J Clin Nutr* 75(3):484, 2002.
6. Psota TL and others: Dietary omega-3 fatty acid intake and cardiovascular risk, *Am J Cardiol* 98(4A):3i, 2006.
7. dos Santos RE and others: Relationship of body fat distribution by waist circumference, dual-energy x-ray absorptiometry and ultrasonography to insulin resistance by homeostasis model assessment and lipid profile in obese and non-obese postmenopausal women, *Gynecol Endocrinol* 21(5):295, 2005.
8. Grundy SM and others: Implications of recent clinical trials for the National Cholesterol Education Program Adult Treatment Panel III guidelines, *Circulation* 110:227, 2004.
9. National Cholesterol Education Program: *Third report of the NCEP Expert Panel on Detection, Evaluation, and Treatment of High Blood Cholesterol in Adults (Adult Treatment Panel III),* Washington, DC, 2002, National Institutes of Health.
10. The ESHRE Capri Workshop Group: Hormones and cardiovascular health in women, *Hum Reprod Update* 12(5):483, 2006.
11. McNeill AM and others: Metabolic syndrome and cardiovascular disease in older people: the cardiovascular health study, *J Am Geriatr Soc* 54:1317, 2006.
12. Guzder RN and others: Impact of metabolic syndrome criteria on cardiovascular disease risk in people with newly diagnosed type 2 diabetes, *Diabetologia* 49:49, 2006.
13. Mead A and others: Dietetic guidelines on food and nutrition in the secondary prevention of cardiovascular disease—evidence from systematic reviews of randomized controlled trials (second update, January 2006), *J Hum Nutr Diet* 19(6):401, 2006.
14. Mackay J, Mensah GA: *The atlas of heart disease and stroke,* Geneva, 2004, World Health Organization.
15. United States Department of Agriculture/Economic Research Service: *Diet and health: food consumption and nutrient intake tables, www.ers.usda.gov/Briefing/DietAndHealth/data/nutrients/table1.htm,* accessed March 2007.
16. Elmer PJ and others: Effects of comprehensive lifestyle modification on diet, weight, physical fitness, and blood pressure control: 18-month results of a randomized trial, *Ann Intern Med* 144:485, 2006.
17. Appel LJ and others: Dietary approaches to prevent and treat hypertension, a scientific statement from the American Heart Association, *Hypertension* 47:296, 2006.
18. Franco V, Oparil S: Salt sensitivity, a determinant of blood pressure, cardiovascular disease and survival, *J Am Coll Nutr* 25(3):247S, 2006.
19. Appel LJ and others: A clinical trial of the effects of dietary patterns on blood pressure. DASH Collaborative Research Group, *N Engl J Med* 336(16):1117, 1997.

20. Sacks FM and others: Effects on blood pressure of reduced dietary sodium and the Dietary Approaches to Stop Hypertension (DASH) diet, *N Engl J Med* 344:3, 2001.
21. Harsha DW and others: Effect of dietary sodium intake on blood lipids, results from the DASH-sodium trial, *Hypertension* 43(2):393, 2004.
22. National Institutes of Health, National Heart, Lung, and Blood Institute National High Blood Pressure Education Program: *The seventh report of the Joint National Committee on Prevention, Detection, Evaluation, and Treatment of High Blood Pressure,* NIH Publication No. 04-5230, Bethesda, MD, 2004, National Institutes of Health.

FURTHER READING AND RESOURCES

American Heart Association: *www.americanheart.org*

NCEP: *www.nhlbi.nih.gov/chd*

NCEP *Risk Assessment Tool for Estimating 10-Year Risk of Developing Coronary Heart Disease: http://hp2010.nhlbihin.net/atpiii/calculator.asp?usertype=prof*

National Center for Chronic Disease Prevention and Health Promotion, Heart Disease Prevention; *What You Can Do: www.cdc.gov/HeartDisease/prevention.htm*

These organizations are valuable sources of information on the most current recommendations for healthy lifestyles to prevent and treat heart disease. The Web sites also provide educational materials for health care professionals.

De Caterina R and others: Nutritional mechanisms that influence cardiovascular disease, *Am J Clin Nutr* 83:421S, 2006.

Grundy SM and others: Implications of recent clinical trials for the National Cholesterol Education Program Adult Treatment Panel III Guidelines, *Circulation* 110:227, 2004.

As large-scale research studies continue to uncover the underlying factors associated with heart disease, the national recommendations for preventative measures are continually updated. This report outlines the most recent recommendations for preventing and treating high blood pressure.

CHAPTER 20

Diabetes Mellitus

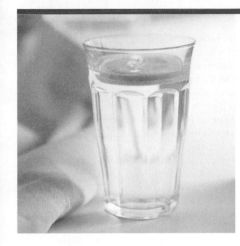

KEY CONCEPTS

- Diabetes mellitus is a metabolic disorder of glucose metabolism with many causes and forms.
- A consistent, sound diet is a major keystone of diabetes care and control.
- Daily self-care skills enable a person with diabetes to remain healthy and reduce risks for complications.
- Blood glucose monitoring is a critical practice for blood glucose control.
- A personalized care plan balancing food intake, exercise, and insulin regulation is essential to successful diabetes management.

The CDC estimates that 20.8 million Americans have diabetes (7% of the total U.S. population), and an additional 54 million have a condition known as prediabetes.[1] Diabetes currently is the seventh-ranking cause of death in the United States.[2]

Historically diabetes mellitus claimed the lives of its victims at a young age. Greater knowledge of the disease and proper self-care practices have enabled persons with diabetes to live long and fulfilling lives. However, diabetes has no cure and individuals without health care and access to proper medication continue to die early in life. With professional guidance and support, individuals with diabetes can remain in a state of good health and reduce the risk of long-term complications by consistently practicing good self-care skills.

This chapter examines the nature of diabetes and details why daily self-care is essential for health.

NATURE OF DIABETES
Defining Factor

Glucose is the primary, and preferred, source of energy for the body. As discussed in Chapter 2, carbohydrate foods break down during digestion in the GI tract and are absorbed into the blood stream mainly as glucose. Glucose is then transported throughout the body to be used as energy. However, for glucose to be used by the cells in the body, it first has to be taken out of the blood and transported into the cells. For this process to happen in most cells, the hormone insulin must be present. Insulin is produced by the β cells of the pancreas (see the For Further Focus box, "The History and Discovery of Insulin"). Individuals with diabetes either do not produce insulin or cannot effectively use the insulin produced. Without insulin, glucose accumulates in the bloodstream. The Expert Committee on the Diagnosis and Classification of Diabetes Mellitus defines diabetes as "a group of metabolic dis-

---

insulin a hormone produced by the pancreas that attaches to insulin receptors on cell membranes and allows absorption of glucose into the cell.

FOR FURTHER FOCUS

THE HISTORY AND DISCOVERY OF INSULIN

Early History and Name

The symptoms of diabetes were first described on an Egyptian papyrus, the Ebers Papyrus, which dates to approximately 1500 BC. In the first century the Greek physician Areatus wrote of a malady in which the body "ate its own flesh" and gave off large quantities of urine. He named it *diabetes*, from the Greek word meaning siphon or to pass through. In the seventeenth century the word *mellitus*, from the Latin word meaning honey, was added because of the sweetness of the urine. The addition of *mellitus* distinguished the disorder from another disorder, *diabetes insipidus*, in which large urine output also was observed. However, diabetes insipidus is a much rarer and quite different disease caused by lack of the pituitary antidiuretic hormone. Today, the simple term *diabetes* refers to diabetes mellitus.

Diabetic Dark Ages

Throughout the Middle Ages and the dawning of the scientific era, many early scientists and physicians continued to puzzle over the mystery of diabetes, but the cause remained obscure. For physicians and their patients these years could be called the Diabetic Dark Ages. Patients had short life spans and were maintained on a variety of semistarvation and high-fat diets.

Discovery of Insulin

The first breakthrough came from a clue pointing to involvement of the pancreas in the disease process. This clue was provided by a young German medical student, Paul Langerhans (1847-1888), who found special clusters of cells scattered about the pancreas forming little islands of cells. Although he did not yet understand their function, Langerhans could see that these cells were different from the rest of the tissue and assumed they must be important. When his suspicions later proved true, these clusters of cells were named for their young discoverer, *the islets of Langerhans*. In 1922, using this important clue, two Canadian scientists, Frederick Banting and his assistant, Charles Best, together with two other research team members, physiologists J.B. Collip and J.J.R. Macleod, extracted the first insulin from animals. It proved to be a hormone that regulates the oxidation of blood glucose and helps convert it to heat and energy. They called the hormone *insulin,* from the Latin word *insula,* meaning island. Insulin did prove to be the effective agent for treating diabetes. The first child treated in January 1922, Leonard Thompson, lived to adulthood but died at age 27 years, not from his diabetes but from coronary heart disease caused by the diabetic diet of the day, which was based on 70% of its total kilocalories from fat. Unsurprisingly, his autopsy showed marked atherosclerosis.

Successful Use of Diet and Insulin

The insulin discovery team was more successful on their third try with a young girl diagnosed as having diabetes at age 11 years. She initially had been put on a starvation diet, and her weight fell from 75 to 45 pounds (34 to 21 kg) over a 3-year period. However, the medical research team fortunately had learned the importance of a well-balanced diet for normal growth and health. Thus with a good diet and the new insulin therapy, this child, Elizabeth Hughes, gained weight and vigor and lived a normal life. She married, had three children, took insulin for 58 years, and died at age 73 years of heart failure.

---

eases characterized by hyperglycemia resulting from defects in insulin secretion, insulin action, or both."[3]

Classification of Diabetes Mellitus and Glucose Intolerance

Various types of diabetes mellitus are classified according to the pathogenic process of the disease.

Type 1 Diabetes Mellitus

Type 1 diabetes mellitus accounts for 5% to 10% of all cases of diabetes. Previously called *insulin-dependent diabetes* or *juvenile-onset diabetes,* type 1 diabetes develops rapidly and tends to be more severe and unstable than other types of diabetes. This form of diabetes is caused by an autoimmune destruction of the β cells in the pancreas. At least four different autoantibodies have been identified as the cause for destruction (islet cell autoantibodies, autoantibodies to insulin, autoantibodies to glutamic acid decarboxylase, and autoantibodies to the tyrosine phosphatases IA-2 and IA-2β). The rate of destruction determines the onset of diabetes. The initial onset of type 1 diabetes occurs rapidly in children and adolescents, hence the former name of juvenile-onset diabetes, but it can occur at any age. For some individuals the rate of destruction is slower and may not present symptoms until adulthood. Individuals with this type of diabetes rely on exogenous insulin for survival (source of the former name insulin-dependent diabetes). Persons with type 1 diabetes usually are underweight and at higher risk for acidosis at the time of diagnosis.

Type 2 Diabetes Mellitus

Approximately 90% to 95% of the individuals with diabetes have type 2 diabetes. This form has a strong genetic link and is more prevalent in older, obese individuals.[3] Box 20-1 lists additional risk factors for the development of type 2 diabetes. Unlike type 1 diabetes, type 2 is not

BOX 20-1

RISK FACTORS FOR TYPE 2 DIABETES MELLITUS

- A family history of diabetes
- Age 45 years or older
- Overweight (BMI $\geq$25 kg/m^2)
- Not physically active on a regular basis
- Race/ethnicity (African American, Hispanic American, Native American, Asian American, and Pacific Islander)
- History of gestational diabetes mellitus
- Woman who has delivered an infant weighing more than 9 pounds
- Previously identified as impaired glucose tolerance

caused by an autoimmune response. This form of diabetes results from an insulin resistance or insulin defect—the body is either not producing enough insulin or the insulin it is producing cannot be used. These individuals usually do not need exogenous insulin for survival, but rather rely on diet, exercise, and (usually) oral medications for disease management. This form of diabetes, previously called *adult-onset* or *non-insulin-dependent diabetes,* has an onset primarily in adults older than 40 years. However, as American children get heavier, the occurrence of type 2 diabetes in young people is on the rise (1.82 cases per 1000 youth younger than 20 years).[4] The Cultural Considerations box, "Risk Factors for Diabetes: Genetic versus Environmental," discusses this issue in more depth. Many adults and children with type 2 diabetes can improve or reduce their symptoms with weight loss and thus require only diet therapy and balanced exercise programs. Table 20-1 summarizes the differences between type 1 and type 2 diabetes mellitus.

Gestational Diabetes

Gestational diabetes mellitus (GDM) is a temporary form of diabetes occurring during pregnancy, with normal blood glucose control usually recovered after delivery. Women who have diabetes before conception (type 1 or 2) are considered to have pregestational diabetes and do not fall into this category during pregnancy. GDM can present complications for both mother and infant if not carefully monitored and controlled. Persistent hyperglycemia is associated with an increased risk of intrauterine fetal death and macrosomia.

GDM develops in approximately 4% of all pregnant women.[3] Risk factors for GDM are the same as for type 2 diabetes (see Box 20-1). Pregnant women at high risk for developing GDM should be screened with a glucose tolerance test as soon as possible. Women who do not have

multiple risk factors but who are at moderate risk undergo screening at 24 to 28 weeks of gestation. The American Diabetes Association does not recommend screening women unlikely to develop GDM because it is not cost effective. The low-risk group is defined by the following criteria[3]:

- Younger than 25 years of age
- Normal body weight
- No family history (i.e., first-degree relative) of diabetes
- No history of abnormal glucose metabolism
- No history of poor obstetric outcome
- Not members of an ethnic or racial group with a high prevalence of diabetes (e.g., Hispanic American, Native American, Asian American, African American, Pacific Islander)

Screening for GDM should follow one of the following two approaches:

1. *One-step approach:* 100-g oral glucose tolerance test (OGTT). In this test the patient is given a 100-g solution of glucose; the venous blood glucose level is then measured at 1, 2, and 3 hours after administration to monitor response. The test must be given in the morning after an overnight fast (8 to 14 hours of nothing to eat) and after at least 3 days of unrestricted diet and physical activity. If two or more of the following criteria are met, the individual is diagnosed with GDM:
   - Fasting glucose: $\geq$95 mg/dl
   - Glucose after 1 hour: $\geq$180 mg/dl
   - Glucose after 2 hours: $\geq$155 mg/dl
   - Glucose after 3 hours: $\geq$140 mg/dl
2. *Two-step approach:* 50 g oral glucose challenge test and OGTT. The patient is first screened for glucose intolerance with the 50-g oral glucose challenge test (using the same protocol as for the 100-g OGTT). If blood glucose levels do not fall below 140 mg/dl within 1 hour after administration, an OGTT is then performed. The American Diabetes Association states that the threshold value of 140 mg/dl cutoff point identifies 80% of women with GDM.[3]

If a fasting plasma glucose test meets the general diagnostic criteria for diabetes, a glucose tolerance test may not be necessary for diagnosis of GDM.

hyperglycemia blood glucose elevated above normal.

exogenous originating from outside the body.

macrosomia excessive fetal growth resulting in an abnormally large infant; carries high risk for perinatal death.

CULTURAL CONSIDERATIONS

RISK FACTORS FOR TYPE 2 DIABETES: GENETIC VERSUS ENVIRONMENTAL

Type 2 diabetes has been known for years as adult-onset diabetes because it rarely affected anyone younger than 40 years. However, this form of diabetes is rapidly becoming a health care concern in children and adolescents. As with the occurrence of type 2 diabetes in adults, it has been reported in all races and ethnic populations, with a disproportionate burden on minority groups. In an effort to define the contributing factors responsible for the increased prevalence of type 2 diabetes, researchers are considering in utero exposure to diabetes from mother to fetus and shared maternal-child environmental factors.

A positive association between family history of type 2 diabetes and insulin resistance in adults has been well accepted. However, this association has not been fully researched in children with a family history. A study by Goran and colleagues evaluated the influence of family history on insulin sensitivity in children.* The researchers in this study controlled for other factors known to increase the risk for type 2 diabetes (increased body fat, ethnicity, and onset of puberty). African-American, Hispanic, and Native American children have a higher risk for developing type 2 diabetes than Caucasian children. Although this was a small study (21 paired children), the results indicate that family history may not influence insulin resistance during childhood. Such findings indicate that the environmental factor associated within family settings could be more influential at this point of development in children than genetic factors.

Regardless of cause, diabetes, IGT, obesity, and even CVD are beginning to plague the children of Americans in a similar fashion as adults. Ethnic groups with pronounced risk are African Americans, Hispanic and Latino Americans, Native Americans, and some Asian Americans and Native Hawaiians or other Pacific Islanders. The estimated prevalence of type 2 diabetes in children (younger than 20 years) is 1.82 cases per 1000 youth.† As research continues to uncover the pathophysiology, risk factors, and methods of prevention and treatment, hopefully this trend in disease progression will slow or come to a halt.

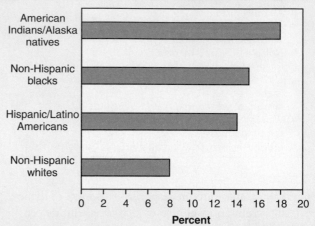

Prevalence of diabetes in adults. For Native Americans and Alaska Natives, the estimate of total prevalence was calculated using the estimate of diagnosed diabetes from the 2003 outpatient database of the Indian Health Service and the estimate of undiagnosed diabetes from the 1999-2002 National Health and Nutrition Examination Survey. For the other groups, 1999-2002 National Health and Nutrition Examination Survey estimates of total prevalence (both diagnosed and undiagnosed diabetes) were projected to year 2005. (From Centers for Disease Control and Prevention: *National diabetes fact sheet, www.cdc.gov/diabetes/pubs/pdf/ndfs_2005.pdf*, accessed April 2007.

*Goran MI and others: Influence of family history of type 2 diabetes on insulin sensitivity in prepubertal children, *J Clin Endocrinol Metab* 88(1):192, 2003.
†SEARCH for Diabetes in Youth Study Group: The burden of diabetes mellitus among US youth: prevalence estimates from the SEARCH for Diabetes in Youth Study, *Pediatrics* 118(4):1510, 2006.

Women with GDM have their blood glucose levels carefully monitored and are taught to follow a tightly managed program of diet and self-testing of blood glucose, blood pressure, and urinary protein. For women who are unable to maintain blood glucose levels within an acceptable range (≤95 mg/dl fasting, ≤140 mg/dl 1 hour postprandial, or ≤120 mg/dl 2 hours postprandial), insulin therapy is recommended. Oral hypoglycemic agents were not used for GDM in the past for fear of teratogenic effects. How-

ever, recent research indicates that selective oral hypoglycemic agents may be appropriate for use in this population.[5]

Complications of GDM for mother and child are greatly reduced, if not eliminated, by tight control of blood glucose levels. Women with GDM also are advised to maintain a balanced diet, regular exercise schedule, a healthy BMI, and follow-up visits with their physician. The risk for developing type 2 diabetes is significantly higher in women with a history of GDM.[6]

TABLE 20-1

DIFFERENTIATING TYPE 1 AND TYPE 2 DIABETES MELLITUS

FACTOR	TYPE 1	TYPE 2
Ethnicity	Increased rates among persons with Northern European heritage	Increased rate among persons with heritage from equatorial countries; highest rates found with Native American, Hispanic, African-American, Asian, Pacific Islander, and Mediterranean heritage
Age of onset	Generally younger than 30 years, with peak onset before puberty	Generally older than 40 years, although genetic predisposition and obesity may cause onset to occur at younger ages
Weight	Usually normal or underweight; unintentional weight loss often precedes diagnosis	Usually overweight but may be of normal weight
Treatment	Insulin injections are necessary to prevent death; food and exercise must be balanced with insulin injections	Weight loss usually is the first goal; reduction in sugar and fat and increase in fiber (soluble) are helpful; oral hypoglycemic agents or insulin or both may be necessary for good blood glucose management but are not necessary to prevent imminent death; exercise is important
β cell functioning	Totally absent (no insulin produced) after the "honeymoon period"; residual insulin produced for approximately 1 year after diagnosis	Excess insulin production usually evident (hyperinsulinemia), but insulin resistance occurs at the cell level; insulin production also may be normal or below normal

Reprinted from Peckenpaugh NJ: *Nutrition essentials and diet therapy*, ed 9, Philadelphia, 2003, Saunders.

Other Types of Diabetes

Secondary diabetes may be caused by a number of conditions or agents affecting the pancreas, including the following:

- *Genetic defects:* Defects in the β cells or insulin action may result in several forms of diabetes. These forms are not characteristic of the autoimmune destruction found in type 1 diabetes. Mutations on at least six genetic loci have been identified, resulting in impaired insulin secretion (although not the action of the insulin). Other less-common defects in the action of the insulin (but not the amount secreted) also result in hyperglycemia and diabetes. Two such syndromes identified in the pediatric population are leprechaunism and Rabson-Mendenhall syndrome.[3]
- *Pancreatic conditions or disease:* Any condition causing damage to the pancreatic cells can result in diabetes. Such conditions include tumors affecting the islet cells; acute viral infection by a number of agents, such as the mumps virus; acute pancreatitis from biliary disease and gallstones; chronic pancreatic insufficiency, such as that occurring in cystic fibrosis; pancreatic surgery, which may occur in cancer of the pancreas; and severe traumatic abdominal injury. One of the most common causes of chronic pancreatitis is alcohol abuse. Approximately one third to one half of patients with acute pancreatitis develop disorders such as diabetes and steatorrhea.[7]
- *Endocrinopathies:* Insulin works in conjunction with several other hormones in the body. Hormones such as growth hormone, cortisol, glucagon, and epinephrine are all antagonistic to the functions of insulin. Therefore in disorders in which excessive amounts of these antagonistic hormones are produced, the action of insulin is hindered and hyperglycemia ensues. Cushing's syndrome, glucagonoma, pheochromocytoma, hyperthyroidism, and aldosteronoma are examples of endocrinopathies that ultimately cause symptoms of diabetes. When the primary disorder

---

Cushing's syndrome excess secretion of glucocorticoids from the adrenal cortex. Symptoms and complications include protein loss, obesity, fatigue, osteoporosis, edema, excess hair growth, diabetes, and skin discoloration.

pheochromocytoma tumor of the adrenal medulla or the sympathetic nervous system in which the affected cells secrete increased amounts of epinephrine or norepinephrine and cause headache, hypertension, and nausea.

aldosteronoma excess secretion of aldosterone from the adrenal cortex. Symptoms and complications include sodium retention, potassium wasting (loss in the urine), alkalosis, weakness, paralysis, polyuria, polydipsia, hypertension, and cardiac arrhythmias.

(excessive antagonistic hormone secretion) is removed, the resulting hyperglycemia usually is resolved.

- *Drug- or chemical-induced diabetes:* Certain drugs and toxins can impair insulin secretion or insulin action. The following drugs and toxins have been linked to impaired glucose tolerance (IGT) and diabetes: vacor (rat poison), pentamidine, nicotinic acid, glucocorticoids, thyroid hormone, diazoxide, thiazides, diazoxide, phenytoin (Dilantin), β-adrenergic agonist, and α-interferon.[3]

Impaired Glucose Tolerance

Individuals whose fasting blood glucose is above normal (≥110 mg/dl) but not high enough for diagnosis of diabetes (>126 mg/dl) fall into the IGT classification, also referred to as prediabetes. IGT is a risk factor for developing type 2 diabetes. Treatment guidelines follow those designed for type 2 diabetes and can help prevent or prolong the progression into full-blown diabetes. Individuals with IGT often have a complicated assortment of underlying conditions (e.g., hypercholesterolemia, obesity, hypertension) that build on one another to create the condition known as syndrome X, or metabolic syndrome. A recent study found that the prevalence of CVD at diagnosis of type 2 diabetes in patients with metabolic syndrome was 20.1%, and metabolic syndrome is thought to be an independent risk factor for CVD.[8] See Table 19-2 for diagnostic criteria of metabolic syndrome.

Symptoms of Diabetes

Initial Signs

Early signs of diabetes include three primary symptoms: (1) increased thirst (polydipsia), (2) increased urination (polyuria), and (3) increased hunger (polyphagia). Unintentional weight loss may occur with type 1 diabetes and weight gain with type 2.

Laboratory Test Results

Various laboratory tests show glucosuria (sugar in the urine), hyperglycemia (elevated blood sugar), and abnormal glucose tolerance tests. Although urinary excretion of glucose is correlated to increasing levels of blood glucose, it is not as sensitive when blood glucose levels are returning to normal. In other words, glucosuria remains elevated after blood glucose levels drop following a hyperglycemic period.[9]

Other Possible Symptoms

Additional signs include blurred vision, dehydration, skin irritation or infection, and general weakness and loss of strength. Older adults also may demonstrate poor wound healing.

Progressive Results

If the disease is left uncontrolled, chronic hyperglycemia causes progressive deterioration. These results may include water and electrolyte imbalance, ketoacidosis, and coma.

THE METABOLIC PATTERN OF DIABETES

Energy Balance and Normal Blood Glucose Controls

Energy Balance

Diabetes has been called a disease of carbohydrate metabolism, but it is a general metabolic disorder involving all three of the energy nutrients: carbohydrate, fat, and protein. Diabetes is especially related to the metabolism of the two main fuels, carbohydrate and fat, in the body's overall energy system. The following three basic stages of normal glucose metabolism are illustrated in Figure 20-1:

- Initial interchange with glycogen (glycogenolysis) and reduction to a smaller central compound (glycolysis pathway)
- Joining with the other two energy nutrients fat and protein (pyruvate link)
- Final common energy production (citric acid cycle)

Normal Blood Glucose Balance

Control of blood glucose within its normal range of 70 to 110 mg/dl is important for general health. Normal control mechanisms ensure sufficient circulating blood glucose to meet the constant energy needs—even the basal metabolic energy needs during sleep—because glucose is the body's preferred fuel. Figure 20-2 shows the balanced sources and uses of blood glucose.

Sources of Blood Glucose. To ensure a constant supply of the body's main fuel, the body obtains blood glucose from the following two sources:

- *The diet:* the energy nutrients in food (dietary carbohydrate, fat and, as needed, protein)
- *Glycogen:* the backup source from constant turnover of stored glycogen in liver and muscles (glycogenolysis)

Uses of Blood Glucose. To prevent blood glucose from continually rising above a normal range, the body uses glucose as needed by the following actions:

- Burning it during cell oxidation for immediate energy needs (glycolysis)
- Changing it to glycogen (glycogenesis), which is briefly stored in muscles and liver, then withdrawn

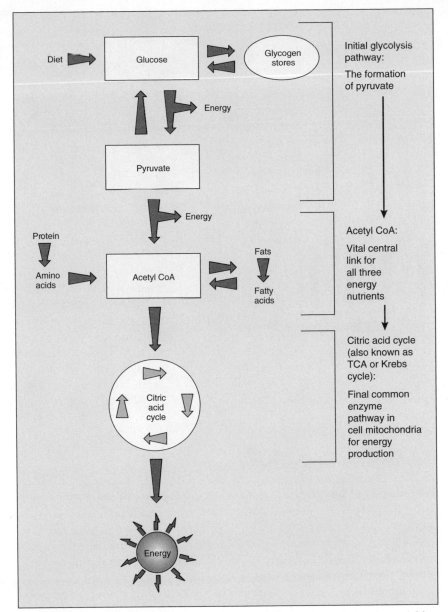

Figure 20–1 Basic glucose metabolism and interaction with fat and protein to yield energy.

and changed back to glucose for short-term energy needs when needed

- Changing it to fat, which is stored for longer periods in adipose tissue (lipogenesis)

Figure 20-3 summarizes the pathways involved in glucose metabolism.

Pancreatic Hormonal Control

The specialized cells of the islets of Langerhans in the pancreas provide three hormones that work together to regulate blood glucose levels: insulin, glucagon, and somatostatin. The specific arrangement of human islet cells is illustrated in Figure 20-4.

Insulin. Insulin is the major hormone controlling the level of blood glucose. It accomplishes this through the following metabolic actions:

- Helping transport circulating glucose into cells by activating insulin receptors
- Stimulating glycogenesis

ketoacidosis excess production of ketones; a form of metabolic acidosis as occurs in uncontrolled diabetes or starvation from burning body fat for energy fuel; a continuing, uncontrolled state can result in coma and death.

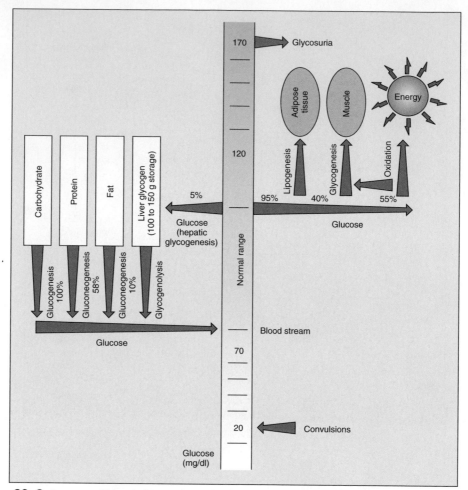

Figure 20–2 Sources of blood glucose (e.g., food and stored glycogen) and normal routes of control.

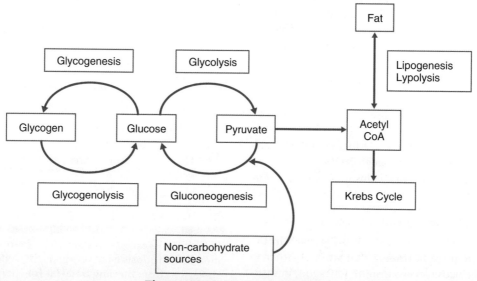

Figure 20–3 Glucose metabolism.

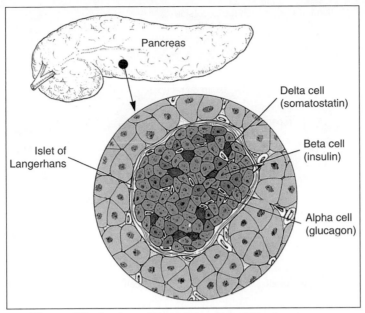

Figure 20–4 Islets of Langerhans, located in the pancreas.

- Stimulating lipogenesis
- Inhibiting breakdown of tissue fat (lipolysis) and protein degradation
- Promoting uptake of amino acids by skeletal muscles, increasing tissue protein synthesis
- Influencing the burning of glucose for constant energy as needed

Insulin is produced in the β cells of the islets, which fill its central zone and make up about 60% of each islet gland (Figure 20-4).

Glucagon. Glucagon is a hormone that acts in an opposite manner of insulin to balance the overall blood glucose control. It can rapidly break down stored glycogen. This action raises blood glucose concentrations as needed to protect the brain and other tissues during sleep or fasting. Glucagon is produced in the α cells of the pancreatic islets, which are arranged around the outer rim of each of these glands, making up about 30% of its total cell mass.

Somatostatin. Somatostatin is the pancreatic hormone that acts as a referee for several other hormones affecting blood glucose levels. Somatostatin is produced in the δ cells of the pancreatic islets, scattered between the α and β cells and making up approximately 10% of each islet's cells. Somatostatin inhibits the secretion of insulin, glucagon, and other GI hormones such as gastrin and cholecystokinin. Because it has more generalized functions in the regulation of circulating blood glucose, somatostatin also is produced in other parts of the body (e.g., the hypothalamus).

Abnormal Metabolism in Uncontrolled Diabetes

When insulin activity is lacking, such as in uncontrolled diabetes, the normal controls for blood glucose levels do not function properly. As a result, abnormal metabolic changes and imbalances occur among the three energy nutrients.

Glucose

Glucose cannot enter cells for oxidation through its normal cell pathways to produce energy without the action of insulin (Figure 20-5). Thus it builds up in the blood, creating hyperglycemia. During hyperglycemia, cells are effectively starved for glucose. (See the Drug-Nutrient Interaction box, "Insulin Abuse," for an example of intentional hyperglycemia.)

---

glucagon a hormone secreted by the α cells of the pancreatic islets of Langerhans in response to hypoglycemia; it has an opposite balancing effect to that of insulin, raising the blood glucose concentration, and thus is used as a quick-acting antidote for a low blood glucose reaction of insulin. It also counteracts the overnight fast during sleep by breaking down liver glycogen to keep blood glucose levels normal and maintain an adequate energy supply for normal nerve and brain function.

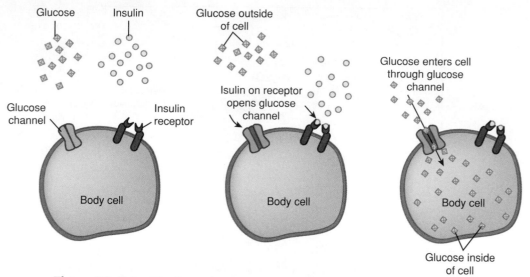

Figure 20–5 Insulin allows glucose to enter the cell through the glucose channel.

Fat

In the absence of functioning insulin, fat tissue formation (lipogenesis) decreases and fat tissue breakdown (lipolysis) increases. However, normal lipolysis requires an adequate supply of glucose, which in turn relies on the help of insulin to accept glucose into the cell. Therefore intermediate products of fat breakdown, called ketones, accumulate in the body. Ketones are acids; therefore increased fat breakdown leads to excess formation of ketones, causing ketoacidosis. The appearance of one of these ketones, acetone, in the urine is one indicator of the adverse development of ketoacidosis.

Protein

Protein tissues also are broken down in the body's effort to secure energy sources, causing weight loss, muscle weakness, and urinary nitrogen loss.

Long-Term Complications

The long-term complications associated with diabetes result from continuous hyperglycemia. These health problems mainly relate to microvascular and macrovascular dysfunction in vital organs. Individuals with good blood glucose control can avoid many such complications.

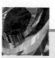 # DRUG-NUTRIENT INTERACTION

INSULIN ABUSE

People of all age groups want to fit in and feel a sense of belonging, and this desire is especially evident during adolescence. Situations that make teenagers feel different and therefore separated from a social group often are resented. One such situation may be type 1 diabetes and its associated need for insulin injections and carbohydrate counting. When this resentment about being different is coupled with the societal pressure of being thin, the result may be insulin abuse.

Individuals with type 1 diabetes rely on exogenous insulin. Insulin opens channels in the cell membrane that allow glucose to enter the cell. Injecting less insulin than is prescribed means the individual will not absorb all the carbohydrate calories into the cell. Some individuals may perceive this to be an easy way to stay thin or lose weight.

The harmful effects associated with this insulin-glucose interaction are not immediately felt and may not be apparent for years. If a patient talks often about weight, has friends who abuse insulin, or has a high HbA1c test that does not match a food and insulin diary, careful questioning of insulin use may be warranted.

When speaking with these individuals, keep the following tips in mind:

- Do not begin a conversation with an accusation. Instead, explain the effect of prolonged high blood glucose levels as with every patient.
- Give them options so they feel in control. Review their diet with them and talk about ways they could maintain or lose weight without abusing insulin.
- Refer back to the endocrinologist. Long-term abuse can lead to chronic complications. All health care providers should be involved and aware of the situation.

Sara Oldroyd

Retinopathy

Retinopathy involves small hemorrhages from broken arteries in the retina, with yellow, waxy discharge or retinal detachment. Diabetic retinopathy is the leading cause of new cases of blindness in adults ages 20 to 74 years.[1] The risk for retinopathy significantly increases with incessant hyperglycemia (fasting blood glucose ≥120 mg/dl). Retinopathy has few warning signs; however, nearly all patients with type 1 diabetes develop some degree of retinopathy, and up to 21% of patients with type 2 diabetes have retinopathy at the time of diagnosis.[10] Some treatment modalities (e.g., laser photocoagulation therapy) can prevent, or at least delay, the onset; thus ongoing eye evaluations are an important part of the care plan. The American Diabetes Association position statement on diabetic retinopathy recommends individuals with type 1 diabetes go for a first-time eye examination within 3 to 5 years after diagnosis and those with type 2 diabetes have their first eye examination shortly after diagnosis. Examinations with dilation should continue on a yearly basis from that point forward.[11] Studies indicate that strict control of blood glucose and intensive intervention can reduce retinopathy progression by 65% and decrease the development of severe diabetic retinopathy by 47%.[12]

Retinopathy should not be confused with the blurry vision that sometimes occurs as one of the first signs of diabetes. Blurry vision is caused by the increased glucose concentration in the fluids of the eye, bringing brief changes in the curved, light-refracting surface of the eye.

Nephropathy

Diabetes is the leading cause of end-stage renal disease in the United States, which affects 20% to 40% of all patients with diabetes.[11] As with retinopathy, nephropathy is exacerbated by poor blood glucose control. The primary symptom is microalbuminuria (low but abnormal levels of albumin in the urine). Nephropathy and end-stage renal disease cannot be cured, but with better blood glucose control and antihypertensive therapy disease progression can be slowed. Recommendations for screening are the same as for retinopathy—within 5 years of diagnosis for type 1 and at diagnosis for type 2, with annual follow-up.

Neuropathy

Current statistics indicate that approximately 50% of people with diabetes have mild to severe forms of nervous system damage.[13] Changes in the nerves involve injury and disease in the peripheral nervous system, especially in the legs and feet, causing prickly sensations, increasing pain, and eventual loss of sensation resulting from damaged nerves. The loss of nerve reaction can lead to further tissue damage and infection from unfelt foot injuries such as bruises, burns, and deeper cellulitis. Amputations and foot ulcerations are the most common results of severe neuropathy. The risk for such complications is increased for individuals who have had diabetes for more than 10 years; are male; have poor glucose control; or have concurrent complications such as cardiovascular, retinal, or renal disease.[14] Diabetic neuropathy also is linked to chronic problems such as motor deficits, cardiac ischemia, hypotension, gastroparesis, bladder dysfunction, and sexual dysfunction.

Heart Disease

CVD is a major cause of death for persons with diabetes and occurs more often in this population than in the general population. The standards of medical care for individuals with diabetes include recommendations for the prevention and management of CVD, specifically aimed at blood lipid levels, blood pressure, aspirin use, and smoking cessation.[11] Glycemic control is not as strongly related to dyslipidemia and hypertension as it is to other long-term complications of diabetes (e.g., retinopathy, nephropathy, and neuropathy). However, the comorbid conditions (hyperglycemia and dyslipidemia) greatly increase the risk of CVD; thus evaluation and treatment must be part of the overall health care plan for individuals with diabetes.

Dyslipidemia. Elevated triglyceride levels and decreased HDL cholesterol are characteristic of dyslipidemia in patients with type 2 diabetes. Management of dyslipidemia is prioritized as (1) lifestyle modification focusing on the reduction of saturated fat, *trans* fat, and cholesterol intake; weight loss (if indicated); and increased physical activity; (2) lower LDL cholesterol; (3) raise HDL cholesterol; and (4) lower triglycerides. Recommendations for lipid profiles for adults with diabetes are as follows[11]:

- LDL cholesterol: less than 100 mg/dl; if patients have advanced CVD, reduce LDL cholesterol to less than 70 mg/dl

---

ketones chemical name for a class of organic compounds, including three ketoacid bases that occur as intermediate products of fat metabolism, one of which is acetone.

acetone a major ketone compound that results from fat breakdown for energy in uncontrolled diabetes; persons with diabetes periodically take urinary acetone tests to monitor the status of their diabetes control.

cellulitis diffuse inflammation of soft or connective tissues (e.g., in the foot) from injury, bruises, or pressure sores that leads to infection; poor care may result in ulceration and abscess or gangrene.

- HDL cholesterol: greater than 40 mg/dl for men and greater than 50 mg/dl for women
- Triglycerides: less than 150 mg/dl

A recent study evaluating the efficacy of intensive glycemic treatment on development of coronary artery calcification, an index of atherosclerosis, found individuals undergoing intensive treatment and exhibiting good glucose control had less atherosclerosis.[15]

Hypertension. Depending on other risk factors, such as obesity, ethnicity, and age, hypertension affects between 20% and 60% of individuals with diabetes and is a major comorbid complication.[16] The risk for CVD is doubled for people with both diabetes and hypertension, making blood pressure evaluation and treatment an important part of the health care plan. The recommendation for blood pressure in adults with diabetes is less than 130/80 mm Hg.

GENERAL MANAGEMENT OF DIABETES

Early Detection and Monitoring

The guiding principles for the treatment of diabetes are early detection and prevention of complications. Community screening programs and annual physical examinations help identify persons with elevated blood glucose levels who may benefit from a glucose tolerance test (e.g., fasting and 2-hour tests with a measured glucose dose) and medical evaluation. An additional monitoring aid is the glycosylated hemoglobin A1c assay (HbA1c; normal range, 4% to 6%), which provides an effective tool for evaluating long-term management of diabetes and degree of control. Because glucose attaches itself to the hemoglobin molecule over the life of the RBC, this test reflects the level of blood glucose over the preceding 3 months. Other tests such as fructosamine (an amino sugar formed from glucosamine) or C-peptide (an antibody radioimmunoassay after a special test meal to determine the type of diabetes) are sometimes used for diagnostic purposes. However, HbA1c currently is the most accurate assessment for monitoring ongoing blood glucose control. Box 20-2 outlines the criteria for diagnosis of diabetes mellitus, and Table 20-2 gives the correlation between HbA1c values and plasma glucose. HbA1c is closely associated with complications of diabetes. For example, a 10% reduction in HbA1c provides approximately a 40% reduction in the risk of retinopathy.[12]

Basic Goals of Care

General Overall Objectives

The health care team is guided by three basic objectives when working with patients with diabetes.

BOX 20-2

CRITERIA FOR THE DIAGNOSIS OF DIABETES MELLITUS

- Symptoms of diabetes plus casual plasma glucose concentration ≥200 mg/dl
  - Casual is defined as any time of day without regard to time since the last meal. The classic symptoms of diabetes include polyuria, polydipsia, and unexplained weight loss.
- Fasting plasma glucose ≥126 mg/dl
  - Fasting is defined as no caloric intake for at least 8 hours.
- Two-hour plasma glucose ≥200 mg/dl during an OGTT
  - The OGTT should be performed using a glucose load equivalent of 75 g anhydrous glucose dissolved in water.

In the absence of unequivocal hyperglycemia with acute metabolic decompensation, these criteria should be confirmed by repeat testing on a different day. The third measure (OGTT) is not recommended for routine clinical use.

Reprinted from The Expert Committee on the Diagnosis and Classification of Diabetes Mellitus: Position statement of the Expert Committee on the Diagnosis and Classification of Diabetes Mellitus, *Diabetes Care* 30(1 suppl):S42, 2007.

TABLE 20-2

CORRELATION BETWEEN HbA1c AND PLASMA GLUCOSE LEVELS

HbA1c	MEAN PLASMA GLUCOSE	
	mg/dL	mmol/L
6	135	7.5
7	170	9.5
8	205	11.5
9	240	13.5
10	275	15.5
11	310	17.5
12	345	19.5

Maintaining Optimal Nutrition. The first objective is to sustain a high level of nutrition for general health promotion, adequate growth and development, and maintenance of an appropriate lean weight.

Avoiding Symptoms. This objective seeks to keep a person relatively free from symptoms of hyperglycemia, hypoglycemia, and glycosuria, which indicate poor blood glucose control.

Preventing Complications. Consistent control of blood glucose levels helps reduce the risks of chronic complications. Table 20-3 summarizes recommendations for adults with diabetes as defined by the American Diabetes Association.

TABLE 20-3

SUMMARY OF RECOMMENDATIONS FOR ADULTS WITH DIABETES

Parameter	Recommendation
HbA1c	<7.0%*
Preprandial capillary plasma glucose	90-130 mg/dl (5.0-7.2 mmol/L)
Peak postprandial capillary plasma glucose†	<180 mg/dl (<10.0 mmol/L)
Blood pressure	<130/80 mm Hg
Lipids‡	
LDL	<100 mg/dl (<2.6 mmol/L)
Triglycerides	<150 mg/dl (<1.7 mmol/L)
HDL	>40 mg/dl (>1.0 mmol/L)§

Key concepts in setting glycemic goals: (1) HbA1c is the primary target for glycemic control. (2) Goals should be individualized. (3) Certain populations (children, pregnant women, and elderly) require special considerations. (4) More stringent glycemic goals (e.g., normal HbA1c, <6%) may further reduce complications at the cost of increased risk of hypoglycemia. (5) Less-intensive glycemic goals may be indicated in patients with severe or frequent hypoglycemia. (6) Postprandial glucose may be targeted if HbA1c goals are not met despite reaching preprandial glucose goals.

Reprinted from American Diabetes Association: Position statement on standards of medical care in diabetes—2007, *Diabetes Care* 30(1): S4, 2007.

*Referenced to a nondiabetic range of 4.0% to 6.0% using a DCCT-based assay.

†Postprandial glucose measurements should be made 1 to 2 hours after the beginning of the meal, generally the peak level in patients with diabetes.

‡Current NCEP/ATP III guidelines suggest that in patients with triglycerides ≥200 mg/dl, the non-HDL cholesterol (total cholesterol minus HDL), be used. The goal is ≤130 mg/dl.

§For women, an increase in the HDL goal by 10 mg/dl has been suggested.

Importance of Good Self-Care Skills

To accomplish these objectives, a person with diabetes must learn and regularly practice good self-care. Daily self-discipline and informed self-care are necessary for sound diabetes management because all persons with diabetes must ultimately treat themselves, with the support of a good health care team. More emphasis is now being given to comprehensive diabetes education programs that encourage more self-care responsibility.

Basic Elements of Diabetes Management

Balancing three basic elements is essential in good control of blood glucose levels. First, the healthy diet described here is essential for good glucose management. Second, physical exercise provides an important balance to maintain good blood glucose control. Third, to ensure adequate insulin activity, some persons need medications

(e.g., insulin injections or oral hypoglycemic agents). However, a fourth element, stress-coping skills, may well be added in today's stressful world.

Special Objectives in Pregnancy

When a woman with diabetes becomes pregnant or the pregnancy induces GDM, her body metabolism changes to meet the increased physiologic needs of the pregnancy while battling the manifestations of diabetes (see Chapter 10). A team of specialists usually works closely with the mother. Careful team monitoring of the mother's diabetes management is essential to ensure her health and the health of her baby. Potential problems of fetal damage, perinatal death, stillbirth, prematurity, or delivery of a very large baby (macrosomia) are serious concerns during this time.

MEDICAL NUTRITION THERAPY FOR INDIVIDUALS WITH DIABETES

The Diabetes Control and Complications Trial

The need for a more comprehensive program of care for diabetes triggered a large-scale U.S. clinical research study supported by the NIH. This project (the Diabetes Control and Complications Trial [DCCT]) compared the effects of intensive insulin therapy aimed at achieving blood glucose levels as close as possible to the normal nondiabetic range with the effects of conventional therapy on early microvascular complications of type 1 diabetes mellitus. The positive results of this study, supported by both the ADA and the American Diabetic Association, remain highly significant. A decrease of approximately 60% in the risk of retinopathy, nephropathy, and neuropathy occurred in the individuals who underwent intensive treatment and rigorous control of blood glucose levels.[17] Results from DCCT confirmed the association between long-term complications of diabetes and blood glucose control and provided support for the development of the current standards of medical care.

Application in Clinical Practice

Recommendations

The American Diabetes Association's position paper on nutrition recommendations and interventions for diabetes state the following as the goal of medical nutrition therapy:

- For individuals at risk for type 2 diabetes or with prediabetes: decrease the risk of diabetes and CVD by promoting healthy food choices and physical activity, leading to maintained moderate weight loss.

For individuals with diabetes:

1. Achieve and maintain:
   - Blood glucose levels in the normal range or as close to normal as is safely possible
   - A lipid and lipoprotein profile that reduces the risk for vascular disease
   - Blood pressure levels in the normal range or as close to normal as is safely possible
2. Prevent, or at least slow, the rate of development of the chronic complications of diabetes by modifying nutrient intake and lifestyle
3. Address individual nutrition needs, taking into account personal and cultural preferences and willingness to change
4. Maintain the pleasure of eating by only limiting food choices when indicated by scientific evidence

Goals of medical nutrition therapy that apply to specific situations include the following:

1. For youth with type 1 diabetes, youth with type 2 diabetes, pregnant and lactating women, and older adults with diabetes: meet the nutrition needs of these unique times in the life cycle
2. For individuals treated with insulin or insulin secretagogues: provide self-management training for safe conduct of exercise, including the prevention and treatment of hypoglycemia and diabetes treatment during acute illness

Core Focus

The primary focus in diabetes care is glycemic control, the regulation of the body's primary fuel, blood glucose. The concept of balance promotes the following three main principles of nutrition therapy:

- Total energy balance
- Nutrient balance (macronutrients and micronutrients)
- Food distribution balance

Personal diet is then expressed in terms of the following:

- Total kilocalories necessary for energy balance
- Ratio of these kilocalories in relative amounts of the three energy nutrients: carbohydrate, fat, and protein
- A food distribution pattern for the day

A fundamental personal principle underlies the whole plan. The diet for any person with diabetes is always based on the normal nutrition needs of that person for positive health.

Total Energy Balance

Normal Growth and Weight Management

Because type 1 diabetes usually begins in childhood (typically before puberty), the normal height/weight charts for children provide a standard for adequate growth and development. During adulthood, maintaining a lean weight continues to be a basic goal. Because type 2 diabetes usually occurs in overweight adults, the major goal is weight reduction and control.

Energy Intake

The total energy value of the diet for a person with diabetes should be sufficient to meet individual needs for normal growth and development, physical activity and exercise, and maintenance of a desirable lean weight. Exercise is always an important factor in diabetes control because it improves the body's ability to uptake glucose in cells. Energy intake in the diet is constantly balanced with energy output in work and exercise and metabolic body work. The DRIs for children and adults (see inside cover of text) can serve as a guide for total energy needs, with appropriate reductions in kilocalories for overweight adults (see Chapter 15).

Nutrient Balance

The ratios of carbohydrate, fat, and protein in the diet are based on current recommendations for ideal glucose regulation and lower fat intake to reduce risks of cardiovascular complications.

Carbohydrate

The American Diabetes Association recommends a diet including carbohydrates from fruits, vegetables, whole grains, legumes, and low-fat milk for good health (Box 20-3). Low-carbohydrate diets, with fewer than 130 g/day total carbohydrate, are not recommended in the management of diabetes.

Starch and Sugar. A food's glycemic index is determined by measuring the increase in blood glucose after ingestion of a 50-g carbohydrate sample of the food compared with a 50-g sample from a known source, usually white bread or pure glucose. The rate of digestion and absorption determines the glycemic index value. The glycemic index theory of carbohydrate foods indicates that starchy foods greatly differ from one another in their ability to raise plasma glucose levels, thus contradicting the notion that all complex carbohydrates are created equal.

BOX 20-3

NUTRITION RECOMMENDATIONS FOR MANAGEMENT OF DIABETES

Carbohydrate

- A dietary pattern that includes carbohydrate from fruits, vegetables, whole grains, legumes, and low-fat milk is encouraged for good health.
- Low-carbohydrate diets, restricting total carbohydrate to <130 g/day, are not recommended in the management of diabetes.
- Monitoring carbohydrate, whether by carbohydrate counting, exchanges, or experienced-based estimation, remains a key strategy in achieving glycemic control.
- Use of the glycemic index and load, in conjunction with carbohydrate counting, may provide a modest additional benefit over that observed when total carbohydrate is considered alone.
- Sucrose-containing foods can be substituted for other carbohydrates in the meal plan or, if added to the meal plan, covered with insulin or other glucose-lowering medication. Care should be taken to avoid excess energy intake.
- As for the general population, people with diabetes are encouraged to consume a variety of fiber-containing foods. However, evidence is lacking to recommend a higher fiber intake than for the population as a whole.
- Sugar alcohols and nonnutritive sweeteners are safe when consumed within the daily intake levels established by the FDA.

Fat

- Limit saturated fat to less than 7% of total calories.
- Intake of *trans* fat should be minimized.
- In individuals with diabetes, limit dietary cholesterol to less than 200 mg/day.
- Two or more servings of fish per week (with the exception of commercially fried fish filets) provide n-3 polyunsaturated fatty acids and are recommended.

Protein

- For individuals with diabetes and normal renal function, evidence is insufficient to suggest that usual protein intake (15% to 20% of energy) should be modified.

- In individuals with type 2 diabetes, ingested protein can increase insulin response without increasing plasma glucose concentrations. Therefore protein should not be used to treat acute or prevent nighttime hypoglycemia.
- High-protein diets are not recommended as a method for weight loss. The long-term effects of protein intake greater than 20% of calories on diabetes management and its complications are unknown. Although such diets may produce short-term weight loss and improved glycemic control, these benefits have not been established to be long term.

Alcohol

- If adults with diabetes choose to drink alcohol, daily intake should be limited to a moderate amount (one drink per day or less for women and two drinks per day or less for men).
- To reduce risk of nocturnal hypoglycemia in individuals using insulin or insulin secretagogues, alcohol should be consumed with food.
- In individuals with diabetes, moderate alcohol consumption (when ingested alone) has no acute effect on glucose and insulin concentrations, but carbohydrate ingested with alcohol (as in a mixed drink) may raise blood glucose.

Micronutrients

- No clear evidence shows a benefit from vitamin or mineral supplementation in people with diabetes (compared with the general population) who do not have underlying deficiencies.
- Routine supplementation with antioxidants, such as vitamins E and C and carotene, is not advised because of lack of evidence of efficacy and concern related to long-term safety.
- Benefit from chromium supplementation in individuals with diabetes or obesity has not been clearly demonstrated and therefore cannot be recommended.

Reprinted from American Diabetes Association: Nutrition recommendations and interventions for diabetes, *Diabetes Care* 30(1 suppl):S48, 2007.

Although carbohydrates differ in their ability to raise blood glucose, no clear trend separates simple sugars from complex carbohydrates (see Chapter 2). For example, potatoes and white bread—both complex carbohydrates—have a similar glycemic index to pure glucose. Current recommendations for carbohydrate intake are based on studies in which the glycemic response of individuals with diabetes was not significantly different when consuming either complex carbohydrates or simple sug-

secretagogue a substance, such as a hormone or medication, that causes another substance to be secreted; sulfonylureas, for example, are medications used to increase the secretion of insulin from β cells in the pancreas.

glycemic index the increase above fasting in the blood glucose area more than 2 hours after ingestion of a constant amount of that food divided by the response to a reference food.

ars as long as the total amount of carbohydrate was the same.[19]

Fiber. As with all people, consumption of dietary fiber is encouraged. No reasons exist for individuals with diabetes to consume greater amounts than what is recommended for the general public (approximately 25 to 30 g/day).

Sugar Substitute Sweeteners. Nutritive and nonnutritive sweeteners may be used in the diet in moderation. Various sugar substitutes are available. Approved noncaloric sweeteners include products such as saccharin, neotame, aspartame, acesulfame-K, and sucralose. Aspartame is made from two amino acids, phenylalanine and aspartic acid, and is metabolized as such. Small amounts of caloric sweeteners, such as sucrose, fructose, and sorbitol must be accounted for in a meal. However, many persons cannot tolerate sorbitol and have significant diarrhea when it is used in excess. Nutritive and nonnutritive sweeteners are safe to consume in moderation and as part of a nutritious and well-balanced diet.

Protein

Normal age requirements, as outlined in the DRIs, can be a guide for protein intake. In general approximately 15% to 35% of the total energy as protein is sufficient to meet growth needs in children and maintain tissue integrity in adults. High protein intake generally is not recommended because of saturated fat content and unnecessary stress on the kidneys from the excretion of excess nitrogen.

Fat

No more than 25% to 30% of the diet's total kilocalories should come from fat, with saturated fat less than 7%. Lower cholesterol intake—no more than 200 mg/day—also is recommended. Control of fat-related foods, which contribute to the development of atherosclerosis and coronary heart disease, helps lessen the increased risk for CVD. An emphasis is placed on polyunsaturated fats (such as fish oil) and avoidance of trans fats.

Guidelines for macronutrient, micronutrient, and alcohol intake are based on the recommendations from the American Diabetes Association position statement and are outlined in Box 20-3.

Food Distribution

As a general rule, fairly even amounts of food should be eaten at regular intervals throughout the day, adjusted to blood glucose self-monitoring. This basic pattern helps provide a more even blood glucose supply and prevent extremes in high and low levels, which is damaging to blood vessels. Snacks between meals may be needed.

Daily Activity Schedule

Food distribution must be planned ahead, especially when using insulin, and adjusted according to each day's scheduled activities and blood glucose monitoring to prevent episodes of hypoglycemia from insulin reactions. Careful distribution of food and snacks is especially important for children and adolescents with diabetes to balance with insulin during growth spurts and changing hormone patterns of puberty. Practical consideration should be given to school and work schedules and demands, athletics, social events, and stress periods. A stressful event caused by any source (e.g., injury, anxiety, fear, or pain) brings an adrenaline (epinephrine) rush. This fight-or-flight effect counteracts insulin activity and can contribute to a glycemic response.

Exercise

For persons using insulin, any exercise or additional physical activity must be covered in the food distribution plan (Table 20-4). The energy demands of exercise are discussed in Chapter 16.

The American Diabetes Association position statement on physical activity and exercise and diabetes recommends the following guidelines for regulating the glycemic response to exercise[20]:

- Achieve metabolic control before physical activity.
- Avoid physical activity if fasting glucose levels are higher than 250 mg/dl and ketosis is present, and use caution if glucose levels are higher than 300 mg/dl and no ketosis is present.
- Ingest added carbohydrate if glucose levels are less than 100 mg/dl.
- Monitor blood glucose before and after physical activity.
- Identify when changes in insulin or food intake are necessary.
- Learn the glycemic response to different physical activity conditions.
- Monitor food intake.
- Consume added carbohydrate as needed to avoid hypoglycemia.
- Carbohydrate-based foods should be readily available during and after physical activity.

For adults with type 2 diabetes, regular exercise is an essential part of successful weight management and glucose control programs. Regular, moderate-intensity exercise programs help individuals with type 2 diabetes control blood glucose and reduce the risk of cardiovascular disease, hyperlipidemia, hypertension, and obesity.

TABLE 20-4

MEAL PLANNING GUIDE FOR ACTIVE PEOPLE WITH TYPE 1 DIABETES

ACTIVITY LEVEL	EXCHANGE NEEDS	SAMPLE MENUS
Moderate		
30 minutes	1 bread or 1 fruit	1 bran muffin or 1 small orange
1 hour	2 bread + 1 meat or 2 fruit + 1 milk	Tuna sandwich or ½ cup fruit salad + 1 cup milk
Strenuous		
30 minutes	2 fruit or 1 bread + 1 fat	1 small banana or ½ bagel + 1 tsp cream cheese
1 hour	2 bread + 1 meat + 1 milk or 2 bread + 2 meat + 2 fruit	Meat and cheese sandwich + 1 cup milk or Turkey sandwich + 1 cup orange juice

TABLE 20-5

DIETARY STRATEGIES FOR TYPE 1 AND TYPE 2 DIABETES MELLITUS

DIETARY STRATEGY	TYPE 1	TYPE 2
Decrease energy intake (kilocalories)	No	Yes, if weight loss is recommended
Increase frequency and number of feedings	Yes	Usually no
Have regular daily intake of kilocalories from carbohydrate, protein, and fat	Very important	Yes
Plan consistent daily ratio of protein, carbohydrate, and fat for each feeding	Desirable	Yes, but not as tightly controlled
Use extra or planned food to treat or prevent hypoglycemia	Very important	Usually not necessary
Plan regular times for meals and snacks	Very important	Yes
Use extra food for unusual exercise	Yes	Usually not necessary
During illness, use small, frequent feedings of carbohydrates to prevent starvation ketoacidosis	Important	Usually not necessary because of resistance to ketoacidosis

Drug Therapy

The food distribution pattern also is influenced by any form of drug therapy (type, amount, and dose schedule of insulin or oral hypoglycemic agent) necessary for control of the diabetes. Successful self-care means the patient can adjust diet, medications, and exercise on the basis of blood glucose monitoring results.

Diet Management

General Planning According to Type of Diabetes

Because forms of diabetes vary widely, the nature of an individual's diabetes and its treatment regime largely determine the necessary personal diet management. Table 20-5 provides guidelines for diet strategies necessary for diabetes types 1 and 2.

Individual Needs

Every person with diabetes is unique, with a particular form and degree of diabetes as well as a different living situation, background, and food habits. All these personal needs must be considered, as discussed in Chapters 14 and 17, if appropriate and realistic care is to be planned. The nutrition counselor, who usually is the clinical dietitian, should determine these various needs in a careful initial nutrition assessment that includes medical and

hypoglycemia low blood glucose; a serious condition in type 1 diabetes management that requires immediate sugar intake to counteract, followed by a snack of complex carbohydrate food (e.g., bread or crackers) and a protein (e.g., lean meat, peanut butter, or cheese) to maintain normal blood glucose.

psychosocial needs as well as personal lifestyle characteristics. This information provides the basis for determining the diet prescription.

A major principle of diabetes management is the variety of methods and dietary guidelines that the clinical dietitian, assisted by the nutrition team, can use in planning and supporting patients. Among these dietary guides, the familiar food exchange method, tailored to meet individual needs, remains a commonly used approach. Materials used for planning the diet are available from the ADA and the American Diabetes Association in English and Spanish.

Food Exchange System

The dietitian uses the food exchange system to calculate the patient's energy and nutrient needs as well as distribute foods in a balanced meal and snack pattern. The food exchange system is called as such because persons with diabetes use the system to select a variety of foods from the various food groups according to their personal diet plan.

In this system commonly used foods are grouped into three basic exchange lists according to roughly equal food values in the portions indicated. Thus a variety of foods may be chosen from these lists to fulfill the basic food plan while the basic diet prescription of total energy and bal-

anced ratio of nutrients is maintained. The designated food values for each of the food exchange groups are shown in Table 20-6. The booklet "Choose Your Foods: Exchange Lists for Diabetes" is available from the American Diabetes Association (www.diabetes.org/nutrition-and-recipes/nutrition/exchangelist.jsp). Its colorful illustrations, clear content, and style provide a helpful tool for patient and client education. These exchange lists are included in Appendix E. Table 20-7 illustrates a calculated 2200-kcal diet and food pattern using the exchange system, and Box 20-4 outlines a sample menu based on this pattern.

Carbohydrate Counting

Carbohydrate counting is a way to balance carbohydrate intake with insulin injections. Patients count the total number of carbohydrates for a meal and then inject an appropriate amount of insulin to process the carbohydrates. Insulin may be injected manually or with the insulin pumps (see Figures 20-6 and 20-7). Helpful books list grams of carbohydrates for thousands of foods. One benefit of carbohydrate counting is that meal plans are much less stringent and flexibility is more easily accommodated. For this type of meal and insulin planning to work, the patient must be well versed in calculating the total number of carbohydrate grams consumed per meal or snack.

TABLE 20-6

AMOUNT OF NUTRIENTS IN ONE SERVING FROM EACH EXCHANGE LIST

FOOD LIST	CARBOHYDRATE (g)	PROTEIN (g)	FAT (g)	CALORIES (g)
Carbohydrates				
Starch: breads, cereals and grains; starchy vegetables; crackers and snacks; and beans, peas, and lentils	15	0-3	0-1	80
Fruits	15	—	—	60
Milk				
Fat free, low fat, 1%	12	8	0-3	100
Reduced fat, 2%	12	8	5	130
Whole	12	8	8	150
Sweets, desserts, and other carbohydrates	15	Varies	Varies	Varies
Nonstarchy vegetables	5	2	—	25
Meat and Meat Substitutes				
Lean	—	7	0-3	45
Medium fat	—	7	4-7	75
High fat	—	7	8+	100
Plant-based proteins	Varies	7	Varies	Varies
Fats	—	—	5	45
Alcohol	Varies	—	—	100

Reprinted from American Diabetes Association, American Dietetic Association: *Choose your foods: exchange lists for meal planning*, Chicago/Alexandria, VA, 2007, American Diabetes Association, American Dietetic Association.

TABLE 20-7

CALCULATION OF DIABETIC DIET USING EXCHANGE SYSTEM (2200 KCAL)

FOOD GROUP	TOTAL DAY'S EXCHANGES	CARBOHYDRATES: 275 g (50% kcal)	PROTEIN: 110 g (20% kcal)	FAT: 75 g (30% kcal)	BREAKFAST	LUNCH	DINNER	SNACKS Afternoon	SNACKS Bedtime
Carbohydrates									
Fruit	3	45	–	–	1	1		1	
Vegetable	4	20	8	–		2	2		
Other carbohydrates	1	15	Varies	Varies			1		
Milk									
Fat free	2	24	16	–	1				1
Reduced fat	–	–	–	–					–
Whole	–	–	–	–					
Starch	11.5	172	34.5	–	3	3	3	1	1.5
Meat and Meat Substitutes									
Very lean	2	–	14	0-1				1	1
Lean	3	–	21	9			3		
Medium fat	2	–	14	10	1	1			
High fat	–	–	–	–				–	
Fat	11	–	–	55	3	3	3	1	1
Total grams		276	107.5	75					

BOX 20-4

SAMPLE MENU PRESCRIPTION: 2200 KCAL

- 275 g carbohydrate (50% kcal)
- 110 g protein (20% kcal)
- 75 g fat (30% kcal)

Breakfast
- 1 medium fresh peach
- 1 serving shredded wheat cereal
- 1 poached egg on whole-grain toast
- 1 bran muffin
- 1 tsp margarine
- 1 cup low-fat milk
- Coffee or tea

Lunch
- Vegetable soup with wheat crackers
- Tuna sandwich on whole-wheat bread
  - Tuna (½ cup, drained)
  - Mayonnaise (2 tsp)
  - Chopped dill pickle
  - Chopped celery
- 1 Fresh pear

Dinner
- Pan-broiled pork chop (well trimmed)
- 1 cup brown rice
- ½ cup green beans
- Tossed green salad
  - Italian dressing (1 to 2 Tbsp)
- ½ cup applesauce
- 1 bran muffin

Afternoon Snack
- 10 crackers with 2 Tbsp peanut butter
- 1 medium orange

Evening Snack
- 3 cups popped, plain popcorn
- 1 oz cheese
- 1 cup low-fat milk

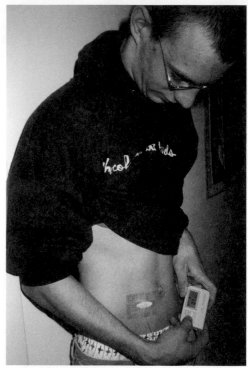

Figure 20–6 Insulin injection with an insulin pump (Reprinted from Peckenpaugh NJ: *Nutrition essentials and diet therapy,* ed 9, Philadelphia, 2003, Saunders.)

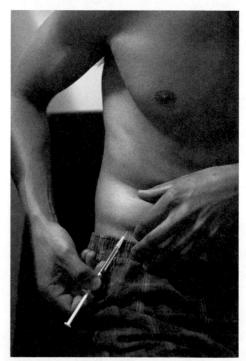

Figure 20–7 Man with diabetes injecting himself with insulin. (Copyright PhotoDisc.)

Additional information and tool kits about dietary planning based on carbohydrate counting can be found on the American Diabetes Association Web site *(www.diabetes.org/for-parents-and-kids/diabetes-care/carb-count.jsp).*

Special Concerns

Special concerns come up in daily living and become an important part of ongoing dietary counseling. Some suggestions for these concerns are given below.

Special Diet Food Items. Little need exists for special "diabetic" foods. Persons with diabetes should eat the regular, well-balanced diet recommended for the general population to promote health and prevent disease. This kind of a healthful diet primarily uses regular fresh foods from all the basic food groups, with limited use of processed foods (noting the grams of carbohydrate per serving on the label) and more use of nonfat seasonings. The simple principles of moderation and variety guide food choices and amounts.

Alcohol. Occasional use of alcohol in an adult diabetic diet can be planned, but caution must be the guide. Individuals with type 1 diabetes who consume alcohol must be reminded of the following: (1) to eat when they drink and (2) to not increase insulin dose because the overall effect of alcohol is to lower the blood glucose level. Occasional use is defined as moderate intake (e.g., less than 6% of the total energy on a given day) and not more than 1 or 2 equivalent portions once or twice a week. An equivalent portion is 1 oz of liquor, 4 oz of wine, or 12 oz of beer. The same precautions for the use of alcohol that apply to the general public apply to people with diabetes.

When a person with type 1 diabetes drinks alcohol, it should not be substituted for food exchanges in the diet, but only used in addition, to avoid the possibility of hypoglycemic reactions. When a person's blood glucose levels begin to drop, the liver typically responds to the hormone glucagon and releases glucose into the blood to reestablish normal blood glucose levels. However, when alcohol is in the system, the liver's primary role is to detoxify the blood of alcohol, and it will not respond to impending hypoglycemia until the alcohol is cleared. Therefore alcohol should only be consumed in moderation and in conjunction with food. Alcohol may be used in cooking as desired because it vaporizes in the cooking process and only contributes its flavor to the finished product.

Hypoglycemia. Persons with diabetes must learn how to avoid bouts of hypoglycemia. The body's vital "brain food" is glucose. The brain depends on a constant supply of glucose for metabolism and proper function; a prolonged lack of glucose can lead to permanent brain damage. Hypoglycemia can occur from too high a dose of insulin or from oral hypoglycemic drugs that act by stimulating the islet cells in the pancreas to secrete more insulin. Hypoglycemia also can occur if a person with diabetes delays a meal or snack, does not eat enough carbohydrate, or exercises too much without sufficient food. Table 20-8 lists symptoms of both hyperglycemia and hypoglycemia. Because behavior often is irrational and movements are uncoordinated, this state may be mistaken for drunkenness, and the person may lapse into coma. Thus an identification bracelet or pendant is an important means of informing others of the true condition so that proper treatment—a glucose

TABLE 20-8

SYMPTOMS OF HYPERGLYCEMIA AND HYPOGLYCEMIA

FACTOR	HYPERGLYCEMIA	HYPOGLYCEMIA
Cause	Too much food, not enough insulin, illness, or stress	Not enough food, too much insulin, or too much exercise
Symptoms	Polydipsia	Sudden shaking
	Polyuria	Rapid heartbeat
	Polyphagia	Sweating
	Dry skin	Anxiety and irritability
	Blurred vision	Dizziness
	Drowsiness	Polyphagia
	Nausea	Impaired vision
		Weakness
		Headache

replacement in food or beverage or an injection of glucagon—can be given. (Note the 15-g carbohydrate replacement portions listed in the bread/cereal (starch) and fruit exchange groups [see Table 20-6 and Appendix E].) Persons with type 1 diabetes should always carry a convenient form of sugar (e.g., sugar lumps or glucose tablets) with them to take at the first sign of a hypoglycemic attack, and then follow this sugar as soon as possible with a snack of complex carbohydrate and protein (e.g., peanut butter crackers, granola bar and yogurt, ham and cheese sandwich).

Illness. When general illness occurs, food and insulin should be adjusted accordingly. The texture of the food can be modified to use easily digested and absorbed liquid foods (Table 20-9). This type of liquid substitution can be used for meals not eaten. In general, persons with diabetes who are ill should do the following:

- Maintain food intake every day; do not skip meals.
- Do not omit insulin; follow an adjusted dosage if needed.
- Replace carbohydrate solid foods with equal liquid or soft foods.
- Monitor blood glucose level frequently.
- Contact a physician if the illness lasts more than a few days.

Travel. When a trip is planned, the diet counselor and the client should confer to decide on food choices depending on what will be available to the traveler. In general, preparation activities can include the following:

- Review meal planning skills, the number and type of exchanges at each meal, basic portion sizes, and tips on eating out.

TABLE 20-9

MODIFYING A DIABETIC MEAL PLAN FOR ILLNESS

FOOD INTAKE	EXCHANGE	CARBOHYDRATE (G)
Usual Intake		
½ chicken breast, roasted	3 meat	0
1 tsp margarine	1 fat	0
½ cup rice	1 bread	15
Tossed green salad, lemon wedge	Free food	0
¾ cup strawberries	1 fruit	10
1 cup skim milk	1 milk	12
TOTAL		37
Sick-Day Intake*		
2 cups broth	Free food	0
1 cup gelatin	1 other carbohydrate	15
1 cup ginger ale (regular)	1 other carbohydrate	15
2 cups herbal tea	Free food	0
TOTAL		30

*Objective: To provide adequate amounts of carbohydrate for times when the person with diabetes has a poor appetite.

- Learn about foods that will be available (e.g., ordering a diabetic diet ahead from airlines).
- Select appropriate snacks to carry and plan time intervals for their use.
- Plan for time zone changes in regard to medication, exercise, and diet routine.
- Carry some quick-acting form of carbohydrate (e.g., sugar lumps or glucose tablets) at all times and tell companions about signs, symptoms, and treatment of hypoglycemia.
- Wear an identification bracelet or pendant.
- Secure a physician's letter concerning syringes and insulin prescription.

Eating Out. In general, persons with diabetes should plan ahead so that food eaten at home before and after a meal out can be accommodated to maintain the continuing day's balance. Choosing restaurants with appropriate food also makes menu selection easier. Timing insulin doses to food arrival is important because taking insulin too long before eating will result in hypoglycemia.

Stress. Any form of physiologic or psychosocial stress affects diabetes control because of the hormonal responses that are antagonistic to insulin. Persons with diabetes, especially those using insulin, should learn useful stress reduction exercises and activities as part of their

self-care skills and practices. Stress-reducing activities can vary greatly from one person to the next (e.g., running, yoga, journaling, playing music). Finding the best coping mechanism may require trial and error.

DIABETES EDUCATION PROGRAM
Goal: Person-Centered Self-Care

In the past few years the traditional roles of health care professionals and their patients have been changing. Patients are taking a much more active and informed role in their own health care. This action is especially true in the case of persons with diabetes. By the nature of the disease process and the necessity of daily survival skills, persons with diabetes must practice regular, daily self-care (see the Clinical Applications box, "Case Study: Richard Manages His Diabetes"). Thus any effective and successful diabetes education program must focus on personal needs and informed self-care skills.

Content: Tools for Self-Care
Necessary Skills

Diabetes educators and the American Diabetes Association have developed guidelines for diabetes education based on the learning needs and skills and content areas necessary for self-care of diabetes. Persons with diabetes must have essential skills for the best possible control as well as favorable surrounding factors related to life situations and psychosocial needs. The tools for self-care involve seven basic content areas.

Nature of Diabetes. Patients should have a general knowledge of the nature of diabetes and how their individual form and degree of diabetes relate to this process. This means comparing the big picture with their particular situation. Such a comparison includes evaluating initial basic survival needs and fulfilling their own fundamental needs, especially support for personal concerns and feelings, in dealing with their diabetes.

Nutrition. Together with their dietitians, persons with diabetes should develop a sound food plan based on individual nutrition needs, living and working situations, and food habits. Such planning includes understanding how the food plan relates to maintaining good blood glucose control and promoting positive health.

Insulin. According to their treatment plan, persons with diabetes should understand the following about their medications:

1. Insulin types and duration of action (Table 20-10), as well as combinations of insulin use (see the For Further Focus box, "Comparative Types of Insulin"), which includes learning how insulin works in the

CLINICAL APPLICATIONS

CASE STUDY: RICHARD MANAGES HIS DIABETES

Richard Smith, age 21 years, has type 1 diabetes mellitus. He gives himself two injections a day, each a combination of medium-acting insulin and regular short-acting insulin. He takes one injection before breakfast and one before dinner and usually tests his blood glucose level before each meal and at bedtime. Richard is a college student who usually is active in athletics.

However, this is final exam week and Richard's schedule is irregular. He is putting in long hours of study and is under considerable stress. On the day before a particularly difficult examination, he is reviewing his study materials at home and forgets to check his blood glucose or eat lunch. During mid-afternoon, he begins to feel faint and realizes that his blood glucose is low and an insulin reaction is imminent if he does not get a quick source of energy. He looks in the kitchen, but all he can find is orange juice, milk, a loaf of bread, and a jar of peanut butter.

Questions for Analysis

1. Which of the foods should Richard eat immediately? Why?
2. Later, when he is feeling better, Richard makes a peanut butter sandwich, pours a glass of milk, and eats his snack while he continues studying. What carbohydrate food sources of energy are in his snack?
3. Are these carbohydrate sources in a form that the cells can burn for energy? What changes must Richard's body make in these sources to get them into the basic carbohydrate fuel form? What is the complex form of carbohydrate in his snack? Why is this a valuable form of carbohydrate in his diet? What is the basic form of carbohydrate fuel circulating in the blood for use by the cells?
4. If Richard did not take his insulin to provide the necessary control agent for metabolizing the carbohydrate, what would happen to him as the result of improper handling of fat and accumulation of ketones?

body and how its action relates to the food plan. Learning good insulin injection technique also is an important part of the treatment plan. In addition to the standard injections, insulin also can be administered with a pump (see Figure 20-6). Newer forms of insulin pump therapy continuously deliver insulin to the body in response to a programmed basal rate (Figure 20-8). Fast-acting insulin can then be delivered in bolus immediately after a meal based on the number of carbohydrates the meal contained.

2. Oral hypoglycemic agents that stimulate insulin activity, their comparative types and effects (Table 20-11), and how to regulate them are key points that should be well understood by the patient and/or caretaker.

Monitoring Glucose Levels. Monitoring blood glucose levels as well as urinary acetone to note possible ketoacidosis is vital. This monitoring includes learning accurate self-testing procedures as well as understanding the meaning of the results and knowing what action to take in relation to food, insulin, or exercise. A variety of self-tests are now available for quick blood glucose monitoring. Small glucose testing kits can fit into purses, backpacks, and glove compartments for easy access and convenience. Some insulin pumps provide continuous interstitial blood glucose monitoring. Techniques now exist that use very small amounts of blood from the finger or arm, and more advanced methods using oil secretions on the skin currently are under evaluation for accuracy.

TABLE 20-10

TYPES OF INSULIN

TYPE	EXAMPLES	ONSET OF ACTION	PEAK ACTION	DURATION OF ACTION
Rapid acting	Humalog (Lispro)	5-15 min	30-90 min	3-5 h
	NovoLog (Aspart)	15 min	40-50 min	
Short acting (regular)	Humulin R	30-60 min	60-120 min	5-8 h
	Novolin R			
Intermediate acting*	Humulin N	1-3 h	8 h	20 h
	Novolin N			
	Humulin L	1-2.5 h	7-14 h	18-24 h
	Novolin L			
Long acting	Ultralente	4-8 h	8-12 h	36 h
	Lantus (Glargine)	1 h	None	24 h

*Intermediate and short-acting mixtures also are available.

FOR FURTHER FOCUS

COMPARATIVE TYPES OF INSULIN

A common method of insulin use is a mixture of short-acting and longer acting types injected twice a day (see figure below). Persons with unstable diabetes or irregular mealtimes may inject short-acting insulin before each meal or snack and use a longer acting type of insulin once or twice a day. Many experienced patients self-test their blood glucose levels with finger pricks and glucose monitors. These patients have learned to adjust their insulin dosage to their test results; food pattern; work, school, and social activities; and exercise schedule. In difficult cases, a device that continuously delivers insulin into the bloodstream, an insulin pump, may be used to maintain a finer control over the body's varying insulin needs.

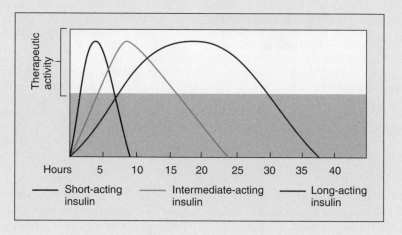

Controlling Emergencies. Persons should recognize the early signs of hypoglycemia and its causes and treatment. This recognition includes (1) knowledge of hypoglycemia's relation to the interactive balances among insulin, food, and exercise as the basis of the diabetes care plan (Figure 20-9); (2) daily diabetic care and how to prevent such episodes; (3) the immediate emergency treatment with some form of quick-acting simple carbohydrate to counteract it; and (4) the need to follow the emergency sugar with a snack of complex carbohydrate and protein as soon as possible to sustain a normal blood glucose.

Illness and Special Needs. Persons with diabetes should learn how to deal with illness and other special needs, several of which have been discussed. This knowledge includes how to adjust diet and insulin and plan ahead for events of daily living such as travel, eating out, exercise, and stress.

Personal Identification. It is also helpful for patients to obtain a personal identification bracelet or pendant. Obtaining such identification should entail an understanding of why having it at all times is important, especially for patients using insulin.

Resources

A number of useful resources are available from health agencies such as the American Diabetes Association and the American Heart Association, including informational materials and useful cookbooks with nutritional values of

Figure 20–8 Insulin pump with optional continuous glucose monitoring functionality (Courtesy DexCom, Inc., San Diego, Calif.)

TABLE 20-11

ORAL HYPOGLYCEMIC MEDICATIONS

CATEGORY OF MEDICATION	EXAMPLES	ACTION
α-Glucosidase inhibitor	Acarbose (Precose) Miglitol (Glyset)	Slows breakdown of starches, delaying the rise in blood glucose after a meal
Biguanide	Metformin (Glucophage)	Increases sensitivity of endogenous insulin
Meglitinide	Nateglinide (Starlix) Repaglinide (Prandin)	Stimulates release of insulin from β cells
Sulfonylurea	Acetohexamide (Dymelor) Chlorpropamide (Diabinese) Glimepiride (Amaryl) Glipizide (Glucotrol) Glyburide (DiaBeta, Micronase, Glynase) Tolazamide (Tolinase) Tolbutamide (Orinase)	Stimulates release of insulin from β cells
Thiazolidinedione	Pioglitazone (Actos) Rosiglitazone (Avandia)	Increases insulin sensitivity in muscle and fat

recipes. More cookbooks on light cooking that reduces fat, sugar, and salt and suggests many alternative seasonings and methods of preparation also are available. In addition, resource persons include hospital and clinic dietitians, dietitians in private practice, public health nutritionists, and local chapters of the American Diabetes Association. Any resource materials used must be evaluated in terms of individual needs.

Staff Education

In the final analysis, the success of the diabetes education program in any health care facility depends on the sensitivity and training of the staff conducting the program. Continuing education is essential for all professionals and their assistants. Educational games often are useful tools as part of the staff education program, which the staff can then use in teaching their patients and clients.

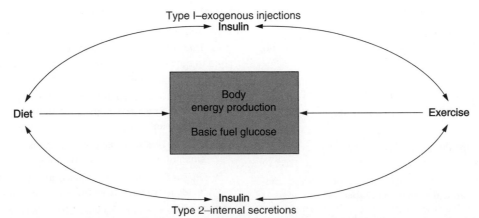

Figure 20–9 Basis of diabetes management: body energy balance. Interacting relations among diet (energy source), insulin (hormone controlling body use of glucose), and exercise (physical activity using blood glucose).

SUMMARY

Diabetes mellitus is a syndrome of varying forms and degrees that has the common characteristic of hyperglycemia. Its underlying metabolic disorder involves all three of the energy nutrients—carbohydrate, fat, and protein—and influences energy balance. The major controlling hormone involved is insulin from the pancreas, and persons with diabetes have either a lack of insulin or a resistance to its action.

Type 1 diabetes affects approximately 5% to 10% of all persons with diabetes; it usually presents itself first during childhood and is more severe and unstable. Treatment of type 1 diabetes involves regular meals and snacks balanced with insulin and exercise. Self-monitoring of blood glucose levels is an important part of disease management.

Type 2 diabetes occurs mostly in adults, especially those who are overweight. Acidosis is rare. Treatment involves weight reduction and maintenance along with regular exercise. Medications may or may not be needed.

A significant keystone of care for all forms of diabetes is sound diet therapy. The basic food plan should be rich in complex carbohydrates and dietary fiber; low in simple sugars, fats (especially saturated fats), and cholesterol; and moderate in protein. Food should be distributed throughout the day in fairly regular amounts and at regular times and tailored to meet individual needs.

CRITICAL THINKING QUESTIONS

1. Define diabetes mellitus. Describe the nature of the underlying metabolic disorder. What is the one common characteristic of all forms of diabetes mellitus?
2. Describe the major characteristics of the two main types of diabetes mellitus. Explain how these characteristics influence nutrition therapy.
3. Identify and explain symptoms of uncontrolled diabetes mellitus. How would you explain to a patient the differences between hyperglycemia and hypoglycemia and how to recognize and treat these symptoms?
4. Describe the possible long-term complications of poorly controlled diabetes mellitus. Can these complications be avoided? If so, how?
5. In terms of the balance concept, describe the principles of a sound diet for a person with diabetes mellitus.

CHAPTER CHALLENGE QUESTIONS

True-False
Write the correct statement for each statement that is false.

1. *True or False:* Most persons with type 2 diabetes are underweight when the disease is discovered.
2. *True or False:* The two nutrients whose metabolism is most directly affected in diabetes are fat and protein.
3. *True or False:* Insulin is a hormone produced by the pituitary gland.
4. *True or False:* Insulin action is influenced by both glucagon and somatostatin.
5. *True or False:* Acetone in the urine of a person with diabetes usually indicates that the diabetes is in poor control.
6. *True or False:* Persons with type 1 diabetes usually are taught to test their own blood glucose daily and regulate their insulin, food, and exercise accordingly.
7. *True or False:* Coronary artery disease occurs in persons with diabetes at a higher rate than that of the general population.
8. *True or False:* Chronic complications occur in a relatively small number of persons with diabetes.
9. *True or False:* A diabetic diet is a combination of specific foods that should remain constant.
10. *True or False:* Persons with unstable type 1 diabetes should follow a low-carbohydrate diet for better control.

Multiple Choice

1. The caloric value of the diet for a person with diabetes should be

a. increased above normal requirements to meet the increased metabolic demand.

b. decreased below normal requirements to prevent glucose formation.

c. sufficient to maintain the person's appropriate lean weight.

d. contributed mainly by fat to spare the carbohydrate for energy needs.

2. The exchange system of diet control is based on which of the following principles? *(Circle all that apply.)*

a. Equivalent food values

b. Variety of food choices

c. Nutritional balance

d. High fat content

3. Oral hypoglycemic agents are used for individuals with which kind of diabetes?

a. Type 1 diabetes

b. Type 2 diabetes

c. Prediabetes

d. All the above

4. Which of the following conditions are potential long-term complications of uncontrolled diabetes? *(Circle all that apply.)*

a. Retinopathy

b. Nephropathy

c. Neuropathy

d. Heart disease

---

evolve **Please refer to the Students' Resource section of this text's Evolve Web site for additional study resources.**

REFERENCES

1. Centers for Disease Control and Prevention: National diabetes fact sheet, *www.cdc.gov/diabetes/pubs/pdf/ndfs_2005. pdf*, accessed April 2007.

2. National Center for Health Statistics: *Health, United States, 2006 with chartbook on trends in the health of Americans,* Hyattsville, MD, 2006, U.S. Government Printing Office.

3. The Expert Committee on the Diagnosis and Classification of Diabetes Mellitus: Position statement of the Expert Committee on the Diagnosis and Classification of Diabetes Mellitus, *Diabetes Care* 30(1 suppl):S42, 2007.

4. SEARCH for Diabetes in Youth Study Group: The burden of diabetes mellitus among US youth: prevalence estimates from the SEARCH for Diabetes in Youth Study, *Pediatrics* 118(4):1510, 2006.

5. Homko CJ, Reece EA: Insulins and oral hypoglycemic agents in pregnancy, *J Matern Fetal Neonatal Med* 19(11):679, 2006.

6. Lee AJ and others: Gestational diabetes mellitus: clinical predictors and long-term risk of developing type 2 diabetes: a retrospective cohort study using survival analysis, *Diabetes Care* 30(4):878, 2007.

7. Sekimoto M and others: JPN guidelines for the management of acute pancreatitis: epidemiology, etiology, natural history, and outcome predictors in acute pancreatitis, *J Hepatobil Pancreat Surg* 13(1):10, 2006.

8. Guzder RD and others: Impact of metabolic syndrome criteria on cardiovascular disease risk in people with newly diagnosed type 2 diabetes, *Diabetologia* 49:49, 2006.

9. Rave K and others: Renal glucose excretion as a function of blood glucose concentration in subjects with type 2 diabetes—results of a hyperglycaemic glucose clamp study, *Nephrol Dial Transplant* 21(8):2166, 2006.

10. Fong DS and others: Diabetic retinopathy, *Diabetes Care* 26(1 suppl):99, 2003.

11. American Diabetes Association: Position statement on standards of medical care in diabetes—2007, *Diabetes Care* 30(1):S4, 2007.

12. Genuth S: Insights from the diabetes control and complications trial/epidemiology of diabetes interventions and complications study on the use of intensive glycemic treatment to reduce the risk of complications of type 1 diabetes, *Endocr Pract* 12(1 suppl):34, 2006.

13. Aring AM and others: Evaluation and prevention of diabetic neuropathy, *Am Fam Physician* 71(11):2123, 2005.

14. American Diabetes Association: Preventive foot care in people with diabetes, *Diabetes Care* 26(1 suppl):78, 2003.

15. Cleary PA and others: The effect of intensive glycemic treatment on coronary artery calcification in type 1 Diabetes Control and Complications Trial/Epidemiology of Diabetes Interventions and Complications (DCCT/EDIC) study, *Diabetes* 55:3556, 2006.

16. American Diabetes Association: Treatment of hypertension in adults with diabetes, *Diabetes Care* 26(1 suppl):83, 2003.

17. American Diabetes Association: Implications of the diabetes control and complications trial, *Diabetes Care* 26(1 suppl):25, 2003.

18. American Diabetes Association: Nutrition recommendations and interventions for diabetes, *Diabetes Care* 30(1 suppl):S48, 2007.

19. Sheard NF and others: Dietary carbohydrate (amount and type) in the prevention and management of diabetes: a statement of the American Diabetes Association, *Diabetes Care* 27:2266, 2004.

20. American Diabetes Association: Physical activity/exercise and diabetes mellitus, *Diabetes Care* 26(1 suppl):73, 2003.

FURTHER READING AND RESOURCES

American Diabetes Association: *www.diabetes.org*

American Diabetes Association, Diabetes Risk Test: *www. diabetes.org/risk-test.jsp*

Diabetes.com: *www.diabetes.com*

Medical journals on diabetes, including: Diabetes, Diabetes Care, Clinical Diabetes, Diabetes Spectrum: *http://diabetes. diabetesjournals.org*

National Institute of Diabetes and Digestive and Kidney Diseases: *www.niddk.nih.gov*

> *The preceding organizations are dedicated to providing the most current information on evaluation, treatment, and prevention of diabetes. These web sites are excellent resources for health care professionals and patients.*

American Diabetes Association: Nutrition recommendations and interventions for diabetes, *Diabetes Care* 30(1 suppl):S48, 2007.

> *A thorough review of the literature regarding nutrition recommendations and intervention is summarized in this position statement by the American Diabetes Association.*

CHAPTER 21

Kidney Disease

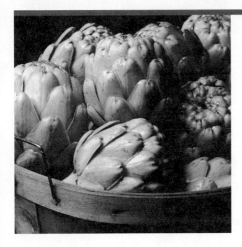

KEY CONCEPTS

- Kidney disease interferes with the normal capacity of nephrons to filter waste products of body metabolism.
- Short-term kidney disease requires basic nutrition support for healing rather than dietary restriction.
- The progressive degeneration of chronic kidney disease requires dialysis treatment and nutrient modification according to individual disease status.
- Current therapy for kidney stones depends more on basic nutrition and health support for medical treatment than on major food and nutrient restrictions.

More than 3.8 million Americans have been diagnosed with some form of kidney disease, resulting in more than 42,000 deaths per year.[1] Decreased kidney function often goes undiagnosed. A review of the National Health and Nutrition Examination Survey found less than 10% of individuals with compromised kidney function were aware of their condition.[2] These kidney problems are costly in lost work, time, and pay as well as in personal quality of life.

This chapter looks at the nutrition care of people with kidney disease, mainly the extensive problem of chronic kidney disease (CKD). Although dialysis extends the lives of patients with this irreversible disease, it does so at tremendous emotional, physical, and financial cost.

BASIC STRUCTURE AND FUNCTION OF THE KIDNEY

Tremendous quantities of fluid (approximately 1.2 L) are filtered through the kidneys every minute. Most of this fluid is reabsorbed back into the vascular system to maintain circulating blood volume. As the blood circulates through the kidneys, these twin organs repeatedly "launder" it to monitor and maintain its quantity and quality. Indeed, the composition of various body fluids is determined not as much by what the mouth takes in as by what the kidneys keep; they are the master chemists of the internal environment.

Structures

The basic functional unit of the kidney is the nephron. Each human kidney is made up of approximately 1 million nephrons, all of which are independently capable of forming urine. Key parts of the nephron include the glomerulus and the different tubules (Figure 21-1).

---

nephron microscopic anatomic and functional unit of the kidney that selectively filters and reabsorbs essential blood factors, secretes hydrogen ions as needed to maintain acid-base balance, reabsorbs water to protect body fluids, and forms and excretes a concentrated urine for elimination of wastes. Each kidney contains approximately 1 million nephrons.

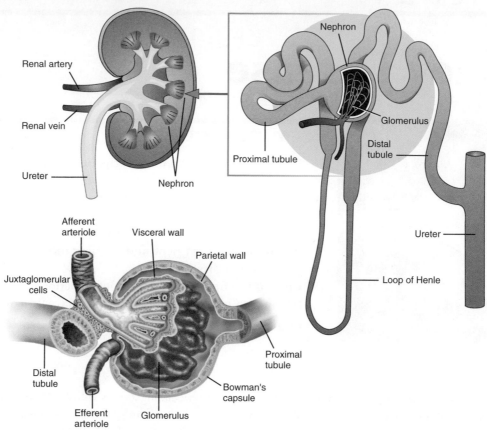

Figure 21–1 Anatomy of the kidney. (*Top,* Reprinted from Peckenpaugh NJ: *Nutrition essentials and diet therapy,* ed 10, Philadelphia, 2002, Saunders; *bottom,* reprinted from Thibodeau GA, Patton KT: *Anatomy & physiology,* ed 6, St Louis, 2007, Mosby.)

Glomerulus

At the head of each nephron, a cup-shaped membrane holds the entering blood capillary and its branching tuft of smaller vessels. This cup-shaped capsule is Bowman's capsule, named for the English physician Sir William Bowman, who in 1843 first established the basis of plasma filtration and consequent urine secretion on the relation of the blood-filled glomeruli and the filtration across the enveloping membrane. Within Bowman's capsule, the afferent arteriole branches into a cluster of capillaries forming the glomerulus (see Figure 21-1). Only the larger blood proteins and cells remain behind in the circulating blood as it leaves the glomerulus in the efferent arteriole. The rate at which blood is filtered through the glomerulus, the glomerular filtration rate (GFR), is the preferred method for monitoring kidney function and defining stages of kidney disease. CKD is defined as a GFR less than 60 ml/min (adjusted to a standard body surface area of 1.73 m^2) for 3 or more months.[3] Diet therapy often is based on a patient's GFR.

Tubules

From the cupped head of each nephron, a small tubule carries the filtered fluid through its winding pathway and empties into the central area of the kidney medulla. Specific substances are reabsorbed and secreted along the way in each of the four parts of these tubules (Table 21-1).

Proximal Tubule. Most of the needed nutrients are reabsorbed in this first part of the tubule and returned to the blood. The surface area of the tubule is greatly increased by a brush border membrane with thousands of microvilli. Glucose and amino acids, as well as approximately 80% of the water and other substances, usually are reabsorbed here. Approximately 20% of the filtered fluid remains to enter the next section of the tube.

Loop of Henle. The tubule's midsection narrows and dips down into the central part of the kidney. Here, the important exchange of sodium, chloride, and water occurs. This fluid environment maintains the necessary osmotic pressure to concentrate the urine as it passes through the

TABLE 21-1

REABSORPTION AND SECRETION IN PARTS OF THE NEPHRON

PART	FUNCTION	SUBSTANCE MOVED
Proximal tubule	Reabsorption (active)	Sodium, glucose, amino acids
	Reabsorption (passive)	Chloride, phosphate, urea, water, other solutes
Loop of Henle		
Descending limb	Reabsorption (passive)	Water
	Secretion (passive)	Urea
Ascending limb	Reabsorption (active)	Sodium
	Reabsorption (passive)	Chloride
Distal tubule	Reabsorption (active)	Sodium
	Reabsorption (passive)	Chloride, other anions, water (in the presence of antidiuretic hormone)
	Secretion (passive)	Ammonia
	Secretion (active)	Potassium, hydrogen, some drugs
Collecting duct	Reabsorption (active)	Sodium
	Reabsorption (passive)	Urea, water (in the presence of antidiuretic hormone)
	Secretion (passive)	Ammonia
	Secretion (active)	Potassium, hydrogen, some drugs

Modified from Thibodeau GA, Patton KT: *Anatomy and physiology*, ed 6, St Louis, 2007, Mosby.

distal tubule and ureter on its way to the bladder for elimination.

Distal Tubule. The latter part of the tubule winds back up into the outer area of the kidney cortex. Here, secretion of hydrogen ions occurs as needed to control acid-base balance. Sodium also is reabsorbed as needed under the influence of the adrenal hormone aldosterone.

Collecting Tubule. In this final section of the tubule, concentrated urine is produced by the following important water-reabsorbing actions: (1) influence of the pituitary hormone antidiuretic hormone, also called *vasopressin*, and (2) the osmotic pressure from the more dense surrounding fluid in the central area of the kidney. The urine, which is now concentrated and ready for excretion, only amounts to 0.5% to 1% of the original fluid and materials filtered through the glomerulus.

Function

Nephron structure has adapted in fine detail to balance internal fluids necessary for life. At birth, each person has far more nephrons than actually needed, but they are gradually lost after approximately age 30 years. Diabetes and high-protein diets tend to exacerbate damage to the glomerulus in the nephron and increase the rate of lost functioning nephrons.[4]

Excretory and Regulatory Functions

The following tasks are performed while blood flows through the nephron:

- *Filtration:* Most particles in blood are filtered out except for the larger components of RBCs and proteins.
- *Reabsorption:* As the filtrate continues through the winding tubules, substances the body needs are selectively reabsorbed and returned to the blood to maintain electrolyte, acid-base, and fluid balance.
- *Secretion:* Along the tubules, additional hydrogen ions are secreted as needed to maintain acid-base balance.
- *Excretion:* Waste materials are excreted in the now-concentrated urine.

glomerular filtration rate (GFR) volume of fluid filtered from the renal glomerular capillaries into Bowman's capsule per unit of time; used clinically as a measure of kidney function.

aldosterone a potent hormone of the outside layer of the adrenal glands that acts on the distal nephron tubule to stimulate reabsorption of sodium in an ion exchange with potassium. The aldosterone mechanism is essentially a sodium-conserving mechanism but also indirectly conserves water because water absorption follows sodium resorption.

antidiuretic hormone a hormone of the pituitary gland that acts on the distal nephron tubule to conserve water by reabsorption; also called vasopressin.

glomerulus the first section of the nephron, a cluster of capillary loops cupped in the nephron head that serves as an initial filter.

Endocrine Functions

In addition to major functions in regulating blood constituents and making and excreting concentrated urine, the kidneys perform the following other functions:

- *Renin secretion:* When the arteriole pressure falls, the kidneys activate and secrete renin, an enzyme that initiates the renin-angiotensin-aldosterone mechanism to reabsorb sodium and maintain hormonal control of body water balance (see Chapter 9).
- *Erythropoietin secretion:* The kidneys are responsible for producing the body's major supply (80% to 90%) of erythropoietin, a circulating hormone that is the principal factor in stimulating RBC production within bone marrow in response to decreased tissue oxygen.
- *Vitamin D activation:* The kidneys convert an intermediate inactive form of vitamin D to the final active vitamin D hormone in the proximal tubules of the nephrons (see Chapter 7). This action is stimulated by the parathyroid hormone.

DISEASE PROCESS AND DIETARY CONSIDERATIONS

General Causes of Kidney Disease

Several disease conditions may interfere with the normal functioning of nephrons, resulting in kidney disease.

Infection and Obstruction

Symptoms of bacterial urinary tract infection may range from the mild discomfort of bladder infections to more involved chronic disease and obstruction from kidney stones. Obstruction anywhere in the urinary tract blocks drainage and may cause further infection and general tissue damage.

Damage from Other Diseases

Circulatory disorders such as prolonged, poorly controlled hypertension can cause degeneration of the small arteries within the kidney and interfere with normal nephron function. More than 80% of patients with CKD have hypertension.[5] Increased demand on other nephrons may in turn cause more hypertension and additional damage to nephrons. Diabetes mellitus is the leading cause of end-stage renal disease (ESRD) in the United States.[6] Other major causes are glomerulonephritis and cystic kidney disease (Figure 21-2). Hyperglycemia and hypertension associated with diabetes can damage small renal arteries, leading to glomerulosclerosis (loss of functioning nephrons) and eventual CKD.[7,8] Autoimmune diseases such as systemic lupus erythematosus also may lead to compromised function or kidney disease.

Toxins

Various environmental agents (e.g., chemical pesticides, solvents, and similar materials), animal venom, certain plants, heavy metals, and some drugs (e.g., NSAIDs, aminoglycoside antibiotics, radiographic contrast dye) are nephrotoxic and can cause kidney damage.

Genetic Defects

Congenital abnormalities of both kidneys can contribute to kidney disease with extensive distortion of kidney structure. Cystic diseases (e.g., polycystic kidney disease, medullary cystic disease) are genetically linked kidney diseases that can lead to ESRD later in life.[9] Individuals born with only one kidney do not necessarily have kidney disease or even impaired function. People with a single kidney often are unaware that they have only one kidney and lead a full life without decreased kidney function.

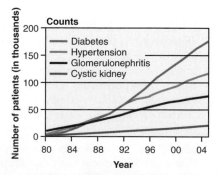
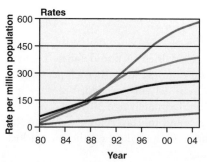

Figure 21-2 Prevalence of chronic kidney disease by primary diagnosis. (Reprinted from U.S. Renal Data System: *USRDS 2007 annual data report: atlas of chronic kidney disease and end-stage renal disease in the United States,* Bethesda, MD, 2007, National Institutes of Health.)

Risk Factors

Risks for CKD are higher in individuals who are older than 60 years and those with a family history of kidney disease. Malnutrition can exacerbate the rate of renal tissue destruction and increase susceptibility to infection. A marked difference in prevalence of CKD exists between ethnic groups. African Americans have a 3.7 times greater incidence of ESRD than Caucasians. The incidence for other minority groups are 1.9 times greater for Native Americans, 1.3 times greater for Asians, and 1.5 times greater for Hispanics (see the Cultural Considerations box, "Prevalence of Kidney Disease among Ethnic Groups in the United States").[6] Box 21-1 lists risk factors and common causes of kidney disease.

Medical Nutrition Therapy in Kidney Disease

In the treatment of kidney disease, appropriate medical nutrition therapy is based on the severity of the disease, GFR, metabolic abnormalities, and medical treatment.

BOX 21-1

RISK FACTORS AND COMMON CAUSES OF KIDNEY DISEASE

Sociodemographic Factors
- Older age
- Member of racial or ethnic minority
- Exposure to certain chemical and environmental conditions
- Low income or education level

Clinical Factors
- Poor glycemic control in diabetes
- Hypertension
- Autoimmune disease
- Systemic infection
- Urinary tract infection
- Urinary stones
- Lower urinary tract obstruction
- Neoplasia
- Family history of CKD
- Recovery from acute kidney failure
- Reduction in kidney mass
- Exposure to certain nephrotoxic drugs
- Low birth weight

Reprinted from Eknoyan G, Levin NW: K/DOQI clinical practice guidelines for CKD: evaluation, classification, and stratification, *Am J Kidney Dis* 39(2 suppl):1, 2002. Copyright National Kidney Foundation.

Length of Disease

In short-term acute disease from infection, drug therapy with antibiotics usually controls the disease. Nutrition therapy is aimed at optimal nutrition support for healing and normal growth. More specific nutrient modifications may be necessary if the patient is a child or if the disease is chronic.

Degree of Impaired Kidney Function and Clinical Symptoms

In milder acute disease with few nephrons involved, less interference occurs with general kidney function because the large number of backup nephrons can meet basic needs. However, in progressive chronic disease more and more nephrons become involved, resulting in CKD. In such cases extensive medical nutrition therapy is required to help maintain kidney function as long as possible. In continuing disease, nutrient modifications are designed to meet individual needs according to clinical symptoms. Working closely with an RD for personalized nutrition therapy is especially important when advanced kidney disease is treated with dialysis.

This chapter's discussion focuses primarily on the more serious degenerative process of CKD and dialysis that requires medical nutrition therapy. Clinical practice guidelines are discussed for each type of kidney disease in the following sections.

NEPHRON DISEASES

Acute Glomerulonephritis or Nephritic Syndrome

Disease Process

This inflammatory process affects the glomeruli, the small blood vessels in the cupped membrane at the head of the nephron. Glomerulonephritis is one of the three most common causes of stage 5 CKD (also known as ESRD).[6]

---

arteriole smallest branch of an artery, connects with capillaries.

erythropoietin hormone that stimulates the production of RBCs in the bone marrow.

nephrotoxic poisonous to the kidney.

CULTURAL CONSIDERATIONS

PREVALENCE OF KIDNEY DISEASE AMONG ETHNIC GROUPS IN THE UNITED STATES

According to the U.S. Renal Data System Annual Report, the incidence of kidney disease continues to rise at a rate of approximately 1% per year.* Part of this occurrence results from the average increase in age of the population and the high prevalence of diabetes in the elderly (diabetes is the leading cause of kidney disease). These estimates only consider patients who meet the clinical definition of CKD: structural or functional abnormalities of the kidney for at least 3 months, most often defined as decreased GFR less than 60 ml/min per 1.73 m². Decline in kidney function goes largely unnoticed and untreated. When researchers evaluated GFR in adults participating in the National Health and Nutrition Examination Survey (1999 to 2000), an additional 36.3% of the population had a mild reduction in GFR (60 to 89 ml/min per 1.73 m²).† In addition, less than one fifth of the population with moderately decreased kidney function (30 to 59 ml/min per 1.73 m²) reported awareness and prior knowledge of their condition.†

Many factors increase a person's risk for CKD, such as diabetes, hypertension, age, and ethnicity. Minority groups historically have had a higher incidence of CKD than Caucasians (see figure below). Recent studies have evaluated causes of CKD in various ethnic groups in an attempt to identify and explain this racial disparity. One study found that the primary cause of ESRD in African Americans was hypertension, whereas the highest cause in Native Americans was diabetes.‡ In addition, patients from minority groups tend to have lower quality health care and seek treatment later in the progression of CKD. Such findings lend important information to health care providers regarding prevention and treatment of CKD. Although these factors do not account for all causes of racial disparity, they are modifiable and therefore achievable in terms of goals for reducing the risk of CKD.

The health-related quality of life (HRQOL) questionnaire assesses each patient on a mental, physical, and disease process level and is associated with mortality rate. Recent studies evaluated the HRQOL and associated outcomes among patients of different ethnicities undergoing hemodialysis in the United States.§¶ Questions about symptoms, effects of disease on daily life, burden of disease, work status, cognitive function, quality of social interaction, sexual function, sleep, social support, staff encouragement, and patient satisfaction also were considered. Mortality risk in CKD is significantly higher in Caucasians than African Americans and is attenuated with low HRQOL scores. African Americans treated by dialysis scored higher than Caucasians in several components of the questionnaire.

Although African Americans are at greater risk for developing CKD, their HRQOL remains higher than Caucasians with CKD. Caucasians on dialysis do not cope as well in terms of quality of life. As research continues to advance, perhaps the disparities between ethnicity and disease outcome will become clearer, making more prevention or treatment mechanisms available.

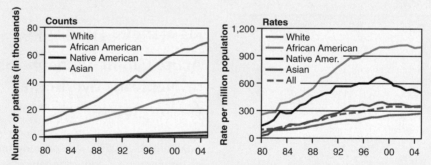

Incident counts and adjusted rates, by race of ESRD. (Reprinted from U.S. Renal Data System: *USRDS 2007 annual data report: atlas of chronic kidney disease and end-stage renal disease in the United States,* Bethesda, MD, 2007, National Institutes of Health.)

*U.S. Renal Data System: *USRDS 2007 annual data report: atlas of chronic kidney disease and end-stage renal disease in the United States,* Bethesda, MD, 2007, National Institutes of Health.

†Coresh J and others: Chronic kidney disease awareness, prevalence, and trends among U.S. adults, 1999 to 2000, *J Am Soc Nephrol* 16(1):180, 2005.

‡Lopes AA: Relationship of race and ethnicity to progression of kidney dysfunction and clinical outcomes in patients with chronic kidney failure, *Adv Ren Replace Ther* 11(1):14, 2004.

§Lopes AA and others: Health-related quality of life and associated outcomes among hemodialysis patients of different ethnicities in the United States: the Dialysis Outcomes and Practice Patterns Study (DOPPS), *Am J Kidney Dis* 41(3):605, 2003.

¶Unruh M and others: Racial differences in health-related quality of life among hemodialysis patients, *Kidney Int* 65:1482, 2004.

Clinical Symptoms

Classic symptoms include hematuria and proteinuria, although edema and mild hypertension also may occur. These patients usually have little appetite, which contributes to feeding problems and malnutrition. If the disease progresses to more kidney involvement, signs of oliguria or anuria may develop. Table 21-2 outlines the five glomerular syndromes and their respective clinical manifestations.

Medical Nutrition Therapy

General care in uncomplicated disease focuses mainly on bed rest and antibiotic drug therapy. Pediatricians and dietitians favor overall optimal nutrition support for growth with adequate protein. Diet modifications are not crucial in most patients with acute, short-term disease. Fluid intake is adjusted to output and insensible losses.

Nephrotic Syndrome

Disease Process

Nephrotic syndrome, or nephrosis, results from nephron tissue damage to the major filtering membrane of the glomerulus, allowing large amounts of protein to pass into the tubule. This high-protein concentration then may cause further damage to the tubule. Both filtration and reabsorption functions of the nephron are disrupted. Nephrosis may be caused by progressive glomerulonephritis or diseases such as diabetes, systemic lupus erythematosus, and connective tissue disorders (e.g., collagen disease).

TABLE 21-2

GLOMERULAR SYNDROMES

SYNDROME	CLINICAL MANIFESTATIONS
Acute nephritic syndrome	Hematuria, azotemia, variable proteinuria, oliguria, edema, and hypertension
Rapidly progressive glomerulonephritis	Acute nephritis, proteinuria, and acute kidney failure
Nephrotic syndrome	>3.5 g proteinuria, hypoalbuminemia, hyperlipidemia, lipiduria
Chronic kidney failure	Azotemia, uremia progressing for years
Asymptomatic hematuria or proteinuria	Glomerular hematuria, subnephrotic proteinuria

Reprinted from Kumar V and others: *Robbins and Cotran pathologic basis of disease*, ed 7, Philadelphia, 2005, Saunders.

Clinical Symptoms

Nephrotic syndrome is characterized by a group of symptoms resulting from the nephron tissue damage and impaired function. The large protein losses (>3.5 g/day in adults) lead to hypoalbuminemia, edema, and ascites. The abdomen becomes distended as fluid accumulates, and plasma protein level is greatly reduced because of large losses in the urine. As protein loss continues, tissue proteins are broken down and general malnutrition follows. Severe edema and ascites often mask the extent of body tissue wasting. Other clinical manifestations include hyperlipidemia and lipiduria.

Medical Nutrition Therapy

The former standard recommendation for patients with nephrotic syndrome was a high-protein diet, sometimes as high as 1.5 g/kg body weight per day. However, current evidence indicates that high-protein diets may accelerate loss of kidney function and moderately low-protein diets

hematuria the abnormal presence of blood in the urine.

proteinuria an abnormal excess of serum proteins (e.g., albumin) in the urine.

edema excess accumulation of fluid in the body tissues.

hypertension high blood pressure.

oliguria the secretion of small amounts of urine in relation to fluid intake (≤ 0.5 ml/kg per hour).

anuria the absence of urine production; indicates kidney shutdown or failure.

nephrosis a nephrotic syndrome caused by degenerative lesions of the renal tubules of the nephrons, especially the thin basement membrane of the glomerulus that helps support the capillary loops; marked by edema, albuminuria, and decreased serum albumin.

collagen disease a disease attacking collagen tissues, the protein substance of the white fibers (collagenous fibers) of skin, tendon, bone, cartilage, and other connective tissues; any of a group of diseases that cause widespread changes in the connective tissue (e.g., rheumatoid arthritis, lupus erythematosus, scleroderma, and rheumatic fever).

ascites outflow and accumulation of serous fluid (blood and lymph serum) in the abdominal cavity; also known as abdominal or peritoneal dropsy.

lipiduria lipid droplets found in the urine composed mostly of cholesterol esters.

reduce albuminuria and albumin catabolism, with no change in the GFR. Nutrition therapy is now directed toward controlling major symptoms (e.g., edema and malnutrition) resulting from the massive protein losses. Therefore physicians and dietitians manage these patients with diets containing less protein, as follows:

- *Protein:* The diet usually is moderate in protein (0.8 g/kg ideal body weight), with the majority of the protein from high biologic value sources. Total protein amounts may be modified on the basis of blood urea nitrogen (BUN) and GFR results. If BUN is elevated and urine output is decreased, dietary protein may be restricted.
- *Carbohydrate:* To provide sufficient energy in kilocalories, carbohydrates should be given liberally, which also helps combat catabolism of tissue protein and prevent starvation ketosis.
- *Lipids:* Decreasing dietary intake of fat and cholesterol may help alleviate hypercholesterolemia and the resulting risk for CVD.
- *Sodium:* Edema is common in glomerular diseases. Sodium overload is difficult to treat because of the characteristic hypoalbuminuria and hypotension. To avoid attenuating hypotension, only modest sodium restriction (approximately 3 g/day) is recommended so that additional sodium and water are not lost.
- *Potassium:* If oliguria becomes severe, renal clearance of potassium is impaired. Thus potassium intake must be monitored and carefully adjusted according to individual needs.
- *Water:* Fluid intake is restricted according to urine output and insensible losses. If restriction is not indicated, fluids can be consumed as desired.

KIDNEY FAILURE

The two types of kidney failure, acute and chronic, have a number of symptoms that reflect interference with normal nephron functions in nutrient metabolism. Both forms have similar nutrition therapy depending on the extent of renal tissue damage and treatment.

Acute Kidney Failure

Disease Process

Kidney function in healthy kidneys may suddenly shut down after metabolic insult or traumatic injury, causing a life-threatening situation. This is a medical emergency in which the dietitian and nurse play important supportive roles. The following causes may lead to acute kidney failure:

- *Prerenal:* severe dehydration, circulatory collapse

- *Intrinsic:* acute tubular necrosis from trauma, surgery, or septicemia; nephrotoxicity from antibiotics, antimicrobial agents, or other drugs; vascular disorders such as bilateral renal infarction; acute glomerulonephritis
- *Postrenal obstruction:* benign prostatic hypertrophy with urinary retention, carcinoma of the bladder or prostate, retroperitoneal or pelvic cancer, bilateral ureteral stones, and obstruction[10]

Acute kidney failure can last from days to weeks, with normal function returning when the condition causing the failure is resolved. Depending on the extent of renal tissue damage, regaining full function may take months. However, some individuals do not regain normal kidney function, and the disease progresses to CKD. Predisposing risk factors for acute kidney failure include older age, diabetes, underlying renal insufficiency, and heart failure.[11]

Clinical Symptoms

The major sign of acute kidney failure is oliguria, which is caused when cellular debris from the tissue damage blocks the tubules. Diminished urine output often is accompanied by proteinuria or hematuria. Other symptoms include nausea and vomiting, fatigue and muscle weakness, swelling in the lower extremities, itchy skin, and confusion. Water balance becomes a crucial factor. Short-term dialysis may be needed to support kidney function.

Medical Nutrition Therapy

The major challenge during acute kidney failure is to improve or maintain nutrition status while the patient is faced with marked catabolism. Loss of appetite is common, and enteral nutrition may be required (see Chapter 22). If enteral nutrition is not appropriate or well accepted, parenteral nutrition may then be necessary. Recommendations for protein intake during acute kidney failure have been debated over the years. Current standards indicate the need for highly individualized therapy based on the patient's kidney function, as indicated by the GFR.

Preventing protein catabolism, electrolyte and hydration disturbances, acidosis, and uremic toxicity through individualized medical nutrition therapy is thought to play a role in maintaining kidney function while reducing the complications of CVD and progressive kidney deterioration.[12] General recommendations for acute kidney failure are presented in Table 21-3, keeping in mind that kidney function and treatment modality may vary greatly between patients; thus medical nutrition therapy should be adjusted accordingly.

TABLE 21-3

SUMMARY OF MEDICAL NUTRITION THERAPY FOR ACUTE KIDNEY FAILURE

NUTRIENT	AMOUNT
Calories	30-40 kcal/kg body weight
Protein	0.8-1.0 g/kg ideal body weight increasing as GFR returns to normal; 60% should be high biologic value protein
Sodium	20-40 mEq/day in oliguric phase (depending on urinary output, edema, dialysis, and serum sodium level); replace losses in diuretic phase
Potassium	30-50 mEq/day in oliguric phase (depending on urinary output, dialysis, and serum potassium level); replace losses in diuretic phase
Phosphorus	Limit as needed
Fluid	Replace output from the previous day (vomitus, diarrhea, urine) plus 500 ml

Reprinted from Mahan LK, Escott-Stump S: *Krause's food and nutrition therapy,* ed 12, Philadelphia, 2008, Saunders.

Chronic Kidney Disease

Disease Process

CKD, or chronic renal insufficiency, is caused by the progressive breakdown of kidney tissue, which impairs all kidney functions. Few functioning nephrons remain and then gradually deteriorate. CKD develops slowly and no cure exists. Kidney transplantation, another treatment modality, improves survival rate and is more cost effective than maintenance dialysis; however, waiting lists can be long and donor matches difficult to find.[13] Patients undergoing transplantation have significantly lower rates of CVD progression despite the disadvantages of immunosuppressive therapy (see the Drug-Nutrient Interaction box, "Corticosteroid Use and Kidney Transplantation").

Chronic kidney disease may result from the following diseases involving the nephrons:

- Primary glomerular disease
- Metabolic disease with kidney involvement (e.g., diabetes)
- Renal vascular disease
- Renal tubular disease
- Congenital abnormality of both kidneys
- Hypertension
- Heart or lung disease

Modifiable risk factors include control of blood pressure, proteinuria or albuminuria, and HbA1c level.[14]

Clinical Symptoms

Depending on the nature of the underlying kidney disease, chronic kidney changes may involve extensive scarring of renal tissue, which distorts the kidney structure and brings vascular changes from prolonged hypertension. As nephrons are lost one by one, the remaining nephrons gradually lose their ability to sustain metabolic balances.

Water Balance. In the beginning stages of chronic kidney failure the kidneys are unable to reabsorb water and properly concentrate urine. Therefore large amounts of dilute urine are produced (polyuria). Dehydration is a risk factor at this point and may become critical. As the disease progresses, urine production declines to a point of oliguria and finally anuria. Without urinary excretion of waste products, dangerous levels of urea accumulate in the blood.

Electrolyte Balance. Several imbalances among electrolytes result from decreasing nephron function. The failing kidney cannot appropriately maintain the vital sodium-potassium balance that guards body water (see Chapter 9). A concentration of materials (e.g., phosphate, sulfate, and organic acids) is produced by the metabolism of food. Without appropriate filtering, these materials accumulate in the blood, causing metabolic acidosis. The disturbed metabolism of calcium and phosphate from lack of activated vitamin D, a process that occurs in the kidneys, leads to bone pain, abnormal bone metabolism, and osteodystrophy.[15]

Nitrogen Retention. Increasing loss of nephron function results in elevated amounts of nitrogenous metabolites, such as urea and creatinine.

Anemia. The damaged kidney cannot accomplish its normal initiation of RBC production through erythro-

blood urea nitrogen (BUN) a basic test of nephron function by measuring its ability to normally filter urea nitrogen, a product of protein metabolism, from the blood.

ketosis the accumulation of ketones, intermediate products of fat metabolism, in the blood.

hypotension low blood pressure.

osteodystrophy bone disease resulting from defective bone formation. The general term dystrophy applies to any disorder arising from faulty nutrition.

urea chief nitrogen-carrying product of dietary protein metabolism; appears in blood, lymph, and urine.

creatinine nitrogen-carrying product of normal tissue protein breakdown; excreted in the urine.

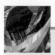

DRUG-NUTRIENT INTERACTION

CORTICOSTEROID USE AND KIDNEY TRANSPLANTATION

Kidney transplantation is the most common type of solid organ transplant.* One of the greatest concerns after transplantation is rejection of the kidney. This occurs when the immune system attacks the new kidney because it is recognized as foreign.

Corticosteroids act by suppressing the immune system and therefore decrease the risk of rejection. The amount of corticosteroid prescribed decreases over time until the patient is weaned from the drug.

Over this time, however, corticosteroids can have the following side effects:

- Peptic ulcer disease
- Hypertension
- Hyperglycemia
- Hyperlipidemia
- Bone disease
- Increased appetite and weight gain
- Growth retardation (in children)

Corticosteroids also increase the excretion of key nutrients. Increased amounts of protein, potassium, calcium, magnesium, zinc, vitamin C, and vitamin B_6 are sometimes needed. However, some of these nutrient losses are counteracted when other drugs are prescribed in addition to corticosteroids. Cyclosporine is one such drug; it may lead to hyperkalemia, in which case increasing potassium intake from food should be avoided. Monitoring serum electrolyte levels, blood pressure, and lipid profiles is vital for transplant recipients. Ensuring these are within normal levels, as well as watching for deficiency symptoms of the other nutrients, is part of optimal care of the patient.

Some of the other drugs used to prevent organ rejection include tacrolimus (Prograf), azathioprine (Imuran), and sirolimus (Rapamune). The side effects of each drug vary when used separately and/or concomitantly with corticosteroids.† Because these side effects often are quite severe, development of new administration strategies is under way. For example, recent research shows that some patients on a lower, less-frequent dose of corticosteroids can recover as well as those on the typical protocol. A few studies also have indicated that some patients recover just as well without corticosteroid use (using other types of drugs instead, such as those listed above), but this method is not supported by medical professionals because of a lack of evidence. ‡

Sara Oldroyd

*Merck Manuals Online Medical Library: *Kidney transplantation, www.merck.com/mmpe/print/sec13/ch166/ch166e.html,* accessed March 2007.
†Peters TG: *Transplant drugs: medicines that prevent rejection, www.aakp.org/aakp-library/Transplant-Drugs,* accessed September 2007.
‡Curtis J: Corticosteroids and kidney transplantation, *Clin J Am Soc Nephrol* 1:907-908, 2006.

poietin. Therefore fewer RBCs are produced, and those that are produced have a decreased survival time.

Hypertension. When blood flow to kidney tissue is increasingly impaired, renal hypertension develops. In turn, hypertension causes cardiovascular damage and further deterioration of the kidneys.

Azotemia. Elevated BUN, serum creatinine, and serum uric acid levels are reflected in the characteristic laboratory finding of azotemia.

In its clinical practice guidelines, the National Kidney Foundation categorizes CKD into five stages based on GFR (Table 21-4).[9]

General Signs and Symptoms

Increasing loss of kidney function causes progressive weakness, shortness of breath, general lethargy, and fatigue. Thirst, anorexia, weight loss, diarrhea, and vomiting may occur. Increasing capillary fragility may cause skin, nose, oral, and GI bleeding. Nervous system involvement brings muscular twitching, burning sensations in the extremities, or convulsions. Irregular cyclic breathing (i.e., Cheyne-Stokes respiration) indicates acidosis. Acidosis may cause mouth ulcers, a foul taste, and bad breath in the patient. Malnutrition lowers resistance to infection. Bone and joint pain continue.

TABLE 21-4

STAGES OF CKD

STAGE	DESCRIPTION	GFR (ml/min/1.73 m²)
1	Kidney damage, with normal or elevated GFR	≥90
2	Kidney damage, with mild decrease in GFR	60-89
3	Moderate decrease in GFR	30-59
4	Severely decreased GFR	15-29
5	Kidney failure	<15 (or dialysis)

CKD is defined as either kidney damage or GFR <60 ml/min per 1.73 m² for 3 or more months. Kidney damage is defined as pathologic abnormalities or markers of damage, including abnormalities in blood or urine tests or imaging studies.
Reprinted from Eknoyan G, Levin NW: K/DOQI clinical practice guidelines for chronic kidney disease: evaluation, classification, and stratification, *Am J Kidney Dis* 39(2 suppl):1, 2002. Copyright National Kidney Foundation.

Medical Nutrition Therapy

Basic Objectives. Treatment must always be individual and adjusted according to progression of the illness, the type of treatment, and the patient's response. The Kidney Disease Outcomes Quality Initiative dietary guidelines

TABLE 21-5

SELECTED NUTRITION PARAMETERS FOR VARIOUS LEVELS OF KIDNEY FAILURE*

PARAMETER	NORMAL KIDNEY FUNCTION	STAGES 1-4 CKD	STAGE 5 HEMODIALYSIS	STAGE 5 PERITONEAL DIALYSIS	TRANSPLANT
Calories (kcal/kg/day)	30-37	35 kcal/kg if < 60 years 30-35 kcal/kg if ≥ 60 years	35 kcal/kg if < 60 years 30-35 kcal/kg if ≥ 60 yrs	35 kcal/kg if < 60 years 30-35 kcal/kg if ≥ 60 years; include calories from dialysate	30-35 kcal/kg initial 25-30 kcal/kg for maintenance
Protein (g/kg/day)	0.8	0.6-0.75 50% HBV	1.2 50% HBV	1.2-1.3 50% HBV	1.3-1.5 initial 1.0 for maintenance
Fat (% total kcal)	30%-35%	Patients considered at highest risk for CVD; emphasis on PUFA, MUFA, 250-300 mg cholesterol/day			<10% saturated fat
Sodium (mg/day)	Unrestricted	2000	2000	2000	Unrestricted; monitor medication effect
Potassium (mg/day)	Unrestricted	Correlated to laboratory values	2000-3000 (8-17 mg/kg/day)	3000-4000 (8-17 mg/kg/day)	Unrestricted; monitor medication effect
Calcium (mg/day)	Unrestricted	1200	≤2000 from diet and medications	≤2000 from diet and medications	1200
Phosphorus (mg/day)	Unrestricted	Correlated to laboratory values	800-1000	800-1000	Unrestricted unless indicated
Fluid (ml/day)	Unrestricted	Unrestricted with normal urine output	1000 + urine output	Monitored; 1500-2000	Unrestricted unless indicated

*These are guidelines for initial assessment only; individualization to the patient's own metabolic status and coexisting metabolic conditions is essential for optimal care.

HBV, High biologic value; *PUFA*, polyunsaturated fatty acids; *MUFA*, monounsaturated fatty acids.

Reprinted from Beto JA, Bansal VK: Medical nutrition therapy in chronic kidney failure: integrating clinical practice guidelines, *J Am Diet Assoc* 104:404, 2004.

recommend monitoring nutrition status of patients with CKD at regular intervals: every 1 to 3 months for patients with a GFR less than 30 ml/min per 1.73 m^2 and every 6 to 12 months for patients with a GFR of 30 to 59 ml/min per 1.73 m^2 to identify anorexia and help prevent malnutrition.[9] Following are basic therapy objectives in the care of patients with CKD:

- Reduce protein breakdown
- Avoid dehydration or excess hydration
- Correct acidosis
- Correct electrolyte imbalances
- Control fluid and electrolyte losses from vomiting and diarrhea
- Maintain optimal nutrition status
- Maintain appetite, general morale, and sense of well-being
- Control complications of hypertension, bone pain, and nervous system involvement

- Slow the rate of kidney failure, postponing the ultimate need for dialysis

Principles. Nutrition for chronic kidney failure involves variable nutrient adjustments according to individual need. Table 21-5 outlines the nutrition parameters for varying levels of kidney function.[14]

- *Calories:* Carbohydrate and fat must provide sufficient nonprotein kilocalories to supply energy and spare protein for tissue synthesis. For individuals younger than 60 years with CKD and a GFR less than 25 ml/min, the recommended energy intake is 35 kcal/kg body weight per day. Energy needs are less for individuals aged 60 years or older (30 to 35 kcal/kg per day). Because CVD is accelerated in CKD, the remain-

azotemia an excess of urea and other nitrogenous substances in the blood.

ing calories should support cardiovascular health principles (e.g., substitute monounsaturated and polyunsaturated fats for saturated and trans fats, reduce total cholesterol intake; see Chapter 19).

- *Protein:* The goal is to provide adequate protein to maintain tissue integrity while avoiding excess. Protein generally is limited to 0.6 to 0.75 g/kg body weight per day for individuals not on dialysis with a GFR less than 25 ml/min. At least 50% of this amount should come from high biologic value protein (see Chapter 4) to ensure an adequate intake of essential amino acids. Mixtures of essential amino acids or amino acid precursors provide necessary protein supplementation for low-protein diets. Other supplements are made up of nitrogen-free "copies" of essential amino acids called *analogs*.
- *Sodium:* The need for sodium varies. If hypertension and edema are present, sodium intake must be restricted. Sodium intake usually is limited to 2000 mg/day.
- *Potassium:* The damaged kidney cannot adequately clear potassium, so dietary intake is determined by assessing laboratory values.
- *Phosphate and calcium:* Inappropriate blood phosphorus and calcium levels negatively affect bone composition. As the kidney loses function, activation of vitamin D and control of blood calcium levels decline. This problem is worsened by excess blood phosphorus, which results in calcium resorption from the bone. Thus moderate dietary phosphorus restriction depends on laboratory values in the patient not undergoing di-

alysis and generally is limited to 800 to 1000 mg/day in patients undergoing dialysis treatment. A calcium supplement may be used to correct hypocalcemia.

- *Vitamins:* A multivitamin supplement specifically formulated for kidney disease usually is added to the diet of patients on protein and mineral restriction. A diet of up to 40 g of protein does not contribute the full daily requirement of all the vitamins (see the Clinical Applications box, "Case Study: The Patient with CKD"). Fat-soluble vitamins A and E are not recommended because they may accumulate to toxic levels in kidney failure. Excess of vitamins D and K are contraindicated because the kidney cannot convert vitamin D to its active form and vitamin K can adversely affect clotting time.
- *Water:* Fluid intake should be sufficient to maintain adequate urine volume in patients not undergoing dialysis,. Intake usually is balanced with output.

End-Stage Renal Disease

Disease Process

When CKD advances to an end stage, life-support decisions face the patient, family, and physician. ESRD occurs when the patient's GFR decreases to 15 ml/min. This decrease is caused by irreversible damage to a majority of the kidneys' nephrons. At this point the patient has two options: long-term kidney dialysis or kidney transplantation. The lives of an estimated 500,000 persons in the

CLINICAL APPLICATIONS

CASE STUDY: THE PATIENT WITH CKD

Gary B., age 49 years, is an active man working at a large company who has begun to tire more easily. He has little appetite and generally feels ill most of the time. He recently noticed some ankle swelling and some blood in his urine. At his wife's insistence, he finally decided to see his physician.

After a complete workup, his physician's findings included the following:

- No prior illness except a case of the flu with a throat infection during his overseas service in the Army
- Laboratory tests: albumin, RBCs, and white blood cells in the urine; abnormal BUN and low GFR (20 ml/min per 1.73 m²)
- Other symptoms: hypertension, edema, headache, occasional vision blurring, and low-grade fever

The physician discussed the findings and the serious prognosis of CKD (stage 4) with Gary and his wife, and together they explored the immediate medical and nutrition needs for treatment. They also discussed the ultimate need for medical management with dialysis. The physician prescribed medications to control Gary's growing symptoms and discomfort.

Over the next 10 months Gary's symptoms worsened. He lost more weight, became anemic, and had increased bone and joint pain and GI bleeding. Nausea increased, and he had occasional muscle twitching or spasms. Small mouth ulcers made eating a painful effort. Gary and his wife were referred to an RD to learn how to manage his present predialysis diet at home.

Questions for Analysis

1. What metabolic imbalances in CKD do you think account for Gary's symptoms?
2. What are the objectives of treatment in CKD?
3. What are the basic principles of Gary's predialysis diet? Describe this type of diet. What foods would be included? Plan a 1-day menu for Gary using the dietary analysis program included with this text.
4. What nutrient-related medications and supplements would Gary's physician and clinical dietitian probably use in his treatment plan? Why?

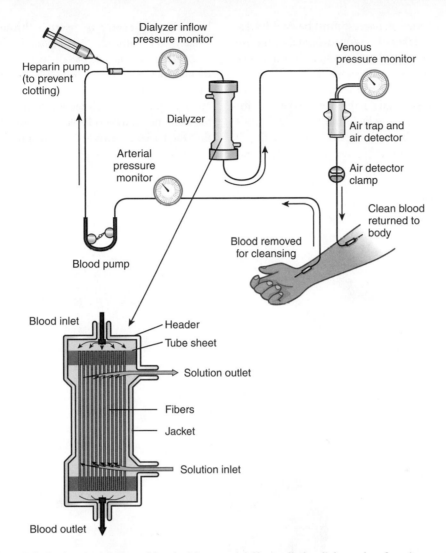

Figure 21-3 Hemodialysis cleans and filters blood with a special filter called a dialyzer that functions as an artificial kidney. Blood travels through tubes into the dialyzer, which filters out wastes and extra water. Then the cleaned blood flows through another set of tubes back into the body. (Modified from National Institute of Diabetes and Digestive and Kidney Diseases: *Treatment methods for hemodialysis,* NIH publication No. 07-4666, 2006, Bethesda, MD, National Institute of Health.)

United States have been prolonged by dialysis and/or kidney transplants.[6] Kidney transplantation has several advantages. Current advances in surgical techniques, immunosuppressive drugs to prevent rejection, and antibiotics to control infection have helped ensure successful outcomes. A successful kidney transplant can provide an improved quality of life and is more cost effective than dialysis. Long-term effects of dialysis include bone disorders, malnutrition, anemia, and hormonal imbalances as well as psychological depression and diminished quality of life from constant dependence on treatments. However, dialysis has become the major treatment for advanced kidney disease. Two forms of dialysis are used: hemodialysis and peritoneal dialysis.

Types of Therapy and Respective Medical Nutrition Therapy

Hemodialysis. Hemodialysis is the use of an artificial kidney machine to remove toxic substances from the blood and help restore nutrients and metabolites to normal blood levels (Figure 21-3). To prepare a patient for

dialysis the process of separating crystalloids (crystal-forming substances) and colloids (gluelike substances) in solution by the difference in their rates of diffusion through a semipermeable membrane; crystalloids (e.g., blood sugar and other simple metabolites) pass through readily and colloids (e.g., plasma proteins) pass through slowly or not at all.

hemodialysis therapy, vascular access must be established. This procedure ideally takes place approximately 1 month before treatments begin to allow adequate healing. The three basic kinds of vascular access for hemodialysis are arteriovenous (AV) fistula, AV graft, and a venous catheter (Figure 21-4). An AV fistula is the preferred access for long-term dialysis and is made by joining an artery and a vein on the forearm just beneath the skin. After the fistula has healed, a needle is inserted through the tissue and connected by tubes to the dialysis machine.

A patient with CKD usually requires two to three treatments per week, each of which lasts 3 to 4 hours. During each treatment the patient's blood makes several complete cycles through the dialyzer, which removes excess waste to maintain normal blood levels of life-sustaining substances that the patient's own kidneys can no longer accomplish.

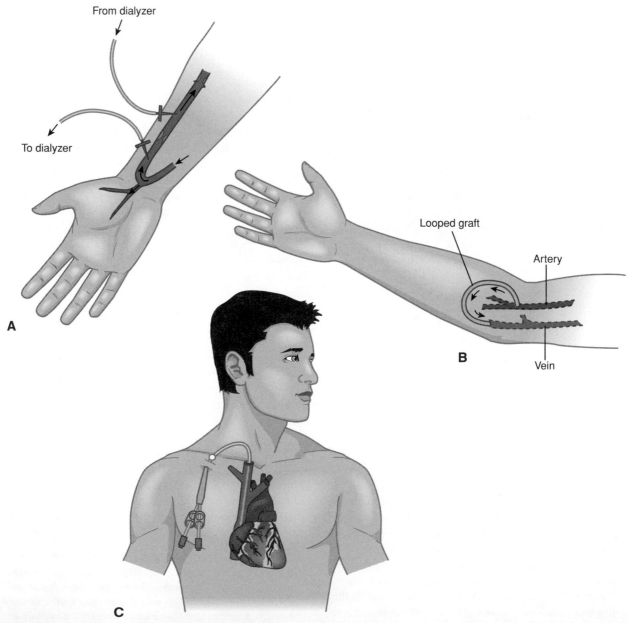

Figure 21–4 Types of access for hemodialysis. **A,** Forearm AV fistula. **B,** Artificial loop graft. **C,** Venous catheter for temporary hemodialysis access. (Modified from National Institute of Diabetes and Digestive and Kidney Diseases: *Kidney failure: choosing a treatment that's right for you,* NIH publication No. 00-2412, 2007, Bethesda, MD, National Institute of Health.)

Two compartments in the machine are separated by a filter. One compartment contains blood from the patient that contains all the excess fluids and waste; the other contains the dialysate, which is a type of "cleaning fluid." As in normal capillary filtration, the blood cells are too large to pass through the pores in the filter. However, the remaining smaller molecules in the blood pass through the filter and are carried away by the dialysate. If the patient's blood is deficient in certain materials, these may be added to the dialysate.

Medical Nutrition Therapy for Hemodialysis. The diet of a patient undergoing hemodialysis is an important aspect of maintaining biochemical control. RDs are heavily involved with meal planning and diet education. Several basic objectives govern an individual's diet and are designed to perform the following four tasks:

1. Maintain protein and energy balance
2. Prevent dehydration or fluid overload
3. Maintain normal serum potassium and sodium levels
4. Maintain acceptable phosphate and calcium levels

Controlling infection is always an underlying goal. In most cases nutrition therapy can be planned with more liberal nutrient allowances, as follows:

- *Calories:* Interestingly, the mortality rate decreases as BMI increases to 25 to 28 kg/m^2 because of the association between malnutrition and clinical outcomes.[16] The unfortunate combination is that CKD is closely related to a decrease in appetite when GFR falls below 60 ml/min.[9] A generous amount of carbohydrates with some fat continues to supply needed kilocalories for energy and protein sparing. An intake of 35 kcal/kg of lean body weight helps avoid catabolism, which would further complicate kidney function.
- *Protein:* Protein energy malnutrition is a major concern in patients on dialysis and is considered one of the most significant predictors of adverse outcomes. Patients undergoing hemodialysis typically consume less protein on treatment days than other days of the week, and middle-aged (50 to 64 years) and older patients (>65 years) may be at greater risk for developing protein energy malnutrition than are patients younger than 50 years.[17,18] For most adult patients on dialysis, a protein allowance of 1.2 g/kg lean body weight is the goal to prevent protein malnutrition. This amount provides nutrition needs, maintains positive nitrogen balance, does not produce excessive nitrogenous waste, and replaces the amino acids lost during each dialysis treatment. At least 50% of this daily allowance should consist of protein foods of high biologic value (e.g., eggs, meat, fish, and poultry).[14]

- *Sodium:* To control body fluid retention and hypertension, sodium is limited to 2000 mg/day. Sodium intake is not as stringently regulated for patients on dialysis as it is for those with CKD and not yet on dialysis because the dialysis process rids the body of excess sodium.
- *Potassium:* To prevent potassium accumulation, which can cause cardiac problems, intake is restricted to 2000 to 3000 mg/day.
- *Vitamins:* A supplement of the water-soluble vitamins (i.e., B complex and C) is given to replace their loss during the dialysis treatment.
- *Water:* Fluid usually is limited to 1000 ml/day plus an amount equal to any urine output.

Peritoneal Dialysis. An alternative form of treatment for some patients is peritoneal dialysis, which has the convenience of mobility. In this process the patient introduces the dialysate solution directly into the peritoneal cavity, where it can be exchanged for fluids that contain the metabolic waste products. Because this form of dialysis is continuous within the body, the process is called *continuous ambulatory peritoneal dialysis.* First, the patient is prepared by surgically inserting a permanent catheter. Treatments are carried out by (1) attaching a disposable bag containing the dialysate solution to the abdominal catheter leading into the peritoneal cavity, (2) allowing 4 to 6 hours for the solution exchange, (3) lowering the bag to allow gravity to pull the waste-containing fluid into it, and (4) repeating the procedure (Figure 21-5). When the bag is empty, it can be folded around the waist or tucked into a pocket, providing the patient mobility. Intermittent use of peritoneal dialysis, self-administered at home, gives the patient a sense of control. An automated device often is used to provide several solution exchanges during sleep hours and one continuous exchange during the day, a technique called *continuous cyclic peritoneal dialysis.*

Medical Nutrition Therapy. A slightly more liberal diet may be used with peritoneal dialysis, as follows[14]:

- *Calories:* Maintain lean body weight by accounting for the energy provided by the dialysate solution into the total meal plan.
- *Protein:* Increase protein intake to 1.2 to 1.3 g/kg body weight.

---

peritoneal cavity a serous membrane lining the abdominal and pelvic walls and undersurface of the diaphragm, forming a sac enclosing the body's vital visceral organs within the peritoneal cavity. Peritoneal dialysis is a form of dialysis through the peritoneum into and out of the peritoneal cavity.

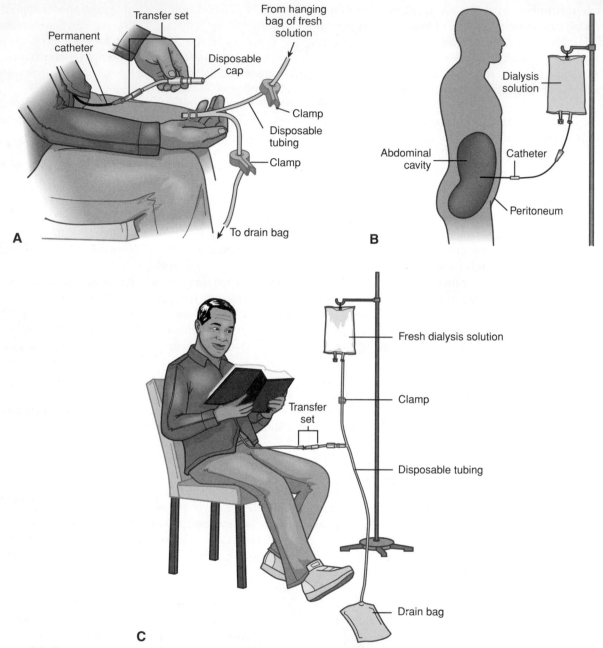

Figure 21–5 Continuous ambulatory peritoneal dialysis. **A,** A soft tube catheter is used to fill the abdomen with a cleansing dialysis solution. **B,** The walls of the abdominal cavity are lined with a peritoneum membrane, which allows waste products and extra fluid to pass from the blood into the dialysis solution. **C,** Wastes and fluid then leave the body when the dialysis solution is drained. Time in which the dialysis solution remains in the abdominal cavity (dwell time) ranges from 4 to 6 hours, and the patient is mobile. An exchange takes approximately 30 to 40 minutes. A typical schedule calls for 4 to 5 exchanges every day. (Modified from National Institute of Diabetes and Digestive and Kidney Diseases: *Treatment methods for kidney failure: peritoneal dialysis,* NIH publication No. 06-4688, 2006, Bethesda, MD, National Institute of Health.)

- *Potassium:* Increase potassium by eating a wide variety of fruits and vegetables each day (3000 to 4000 mg/day).
- *Water:* Increase fluid intake to 1500 to 2000 ml/day to prevent dehydration.

Table 21-5 summarizes the nutrition parameters, and Table 21-6 presents nutrition laboratory parameter outcome goals for patients with CKD on either hemodialysis or peritoneal dialysis.

TABLE 21-6

NUTRITION LABORATORY PARAMETER OUTCOME GOALS FOR STAGE 5 CKD (HEMODIALYSIS AND PERITONEAL DIALYSIS)

NUTRITION LABORATORY PARAMETER	GOAL	OUTCOME PREVENTION FOCUS
Serum albumin (g/dl)	≥4.0 (bromcresol green assay)	Protein energy malnutrition
Serum prealbumin (mg/dl)	>30	Protein energy malnutrition
Predialysis serum creatinine (mg/dl)	>10	Protein energy malnutrition
Serum cholesterol (mg/dl)	>150-180	Protein energy malnutrition
	<200	Hyperlipidemia
Kt/V or urea reduction ratio*	>1.2 or >65%	Dialysis adequacy
Hemodialysis Prognostic Nutrition Index	≥0.8	Increased mortality and morbidity rates
Subjective Global Assessment: 4-item, 7-point scale	≥6-7	Malnutrition
Serum phosphorus (mg/dl)	3.5-5.5	Bone disease
Serum calcium (mg/dl)	8.4-10.5	Bone disease
Serum calcium–phosphorus product	≤55	Bone disease
Serum bicarbonate (mmol/L)	≥22	Metabolic acidosis
Lipid Profile		
LDL (mg/dl)	<100	CVD
HDL (mg/dl)	>40	
Triglycerides (mg/dl)	<150	

Based on Kidney Disease Outcome Quality Initiative recommendations.
Also applicable to stages 1 to 4 CKD with individualization to level of kidney function. Parameters to be monitored monthly with exception of Hemodialysis Prognostic Nutrition Index, Subjective Global Assessment (quarterly or when change indicates), and lipid profile (annually).
*K, Dialyzer clearance of urea; t, dialysis time; V, patient's total body water.
Reprinted from Beto JA, Bansal VK: Medical nutrition therapy in chronic kidney failure: integrating clinical practice guidelines, *J Am Diet Assoc* 104:404, 2004.

Comorbid Complications

Osteodystrophy. Bone disease and disorders are highly prevalent in CKD and are an important cause of morbidity. A combination of factors contributes to osteodystrophy during kidney disease. Decreased activation of vitamin D has a cascade effect, resulting in elevated parathyroid hormone and reduced serum calcium levels. Patients also have elevated serum phosphorus levels combined with the inability of the kidney to excrete phosphorus. This combination causes abnormal changes in bone structure and function. Hyperphosphatemia is associated with increased mortality risk; thus phosphate binders are an important management aspect in CKD. Patients with any level of kidney dysfunction should be evaluated for bone disease and disorders of calcium and phosphorus metabolism.

Neuropathy. Central and peripheral neurologic disturbances are common in patients at the initiation of dialysis and are even more prevalent in patients with diabetes. Symptoms of neuropathy may not be present until GFR falls below 12 to 20 ml/min per 1.73 m^2; however, patients should be periodically assessed for implications of uremia or disease progression.[9]

KIDNEY STONE DISEASE

Disease Process

In the United States approximately 5% of women and 12% of men form kidney stones at some point in their life.[19] The basic cause of kidney stones is unknown, but many factors relating to the nature of the urine itself or conditions of the urinary tract environment contribute to their formation. The major stones are formed from calcium, struvite, and uric acid. Figure 21-6 illustrates the formation of these various stones. In addition, Box 21-2 lists risk factors associated with kidney stone development.

Calcium Stones

A growing number of individuals from all age, gender, and ethnic groups are diagnosed with calcium oxalate stones. This form of kidney stone is the most common type, accounting for approximately 80% of all stones.[19] High levels of urinary oxalate increase the risk of forming a stone. Oxalates are derived from endogenous synthesis (relative to lean body mass) and dietary sources (primarily plants). Oxalic acid is a metabolite of ascorbic acid. Therefore long-term megadosing of vitamin C supple-

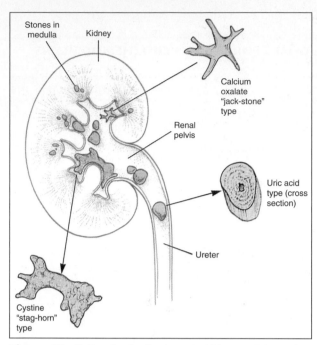

Figure 21–6 Renal calculi: stones in kidney, pelvis, and ureter.

ments (>3 g/day) may pose a potential health risk for kidney stone formation. A small percent of the population are "hyperabsorbers" of dietary oxalate (Box 21-3) and are at higher risk of forming stones.[20]

Imbalances of compounds in the urine may result from the following:

- Excess calcium in the blood (hypercalcemia) or urine (hypercalciuria)
- Excess oxalate in the urine (hyperoxaluria)
- Low levels of citrate in the urine (hypocitraturia)
- Excess animal protein and salt intake
- Prolonged immobilization (withdrawal of bone calcium)
- Infection

Struvite Stones

Struvite stones, accounting for approximately 10% of all stones, are composed of a single compound, magnesium ammonium phosphate ($MgNH_4PO_4$).[19] They often are called *infection stones* because they are mainly caused by urinary tract infections and are not associated with any specific nutrient. Thus no particular diet therapy is involved. Struvite stones usually are large "staghorn" stones that are surgically removed.

Uric Acid Stones

Excess excretion of uric acid may be caused by some impairment with the metabolism of purine, a nitrogen end product of dietary protein from which uric acid is formed. This impairment occurs in diseases such as gout and also can occur in rapid tissue breakdown during wasting disease.

Other Stones

Cystine and xanthine stones are the rarest kidney stones. Cystine stones are caused by a genetic defect in the renal reabsorption of the amino acid cystine, causing an accumulation in the urine (cystinuria). This disorder occurs rarely (one in 15,000 persons). Xanthine stones are associated with treatment for gout and a family history of gout.

General Symptoms and Treatment

Clinical Symptoms

The main symptom of kidney stones is severe pain. Many other urinary symptoms may result from the presence of the stones. General weakness and sometimes fever are present. Laboratory examination of the urine and any passed stones helps determine treatment.

Treatment

General treatment may include several aspects, as discussed below.

Fluid Intake. A large fluid intake helps produce more dilute urine and prevent accumulation of materials that form stones. Exact fluid intake needs vary by patient, but enough fluids, preferably water, should be ingested to produce clear urine.

BOX 21-3

HIGH-OXALATE FOODS AND DRINKS

Drinks
- Beer
- Black tea
- Chocolate milk
- Cocoa
- Instant coffee
- Hot chocolate
- Juice made from high-oxalate fruits (see below)
- Ovaltine
- Soy drinks

Dairy
- Chocolate milk
- Soy cheese
- Soy milk
- Soy yogurt

Fats, Nuts, Seeds
- Nuts
- Nut butters
- Sesame seeds
- Tahini
- Soy nuts

Meat
- None

Starch
- Amaranth
- Buckwheat
- Cereal (bran or high fiber)
- Crispbread (rye or wheat)
- Fruit cake
- Grits
- Pretzels
- Taro
- Wheat bran
- Wheat germ
- Whole-wheat bread
- Whole-wheat flour

Fruit
- Blackberries
- Blueberries
- Canned strawberries
- Carambola
- Concord grapes
- Currants
- Dewberries
- Elderberries
- Figs
- Fruit cocktail
- Gooseberries
- Kiwis
- Lemon peel
- Lime peel
- Orange peel
- Raspberries
- Rhubarb
- Tamarillo
- Tangerines

Vegetables
- Beans (baked, green, dried, kidney)
- Beets
- Beet greens
- Beet root
- Carrots
- Celery
- Chicory
- Collards
- Dandelion greens
- Eggplant
- Escarole
- Kale
- Leeks
- Okra
- Olives
- Parsley
- Peppers (chili and green)
- Pokeweed
- Potatoes (baked, boiled, fried)
- Rutabaga
- Spinach
- Summer squash
- Sweet potato
- Swiss chard
- Zucchini

Condiments
- Black pepper (more than 1 tsp)
- Marmalade
- Soy sauce

Miscellaneous
- Chocolate
- Parsley

High-oxalate foods have more than 10 mg of oxalate per serving.
Reprinted from University of Pittsburgh Medical Center: *Low oxalate diet,* Pittsburgh, PA, 2006, University of Pittsburgh Medical Center.

Stone Composition. In some cases dietary control of the stone constituents may help reduce the recurrence of such stone formation, thus helping prevent the accumulation of these metabolic substances in the urine available for stone formation.

purines nitrogen-containing compounds that yield uric acid as a metabolic end product eliminated in the urine.

Urinary pH. Urinary pH has received much emphasis in relation to diet therapy for kidney stones, but for some years now its importance has been questioned. Research has indicated that dietary attempts to alter urinary pH with acid or alkaline foods are unsuccessful.[21] A desired pH of the urine is better achieved by medical means than by traditional acidic or alkaline diets.

Binding Agents. Materials that bind potential stone elements in the intestine can prevent their absorption and eliminate them from the body. For example, phytate can bind calcium and other cations. Phytates are found in high-fiber plant foods such as whole wheat, bran, and soybeans.

Drug Therapy. A variety of drugs are useful in the treatment of kidney stones in combination with diet therapy. For medications to be most effective, the specific type of stone should be identified. This is not always possible and therefore limits drug therapy in some individuals. Common drugs to treat kidney stones include the following:

- *Calcium stones:* diuretics, citrates, phosphates, thiazides, calcium supplements, and cholestyramine
- *Uric acid stones:* sodium bicarbonate, potassium citrate, and allopurinol
- *Struvite stones:* primarily medications to eliminate the infection and organic acids
- *Cystine stones:* D-penicillamine, captopril, and alpha-mercaptopropionylglycine

Medical Nutrition Therapy

The nutrition care plan mainly relates to the nature of the stone. The diet is designed to reduce intake of nutrients that lead to the formation of a particular type of stone.

Calcium Stones

Historically, individuals who develop calcium oxalate stones were advised to reduce calcium to 400 mg/day. However, recent studies have found that normal calcium intake combined with moderate protein and salt had the most significant reduction in kidney stone recurrence.[22] If a stone is calcium phosphate, additional sources of phosphorus (e.g., meats, legumes, and nuts) should be controlled. If a stone is calcium oxalate, foods high in oxalate (see Box 21-3) should be limited.

Other dietary factors to consider in the case of calcium stones are sodium, fluid, and fiber intake. High salt intake increases the amount of calcium excretion in the urine,

thus precipitating hypercalciuria. General recommendations for individuals at risk for stone formation from hypercalciuria are to restrict sodium intake.[23] Drinking plenty of fluids (2.5 to 3 L/day) is beneficial in preventing all types of kidney stones by diluting the urine.[23] Fiber foods high in phytates help prevent crystallization of oxalate calcium salts.

Uric Acid Stones

Approximately 9% of the total incidence of renal calculi are uric acid stones.[19] Because uric acid is a metabolic product of purines, a low-purine diet sometimes is recommended. If dietary control of purines is desired, the following foods should be limited: organ meats, alcoholic beverages, anchovies, sardines, yeast, legumes, mushrooms, spinach, asparagus, cauliflower, and poultry.

Cystine Stones

Dietary modifications are geared toward reducing urinary cystine concentrations by decreasing intake and diluting the urine. Cystine is derived from the essential amino acid methionine; thus a low-methionine diet sometimes is used. Diluting the urine may require up to 4 L/day of water in adults.[24]

General dietary principles regarding kidney stone disease are summarized in Table 21-7.

TABLE 21-7

SUMMARY OF DIETARY PRINCIPLES IN KIDNEY STONE DISEASE

STONE CHEMISTRY	NUTRIENT MODIFICATION
Calcium	Normal calcium, lower protein and salt
Phosphate	Low phosphorus (1000-1200 mg)
Oxalate	Low oxalate
Struvite	Low phosphorus (1000-1200 mg; associated with urinary infections)
Uric acid	Low purine
Cystine	Low methionine

---

acid and alkaline diets a diet based on the theory that diets high in acidic foods, such as animal protein, caffeine, and simple sugars, will disrupt the body's normal pH balance, which is slightly alkaline.

SUMMARY

The nephrons are the functional units of the kidneys. Through these unique structures the kidney maintains life-sustaining blood levels of materials required for life and health. The nephrons accomplish their tremendous task by constantly cleaning the blood many times each day, returning necessary elements to the blood and eliminating the remainder in concentrated urine. Various diseases that interfere with the vital function of nephrons can cause kidney disease.

At its end stage, CKD is treated by dialysis or kidney transplant. Patients undergoing dialysis require close monitoring for protein, water, and electrolyte balance. Kidney diseases have predisposing factors (e.g., recurrent urinary tract infections may lead to renal calculi, and progressive glomerulonephritis may lead to chronic nephrotic syndrome and kidney failure).

Kidney stones may be formed from a variety of substances. For some patients a change in dietary intake of the identified substance (e.g., fluid, sodium, oxalate, purine) may decrease stone formation.

CRITICAL THINKING QUESTIONS

1. For each of the following conditions, outline the nutrition components of therapy, explaining the effect of each on kidney function: glomerulonephritis, nephrotic syndrome, and CKD.
2. Consider the nutrition factors that must be monitored in persons undergoing kidney dialysis. How would you suggest a client self-monitor fluid intake to meet hydration needs while not exceeding restrictions? Make a general list of dietary sources of fluid.
3. Outline the medical and nutrition therapy for patients on hemodialysis and peritoneal dialysis. What are the critical differences and why?

CHAPTER CHALLENGE QUESTIONS

True-False

Write the correct statement for each statement that is false.

1. *True or False:* The basic functional unit of the kidney is the nephron.
2. *True or False:* Only a few nephrons are present in each kidney, so metabolic stress can easily cause problems.
3. *True or False:* Operation of the nephrons relates little to the rest of the body.
4. *True or False:* The main function of the glomerulus is filtration.
5. *True or False:* The tasks of the various parts of the nephron tubules are reabsorption, secretion, and excretion.
6. *True or False:* Dietary modifications in acute glomerulonephritis usually involve crucial restrictions of protein and sodium.
7. *True or False:* The primary symptom in nephrotic syndrome is massive albuminuria.
8. *True or False:* Nephrotic syndrome is best treated by a very low protein diet.
9. *True or False:* The multiple symptoms of advanced CKD result from metabolic imbalances in the body's inability to handle protein, electrolytes, and water.
10. *True or False:* Prolonged immobilization (e.g., with full body casts or disability) may lead to withdrawal of bone calcium and the formation of calcium kidney stones.

Multiple Choice

1. Acute glomerulonephritis is best treated by which of the following methods? *(Circle all that apply.)*
   a. Reducing protein because filtration is impaired
   b. Using a normal amount of protein for optimal tissue nutrition and growth
   c. Restricting sodium to 1500 mg/day
   d. Allowing moderate salt use in uncomplicated cases

2. Diet therapy in nephrotic syndrome is designed to perform which of the following functions? *(Circle all that apply.)*
   a. Increase protein to replace the massive losses.
   b. Moderately decrease protein to reduce albumin losses.
   c. Increase kilocalories to provide energy and spare protein for tissue needs.
   d. Moderately restrict sodium to help prevent edema.

3. The general diet needs in CKD include which of the following? *(Circle all that apply.)*

a. Reduced protein intake

b. Increased carbohydrate and moderate fat for needed energy

c. Careful control of sodium and potassium according to need

d. Increased fluids to stimulate kidney function

evolve Please refer to the Students' Resource section of this text's Evolve Web site for additional study resources.

REFERENCES

1. U.S. Department of Health and Human Services, Centers for Disease Control and Prevention, National Center for Health Statistics: *Summary health statistics for U.S. adults: National Health Interview Survey, 2005,* DHHS Publication No. (PHS) 2007-1560, Hyattsville, MD, 2006, U.S. Department of Health and Human Services.
2. Coresh J and others: Chronic kidney disease awareness, prevalence, and trends among U.S. adults, 1999 to 2000, *J Am Soc Nephrol* 16(1):180, 2005.
3. Levey AS and others: Definition and classification of chronic kidney disease: a position statement from Kidney Disease: Improving Global Outcomes (KDIGO), *Kidney Int* 67:2089, 2005.
4. Meek RL and others: Amino acids induce indicators of response to injury in glomerular mesangial cells, *Am J Physiol Renal Physiol* 285(1):F79, 2003.
5. Toto RD: Treatment of hypertension in chronic kidney disease, *Semin Nephrol* 25(6):435, 2005.
6. U.S. Renal Data System: *USRDS 2007 annual data report: atlas of chronic kidney disease and end-stage renal disease in the United States,* Bethesda, MD, 2007, National Institutes of Health.
7. American Diabetes Association: Diabetic nephropathy, *Diabetes Care* 26(1 suppl):94, 2003.
8. Kikkawa R and others: Progression of diabetic nephropathy, *Am J Kidney Dis* 41(1 suppl):19, 2003.
9. National Kidney Foundation: K/DOQI Clinical practice guidelines for chronic kidney disease: evaluation, classification and stratification, *Am J Kidney Dis* 39(2 suppl 1):S1, 2002.
10. Mahan LK, Escott-Stump S: *Krause's food, nutrition, and diet therapy,* ed 12, Philadelphia, 2008, Saunders.
11. Leblanc M and others: Risk factors for acute renal failure: inherent and modifiable risks, *Curr Opin Crit Care* 11(6):533, 2005.
12. Moore H and others: National Kidney Foundation Council on renal nutrition survey: past-present clinical practices and future strategic planning, *J Ren Nutr* 13(3):233, 2003.
13. Nolan CR: Strategies for improving long-term survival in patients with ESRD, *J Am Soc Nephrol* 16:S120, 2005.
14. Beto JA, Bansal VK: Medical nutrition therapy in chronic kidney failure: integrating clinical practice guidelines, *J Am Diet Assoc* 104:404, 2004.
15. Moe S and others: Definition, evaluation, and classification of renal osteodystrophy: a position statement from Kidney Disease: Improving Global Outcomes (KDIGO), *Kidney Int* 69(11):1945, 2006.
16. Kalantar-Zadeh K and others: Survival advantages of obesity in dialysis patients, *Am J Clin Nutr* 81(3):543, 2005.
17. Burrowes JD and others: Cross-sectional relationship between dietary protein and energy intake, nutritional status, functional status, and comorbidity in older versus younger hemodialysis patients, *J Ren Nutr* 12(2):87, 2002.
18. Burrowes JD and others: Effects of dietary intake, appetite, and eating habits on dialysis and non-dialysis treatment days in hemodialysis patients: cross-sectional results from the HEMO study, *J Ren Nutr* 13(3):191, 2003.
19. Coe FL and others: Kidney stone disease, *J Clin Invest* 115(10):2598, 2005.
20. Massey LK: Dietary influences on urinary oxalate and risk of kidney stones, *Front Biosci* 8:s584, 2003.
21. Koff SG and others: Comparison between lemonade and potassium citrate and impact on urine pH and 24-hour urine parameters in patients with kidney stone formation, *Urology* 69(6):1013, 2007.
22. Moyad MA: Calcium oxalate kidney stones: another reason to encourage moderate calcium intakes and other dietary changes, *Urol Nurs* 23(4):310, 2003.
23. Finkielstein VA, Goldfarb DS: Strategies for preventing calcium oxalate stones, *CMAJ* 174(10):1407, 2006.
24. Grases F and others: Renal lithiasis and nutrition, *Nutr J* 5:23, 2006.

FURTHER READING AND RESOURCES

National Institute of Diabetes and Digestive and Kidney Diseases: *www.niddk.nih.gov*

National Kidney Foundation: *www.kidney.org*

American Urological Association: *www.auafoundation.org/*

Nephrology Channel: *www.nephrologychannel.com*
These Web sites provide additional information on various forms of kidney disease. Several national organizations provide free education and support for health care providers, patients, and family. Dietary restrictions for patients with kidney disease can sometimes be overwhelming. To fully understand such diets, continuous follow-up and feedback are needed.

Hebert CJ: Preventing kidney failure: primary care physicians must intervene earlier, *Cleve Clin J Med* 70(4):337, 2003.

Coe FL and others: Kidney stone disease, *J Clin Invest* 115(10):2598, 2005.
These articles highlight the risk factors and early signs of decreased kidney function and kidney stone formation. The authors address the important roles of physicians and nurses in identifying such factors.

CHAPTER 22

Surgery and Nutrition Support

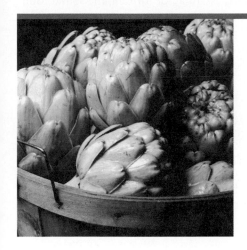

KEY CONCEPTS

- Surgical treatment requires added nutrition support for tissue healing and rapid recovery.
- Nutrition problems related to GI surgery require diet modifications because of the surgery's effect on normal food passage.
- To ensure optimal nutrition for surgery patients, diet management may involve enteral and/or parenteral nutrition support.

Malnutrition continues to occur among hospitalized patients. A review of the literature indicates that 23% of elderly hospitalized patients have clinical signs of malnutrition, which hinders healing.[1] Effective nutrition support must reverse malnutrition, improve prognosis, and speed recovery in a cost-effective manner. The surgical process also places physiologic and psychological stress on patients, bringing added nutrition demands and increased risks for clinical problems.

This chapter looks at the nutrition needs of surgical patients and the enteral and parenteral feeding methods of providing nutrition support. Careful attention to both preoperative and postoperative nutrition support can reduce complications and provide essential resources for healing and health.

NUTRITION NEEDS OF GENERAL SURGERY PATIENTS

A patient undergoing surgery faces large physiologic and psychological stress. As a result, nutrition demands are increased during this period and deficiencies can develop, leading to malnutrition and clinical complications. Therefore careful attention must be given to a patient's nutrition status in preparation for surgery as well as to the individual nutrition needs that follow for wound healing and recovery. A significant amount of research has been dedicated to understanding the association between protein energy malnutrition and clinical outcomes. Although the defining factors for diagnosing protein energy malnu-

---

enteral a mode of feeding that uses the GI tract through oral or tube feeding.

parenteral a mode of feeding that does not use the GI tract but provides nutrition support by IV delivery of nutrient solutions.

trition have varied, poor nutrition status and the following clinical problems are well accepted[2,3]:

- Impaired wound healing
- Increased risk of postoperative infection
- Reduced quality of life
- Impaired function of the GI tract
- Impaired immune system
- Impaired functioning of the cardiovascular and respiratory systems
- Increased hospital stay
- Increased cost
- Increased mortality rate

Preoperative Nutrition Care: Nutrient Reserves

When the surgery is elective (i.e., not necessary or emergency), body nutrient stores can be built up to fortify a patient for the demands of the surgery and the period immediately following, when food intake may be limited. Commercial formulas provide needed nutrition supplementation. Particular needs center on protein, energy, vitamins, and minerals.

Protein

Protein deficiencies among surgical patients on admission are common (see the For Further Focus box, "Protein Energy Malnutrition during Surgery and Illness"). Every patient facing surgery must be equipped with adequate body protein in tissue and plasma to counteract blood losses during surgery and prevent tissue catabolism in the immediate postoperative period. For example, extensive bone healing may be involved in orthopedic surgery. Protein is essential for forming the sound foundation that anchors mineral matter in bone tissue and is especially important with the occurrence of bone fractures in the growing U.S. population of elderly persons, particularly older women.[4]

Energy

Sufficient energy must be provided when increased protein is necessary for tissue building. The increased source of kilocalories supports the added energy demands and spares protein for its tissue-building work. For example, increased carbohydrate intake is needed to maintain optimal glycogen stores in the liver as a necessary resource

---

 ## FOR FURTHER FOCUS

PROTEIN ENERGY MALNUTRITION DURING SURGERY AND ILLNESS

Protein energy malnutrition (PEM) compromises quality of life and the ability to recover from surgery and injury. As general health declines with age and the risk for unplanned surgery increases, so does the prevalence of PEM.* Actively evaluating the nutritional status of older people in the home, hospital, or nursing home may provide valuable information about the preoperative needs of these individuals.† Oral supplements or enteral feedings for malnourished elderly patients before surgery may be a cost-effective way to improve outcome, reduce hospital stay, and reduce the risk of complications associated with surgery.

Even without a formal nutrition assessment, PEM can be identified by monitoring unplanned weight loss. Unplanned weight loss is indicative of PEM and the compromised ability to deal with physiologic stress. An unplanned weight loss of up to 5% over a 1-month period, or 10% over a 6-month period, is considered a significant loss. Unintentional weight loss greater than 5% in 1 month or 10% in 6 months is classified as severe. Identifying and treating those individuals at risk for PEM also may prevent poor outcome in the event of surgery or injury.

The following table provides a quick guide to evaluate weight loss:

Weight Loss (%) and Resulting Weight (lb)		
Initial Weight (lb)	5%	10%
80	76	72
85	81	77
90	86	81
95	90	86
100	95	90
110	105	99
120	114	108
130	124	117
140	133	126
150	143	135
160	152	144
170	162	153
180	171	162

*Crogan NL, Pasvogel A: The influence of protein-calorie malnutrition on quality of life in nursing homes, *J Gerontol A Biol Sci Med Sci* 58(2):159, 2003.
†Guigoz Y: The Mini Nutritional Assessment (MNA) review of the literature—what does it tell us? *J Nutr Health Aging* 10(6):466, 2006.

TABLE 22-1

NONRESIDUE DIET*

FOOD TYPE	FOODS ALLOWED	FOODS NOT ALLOWED
Beverages	Carbonated beverages, coffee, tea	Milk, milk drinks
Bread	Crackers, Melba or Rusk	Whole-grain bread
Cereals	Refined as Cream of Wheat, farina, fine cornmeal, Malt-O-Meal, Pablum, rice, strained oatmeal, cornflakes, puffed rice, Rice Krispies	Whole-grain and other cereals
Cheese		None allowed
Desserts	Plain cakes and cookies, gelatin desserts, water ices, angel food cake, arrowroot cookies, tapioca puddings made with fruit juice only	Pastries, all others
Eggs	As desired, preferably hard cooked	Fried eggs
Fats	Butter or substitute, small amount of cream	All others
Fruits	Strained fruit juices	All others
Meat, fish, poultry	Tender beef, chicken, fish, lamb, liver, veal; crisp bacon	Fried or tough meat, pork
Potatoes or substitute	Only macaroni, noodles, spaghetti, refined rice	Potatoes, corn, hominy, unrefined rice
Soup	Bouillon and broth only	All others
Sweets†	Hard candy, fondant, gumdrops, jelly, marshmallows, sugar, syrup, honey	Other candy, jam, marmalade
Vegetables	Tomato juice	All others
Miscellaneous	Salt	Pepper

*Presurgery nonresidue diet: This diet includes only foods free from fiber, seeds, and skins and with a minimal amount of residue. Fruits and vegetables are omitted except for strained fruit juices. Milk is omitted. The diet is adequate in protein and energy, containing approximately 75 g protein, 100 g fat, 250 g carbohydrate, and 2260 kcal. It is likely to be inadequate in vitamin A, calcium, and riboflavin. If patients are to remain on this diet for a long period, supplementary vitamins and minerals should be administered.
Postsurgical nonresidue diet: This diet is slightly higher in residue but has greater variety, including potatoes (without skin); white bread products (without bran); processed cheeses; sauces; desserts made with milk (but no fruits or nuts); and cream (2 oz) for coffee, cereal, and gravy. The average daily menu contains 85 g protein, 2300 kcal, and slightly more vitamins and minerals.
†Fruit juice and hard candies may be consumed between meals to increase caloric intake.

for immediate energy, thus directing protein to its tissue synthesis task. If a person is underweight, extra energy may be required to increase weight to an ideal maintenance level before surgery. If a person is overweight and the surgery is elective, some weight reduction may help reduce surgical complications.

Vitamins and Minerals

When increased protein and energy are necessary, the appropriate intake of vitamins and minerals involved in protein and energy metabolism (e.g., B vitamins) also must be supplied. Any deficiency state (e.g., iron-deficiency anemia) should be corrected. Electrolyte and water balance are necessary to prevent dehydration.

Immediate Preoperative Period

Usual preparation for surgery calls for nothing to be taken orally for at least 8 hours before the surgery. This preparation is necessary to ensure that the stomach retains no food at surgery, which may cause complications such as aspiration of food particles during anesthesia or recovery from anesthesia. In addition, any food present in the

stomach may interfere with the surgical procedure or increase the risk for postoperative gastric retention and expansion. Before GI surgery, a nonresidue diet may be followed for several days to clear the surgical site of any food residue (Table 22-1). Commercial nonresidue elemental formulas can provide a complete diet in liquid form. These formulas can be administered by tube or made more palatable for oral use with various flavorings.

Emergency Surgery

If the surgery is urgent, no time is available for building up ideal nutrition reserves, which is another reason to maintain good nutrition status through a healthy diet at

catabolism metabolic process of breaking down large substances to yield the smaller building blocks.

elemental formula a nutrition support formula composed of simple elemental nutrient components that require no further digestive breakdown and are thus readily absorbed.

all times. Optimal nutrient reserves are then available to supply needs during times of stress.

Postoperative Nutrition Care: Nutrient Needs for Healing

Adequate nutrition support is necessary to aid recovery from surgery when nutrient losses are great. At the same time, food intake is diminished or even absent for a period. Several nutrients require particular attention during this time.

Protein

Optimal protein intake in the postoperative recovery period is of primary concern for all patients. Protein is needed to replace losses during surgery and supply increased demands for the healing process. During the period immediately after surgery, body tissues usually undergo considerable catabolism, which means that the process of tissue breakdown and loss exceeds the process of tissue buildup. Weight loss and malnutrition are common in patients experiencing catabolic stress. Although maintenance of lean body mass improves survival of catabolic patients, malnutrition or marginal nutritional states are common in hospitalized surgical patients. Some research supports the use of branched-chain amino acids in particular to help alleviate the burden of muscle wasting and increase recovery time during this phase.[5]

In addition to protein losses from tissue breakdown, other losses of protein from the body may occur. These losses include plasma protein loss from hemorrhage, wound bleeding, and various body fluid losses, or exudates. Increased loss of plasma protein from extensive tissue destruction, inflammation, infection, and trauma should be monitored. If any degree of prior malnutrition or chronic infection existed, a patient's protein deficiency could easily become severe and cause complications. Several reasons exist for this increased protein demand.

Building Tissue. The process of wound healing requires building a great deal of new body tissue, which depends on adequate essential amino acids. Necessary amino acids must come from dietary protein (oral or tube feedings) or from parenteral nutrition if a patient cannot eat or tolerate enteral feedings for an extended period. Dietary protein recommendations may increase above normal needs to restore lost protein and build new tissues at the wound site.

Controlling Edema. When serum protein levels are low, osmotic pressure is lost and edema develops. Edema is characterized by puffiness or swelling of the tissue from the excess fluid being held there instead of returning to circulation. Generalized edema may adversely affect heart and lung function. Local edema at the wound site also interferes with closure of the wound and hinders the normal healing process.

Controlling Shock. A sufficient supply of plasma protein, mainly albumin, is necessary to maintain blood volume. If the plasma protein level drops, pressure to keep tissue fluid circulating between the capillaries and cells is insufficient. Without adequate pressure, water leaves the capillaries and cannot be drawn back into circulation resulting in edema. Shock symptoms result from a loss of blood volume and the body's effort to restore it.

Healing Bone. Protein, as well as mineral matter, is essential to the foundation of bone tissue for proper formation and healing. Protein provides a matrix for calcium and phosphorus, which is required for bone callus and strong bones.

Resisting Infection. Protein tissues are the major components of the body's immune system, providing its defense against infection. These defense agents include specialized white cells called *lymphocytes* as well as antibodies and various other blood cells, hormones, and enzymes. Tissue strength is a major defense barrier against infection at all times.

Transporting Lipids. Fat also is an important component of tissue structure, forming the lipid by-layer of cell membranes and participating in many other necessary metabolic activities. Protein is necessary for fat transportation in the bloodstream to all tissues (e.g., lipoproteins). Protein also is necessary to carry fat to the liver for metabolism. Protein in the liver combines with and removes fat, thus avoiding the danger of fatty infiltration, which could lead to liver disease.

Because protein has many important functions during recovery from surgery, protein deficiency at this time can lead to many clinical problems. Such problems include poor wound healing, rupture of the suture lines (dehiscence), delayed healing of fractures, depressed heart and lung function, anemia, failure of GI stomas, reduced resistance to infection, liver damage, extensive weight loss, and increased risk of death.

Water

Surgery induces altered fluid distribution in the patient, which can reduce circulation and hinder recovery.[6] Sufficient fluid intake is necessary to prevent dehydration. Elderly patients, whose thirst mechanism may be depressed, warrant special attention to total intake and hydration status. In patients who have complications or are seriously ill and have extensive drainage, as much as 7 L of fluid daily may be necessary. During the postoperative period, large water losses also may occur from vomiting, hemorrhage, fever, infection, or diuresis. A variety of solutions are available for intravenous (IV) administration depending on the patient's needs. IV fluids after surgery supply some initial hydration needs, but oral intake should begin as soon as possible and be sufficiently maintained.

Energy

As always, when increased protein is demanded for tissue building, enough nonprotein kilocalories must be provided for energy to spare protein for its vital tissue-building function. Therefore the fuel sources, carbohydrate and fat, must be sufficient in the total diet. Because excess fat presents general health problems, carbohydrates become the major source of needed fuel. For adults, a minimum of 130 g carbohydrates must be supplied on a daily basis to spare protein from catabolism.[7] In situations of acute metabolic stress (e.g., in extensive surgery or burns), energy needs may increase to as much as 1.2 to 2 kcal/kg body weight per day over basal energy requirements. Energy requirements can be estimated by first calculating basal energy needs with the Mifflin-St. Jeor equations and then multiplying by an injury factor (1.2 to 2) to meet added energy needs for stress and sepsis:

> Male: BMR = (10 × Weight in kg) +
>   (6.25 × Height in cm) − (5 × Age in yrs) + 5
> Female: BMR = (10 × Weight in kg) +
>   (6.25 × Height in cm) − (5 × Age in yrs) − 161

Energy needs for burn patients depend directly on percent of body surface area (BSA) burned and are calculated as follows[8]:

> Energy needs = 20 kcal/kg + (40 × % of BSA burned)

Carbohydrates spare protein for tissue building and help avoid liver damage by maintaining glycogen reserves in the liver tissue. However, excessive fuel storage as body fat should be avoided because fatty tissue heals poorly and is more susceptible to infection.

Vitamins

Several vitamins require particular attention in wound healing. Vitamin C helps build connective tissue, new capillary walls, and general tissue ground substance. In vitro studies demonstrate that the addition of vitamin C to cell culture media improves the cell's epidermal barrier, metabolic viability, DNA synthesis, and ability to heal.[9] If extensive tissue building is necessary, as much as 1150 to 3000 mg/day vitamin C may be beneficial in the postoperative period.[10,11] (Long-term supplementation at this level is not recommended.) As energy and protein intake are increased, the B vitamins that have important coenzyme roles in protein and energy metabolism (e.g.,

thiamin, riboflavin, and niacin) must be increased. Other B-complex vitamins—folate, B_{12}, pyridoxine, and pantothenic acid—play important roles in building hemoglobin and thus must meet the demands of an increased blood supply and general metabolic stress. Vitamin K, which is essential for blood clotting, usually is present in a sufficient amount because it is synthesized by intestinal bacteria. However, patients treated with antibiotics may have decreased gut flora and vitamin K synthesis.

Minerals

Attention to any mineral deficiencies is essential. Tissue catabolism results in cell potassium and phosphorus loss. Electrolyte imbalances of sodium and chloride also result from fluid imbalances. Iron-deficiency anemia may develop from blood loss or inadequate iron absorption (see the Drug-Nutrient Interaction box, "Aspirin and Iron Absorption"). Another mineral important in wound healing is zinc. An adequate amount of protein usually meets this need because most dietary zinc is found in protein foods of animal origin such as beef, crab, lobster, and oysters. However, suboptimal zinc status is common in elderly patients, young children, and those with inadequate food intake.[12] Recent studies evaluating zinc supplementation in the prevention of diarrhea and respiratory illness in children and infection and oxidative stress

---

exudate various materials such as cells, cellular debris, and fluids, usually resulting from inflammation, that have escaped from the blood vessels and are deposited in or on the surface tissues; protein content is high.

osmotic pressure hydrostatic pressure across a semipermeable membrane necessary to maintain normal movement of fluid between the capillaries and surrounding tissue.

edema an unusual accumulation of fluid in the interstitial (e.g., small structural spaces between tissue parts) spaces of the body.

callus unorganized meshwork of newly grown, woven bone developed on a pattern of the original clot of fibrin, formed after fracture or surgery, and normally replaced in the healing process by hard adult bone.

dehiscence a splitting open; the separation of layers of a surgical wound—partial, superficial, or complete—with total disruption and requiring resuturing.

stoma the opening established in the abdominal wall, connecting with the ileum or colon, for elimination of intestinal wastes after surgical removal of diseased portions of the intestines.

diuresis increased excretion of urine.

DRUG-NUTRIENT INTERACTION

ASPIRIN AND IRON ABSORPTION

Aspirin is one of the most common analgesics used in the United States today. Its use is implicated in other conditions as well, such as transient ischemic attacks (mini strokes), myocardial infarctions, arthritis and other inflammatory diseases, blood clotting disorders, and insomnia.*

Long-term aspirin use may lead to poor iron absorption. The acetylsalicylic acid found in aspirin can irritate the stomach lining and prevent or slow normal excretion of gastric acid. Gastric acid is needed to keep iron in its Fe^{3+} state until absorption can occur in the duodenum. When gastric acid levels are low, iron-deficiency anemia may result.†

For greatest absorption, aspirin should be taken *on an empty stomach with a large glass of water*. This dilutes the acetylsalicylic acid, thereby reducing the erosion of the stomach lining. Aspirin may be taken with other liquids but never with alcohol. It increases the bioavailability of alcohol and thus increases the risk for adverse side effects.

Sara Oldroyd

*Schlenker ED, Long S: *Williams' essentials of nutrition and diet therapy*, ed 9, St Louis, 2007, Mosby.
†Mayoclinic.Com: *Iron deficiency anemia, www.mayoclinic.com/health/iron-deficiency-anemia/ds00323,* accessed March 2007.

TABLE 22-2

DIET PROGRESSION AFTER GASTRIC BYPASS

DIET	AMOUNT	TYPICAL PROGRESSION
Clear liquids	No more than ½ cup total	1 to 2 days after surgery
Full liquids	Gradually increase from ½ cup to no more than ¾ cup total	3 days to 3 weeks after surgery
Pureed	Meals should be from ¾ cup to no more than 1 cup total	3 to 6 weeks after surgery
Regular (small meals and snacks)	No more than 1 cup total; meat should be no more than 2 oz	6 weeks and beyond

General guidelines: (1) Patients need to spread the meal out for 20 minutes or more to avoid bolus eating and allow the feeling of satiety to occur. (2) Food should be well chewed and eaten in small volumes. (3) Liquids should be either ingested well before meals or at least 30 minutes afterwards. (4) Protein should preferably be eaten before fats and carbohydrates, ideally in an amount of at least 60 g daily.
Reprinted from Mahan LK, Escott-Stump S: *Krause's food & nutrition therapy*, ed 12, St Louis, 2008, Saunders; and Marcason W: What are the dietary guidelines following bariatric surgery? *J Am Diet Assoc* 104(3):488, 2004.

in elderly patients concluded that patients receiving supplemental zinc had a significant reduction in illness.[13,14]

Special considerations must be made for patients after bariatric surgery because they typically have deficiencies in macronutrients and micronutrients for an extended period.[15] After gastric bypass, patients progress from a clear liquid diet to a regular diet but are limited to approximately 1 cup of food per meal from that point forward (Table 22-2; see the For Further Focus box, "Nutrient Deficiencies in the Bariatric Patient").

GENERAL DIETARY MANAGEMENT

Initial Intravenous Fluid and Electrolytes

Most general surgical patients can and should progress to oral feedings as soon as possible to provide adequate nutrition. Remember that routine IV fluids are used to supply hydration needs and electrolytes, not to sustain energy and nutrients. For example, a 5% dextrose solution with normal saline (0.9% NaCl solution) contains only 5 g dextrose/dl (approximately 200 kcal/L), although the patient's total energy need is more than 10 times that amount. A rapid return to regular eating should be encouraged and maintained.

Methods of Feeding

The following three basic methods for dietary management are available:

- *Oral:* nourishment through the regular GI route by oral feedings; may include a variety of diet plans, textures, and meal replacement liquid supplements.
- *Enteral:* technically refers to nourishment through the regular GI route either by regular oral feedings or tube feedings. However, in medical nutrition therapy, enteral feedings mean tube feedings.
- *Parenteral:* nourishment through veins, either small peripheral veins or a large central vein.

FOR FURTHER FOCUS

NUTRIENT DEFICIENCIES AFTER BARIATRIC SURGERY

Bariatric surgery for obese patients (defined as a BMI of >30 kg/m²) is becoming more common around the world. Although surgery currently is the most effective means of long-term weight loss and maintenance, it is not without drawbacks. Restrictive eating patterns, dumping syndrome, and nutrition deficiencies from malabsorption are common complications after surgery. The quality of life cost/benefit ratio of surgery is difficult to assess because obesity increases mortality rate, but the complications of surgery can introduce a new set of risks.

The roux-en-Y gastric bypass (see Chapter 15), in which the amount of bowel capable of absorbing nutrients is reduced, is the surgery of choice for obesity in the United States. Obese patients are at increased risk for complications during surgery from comorbid conditions such as diseases of the cardiovascular, endocrine, renal, pulmonary, GI, and musculoskeletal systems.* Therefore special care must be taken in preparing the patient for surgery.

Nutrient deficiencies from malabsorptive procedures, such as gastric bypass and biliopancreatic diversion, warrant mineral and multivitamin supplementation postoperatively.† Following are specific nutrients to be aware of:

- *Roux-en-Y gastric bypass:* iron, vitamin B₁₂, vitamin D, and calcium
- *Biliopancreatic diversion:* protein and fat-soluble vitamins

*Eisenberg D and others: Update on obesity surgery, *World J Gastroenterol* 12(20):3196, 2006.
†Alvarez-Leite JI: Nutrient deficiencies secondary to bariatric surgery, *Curr Opin Clin Nutr Metab Care* 7(5):569, 2004.

When a patient is capable of meeting nutrient needs by oral feedings, and feedings are well tolerated, that is the feeding method of choice. Table 22-3 lists conditions that often require nutrition support by tube feeding or parenteral nutrition. General criteria for selecting the most appropriate nutrition support method are listed in Box 22-1.

Oral Feedings

When the GI tract can be used, it is the preferred route of feeding—orally if possible and by feeding tube if not. Most general surgical patients can and should receive oral feedings as soon as possible. Oral feedings provide needed nutrients and help stimulate normal action of the GI tract. Food usually can be taken orally as soon as peristalsis and passing of flatus return. When oral feedings begin, the patient progresses from clear to full liquids and then to a soft or regular diet as indicated. Examples of these progressive routine house diets used in hospitals are given in Chapter 17. Individual tolerance and needs are always the guide, but encouragement and help should be supplied in the general care of postsurgery patients to facilitate eating as soon as possible. Depending on a patient's condition, a general food supplement formula such as Boost may be added orally, with or between meals. The energy value of foods in the regular diet also may be increased as tolerated with added sauces, dried protein powder, and dressings. More frequent, less-bulky, concentrated small meals may be helpful, making every bite count.

Enteral Feeding

When regular oral feedings are not tolerated, nutrient formulas may be fed by tube. Enteral tube feedings preserve gut function, are noninvasive, and less expensive than parenteral nutrition. The most common route is the nasogastric tube, which is inserted through the nose and down to the stomach. For patients at risk for aspiration, reflux, or continuous vomiting, a nasoduodenal or nasojejunal tube may be more appropriate (Figure 22-1). In both cases, a tube is first inserted through the nose into the stomach. Then it is passed through the stomach and into the appropriate portion of the small intestine by peristaltic activity or endoscopic or fluoroscopic guidance. Correct placement of the tube is verified by radiography, auscultation, or gastric content aspiration. Modern small-bore nasoenteric feeding tubes made of softer, more flexible polyurethane and silicone materials have replaced large-bore, stiff tubing. These feeding tubes are relatively comfortable for the patient and easily carry the variety of nutrient materials available in enteral nutrition support formulas. With the development of improved formulas and feeding equipment, the question of using blender-mixed formulas of regular foods seldom arises. Using pureed table food for tube feedings may present the following problems:

- *Physical form*: Foods broken down and mixed in a blender yield a sticky, larger particle mixture that does not go through the small feeding tubes easily and thus require the more uncomfortable, large-bore tubing.
- *Safety*: Blender-mixed formulas carry problems of bacterial growth and infection as well as inconsistent nutrient composition because the solid components settle out.

auscultation listening to the sounds of the GI tract with a stethoscope.

TABLE 22-3

CONDITIONS OFTEN REQUIRING NUTRITION SUPPORT

RECOMMENDED ROUTE OF FEEDING	CONDITION	TYPICAL DISORDERS
Enteral nutrition	Impaired nutrient ingestion Neurologic disorders	HIV/AIDS Facial trauma Oral or esophageal trauma Congenital anomalies Respiratory failure Cystic fibrosis Traumatic brain injury
	Inability to consume adequate nutrition orally	Hyperemesis of pregnancy Hypermetabolic states such as burns Comatose states Anorexia in congestive heart failure, cancer, chronic obstructive pulmonary disease, eating disorders Congenital heart disease Impaired intake after orofacial surgery or injury Spinal cord injury
	Impaired digestion, absorption, metabolism	Severe gastroparesis Inborn errors of metabolism Crohn's disease Short-bowel syndrome with minimal resection
	Severe wasting or depressed growth	Cystic fibrosis Failure to thrive Cancer Sepsis Cerebral palsy Myasthenia gravis
Parenteral nutrition	GI incompetency Short-bowel syndrome, major resection	Severe acute pancreatitis Severe inflammatory bowel disease Small-bowel ischemia Intestinal atresia Severe liver failure Major GI surgery
	Critical illness with poor enteral tolerance or accessibility	Multiorgan system failure Major trauma or burns Bone marrow transplantation Acute respiratory failure with ventilator dependency and GI malfunction Severe wasting in renal failure with dialysis Small-bowel transplantation, immediately after surgery

Reprinted from Mahan LK, Escott-Stump S: *Krause's food & nutrition therapy,* ed 12, St Louis, 2008, Saunders.

■ *Digestion and absorption*: Pureed food requires a fully functioning GI system to digest the food and absorb its released nutrients. Many patients have GI deficits that require nutrients with varying degrees of predigestion (hydrolysis) or smaller molecular structure.

In comparison, commercial formulas provide a sterile, homogenized solution suitable for the more comfortable, small-bore feeding tubes and ensure a fixed profile of nutrients in intact or elemental form. No matter what type of feeding tube or formula is used to meet a patient's physiologic needs, this feeding method may contribute to a patient's psychological stress. Support for a patient's quality of life is an important part of patient care planning.

Alternative Routes for Enteral Tube Feeding. The nasoenteric route described usually is indicated for short-term therapy (less than 4 weeks) in many clinical situations. For long-term feedings, however, *enterostomies*—surgical placement of the tube at progressive points along the GI tract—provide a more comfortable route, as follows (see Figure 22-1):

■ *Esophagostomy*: A cervical esophagostomy is placed at the level of the cervical spine to the side of the neck after head and neck surgeries for cancer or traumatic injury. This placement removes the discomfort of the nasal route and enables the entry point to be easily concealed under clothing.

- *Percutaneous endoscopic gastrostomy*: A gastrostomy tube may be surgically placed through the abdominal wall into the stomach if a patient is not at risk for aspiration.
- *Percutaneous endoscopic jejunostomy*: A jejunostomy tube is surgically placed through the abdominal wall and passed through the duodenum into the jejunum, the middle section of the small intestine, if the patient is at risk for aspiration. This procedure is indicated for patients who lack a competent gag reflex or have gastric cancer or gastric ulcerative disease.

Tube-Feeding Formula. The tube-feeding formula generally is prescribed by the physician and clinical dietitian according to the patient's nutrition need and tolerance. In any form of tube feeding, the amount of formula and the rate at which it is given must be regulated. Highly concentrated formulas should be started at one quarter to one half of the goal rate of final delivery and advanced every 8 to 12 hours as tolerated. Patients who have not been fed in 5 days will not be able to tolerate large feedings and should start with slow rates (10 ml/hour), with gradual increases to goal rate. In patients fed by tube, diarrhea is the most frequently reported GI complication. Formulas supplemented with soluble fiber (pectin or

BOX 22-1

CRITERIA FOR SELECTING NUTRITION SUPPORT METHOD

Enteral nutrition support is indicated in patients who:
- Have a functional GI tract (at least 2 to 3 ft)
- Have adequate digestive and absorptive capacity of the GI tract but who cannot or will not eat enough to meet needs
- Are at risk for malnutrition without nutrition support

Parenteral nutrition support is indicated in patients who:
- Do not have sufficient GI tract function and need nutrition support for more than 5 days
- Do not have access for feeding tube placement and need nutrition support
- Repeatedly pull out feeding tubes

Peripheral Parenteral Nutrition
- Length of therapy less than 5 to 7 days
- Not hypermetabolic
- No fluid restriction

Central Parenteral Nutrition
- Length of therapy more than 5 to 7 days
- Hypermetabolic
- Fluid restriction
- Intolerance or allergy to IV lipids
- Poor peripheral access
- Central access already in place

Reprinted from Matarese LE, Gottschlich MM: *Contemporary nutrition support practice,* ed 2, St Louis, 2002, Saunders.

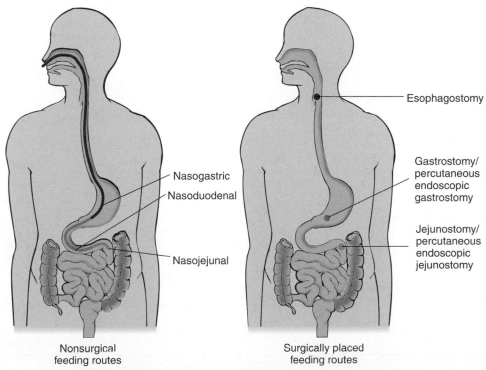

Nasogastric
Nasoduodenal
Nasojejunal

Esophagostomy
Gastrostomy/percutaneous endoscopic gastrostomy
Jejunostomy/percutaneous endoscopic jejunostomy

Nonsurgical feeding routes

Surgically placed feeding routes

Figure 22–1 Types of enteral feeding. (Copyright Rolin Graphics.)

guar gum) may improve bowel function and reduce the incidence of diarrhea.[16] However, fiber-supplemented formulas are contraindicated for patients with impaired gastric emptying. Medications and *Clostridium difficile* enterocolitis are common culprits that cause diarrhea and should be ruled out before further investigation or changes are made.

Several varieties of commercial formulas are available and designed to meet particular needs. These products may be made from *intact nutrients* for use with a fully functioning GI system able to digest and absorb them. Others may be made from predigested *elemental or semielemental nutrients*, which are readily absorbed with only minimal residue. Still others may be formulated for special problems or single-nutrient products (modules) of protein, carbohydrate, and fat mixed together as calculated by the dietitian or pharmacist to meet a patient's specific needs. Commercial enteral formulas have the advantage of standardized composition and are immedi-

ately available for use. These formulas also are sterile and may be stored. Some examples are given in Table 22-4. See the Clinical Applications box, "Calculating a Tube Feeding," for details on setting the rate of administration for a tube feeding.

Tube-fed patients require continuous monitoring for appropriate feeding schedules, tolerance, and potential complications. Box 22-2 provides guidelines for an ideal monitoring schedule, and Table 22-5 gives problem-solving suggestions for common issues encountered with tube feeding.

Parenteral Feedings

Parenteral nutrition refers to any feeding method other than the normal GI route. In current medical terminology, *parenteral nutrition* specifically refers to the special feeding of nutrients directly into the blood circulation through certain veins (i.e., peripheral vein in the arm or the subclavian vein) when the GI tract cannot be used.

TABLE 22-4

EXAMPLES OF ENTERAL FORMULAS AND MACRONUTRIENT COMPONENTS*

BRAND NAME	MANUFACTURER	SOURCES		
		CARBOHYDRATE	PROTEIN	FAT
Standard Complete Diets: Intact Macronutrients				
Ensure	Ross Products (Columbus, OH)	Corn syrup, sucrose	Casein	Soy oil, corn oil
Osmolite	Ross Products	Corn syrup	Casein, soy protein isolate	Canola oil, corn oil, MCT
Jevity (1 Cal)	Ross Products	Maltodextrin, corn syrup	Casein	Canola oil, corn oil, MCT
Standard Complete Diets: Semielemental and Elemental				
Vital HN	Ross Products	Maltodextrin	Whey protein concentrate	Safflower oil, MCT
Optimenal	Ross Products	Maltodextrin, sucrose	Soy protein hydrolysate	Structured lipids
Specialty Diets: Trauma				
Vivonex TEN	Novartis (Basel, Switzerland)	Maltodextrin	Free amino acids	Safflower oil
Promote	Ross Products	Maltodextrin, sucrose	Casein	Safflower oil, canola oil, MCT
Specialty Diets: Cancer, HIV, Renal				
Juven	Ross Products	Sucrose	Arginine, glutamine	None
Ensure Plus	Ross Products	Maltodextrin, sucrose	Casein	Canola oil, corn oil
Suplena	Rose Products	Maltodextrin, sucrose	Casein	Safflower oil, canola oil
Specialty Diets: Children Ages 1 to 10 Years				
PediaSure	Ross Products	Maltodextrin	Casein and whey	Safflower oil, soy oil, MCT
Kindercal	Bristol-Myers Squibb (New York, NY)	Maltodextrin, sucrose	Casein	Canola oil, sunflower oil, corn oil, MCT

*All formulas are enriched with essential micronutrients (vitamins and minerals) as needed.
MCT, Medium-chain triglycerides.

CLINICAL APPLICATIONS

CALCULATING A TUBE FEEDING

To calculate the nutrient needs of a patient, the following information is required:

1. Ideal body weight (IBW) in kilograms (lb/2.2)
   - Female: 100 lb ± 5 lb for every inch above or below 5 feet
   - Male: 106 lb ± 6 lb for every inch above or below 5 feet
2. Energy needs
   - BMR* × Injury factor (depending on the condition of the patient)
3. Total formula needed (Energy need [kcal/day] ÷ Formula [kcal/ml])
4. Feeding schedule (Total formula/Number of feedings)

Sample Calculation†

How much formula (in milliliters) does the following patient need at each feeding?

- 37-year-old woman, 5 feet, 7 inches tall
- Under considerable catabolic stress, with an injury factor of 1.8
- Energy value of formula: 1.5 kcal/ml
- Schedule: 6 feedings per day

1. **IBW**: 100 lb + (7 in × 5 lb) = 135 lb/2.2 = **61.4 kg**
2. **BMR**: (10 × 61.4 kg) + (6.25 × 170.2 cm) − (5 × 37) − 161 = **1332 kcal/day**

   1332 kcal/day × 1.8 = **2398 kcal/day**

3. **Formula**: 2398 kcal/day ÷ 1.5 kcal/ml = **1599 ml/day**
4. **Feeding schedule**: 1599 ml/day ÷ 6 feedings/day = **266.5 ml/feeding**

*As calculated by the Mifflin-St. Jeor equation: Female BMR = (10 × Weight) + (6.25 × Height) − (5 × Age) − 161; Male BMR= (10 × Weight) + (6.25 × Height) − (5 × Age) + 5.
†These equations require the weight in kilograms, the height in centimeters, and the age in years.

BOX 22-2

MONITORING THE PATIENT RECEIVING ENTERAL NUTRITION

- Weight (at least three times per week)
- Signs and symptoms of edema (daily)
- Signs and symptoms of dehydration (daily)
- Fluid intake and output (daily)
- Adequacy of enteral intake (at least twice per week)
- Abdominal distention and discomfort
- Gastric residuals (every 4 hours) if appropriate
- Serum electrolytes, BUN, creatinine (two to three times per week)
- Serum glucose, calcium, magnesium, phosphorus (weekly or as ordered)
- Stool output and consistency (daily)

Reprinted from Mahan LK, Escott-Stump S: *Krause's food & nutrition therapy,* ed 12, St Louis, 2008, Saunders.

Table 22-3 outlines indications for parenteral feedings. Depending on the nutrition support necessary, the following two routes are available:

- *Peripheral parenteral nutrition* is used when a solution of no more than 800 to 900 mOsm/L is sufficient to provide nutrient needs and when feeding is necessary for only a brief period (less than 5-7 days) or as supplemental to enteral feedings. The osmolality (mOsm/L) of a solution depends on the concentration of its total particles, including dextrose, protein, and electrolytes. Small peripheral veins, usually in the arm, are used to deliver the less-concentrated solutions (Figure 22-2). Some catheters allow an extended feeding period in a peripheral vein for individuals with large veins who can tolerate the *extended dwell catheter*.

- *Total parenteral nutrition (TPN)* is used when the energy and nutrient requirement is large or when full nutrition support is needed for longer periods. A large central vein, usually the subclavian vein leading directly into the rapid flow of the superior vena cava to the heart, is used for surgical placement of the catheter. The catheter may access the superior vena cava by (1) direct access (Figure 22-3, *A*), (2) a peripherally inserted central catheter (Figure 22-3, *B*), or (3) a tunneled catheter (Figure 22-3, *C*). Nutrition support solutions of much higher osmolality are tolerated in this vein.

TPN is used in cases of major surgery or complications, especially those involving the GI tract, or when the patient is unable to obtain sufficient nourishment enterally. TPN provides crucial nutrition support from solutions containing large amounts of glucose, amino acids, electrolytes, minerals, and vitamins. Fat in the form of lipid emulsions also is used to supply needed energy and the essential fatty acids. A basic TPN solution may contain between 3.5% and 15% crystalline amino acids and 2.5% to 70% dextrose with added electrolytes, vitamins, and trace elements (Table 22-6). The physician and clinical dietitian on the nutrition support team determine the individual formula needed on the basis of detailed individual nutrition assessment. The pharmacist on the

TABLE 22-5

PROBLEM-SOLVING TIPS FOR PATIENTS RECEIVING ENTERAL NUTRITION

PROBLEM	SUGGESTED SOLUTIONS
Thirst, oral dryness	Lubricate lips Chew sugarless gum Brush teeth Rinse mouth frequently *Caution:* Use lemon drops sparingly because of cariogenic effects; other hard candies are appropriate alternatives
Tube discomfort	Gargle with a mixture of warm water and mouthwash Gently blow nose Clean tube regularly with water or water-soluble lubricant If persistent, gently pull out tube, clean it, and reinsert Request smaller tube
Tension, fullness	Relax, breathe deeply after each feeding
Loud stomach noises	Take feedings in private
Limited mobility	Change positions in bed or chair Walk around the house or hospital corridor
Gustatory Distress*	
General dissatisfaction with feeding	Warm or chill feedings *Caution:* Feedings that are too cold may cause diarrhea Serve favorite foods that have been liquefied
Persistent hunger	Chew a favorite food, then spit it out Chew gum Suck hard candy
Inability to drink	Rinse mouth frequently with water and other liquids

*The frustration experienced when the sense of taste is not satisfied.

TABLE 22-6

EXAMPLE OF BASIC TPN FORMULA COMPONENTS

COMPONENT	AMOUNT
Basic Solution	
Crystalline amino acids	4%
Dextrose	25%
Additives	
Electrolytes	
Na	50 mEq/L
Cl	50 mEq/L
K	40 mEq/L
HPO_4	25 mEq/L
Ca	5 mEq/L
Mg	8 mEq/L
Vitamins	
Multivitamin supplement	1.7 ml/L
Vitamin C (per day)	200 mg
Trace Elements Solution (per Day)	
Zn	3 mg
Cu	0.4 mg
Cr	10 mcg
Se	120 mcg
Mn	2 mcg
I	120 mcg
Fe	1.5 mcg
Other Additives (as Needed)	

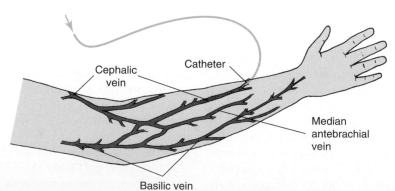

Figure 22–2 Peripheral parenteral nutrition feeding into small veins in the arm.

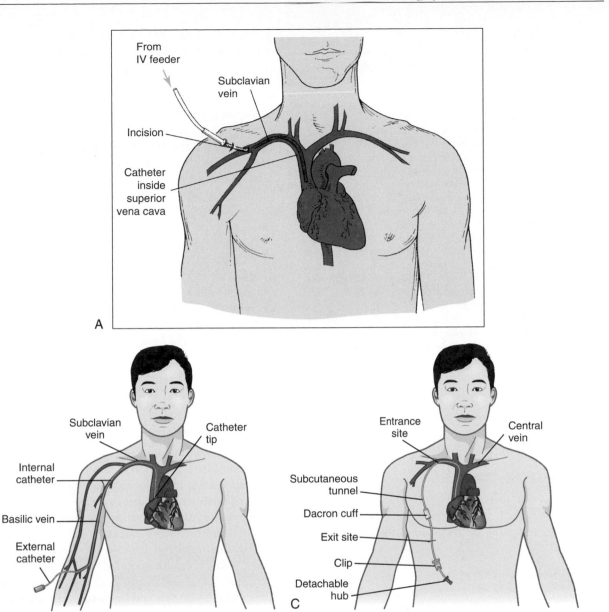

Figure 22–3 Catheter placement for TPN. **A,** Direct line by subclavian vein to superior vena cava. **B,** Peripherally inserted central catheter line. **C,** Tunneled catheter.

nutrition support team mixes the solutions according to the prescription. Administration of the solution is an important nursing responsibility (Box 22-3). Long-term home use of TPN has been a lifesaving measure for many persons but is expensive and requires thorough training.

SPECIAL NUTRITION NEEDS AFTER GASTROINTESTINAL SURGERY

Because the GI system is uniquely designed to handle food, a surgical procedure on any part of this system requires special dietary attention and modification.

Mouth, Throat, and Neck Surgery

Surgery involving the mouth, jaw, throat, or neck requires modification in the mode of eating. A patient usually cannot chew or swallow normally, so accommodations must be made according to individual limitations.

Oral Liquid Feedings

Concentrated liquid feedings should be planned to ensure adequate nutrition in a smaller amount of food. An enriched commercial formula can be used several times a day to supply needed nourishment.

BOX 22-3

ADMINISTRATION OF TPN FORMULA

Careful administration of TPN formulas is essential. Specific protocols vary somewhat but usually include the following points:

- *Start slowly.* Allow time to adapt to the increased glucose concentration and osmolality of the solution.
- *Schedule carefully.* During the first 24 hours, 1 to 2 L is administered by continuous drip, with the slow rate usually regulated by an infusion pump.
- *Monitor closely.* Note the metabolic effects of glucose (not to exceed 200 mg/dl) and electrolytes.
- *Increase volume gradually.* After the first day, increase by 1 L/day to reach the desired daily volume.
- *Make changes cautiously.* Watch the effect of all changes and proceed slowly.
- *Maintain a constant rate.* Keep the correct hourly infusion rate, with no "catch up" or "slow down" effort to meet the original volume order.
- *Discontinue slowly.* Take the patient off the TPN feeding gradually, reducing the rate and daily volume approximately 1 L/day. Patients are given dextrose 10% to help adjust to lower glucose levels.

Mechanical Soft Diets

Mechanical soft diets are used to transition between liquid and regular diets. Whole foods low in fiber and limited seasoning are included as tolerated (see Table 17-3).

Tube Feedings

In cases of radical neck or facial surgery, or when a patient is comatose or severely debilitated, tube feedings may be indicated. For long-term needs, improved equipment and standardized commercial formulas have made continued home tube feeding possible for many patients. A nasogastric tube often is used, but obstruction in the esophagus or other complications require the surgeon to make a gastrostomy at the time of surgery.

Gastric Surgery

Nutrition Problems

Because the stomach is the first major food reservoir in the GI tract, gastric surgery poses special problems in maintaining adequate nutrition. Some of these problems may develop immediately after the surgery, depending on the type of surgical procedure (see Figure 15-7) and

the individual patient's response. Other complications may occur later when the person begins to eat a regular diet.

Immediate Postoperative Period

Serious nutritional deficits may occur immediately after surgery, especially after a total gastrectomy. Increased gastric fullness and distention may result if the gastric resection also involved a vagotomy. Lacking the normal nerve stimulus, the stomach becomes atonic and empties poorly. Food fermentation occurs, producing *flatus*, or gas, and diarrhea. Weight loss is common after extensive gastric surgery.

To cover the immediate postoperative nutrition need after a gastrectomy procedure, surgeons usually prepare a jejunostomy through which the patient can be fed an elemental formula. Frequent small oral feedings are generally resumed according to a patient's tolerance. A typical pattern of simple dietary progression may cover approximately 2 weeks. The basic principles of such general diet therapy for the immediate postgastrectomy period involve the (1) size of meals (small and frequent) and (2) nature of meals (simple, easily digested, bland, and low in bulk).

Dumping Syndrome

Dumping syndrome is a frequently encountered complication after extensive gastric resection. After the initial recovery from surgery, when the patient begins to feel better and eats a regular diet in greater volume and variety, discomfort may occur 30 to 60 minutes after meals. A cramping, full feeling develops, the pulse becomes rapid, and a wave of weakness, cold sweating, and dizziness may follow. Nausea, vomiting, or diarrhea typically terminate the event. These distressing reactions to food increase anxiety. As a result, less and less food is eaten. Weight loss and general malnutrition follow (see the Clinical Applications box, "Case Study: John Has a Gastrectomy").

This complex of symptoms constitutes a shock syndrome that results when a meal containing a large proportion of readily soluble carbohydrates rapidly enters, or dumps, into the small intestine. When the stomach is bypassed, food quickly passes from the esophagus into the small intestine. This rapidly entering food mass is a concentrated solution (higher osmolality) in relation to the surrounding circulation of blood. To achieve an osmotic balance (i.e., a state of equal concentrations of fluids within the small intestine and surrounding blood circulation), water is drawn from the blood into the intestine. This water shift rapidly shrinks the vascular fluid volume, causing shock. Blood pressure drops and signs of rapid heart rate to rebuild the blood volume appear:

CLINICAL APPLICATIONS

CASE STUDY: JOHN HAS A GASTRECTOMY

After a long experience with persistent peptic ulcer disease involving more and more gastric tissue, John and his physician decided that surgery was needed. John then entered the hospital for a total gastrectomy. John weathered the surgery well and received some initial nutrition support from an elemental formula fed through a tube the surgeon had placed into his jejunum. After a few days the tube was removed and, over the next 2-week period, John was gradually able to take a soft diet in small oral feedings. He soon recovered enough to go home and gradually felt his strength returning. He was relieved to be free of his former ulcer pain and began to resume more and more of his usual activities, eating a regular diet of increasing volume and variety.

However, as time went by John began having more discomfort after meals. He felt a cramping sensation and increased heartbeat, and then a wave of weakness with sweating and dizziness. John often would become nauseated and vomit. As his anxiety increased he began to eat less and less and his weight began to drop. He was soon in a state of general malnutrition.

John finally returned to seek medical help. The physician and clinical dietitian outlined a change in his eating habits, and a special food plan was developed for him. Although the diet seemed strange to him, John followed it faithfully because he had felt so ill. To his surprise, he soon found that his previous symptoms after eating had almost completely disappeared. Because he felt so much better on the new diet plan, he formed new eating habits around it. His weight gradually returned to normal, and his state of nutrition markedly improved. John found that he always fared better if he would nibble on food items throughout the day rather than consume large meals as he used to do.

Questions for Analysis

1. What were John's nutrition needs immediately after surgery and over the next 2 weeks? Why did his feedings need to be resumed cautiously?
2. Why is emphasis given to postsurgical protein sources? How should this nutrient be provided?
3. Why must sufficient food for energy be consumed after surgery?
4. Why is fluid therapy important after surgery?
5. What minerals and vitamins are of most concern after surgery? Why?
6. After John began to feel better and resumed eating, why did he become ill? Describe his symptoms and why they developed.
7. Outline the principles of the special diet the dietitian provided to relieve John's symptoms. Plan a day's meal and snack pattern for John with basic instructions and suggestions you would discuss with him.

---

rapid pulse, sweating, weakness, and tremors. In approximately 2 hours a second sequence of events usually follows. The initial concentrated solution of carbohydrate has been rapidly digested and absorbed, resulting in a rapid rise in blood glucose and stimulating an overproduction of insulin. Blood sugar eventually drops below normal, with symptoms of mild hypoglycemia. Careful adherence to the postoperative diet allows dramatic relief from these distressing symptoms as well as gradual stabilization of weight (Table 22-7). Careful reintroduction of milk in small amounts may later be used to test tolerance. Patients also may find that eating slowly, eliminating fluids during meals, and lying down for 15 to 30 minutes after eating help decrease the rate of gastric emptying.

Gallbladder Surgery

For patients with acute gallbladder disease *(cholecystitis)* or gallstones *(cholelithiasis)* (Figure 22-4), the treatment usually is removal of the gallbladder, or *cholecystectomy*. The modern procedure for this removal requires only minimal surgery involving small skin punctures, called *laparoscopic cholecystectomy*, rather than the previous surgery with a transverse right upper quadrant incision. Through these small openings the surgeon can insert needed instruments and a laparoscope fitted with a miniature camera and bright fiberoptic lighting.

Because the function of the gallbladder is to concentrate and store bile, aiding in the digestion and absorption of fat, some moderation in dietary fat usually is indicated. After surgery, control of fat in the diet facilitates wound healing and comfort because the hormonal stimulus for bile secretion still functions in the surgical area, causing pain with high intake of fatty foods. The body also needs a period to readjust to the more dilute supply of bile available to assist fat digestion and absorption directly from the liver. Depending on individual tolerance and response, a low-fat diet may be needed, such as the guide given for gallbladder disease (see Table 18-7).

---

vagotomy cutting of the vagus nerve, which supplies a major stimulus for gastric secretions.

atonic without normal muscle tone.

TABLE 22-7

DIET FOR POSTOPERATIVE GASTRIC DUMPING SYNDROME

MEAL	FOODS
Breakfast	2 scrambled eggs with 1-2 Tbsp butter or margarine ½ to 1 slice bread with butter or margarine or small serving of cereal 1 tsp low-calorie jelly 1 serving solid fruit*
Midmorning snack	Sandwich: 1 slice bread with butter or margarine 2 oz (56 g) lean meat
Lunch	4 oz (112 g) lean meat with 1-2 Tbsp butter or margarine Green or colored vegetable† with butter or margarine ½ to 1 slice bread with butter or margarine ½ banana or other solid fruit*
Midafternoon snack	Same as midmorning snack
Dinner	4 oz (112 g) lean meat or soy product with 1-2 Tbsp butter or margarine Green or colored vegetable† with butter or margarine ½ to 1 slice bread with butter or margarine (or small serving starchy vegetable substitute) 1 serving solid fruit*
Bedtime snack	2 oz (56 g) meat or 2 eggs or 2 oz (56 g) cheese or cottage cheese 1 slice bread or 5 crackers with butter or margarine

General guidelines: (1) Five or six small meals should be administered daily. (2) A relatively high fat content helps slow the passage of food and maintain weight. (3) A high protein content (meat, eggs, cheese) helps rebuild tissue and maintain weight. (4) A relatively low simple carbohydrate content helps prevent rapid passage of quickly absorbed foods. (5) No milk, sugar, sweets, desserts, alcohol, or sweet carbonated beverages are allowed. (6) Fluids should be avoided for at least 1 hour before and after meals and limited to 4 oz during meals. (7) Relatively low-roughage foods are allowed; raw foods are allowed as tolerated. (8) Very hot or very cold foods or liquids should be avoided.
*Fruit choice: applesauce, baked apple, canned fruit (drained), banana, orange, or grapefruit sections.
†Vegetable choice: spinach, green beans, squash, beets, carrots, green peas.

Intestinal Surgery

In cases of intestinal disease involving tumors, lesions, or obstructions, the affected intestinal area may require surgical resection. In complicated cases requiring surgical removal of large sections of the small intestine, nutrition support is difficult. In such cases TPN is used to supply major support, with a small allowance of oral feeding for personal food desires. After general resection for less-severe cases, a diet relatively low in dietary fiber may be briefly used to allow healing and comfort. The surgery sometimes requires making an opening in the abdominal wall to the intestine, called a *stoma,* for the elimination of fecal waste (Figure 22-5). If the opening is in the area of the *ileum,* the last section of the small intestine, it is called an *ileostomy.* In this area the food mass is still fairly liquid and more problems are encountered in management. If the opening is farther along the GI tract in the large intestine, it is called a *colostomy.* In the large intestine the water is predominantly reabsorbed and the remaining feces are more formed, making management easier.

Patients need support and practical help in learning about self-care with an ostomy. A relatively low-fiber diet may be helpful at first, but the goal is to advance to a regular diet as soon as possible. Progression to a regular diet is important for nutritional value and emotional support. Regular food provides psychological comfort to a patient, and dietary adjustments to individual tolerances for specific foods can be made. Patients can occasionally revert to low-fiber intake when diarrhea occurs.

Rectal Surgery

For a brief period after rectal surgery or *hemorrhoidectomy,* a clear fluid or nonresidue diet (see Table 22-1) may be indicated to reduce painful elimination and allow healing. In some cases a nonresidue commercial elemental formula such as Vivonex may be used to delay bowel movements until the surgical area has healed. Return to a regular diet usually is rapid.

SPECIAL NUTRITION NEEDS FOR PATIENTS WITH BURNS

Nutrition Support Base

Treatment and Prognosis

The CDC reports an annual average of 500,000 visits to the emergency department for burn injuries.[17] Treatment of severe burns presents a tremendous nutrition challenge. The following factors influence the plan of care and its outcome:

- *Age:* Elderly persons and very young children are more vulnerable to poor outcome.
- *Health condition:* Any preexisting health problems or other injuries complicate care.
- *Burn severity:* The location and severity of the burns and the time elapsed before treatment are significant.

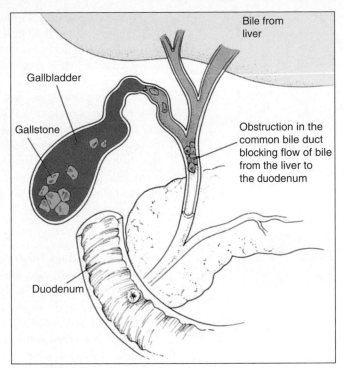

Figure 22–4 Gallbladder with stone (cholelithiasis).

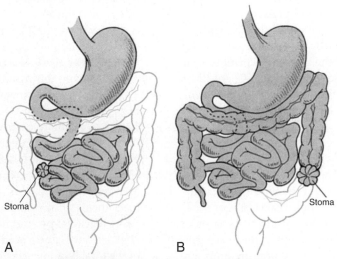

Figure 22–5 A, Ileostomy. B, Colostomy.

Type and Extent of Burns

The depth of the burn affects its treatment and healing process (Figure 22-6). *Superficial* burns only involve cell damage to the *epidermis*. *Superficial partial-thickness* burns involve cell damage to the *dermis*; *deep partial-thickness* burns involve both the first and second layers of skin. *Full-thickness* burns result in complete skin loss, including the underlying fat layer. *Subdermal* burns leave bone and

tendon exposed. In adults, partial-thickness to sub-dermal burns covering at least 15% to 20% of the total BSA are serious and require extensive care. Burns of this severity covering 10% BSA in children and the elderly are categorized as life threatening. Burns of severe depth, covering more than 50% of the BSA, often are fatal. Patients with major burn injuries usually are transferred to a regional burn unit facility for specialized burn team care.

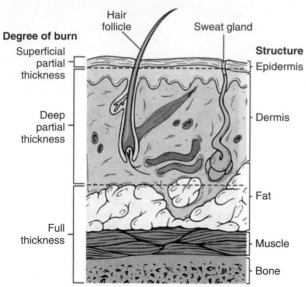

Degree of burn

Superficial partial thickness

Deep partial thickness

Full thickness

Hair follicle

Sweat gland

Structure

Epidermis

Dermis

Fat

Muscle

Bone

Figure 22–6 Depth of skin area involved in burns. (Reprinted from Lewis SM and others: *Medical-surgical nursing: assessment and management of clinical problems,* ed 7, St Louis, 2007, Mosby.)

Stages of Nutrition Care

The nutrition care of adults and children with massive burns presents a great challenge and must be constantly adjusted to individual needs and responses. At each stage critical attention is given to amino acid requirements for tissue rebuilding, fluid/electrolyte balance, and energy (kilocalorie) support. Resting energy expenditure in burned patients can increase in excess of 100% of BMR. Three periods of care generally occur during the immediate shock, recovery, and secondary feeding periods.

Stage 1

Part 1: Immediate Shock Period. From the first hours until approximately the second day after a burn, massive flooding edema occurs at the burn site. Destruction of protective skin leads to immediate losses of water, electrolytes (mainly sodium), and protein. As water is drawn from surrounding blood to replace the losses, general loss continues, blood volume and pressure drop, and urine output decreases. *Cell dehydration* follows as intracellular water is drawn out to balance the loss of tissue fluid. Cell potassium also is withdrawn and circulating serum potassium levels rise.

Immediate IV fluid therapy with a salt solution, such as 6% hetastarch in saline or balanced salt solution, or lactated Ringer's solution replaces water and electrolytes and helps prevent shock.[18] After approximately 12 hours, when vascular permeability returns to normal and losses begin to decrease at the burn site, albumin solutions or plasma can be used to help restore blood volume.

Part 2: Recovery Period. After approximately 48 to 72 hours, tissue fluids and electrolytes are gradually reabsorbed, balance is reestablished, and the pattern of massive tissue loss is reversed. A sudden diuresis occurs, indicating successful initial therapy. Constant attention to fluid intake and output, with checks for any signs of dehydration or overhydration, are essential. Studies evaluating early (within 24 hours) versus delayed (after 48 hours) enteral nutrition support indicate that initiating nutrition support shortly (within 24 hours) after the burn injury may stimulate protein retention, but this has not been associated with an improved recovery rate and thus remains inconclusive.[19]

Stage 2

Part 1: Secondary Feeding Period. Toward the end of the first week after the burn, adequate bowel function returns and a rigorous medical nutrition therapy program must begin. The following three major reasons exist for these increased nutrient and energy demands:

- *Tissue destruction* brings large losses of protein and electrolytes that must be replaced.
- *Tissue catabolism* follows the injury, with further loss of lean body mass and nitrogen.
- *Increased metabolism* brings added nutrition needs to cover the energy costs of infection or fever and the increased protein metabolism of tissue replacement and skin grafting.

Part 2: Medical Nutrition Therapy. Successful nutrition therapy during this critical feeding period is based on vigorous protein and energy intake, as follows:

- *High protein:* Aggressive supplementation of protein is crucial to promote early wound healing and support immune function. Depending on the extent of the burn and catabolic losses, individual protein needs vary from 1.8 to 2.5 g/kg body weight per day.[8] Children may require 2.5 to 3 g/kg body weight per day to meet increased metabolic needs of stress and injury, tissue regeneration, and normal needs of growth.
- *High energy:* Caloric needs are calculated on the basis of the total BSA burned: 20 kcal/kg body weight + (40 × % BSA burned), with a maximum of 50% BSA used.[8] Beyond 50% BSA burned, little increases in total energy needs occur. Overfeeding increases metabolic stress and should be avoided. Such high energy

---

lactated Ringer's solution sterile solution of calcium chloride, potassium chloride, sodium chloride, and sodium lactate in water given to replenish fluid and electrolytes; developed by English physiologist Sidney Ringer (1835-1910).

needs are necessary to spare the protein essential for tissue rebuilding and supply the greatly increased metabolic demands for healing. A liberal portion of the total kilocalories should come from carbohydrate, with a moderate amount of fat (12% to 15%) supplying the remaining needs.

■ *High vitamin, high mineral:* Increased vitamin C, as much as 500 mg twice daily, may be needed as a partner with amino acids for tissue rebuilding. Vitamin A and zinc are specifically important for optimal immune function and often are supplemented. Increased thiamin, riboflavin, and niacin are necessary for increased energy and protein metabolism. Special attention to electrolyte imbalances and calcium/phosphorus ratios in the blood are warranted during this period.

Part 3: Dietary Management. Either enteral or parenteral methods of feeding may be used to meet these crucial nutrient demands. With any method, a careful intake record must be maintained to measure progress toward the increased nutrition goals.

Enteral Feeding. Oral feedings are preferred if well tolerated and needs are met. Concentrated liquids are given with added protein or amino acids. Commercial formulas such as Ensure may be used as added interval nourishment. Solid foods based on individual preferences

usually are tolerated by the second week. However, hypermetabolic states and poor appetite usually make oral feedings difficult for patients with major burns. Patients may require calculated tube feedings to ensure adequate intake in correct nutrient proportions. In such cases, low-bulk defined formula solutions are given through small-bore feeding tubes.

Parenteral Feeding. For some patients oral intake and tube feedings may be inadequate to meet the increased nutrition demands, or enteral feeding may be impossible because of associated injuries or complications. In such cases parenteral feeding can provide essential nutrition support.

Stage 3

Follow-up Reconstruction. Continued nutrition support is essential to maintain tissue strength for successful skin grafting or reconstructive plastic surgery. Patients need the physical rebuilding of body resources that surgery requires as well as personal support to rebuild their will and spirit because disfigurement and disability are possible. Optimal physical stamina gained through persistent supportive medical, nutrition, and nursing care helps patients rebuild the personal resources needed to cope.

SUMMARY

The nutrition demands of surgery begin before a patient reaches the operating table. Before surgery, the task is to correct any existing deficiencies and build nutrition reserves to meet surgical demands. After surgery, the task is to replace losses and support recovery. The additional task of encouraging eating often is necessary during this period of healing.

Postsurgical feedings are given in a variety of ways. The oral route is always preferred. However, the inability to eat or damage to the intestinal tract may require

feeding through a tube or into veins. Special formulas are used for such alternate means of nourishment and are designed to meet individual needs. For patients undergoing surgery to the GI tract, special diets are modified according to the surgical procedure performed. For patients with massive burns, increased nutrition support is necessary in successive stages in response to the burn injury and to continuing tissue rebuilding requirements.

CRITICAL THINKING QUESTIONS

1. Describe the consequences of nutrient imbalances (protein, energy, vitamins, minerals, and fluid) on the preoperative, immediate postoperative, and long-term postoperative periods.
2. Describe appropriate medical nutrition therapy for patients undergoing gastric resection, cholecystectomy, and rectal surgery.
3. Write a 1-day meal plan for a person with postgastrectomy dumping syndrome. What general dietary guidelines are used?
4. How do an ileostomy and a colostomy differ? What are the dietary needs for each?
5. Outline the nutrition care of a burn patient from treatment for immediate shock through recovery and tissue reconstruction.

CHAPTER CHALLENGE QUESTIONS

True-False

Write the correct statement for each statement that is false.

1. *True or False:* Nothing is given by mouth for at least 8 hours before surgery to avoid food aspiration during anesthesia.

2. *True or False:* The most common nutrient deficiency related to surgery is protein.

3. *True or False:* Negative nitrogen balance is a rare finding after surgery.

4. *True or False:* Extensive drainage in complicated surgery cases increases water loss to dangerous levels if constant replacement is not provided.

5. *True or False:* Vitamin C is essential for wound healing because it is involved in building strong connective tissue.

6. *True or False:* Regardless of the type, oral liquid feedings usually provide little nourishment.

7. *True or False:* Tube feedings can only be successfully prepared from complete commercial preparations.

8. *True or False:* After gastrectomy a patient can return to regular eating habits within a few days.

9. *True or False:* After a diseased gallbladder is surgically removed, a patient can freely tolerate any foods containing high amounts of fat.

10. *True or False:* A careful diet record of the total food and liquid intake is important for a burn patient to ensure that increased nutrient and energy demands are met.

Multiple Choice

1. Postsurgical edema develops at the wound site as a result of
   a. decreased plasma protein levels.
   b. excess water intake.
   c. excess sodium intake.
   d. lack of early ambulation and physical exercise.

2. In a postoperative orthopedic patient's diet, protein is essential to
   a. provide extra energy needed to regain strength.
   b. provide a matrix to anchor mineral matter and form bone.
   c. control the BMR.
   d. give more taste to the diet, thus increasing appetite.

3. Complete high-quality protein is essential to wound healing because it
   a. supplies the essential amino acids needed for tissue synthesis.
   b. is used to meet the body's increased energy demands.

   c. is a source of glucose for the body.
   d. provides the most concentrated source of kilocalories.

4. A diet for postgastrectomy dumping syndrome should include which of the following? *(Circle all that apply.)*
   a. Small, frequent meals
   b. No liquid with meals
   c. No milk, sugar, sweets, or desserts
   d. High protein content

5. For a burn patient, a diet high in protein and energy is essential to do which of the following? *(Circle all that apply.)*
   a. Replace the extensive loss of tissue protein at burn sites
   b. Provide essential amino acids for extensive tissue healing
   c. Counteract the negative nitrogen balance from loss of lean body mass
   d. Meet added metabolic demands of infection or fever

evolve Please refer to the Students' Resource section of this text's Evolve Web site for additional study resources.

REFERENCES

1. Guigoz Y: The Mini Nutritional Assessment (MNA) review of the literature—what does it tell us? *J Nutr Health Aging* 10(6):466, 2006.
2. Corish CA: Pre-operative nutritional assessment, *Nutr Soc* 58:821, 1999.
3. Sullivan DH and others: Protein-energy undernutrition and life-threatening complications among the hospitalized elderly, *Gen Intern Med* 17(12):923, 2002.
4. Ilich JZ and others: Bone and nutrition in elderly women: protein, energy, and calcium as main determinants of bone mineral density, *Eur J Clin Nutr* 57(4):554, 2003.
5. Choudry HA and others: Branched-chain amino acid–enriched nutritional support in surgical and cancer patients, *J Nutr* 136(1 Suppl):314S, 2006.
6. Grocott MP and others: Perioperative fluid management and clinical outcomes in adults, *Anesth Analg* 100(4):1093, 2005.
7. Food and Nutrition Board, Institute of Medicine: *Dietary reference intakes for energy, carbohydrate, fiber, fat, fatty acids, cholesterol, protein, and amino acids*, Washington, DC, 2002, National Academies Press.
8. Orr PA and others: Metabolic response and parenteral nutrition in trauma, sepsis, and burns, *J Infus Nurs* 25(1):45, 2002.

9. Boyce ST and others: Vitamin C regulates keratinocyte viability, epidermal barrier, and basement membrane *in vitro*, and reduces wound contraction after grafting of cultured skin substitutes, *J Invest Dermatol* 118:565, 2002.

10. Long CL and others: Ascorbic acid dynamics in the seriously ill and injured, *J Surg Res* 109(2):144, 2003.

11. Rümelin A and others: Metabolic clearance of the antioxidant ascorbic acid in surgical patients, *J Surg Res* 129(1):46, 2005.

12. Briefel RR and others: Zinc intake of the U.S. population: findings from the third National Health and Nutrition Examination Survey, 1988-1994, *J Nutr* 130(5S Suppl):1367S, 2000.

13. Aggarwal R and others: Role of zinc administration in prevention of childhood diarrhea and respiratory illnesses: a meta-analysis, *Pediatrics* 119(6):1120, 2007.

14. Prasad AS and others: Zinc supplementation decreases incidence of infections in the elderly: effect of zinc on generation of cytokines and oxidative stress, *Am J Clin Nutr* 85(3):837, 2007.

15. Virji A, Murr MM: Caring for patients after bariatric surgery, *Am Fam Physician* 73(8):1403, 2006.

16. Rushdi TA and others: Control of diarrhea by fiber-enriched diet in ICU patients on enteral nutrition: a prospective randomized controlled trial, *Clin Nutr* 23(6):1344, 2004.

17. Centers for Disease Control and Prevention, National Center for Health Statistics: *Health data for all ages, www.cdc.gov/nchs/health_data_for_all_ages.htm*, accessed October 2007.

18. Moretti EW and others: Intraoperative colloid administration reduces postoperative nausea and vomiting and improves postoperative outcomes compared with crystalloid administration, *Anesth Analg* 96(2):611, 2003.

19. Wasiak J and others: Early versus delayed enteral nutrition support for burn injuries, *Cochrane Database Syst Rev* 3: CD005489, 2006.

FURTHER READING AND RESOURCES

Burn Foundation: *www.burnfoundation.org*

Choudry HA and others: Branched-chain amino acid–enriched nutritional support in surgical and cancer patients, *J Nutr* 136(1 Suppl):314S, 2006.
  This article highlights the adverse effects of protein energy malnutrition in catabolic patients. It also gives a summary of the role that branched-chain amino acids play in potentially alleviating the burden of catabolism.

Virji A, Murr MM: Caring for patients after bariatric surgery, *Am Fam Physician* 73(8):1403, 2006.
  The authors discuss both short- and long-term complications and risks of bariatric surgery.

CHAPTER 23

Nutrition Support in Cancer and AIDS

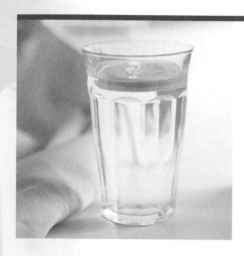

KEY CONCEPTS

- Environmental agents, genetic factors, and weaknesses in the body's immune system can contribute to the development of cancer.
- The strength of the body's immune system relates to its overall nutritional status.
- Nutrition problems affect the nature of the disease process and the medical treatment methods in patients with cancer or AIDS.
- The progressive effects of the human immunodeficiency virus (HIV), through its three stages of white T-cell destruction, have many nutrition implications and often require aggressive medical nutrition therapy.

With the accumulating environmental problems and changing lifestyles of the past several years, cancer has become a more prevalent health problem in the United States. Because cancer generally is associated with aging, the increases in life expectancy have somewhat contributed to this growing incidence. Although cancer and AIDS share a direct relation to the body's immune system and basic nutrition needs, their courses and fatal outcomes are distinct.

This chapter looks at nutrition support in relation to both cancer and AIDS. Both conditions threaten life and have important nutrition connections in prevention and therapy.

SECTION I CANCER

PROCESS OF CANCER DEVELOPMENT

The Nature of Cancer

Multiple Forms

One of the problems in the study and treatment of cancer is that it is not a single problem; it has a highly variable nature and expresses itself in multiple forms. Cancer is a major health problem in the United States. It currently is the second leading cause of death and affects 7.3% of all adults older than 18 years.[1] The general term *cancer* is used to designate a malignant tumor or neoplasm, a term that refers to new growth. The many forms of cancer vary in prevalence worldwide and change as populations migrate to different environments.

Nutrition Relations

No single treatment or special diet for cancer exists despite various fad diets and claims. Instead, relations between nutrition and cancer care focus on the following two fundamental areas:

- *Prevention:* in relation to the environment and the body's natural defense system
- *Therapy:* in relation to nutrition support for medical treatment and rehabilitation

The Normal Cell

Human life results from the process of individual cell growth and reproduction. This process occurs continuously, almost without error, guided by a cell's *genes*. In adults, approximately 3 to 4 million cells complete the life-sustaining process of cell division every second. Cell division is guided by the genetic code contained in the cell nucleus, *deoxyribonucleic acid* (DNA). Each gene carries unique genetic information that controls the synthesis of proteins and transmits genetic inheritance. Thus cells only arise from cell division of preexisting cells and continue in their genetic patterns. Normal cell structure and function operate in an orderly manner under this constant gene control with the aid of regulatory genes.

The Cancer Cell

This orderly cell operation can be lost by a mutation, or changes in the genes, especially in the regulatory genes. Cell growth may form malignant tumors when normal gene control is lost. Thus the misguided cell and its tumor tissue represent normal cell growth that has gone wrong. Cancer tumors are identified by their (1) primary site of origin, (2) stage of tumor size and metastasis, and (3) grade (how aggressive the tumor is). *Sarcomas* arise from connective tissue, *carcinomas* arise from epithelial tissue, and *lymphoma and leukemia* are derived from blood cells.

Carcinogenesis often is described as having three phases: initiation, promotion, and progression. *Initiation* is the point at which a mutagen causes irreversible damage to DNA. *Promotion* is caused by an agent that triggers the mutated cell to grow and reproduce. *Progression* is the phase in which the cancer cells grow, leading to a malignant tumor capable of metastasizing.

Causes of Cancer Cell Development

The underlying cause of cancer is the fundamental loss of cell control over normal cell reproduction. Several factors may contribute to this loss and change a normal cell into a cancer cell.

Mutations

As indicated, mutations are caused by the loss of one or more of the regulatory genes in the cell nucleus or damage to a specific gene. Such a mutant gene may be inherited or arise from an environmental stimulus. Some can-

cers have genetic links (e.g., colorectal cancer, 5% to 10% of gynecologic cancers). Individuals with a predisposition to cancer do not necessarily develop cancer.

Chemical Carcinogens

Agents that cause cancer are called *carcinogens*. Several chemical substances can interfere with the structure or function of regulatory genes. Exposure to such agents may be by individual choice (e.g., cigarette smoking) or result from general exposure to environmental contaminants (e.g., pesticides, fungicides, and industrial chemicals such as dichlorodiphenyltrichloroethane [DDT], tetradifon, and dicofol).[2-4] The actions of such substances may result in gene mutation, damage to gene regulation, or activation of a dormant virus.

Radiation

Radiation damage to genes may come from radiographs, radioactive materials, sunlight, or atomic waste. An estimated 125,000 Americans develop skin cancer every year, and overexposure to the ultraviolet radiation of the sun is the most important environmental factor contributing to this form of cancer.[5] The three major types of skin cancer are associated with the following specific gene mutations:

- *Basal cell carcinoma:* patched gene mutations
- *Squamous cell carcinoma:* p53 gene mutations
- *Melanoma:* p16 gene mutations

Common forms of skin cancer on the head and neck usually are basal cell carcinoma and are relatively easy to remove by surgery.

The most lethal form of skin cancer, *malignant melanoma*, occurs in the skin cells that produce the pigment melanin and accounts for the majority of deaths from skin cancer. Approximately 60,000 cases occur in the United States each year, with 8000 deaths annually (Figure 23-1).[5]

Viruses

Oncogenic, or tumor inducing, viruses that interfere with the function of regulatory genes have been identified in animals and are the focus of much ongoing research. Although oncogenes were first found in viruses, their history indicates that they also function in normal vertebrate

---

neoplasm any new or abnormal cellular growth, specifically one that is uncontrolled and aggressive.

mutation a permanent transmissible change in a gene.

metastasis spread to other tissue.

carcinogenesis development of cancer.

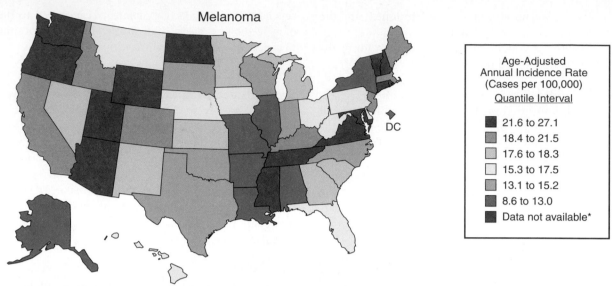

Figure 23–1 Incidence rates for United States. Melanoma of the skin all races (includes Hispanic), both sexes, and all ages from 2001 to 2003 (SEER areas 2000-2004). *NPCR,* National Program of Cancer Registries; *SEER,* Surveillance Epidemiology and End Results. The latest available data vary by geography: 2001-2003 for NPCR areas and 2000-2004 for SEER areas. Incidence rates (cases per 100,000 population per year) are age adjusted to the 2000 U.S. standard population (19 age groups: younger than 1 year, 1-4 years, 5-9 years... 80-84 years, 85+). Rates are for invasive cancer only (except for bladder cancer, which is invasive and in situ) or unless otherwise specified. Rates calculated by using SEER^Stat. Population counts for denominators are based on census populations as modified by NCI. *Data not available for this combination of geography, cancer site, age and race or ethnicity. (Reprinted from National Cancer Institute: *Cancer state profile, http://statecancerprofiles.cancer. gov/map/map.withimage.php?00&001&053&00&0&1&0&1&6&0#map,* accessed October 2007.)

cells. A virus is little more than a packet of a few genes, usually fewer than five, whereas cells of complex organisms such as human beings have thousands. Disease viruses act as parasites, taking over the cell machinery to reproduce themselves.

Epidemiologic Factors

Epidemiology is the study of disease incidence in populations. Studies of cancer distribution involve factors such as race, region, age, heredity, occupation, and diet (see the Cultural Considerations box, "Types and Incidence of Cancer in American Populations"). Incidences of cancer according to race or ethnicity change as population groups migrate to new environments and then acquire the cancer characteristics of the host population—a phenomenon referred to as *acculturation.* One example is the incidence of cancer seen in south Asian populations who have migrated to California. A recent study found that populations who have migrated from south Asian countries have a more similar pattern of cancer incidence and type to Americans than individuals in their land of origin (e.g., India, Pakistan, Bangladesh, Sri Lanka).[6] The incidence of cancer also increases with age.

Stress Factors

Health care professionals recognize psychological stress as a disease risk factor in our complex society, especially in high-risk populations that lack social and economic support. Psychological trauma, especially the loss of central personal relationships, is difficult at best. Studies of people under stress have shown an increased incidence of cancer and reduction of the immune response to disease, especially in natural killer cells.[7] Through their influence on the integrity of the immune system, poor food behaviors, nutrition status, and overall level of oxidative stress make a person more vulnerable to cancer-producing factors.[8]

Dietary Factors

The association between diet and cancer is complex. Although it has been the subject of much research, many questions are still unanswered. Foods contain both carcinogenic and anticarcinogenic compounds. Although studies have found conflicting results about the dietary intake of specific nutrients, general agreement exists in the research community about the preventative role of fruit and vegetable consumption in relation to several

CULTURAL CONSIDERATIONS

TYPES AND INCIDENCE OF CANCER IN AMERICAN POPULATIONS

The prevalence, or number of events in a population at a designated time, of cancer has many variables. The CDC has reported the prevalence of cancer by race, education level, and family income*:

Characteristic	Percent of Population with Any Form of Cancer, Aged 18 Years and Older
Race	
Caucasian	7.9%
Black or African American	3.9%
Native American or Alaska Native	9.2%
Asian	3.6%
Hispanic or Latino	3.9%
Mexican or Mexican American	3.4%
Education	
Less than high school education	6.8%
High school diploma or general equivalency degree	8.1%
Some college	9.3%
Bachelor's degree or higher	9.3%
Family Income	
Less than $20,000	6.8%
$20,000-$54,999	7.6%
$55,000-$74,999	9.6%
$75,000 or more	8.4%

The confounding factors associated with cancer risk are slowly being uncovered and explored. This trend toward prevention ideally will become stronger with advanced research. Identifying high-risk patients and encouraging regular physical examinations is an important aspect of providing general health care as well as a valuable prevention tool.

*Pleis JR, Lethbridge-Çejku M: Summary health statistics for U.S. adults: national health interview survey, 2005, National Center for Health Statistics, *Vital Health Stat* 10(232), 2006.

---

types of cancer. A general consensus also links dietary *deficiencies* of specific nutrients (iron, zinc, folate, and vitamins B_{12}, B_6, and C) with an increased risk of DNA damage and cancer.[9] A recent large-scale study of approximately 500,000 individuals in Europe found that diets high in red and processed meat were positively associated with colorectal cancer, whereas diets high in fish were protective against colorectal cancer.[10]

The Body's Defense System

The body's defense system is remarkably efficient and complex. Special cells protect the body from external invaders such as bacteria and viruses and internal aliens such as cancer cells.

Defensive Cells of the Immune System

Two major cell populations provide the immune system's primary "search and destroy" defense for detecting and killing alien, nonself substances that carry potential disease. These two populations of *lymphocytes*, a special type of white blood cell, develop early in life from a common stem cell in the bone marrow. The two types are *T cells*, derived from thymus cells, and *B cells*, derived from bursal intestinal cells (Figure 23-2). A major function of T cells is to activate the *phagocytes*, cells that destroy invaders and act as killer cells that attack and kill disease-carrying antigens. A major function of B cells is to produce proteins known as antibodies, which also kill antigens.

Specially tailored proteins called *monoclonal antibodies* target cancer cells and stimulate the immune system to produce antibodies against antigens on the surfaces of tumors—essentially acting as a cancer vaccine.[11] Such therapy has proven useful in the treatment of organ transplant rejection, inflammatory disease, colorectal cancer, cardiovascular disease, lymphoma, leukemia, and breast cancer.[12] The difficulty in therapeutic development in this arena is to identify and target antigens that are present only on tumor cells surfaces and not on normal, healthy cells. Clinical trials for cancer vaccines are underway worldwide.

Relation of Nutrition to Immunity

Nutrition support is necessary to maintain the integrity of the human immune system. Severely malnourished persons show changes in the structure and function of their immune system. These changes result from atrophy or losses in the basic tissues involved (e.g., liver, bowel

---

antigen any foreign or non-self substances (e.g., toxins, viruses, bacteria, and foreign proteins) that stimulate the production of antibodies specifically designed to counteract their activity.

antibody any of numerous protein molecules produced by B cells as a primary immune defense for attaching to specific related antigens.

atrophy tissue wasting.

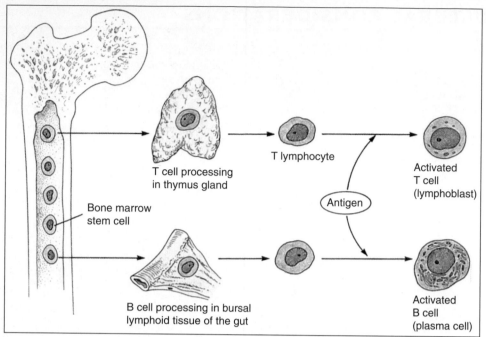

Figure 23–2 Development of the T- and B-cells, lymphocyte components of the body's immune system. (Courtesy Eileen Draper.)

wall, bone marrow, spleen, and lymphoid tissue). Nutrition is fundamental in maintaining normal immunity and combating sustained attacks of diseases such as cancer. The core of the immune system is internally derived proteins—antibodies. A direct and simple example of the important role of nutrition in immunity is the link between protein energy malnutrition and suppressed immune function.

The Healing Process and Nutrition

The strength of any body tissue is maintained through constant synthesis—building and rebuilding—of tissue protein. Such strong tissue is a front line of the body's defense. This process of tissue building and healing requires optimal nutrition intake. Specific nutrients—protein, essential fatty acids, and key vitamins and minerals—must be constantly supplied in the diet. Wise and early use of vigorous medical nutrition therapy for patients with cancer has been shown to provide recovery of normal nutritional status, including immunocompetence, thus improving response to therapy and prognosis.[13]

NUTRITION COMPLICATIONS OF CANCER TREATMENT

Three major forms of therapy are used today as medical treatment for cancer: surgery, radiation, and chemotherapy. Each requires nutrition support.

Surgery

Any surgery, as discussed in Chapter 22, requires nutrition support for the healing process. This requirement is particularly true for patients with cancer because their general condition often is weakened by the disease process and its drain on the body's resources. With early diagnosis and sound nutrition support before and after surgery, many tumors can be successfully removed. Medical nutrition therapy also includes any needed modifications in food texture or specific nutrients, depending on the site of the surgery or the function of the organ involved. Various methods of feeding patients after surgery are reviewed in Chapter 22.

Radiation

Radiation therapy often is used by itself or in conjunction with surgery. This type of therapy involves treatment with high-energy radiography targeted on the cancer site to kill or shrink cancerous cells. Radiation may be administered to the body by an external machine (Figure 23-3) or by implanted radioactive materials at the cancer site. Although the goal is for only the cancer cells to die, other cells within close proximity of the target site and rapidly growing cells often die as well. The site and intensity of the radiation treatment determine the nature of the nutrition problems the patient may encounter. For example, radiation to the head, neck, or esophagus affects the oral

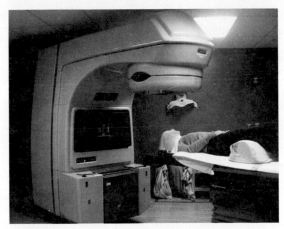

Figure 23–3 Radiation treatment machine. (Courtesy Jormain Cady, Virginia Mason Medical Center, Seattle, WA. In Lewis SM and others: *Medical-surgical nursing: assessment and management of clinical problems*, ed 7, St Louis, 2007, Mosby.)

mucosa and salivary secretions, thus affecting taste sensations and sensitivity to food texture and temperature. Means of enhancing the appetite through food appearance and aroma as well as texture must be explored. Similarly, radiation to the abdominal area affects the intestinal mucosa, causing loss of villi and absorbing surface and possibly malabsorption problems. Ulcers, inflammation, and obstruction, or *fistulas,* also may develop from tissue breakdown. A fistula, from the Latin word for pipe, is an abnormal opening or passageway within the body or to the outside. As such, it interferes with normal functioning of the involved tissue. General malabsorption within the GI tract may be further compounded by a lack of food intake from a loss of appetite and nausea.

Chemotherapy

Chemotherapy drugs kill rapidly growing cancer cells. Unlike radiation therapy, chemotherapy is administered to general circulation by the blood and courses through the entire body. Because these drugs are highly toxic, they also affect normal, healthy cells. This accounts for their side effects on rapidly growing tissues such as those of the bone marrow, GI tract, and hair follicles as well as problems in nutrition management. General complications include the following:

- *Bone marrow effects:* Interference with the production of specific blood factors causes related problems: reduced RBCs, causing anemia; reduced white blood cells, causing lowered resistance to infections; and reduced blood platelets, causing bleeding.
- *GI effects:* Numerous problems may develop that interfere with food tolerance, such as nausea and vomiting,

loss of normal taste sensations, lack of appetite, diarrhea, ulcers, malabsorption, and mucositis.
- *Hair follicle effects:* Interference with normal hair growth results in general hair loss.

Other problems may relate to the use of pretreatment antidepressant drugs that have special blood pressure effects when used with certain tyramine-rich foods. These drugs are the *monoamine oxidase inhibitors;* their use requires a tyramine-restricted diet (Table 23-1). Other antineoplastic drugs have known drug-nutrient interactions that should be addressed with patients on an individual basis. In addition, many patients experiment with herbs that are thought to have a protective role in cancer treatment or prevention. Some of the more commonly used herbs have food-drug interactions that may adversely affect

TABLE 23-1

TYRAMINE-RESTRICTED DIET

Foods to Avoid	Representative Tyramine Values (mcg/g or ml)
Cheeses	
New York state cheddar	1416
Gruyère	516
Stilton	466
Emmenthaler	225
Brie	180
Camembert	86
Processed American	50
Wines	
Chianti	25.4
Sherry	3.6
Beer, Ale (varies by brand)	
Highest	4.4
Average	2.3

The diet was designed for patients taking monoamine oxidase inhibitors, drugs that have been reported to cause hypertensive crises when used with tyramine-rich foods, in which aging, protein breakdown, and putrefaction are used to increase flavor. Studies indicate that as little as 5 to 6 mg tyramine can produce a response and that 25 mg is a dangerous dose. Food sources of other pressor amines, such as histamine, dihydroxyphenylalanine, and hydroxytyramine, should also be limited.
All foods listed should be avoided. Limited amounts of foods with a lower tyramine amount, such as yeast bread, may be included in a specific diet.
Over-the-counter drugs such as decongestants, cold remedies, and antihistamines should be avoided.

immunocompetence the ability or capacity to develop an immune response (i.e., antibody production or cell-mediated immunity) after exposure to an antigen.

mucositis an inflammation of the tissues around the mouth or other orifices of the body.

the patient. Careful questioning will reveal herb use, and any negative potential interactions should be discussed. See the Drug-Nutrient Interaction box, "Drug-Nutrient Interactions with Commonly Used Drugs and Herbs in Patients with Cancer" for a list of possible interactions.

MEDICAL NUTRITION THERAPY IN THE PATIENT WITH CANCER

Problems Related to the Disease Process

General feeding problems pose a great challenge to the clinical dietitian planning care and the nurse providing important supportive assistance. These problems relate to the overall systemic effects of cancer as well as the specific individual responses to the type of cancer involved.

General Systemic Effects

Cancer generally causes the following three basic systemic effects:

- *Anorexia*, or loss of appetite, resulting in poor food intake
- *Increased metabolism*, resulting in increased nutrient and energy needs
- *Negative nitrogen balance*, resulting in more *catabolism*, or breaking down of body tissues

The extent of these effects may vary widely from a mild response to an extreme form of debilitating *cachexia* seen in advanced disease. Extreme weight loss and

DRUG-NUTRIENT INTERACTION

DRUG-NUTRIENT INTERACTIONS WITH COMMONLY USED DRUGS AND HERBS IN PATIENTS WITH CANCER

Drug or Nutrient	Possible Interactions
Antineoplastic Drugs	
Bexarotene (Targretin)	Grapefruit juice may increase drug concentration and toxicities
Methotrexate (Folex, Rheumatrex)	Alcohol may increase hepatotoxicity
Plicamycin (Mithracin)	Supplements containing calcium and vitamin D may decrease effect
Procarbazine (Matulane)	Alcohol may cause disulfiram reaction; caffeine-containing compounds may raise blood pressure
Temozolomide (Temodar)	Food may decrease drug rate and absorption
Herbs	
Black cohosh	May further reduce lipids or blood pressure when combined with prescription medications; may increase antiproliferative effect obtained with tamoxifen
Chamomile	May increase bleeding when used with anticoagulants; may increase sedative effect of benzodiazepines
Dong quai	May increase effects of warfarin
Echinacea	May interfere with immunosuppressive therapy
Garlic	May increase bleeding time with aspirin, dipyridamole, and warfarin; may increase effects and adverse effects of hyperglycemic agents
Ginkgo biloba	May increase bleeding time with aspirin, dipyridamole, and warfarin; may increase blood pressure when used with thiazide diuretics
Ginseng	May adversely affect platelet adhesiveness and blood coagulation; may increase hypoglycemia with insulin; may interfere with antipsychotic drugs; may cause hypertension when used long-term with caffeine
Kava kava	May increase CNS depression when used with alcohol and sedatives; may cause hepatotoxicity
St. John's wort	May cause serotonin syndrome when used with antidepressants and drugs that use p450 microsomal enzyme for metabolism
Ma huang (ephedra)	Increases toxicity with beta-blockers, monoamine oxidase inhibitors, caffeine, and St. John's wort
Yohimbe	Decreases effect of antidepressants, antihypertensives, hyperglycemic agents, monoamine oxidase inhibitors, and St. John's wort

Modified from National Cancer Institute: *Nutrition in cancer care: nutrition implications of cancer therapies, www.cancer.gov/cancertopics/pdq/supportivecare/ nutrition/HealthProfessional/page4,* accessed October 2007.

DRUG-NUTRIENT INTERACTION

CANNABIS (MEDICAL MARIJUANA) AS A TREATMENT FOR ANOREXIA

Both sides of the debate for legalization of medical marijuana have genuine concerns. Proponents argue in favor of the effectiveness marijuana has on relieving nausea from cancer treatment, wasting effects of AIDS, and the pain of glaucoma. Critics cite studies that indicate its addictiveness and link it to cancer and lung damage.

Dronabinol, sold under the brand name Marinol, is a capsule form of marijuana approved by the FDA. It contains tetrahydrocannabinol, or THC, the active ingredient found in plant marijuana, and thus has similar side effects*:

- Dizziness
- Euphoria
- Paranoid reaction
- Somnolence (sleepiness)

Dronabinol is indicated for the treatment of anorexia associated with weight loss in patients with AIDS, and nausea and vomiting associated with cancer chemotherapy in patients who have not adequately responded to conventional antiemetic treatments.†

Dosage should be tightly regulated by the physician because each patient responds to dronabinol differently. Because it is habit forming, the lowest dose needed to produce the desired result is recommended.

Sara Oldroyd

*Goldman, L: Cannabis and clinical RDs: why you need to know about medical marijuana, *ADA Times* 4 (3):5, 2007.
†Seamon MJ and others: Medical marijuana and the developing role of the pharmacist, *Am J Health Syst Pharm* 64(10):1037, 2007.

---

weakness are caused by an inability to ingest or use nutrients, resulting in a patient's body to feed off its own tissue protein.[14,15] Approximately half of all patients with cancer have this debilitating syndrome. An involuntary weight loss of greater than 5% of premorbid weight within a 6-month period is indicative of cachexia. The best way to cure cachexia is to alleviate the cancer. However, because this is not always an immediate possibility, aggressive medical nutrition therapy is the next best option. A variety of drugs are currently in use to increase appetite, decrease nausea, spare protein degradation, and improve caloric intake, such as glucocorticoids, progestational drugs (megestrol), cyproheptadine, prokinetic agents (metoclopramide), branched-chain amino acids, eicosapentaenoic acid, cannabinoids, and 5'-deoxyfluorouridine. See the Drug-Nutrient Interaction box, "Cannabis (Medical Marijuana) as a Treatment for Anorexia," regarding the controversies surrounding the use of cannabis for combating unintended weight loss in cachexic patients.

Specific Effects Related to Type of Cancer

In addition to the primary nutrition problems caused by the disease process itself, secondary problems in eating or nutrient metabolism result from tumors causing obstructions or lesions in the GI tract or surrounding tissue. Such conditions limit food intake and digestion as well as absorption of nutrients. Depending on the nature and location of the tumor as well as the medical treatment of choice, a variety of individual nutrition problems may occur and require personal attention.

Basic Objectives of Medical Nutrition Therapy

Prevention of Catabolism

Every effort is made to meet the increased metabolic demands of the disease process, thus preventing extensive catabolic effects in tissue breakdown. Maintaining nutrition from the beginning is far easier than rebuilding the body after extensive malnutrition. Medical treatment may increase this catabolic effect.

Relief of Symptoms

The symptoms of the disease or side effects of the treatment can be devastating for a patient. Relief requires much individual and family counseling to devise ways of meeting needs and helping the patient eat. The types of foods used, their preparation and service, and the process of feeding should be individualized according to situation, response, and need.

Although the clinical dietitian and the physician have the primary responsibility for planning and managing the nutrition therapy program, a tremendous contribution is made by the nursing staff and other health care personnel in the day-to-day support and counsel in help-

---

cachexia a specific profound syndrome caused by malnutrition and a disturbance in glucose and fat metabolism usually seen in patients with terminal cancer or AIDS; general poor health indicated by an emaciated appearance.

ing the patient eat. This kind of constant care and support often differentiates combating the course of the disease and ensuring the comfort and well-being of the patient.

Principles of Nutrition Care

The basic principles of identifying needs and planning care on the basis of those needs underlie all sound patient care (see Chapter 17).

Nutrition Assessment

Determining and monitoring the nutritional status of each patient is the primary responsibility of the clinical dietitian. Various members of the health care team may take part in body measurements and calculations of body composition, laboratory tests and interpretation of results, physical examination and clinical observations, and dietary analysis. Weight can change rapidly in patients; therefore accurate measurement must be taken instead of reliance on self-reported or estimated values. Severe alterations in weight may change medication dosages and indicate nutrition problems.

Personal Care Plan

On the basis of detailed information gathered about each patient, including living situation and other personal and social needs, the clinical dietitian, in consultation with the physician, develops a personal plan of medical nutrition therapy (MNT) for each patient. This plan should be evaluated on a regular basis with the patient and family and changed as needed to meet the nutrition demands of the patient's condition and individual desires and tolerances.

Nutrition Needs

Although individual needs vary, guidelines for MNT must meet specific nutrient needs and goals related to the accelerated metabolism, which demands increased energy production and protein-tissue synthesis.

Energy

The hypermetabolic nature of cancer and its healing requirements place great energy demands on the patient. Sufficient fuel from carbohydrate and, to a lesser extent, fat must be available to spare protein for vital tissue building. An adult patient with good nutritional status needs between 2000 to 2500 kcal, or 25 to 30 kcal/kg body weight, for maintenance requirements. More kilocalories may be needed according to the degree of individual

stress, amount of tissue synthesis needed, and physical activity. A malnourished patient may require 2500 to 3500 kcal, or 35 to 40 kcal/kg, depending on the degree of malnutrition or extent of tissue injury.

Protein

Essential amino acids and nitrogen are necessary for tissue building, for healing, and to offset tissue breakdown caused by the disease. Efficient protein use depends on an optimal protein/energy ratio to promote tissue building and prevent tissue catabolism. An adult patient with good nutritional status needs approximately 80 to 100 g/day of high-quality protein to meet maintenance requirements. A malnourished patient needs between 100 and 150 g/day to replenish deficits and restore positive nitrogen balance. The patient and dietitian must work together to design a meal plan that meets the high calorie and protein needs while simultaneously dealing with anorexia, nausea, or other intolerances.

Vitamins and Minerals

Key vitamins and minerals help control protein and energy metabolism through their coenzyme roles in specific cell enzyme pathways and also play important roles in building and maintaining strong tissue (see Chapters 7 and 8). Therefore an optimal intake of vitamins and minerals, at least to the DRI standards but more often to higher therapeutic levels, is needed. Vitamin and mineral supplements often are indicated to ensure dietary intake (see the Drug-Nutrient Interaction box, "Antiestrogens and Breast Cancer").

Fluid

Adequate fluid intake must be ensured for the following reasons:

- To replace GI losses from fever, infection, vomiting, or diarrhea
- To help the kidneys dispose of metabolic breakdown products from destroyed cancer cells and the drugs used in chemotherapy

Some chemotherapeutic drugs (e.g., cyclophosphamide [Cytoxan]) require as much as 2 to 3 L of forced fluids daily to prevent hemorrhagic cystitis.

Nutrition Management

Achieving these nutrition objectives and needs in the face of frequent food intolerance, anorexia, or inability to eat presents a great challenge to the nutrition support team and patient. The specific method of feeding depends on the patient's condition. The dietitian and

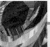

DRUG-NUTRIENT INTERACTION

ANTIESTROGENS AND BREAST CANCER

Tamoxifen citrate is an antiestrogenic drug used to treat breast cancer. Some common symptoms related to nutrition include the following:

- Nausea
- Bone pain
- Fluid retention
- Hot flashes
- Hypercalcemia

Estrogen is needed for bone formation along with vitamin D, calcium, and magnesium. With low levels of estrogen, calcium is taken from the bone and bone resorption may result. Calcium and magnesium supplements can help reduce resorption but should be taken separately from the tamoxifen citrate by at least 2 hours. Grapefruit juice should be avoided because it can interfere with absorption, as can soy supplements and soy-based foods because of their estrogenic effect. Soy products do not contain estrogen but do contain compounds similar in structure to estrogen. Because of the similarity, these estrogenlike compounds may fit into the active site of the drug and therefore act as decoys to the true target estrogen.*

Sara Oldroyd

*Pronsky ZM: Tamoxifen citrate. In *Food medication interactions,* ed 14, Birchrunville, PA, 2006, Food Medication Interactions.

---

physician may manage a patient's nutrition care using either enteral or parenteral modes of feeding (see Chapter 22).

Enteral: Oral Diet with Nutrient Supplementation

An oral diet with supplementation is the most desired form of feeding when tolerated. A personal food plan, based on the nutrition assessment information gathered, must be developed with the patient and family. This food plan must include adjustments in food texture and temperature, food choices, and tolerances and should provide as much energy and nutrient density as possible in smaller volumes of food (see the Clinical Applications box, "Strategies for Improving Food Intake in Patients with Cancer or AIDS"). The plan also must give special attention to eating problems caused by loss of appetite, mouth problems, and GI problems (Table 23-2).

Loss of Appetite. Anorexia is a major problem in patients with cancer and curtails food intake when it is needed most. Anorexia often sets up a vicious cycle that can lead to the gross malnutrition of cancer cachexia. A vigorous program of eating that *does not depend on appetite for stimulus*, must be planned with the patient and family. The overall goal is to provide food with as much nutrient density as possible so that every bite counts.

Mouth Problems. Various problems contributing to eating difficulties may stem from a sore mouth, mucositis, or taste and smell changes. Decreased saliva and sore mouth often result from radiation to the head and neck area or from chemotherapy. Spraying the mouth with

CLINICAL APPLICATIONS

STRATEGIES FOR IMPROVING FOOD INTAKE IN PATIENTS WITH CANCER OR AIDS

Tips for Increasing Energy and Protein Intake
- Fortify foods with high-calorie condiments, sauces, and dressings.
- Add extra ingredients such as dry milk and cream during food preparation.
- Use high-calorie protein drinks between meals for added nutrients.
- Use regular-calorie foods and beverages, not low-calorie substitutes.
- Prepare favorite foods and freeze leftovers in small serving sizes for snacks.

- Eat by the clock: have a meal or snack every 1 or 2 hours.
- Eat more when appetite is good.
- Enjoy meals with pleasant surroundings, company, and music.
- Keep a supply of easy-to-prepare and convenient foods on hand.
- Try mild exercise, according to physical status.
- If mouth is sore, use soft foods, avoid hot and cold temperature extremes, and discuss a topical anesthetic mouth rinse to use before eating with a physician or nurse.

TABLE 23-2

DIETARY MODIFICATIONS FOR NUTRITION-RELATED SIDE EFFECTS OF CANCER AND HIV/AIDS

Symptom	Suggestions
Anorexia	Plan a menu in advance with small, frequent, meals and snacks, including high-calorie, high-protein, nutrient-dense foods.
	Encourage consumption of high-protein foods first.
	Prepare and store small portions of favorite foods.
	Experiment with different foods and seek foods that appeal to the sense of smell.
	Arrange for help in purchasing and preparing food and meals.
Nausea and vomiting	Avoid spicy foods, greasy foods, and foods with strong odors.
	Eat dry, easy-to-digest foods such as crackers, breadsticks, or toast throughout the day and avoid heavy meals.
	Remain upright for at least 1 hour after eating.
	Avoid eating in areas with strong cooking odors or that are too warm.
	Consume liquids between meals.
Taste alterations	Use herbs and seasonings to enhance flavors.
	Try new foods and be flexible with mealtimes.
	Use plastic utensils if foods taste metallic and use gum or mints when experiencing a bitter taste in the mouth.
	Substitute poultry, fish, eggs, tofu, and cheese for red meat.
Xerostomia	Drink plenty of fluids (25-30 ml/kg per day).
	Eat moist foods with extra sauces and gravies.
	Perform oral hygiene at least 4 times per day but avoid rinses containing alcohol.
	Use hard candy, frozen desserts, chewing gum, and ice pops between meals to moisten mouth.
Diarrhea	Avoid greasy foods, hot and cold liquids, and caffeine.
	Stay well hydrated.
	Limit gas-forming foods and beverages such as soda, cruciferous vegetables, legumes and lentils, chewing gum, and milk (if not well tolerated).
	Limit use of sorbitol.
Constipation	Gradually increase fiber consumption to 25 to 30 g/day.
	Drink 8 to 10 cups of fluid each day.
	Maintain regular physical activity.
Mucositis, stomatitis	Eat foods that are soft, easy to chew and swallow, and nonirritating.
	Moisten foods with gravy, broth, or sauces.
	Avoid known irritants such as acidic, spicy, salty, and coarse-textured foods.
	Cut foods into small bites.
	Eat foods at room temperature.
	Supplement meals with high-calorie, high-protein drinks.
	Maintain good oral hygiene.
Neutropenia*	Check expiration dates on food and do not buy or use if the food is out of date.
	Do not buy or use food in cans that are swollen, dented, or damaged.
	Thaw foods in the refrigerator or microwave; never thaw foods at room temperature.
	Cook foods immediately after thawing.
	Refrigerate all leftovers within 2 hours of cooking and eat them within 24 hours.
	Keep hot foods hot and cold foods cold.
	Avoid old, moldy, or damaged fruits and vegetables.
	Avoid tofu in open bins or containers.
	Cook all meat, poultry, and fish thoroughly; avoid raw eggs and fish.
	Buy individually packaged foods.
	Avoid salad bars and buffets when eating out.
	Limit exposure to large groups of people and people with infections.
	Practice good hygiene and wash hands often.
Dehydration	Drink 8 to 12 cups of liquids a day, regardless of thirst.
	Add soup, flavored ice pops, and other sources of fluid to the diet.
	Limit caffeine.
	Drink most fluids between meals.
	Use antiemetics for relief from nausea and vomiting.
Fatigue	Plan for adequate sleep, relaxation, and exercise.
	Address any underlying anxiety, stress, depression, and/or anemia.

*Low white blood count and increased risk for infection.
Modified from National Cancer Institute: *Nutrition in cancer care: nutrition implications of cancer therapies, www.cancer.gov/cancertopics/pdq/supportive-care/nutrition/HealthProfessional/page4,* accessed October 2007.

artificial saliva is helpful. Good oral care habits are important to avoid infection and prevent dental caries—both of which could further inhibit healthy eating. Basic mouth care includes the following:

- Visiting the dentist before treatment begins
- Examining the mouth daily for sores or irritation
- Brushing and flossing regularly with a soft-bristled toothbrush
- Ensuring dentures fit correctly
- Using mouthwash that does not contain alcohol, which dries out the mouth

Frequent small snacks often are better accepted than traditional meals. The treatment may alter the tongue's taste buds, causing taste distortion, taste blindness, and the inability to distinguish sweet, sour, salt, or bitter, resulting in more food aversions. Strong food seasonings (for those who can tolerate them) and high-protein liquid drinks may be helpful. Because the treatment also may alter salivary secretions, foods with a high liquid content are favored. Solid foods may be swallowed more easily with the use of sauces, gravies, broth, yogurt, or salad dressings. A food processor or blender can turn foods into semisolid or liquid forms for easier swallowing. Any dental problems should be corrected to help with chewing.

GI Problems. Chemotherapy often causes nausea and vomiting, which require special individual attention (see Table 23-2). Food that is hot, sweet, fatty, or spicy sometimes exacerbates nausea and should be avoided according to individual tolerances. Small, frequent feedings of soft to liquid cold foods, eaten slowly with rests in between, may be helpful. The physician's use of antinausea drugs such as prochlorperazine (Compazine, Zofran, and Kytril) may help with food tolerances. Surgical treatment involving the GI tract requires related dietary modifications (see Chapter 22). Chemotherapy and radiation treatment can affect the mucosal cells secreting lactase and thus create lactose intolerance. In such cases, a soy-based nutrient supplement (e.g., Ensure [Ross Products, Columbus, Ohio]) may be used.

Pain and Discomfort. Patients are more able to eat if severe pain is controlled and they are positioned as comfortably as possible. The current medical consensus is to administer pain control medication as needed, in close consultation with the patient and family, and carefully monitor responses. This is especially important for children with cancer undergoing painful treatments. Constipation is a common side effect of several pain medications. Preventive therapy to avoid additional discomfort from constipation is important and should focus on adequate fluids, soluble fiber, and regular physical activity (even short walks can help).

Enteral: Tube Feeding

When the GI tract can still be used but the patient is unable to eat and requires more assistance to achieve essential intake goals, tube feeding may be indicated. However, many patients have negative feelings about tube feeding, especially the use of a nasogastric tube. On the other hand, some highly motivated patients are able to place their small-caliber tubes themselves. In some instances patients can be fed by pump-monitored slow drip during the night and be free from the tube during the day. Bolus feedings with percutaneous endoscopic gastrostomy tubes often are used for patients needing long-term nutrition support; they have the benefit of closely resembling normal meal patterns. The use of special formulas and delivery system equipment also has made home enteral nutrition possible and practical.

Parenteral: Peripheral Vein Feeding

When the GI tract cannot be used and nutrition support is vital, IV feeding must be initiated. For brief periods—in cases requiring less-concentrated intakes of energy and nutrients—solutions of dextrose, amino acids, vitamins, and minerals, with concurrent use of lipid emulsions, may be fed into smaller peripheral veins. The use of smaller peripheral veins carries less risk than use of a larger central vein and can supply necessary support when nutrient needs are not excessive. Peripheral vein feeding is combined with tube feeding to supply additional needs in some cases, avoiding the use of a central vein.

Parenteral: Central Vein Feeding

When nutrition needs are greater and must continue over an extended period, central vein feeding often provides a life-saving alternative. This TPN process requires surgical placement of the feeding catheter along with careful assessment, monitoring, and administration. Although TPN carries risks, and thus requires skilled team management, this hyperalimentation process provides a significant means of turning the metabolic status of patients with cancer from catabolism to anabolism, often avoiding the serious development of cancer cachexia. Details of enteral and parenteral methods of feeding are discussed in Chapter 22.

CANCER THERAPY AND PREVENTION

Therapy

Ample evidence currently indicates that vigorous nutrition support increases the chances for successful medical treatments in the care of cancer. Much effort on the part of the health care team, the patient, and the family, all working together, is absolutely necessary for vigorous nutrition support to become a reality.

Prevention

Based on the most current information in cancer research and prevention, the American Cancer Society has issued guidelines to encourage healthy lifestyle choices to reduce the risk of cancer.[16] These guidelines are established by a national panel of experts and are updated every 5 years. In addition, the FDA has defined specific food labeling guidelines linking certain foods and nutrients to decreased cancer risk.[17] A variety of other government and privately funded research studies are ongoing in the hopes of identifying a more specific cause and cure for cancer.

American Cancer Society Guidelines

The most recent publication of the American Cancer Society guidelines for cancer prevention recommend the following[18]:

1. Maintain a healthy weight throughout life by the following actions:
   - Balancing caloric intake with physical activity.
   - Avoiding excessive weight gain throughout the life cycle. Excess weight is believed to increase the risk of several types of cancer (Box 23-1).
2. Achieve and maintain a healthy weight if currently overweight or obese. The American Cancer Society recommends maintaining a BMI between 18.5 and 25.0 kg/m².
3. Adopt a physically active lifestyle.
   - Children and adolescents are encouraged to participate in at least 60 minutes per day of moderate to vigorous physical activity at least 5 days per week.
   - Adults should engage in at least 30 minutes of moderate to vigorous physical activity for a minimum of 5 days per week. Forty-five to 60 minutes of intentional physical activity is preferable.
   - Examples of moderate activity include walking, skating, yoga, softball or baseball, downhill skiing, garden maintenance, and lawn care. Vigorous activities include running, aerobics, fast bicycling, circuit weight training, soccer, singles tennis, basketball, cross-country skiing, and heavy manual labor. Convincing evidence shows that increasing physical activity can produce protective benefits against colorectal and breast cancer.
4. Consume a healthy diet, with an emphasis on plant sources. The American Cancer Society recommends that individuals do the following:
   - Become familiar with standard serving sizes and read food labels to become more aware of actual servings consumed.
   - Eat smaller portions of high-calorie foods. Be aware that "low fat" and "nonfat" do not mean low calorie, and that low-fat cakes, cookies, and similar foods often are high in calories.
   - Substitute vegetables, fruits, and other low-calorie foods and beverages for calorie-dense foods and beverages such as French fries, cheeseburgers, pizza, ice cream, doughnuts, other sweets, and full-calorie sodas.
   - When eating away from home, choose food low in calories, fat, and sugar and avoid large portion sizes.
   - Eat five or more servings of vegetables and fruits every day.
   - Choose whole grains instead of processed (refined) grains and sugars.
   - Choose fish, poultry, and beans as alternatives to beef, pork, and lamb. Select lean cuts and small portions and prepare meat by baking, broiling, or poaching rather than frying.
5. If you drink alcoholic beverages, limit consumption. The USDHHS and the American Cancer Society recommend men and women who drink alcohol limiting their alcohol intake to two drinks per day for men and one drink per day for women.[19] One drink is defined as 12 oz of beer, 5 oz of wine, or 1.5 oz of 80-proof distilled spirits. Limiting alcohol intake is associated with beneficial effects against mouth, pharynx, larynx, esophagus, and liver cancers.

Dietary choices and physical activity are the most modifiable risk factors for cancer development. One third of all cancer deaths in the United States are attributed to poor diet and physical inactivity, including overweight

---

BOX 23-1

OVERWEIGHT AND OBESITY INCREASE THE RISK FOR CERTAIN TYPES OF CANCER

- Breast
- Colon
- Endometrium
- Kidney
- Pancreas
- Gallbladder
- Adenocarcinoma of the esophagus
- Thyroid
- Ovary
- Cervix
- Myeloma
- Hodgkin's lymphoma
- Prostate cancer

and obesity.[18] Thus following the preceding guidelines could make a significant difference in the lives of many individuals.

Food and Drug Administration Health Claims

Health claims approved for use on food labels are regulated by the FDA (see Chapter 13). The qualified health claims about cancer risk for use on food labels in the United States link the following nutrients with reduced risk[17]:

- Tomatoes and/or tomato sauce with prostate, ovarian, gastric, and pancreatic cancer
- Green tea with cancer
- Calcium with colorectal cancer and recurrent colorectal polyps
- Antioxidant vitamins with cancer
- Selenium with cancer

On the basis of these consistent and strong associations, the CDC has developed a program to encourage Americans to eat five or more servings of fruits and vegetables every day, which is one of the nation's health promotion and disease prevention objectives.[20] The Fruits and Veggies Matter program *(www.fruitsandveggiesmatter.gov)* is partnered with the National Cancer Institute, USDA, American Cancer Society, and the FDA. The CDC works closely with the Association of State and Territorial Public Health Nutrition Directors *(www.astphnd.org)*, which is made up of nutrition coordinators, formerly known as "5-A-Day" coordinators.

Ongoing Cancer Research

Many studies have shown that diets low in fat and high in fiber, fruits, and vegetables—major sources of micronutrients and phytochemicals—are associated with decreased incidence and mortality rate from various cancers.[18,21,22] The exact mechanisms by which such diets are protective against cancer are not yet clearly defined for each association and are still under investigation. The protective roles of several food components such as fish oils, garlic, soy products, various teas, and dietary supplements (e.g., folic acid, selenium, and vitamins A, C, and E) have been analyzed for definitive correlations and mechanisms associated with decreased cancer risk. The effect of dietary intervention for cancer survivors is difficult to assess because of a limited number of well-controlled trials.[23] In addition to preventive cancer research, emerging reports are being published on dietary guidelines for cancer survivors and alternative or complementary therapies.[16,24]

The CDC hosts many programs aimed at preventing and controlling cancers as well as researching cause-and-effect relations, including the National Comprehensive Cancer Control Program; National Breast and Cervical Cancer Early Detection Program; National Program of Cancer Registries; and initiatives such as the colorectal cancer prevention and control initiative; prostate cancer control initiative; skin cancer primary prevention education initiative; hematologic cancer initiative; and ovarian, gynecologic, and cervical cancer control initiatives.[25] Many of these programs have nutrition-related objectives.

ACQUIRED IMMUNODEFICIENCY
SECTION 2 SYNDROME

PROCESS OF AIDS DEVELOPMENT

This section looks at acquired immunodeficiency syndrome (AIDS) and compares its relation to the body's immune system and course of development with that of cancer. Similarly, a brief review is presented on the process of AIDS development, its medical treatment, nutrition support, and conclusions about AIDS therapy and prevention.

According to the NCHS, more than 42,000 people are infected with HIV every year in the United States alone (see the Cultural Considerations box, "Types and Incidence of HIV/AIDS in American Populations"). The most recent statistics reported that 73% of the population infected with HIV is male.[26]

CULTURAL CONSIDERATIONS

TYPES AND INCIDENCE OF HIV/AIDS IN AMERICAN POPULATIONS

Just under 1 million cases of AIDS have been diagnosed in the United States from 1981 to 2005.* The largest percent of new HIV infections each year occur from male-to-male sexual contact. Injection drug use and high-risk heterosexual contact are the next most common causes of HIV transmission.

The percentage of new HIV infections according to race is disproportionate to the total U.S. population. For example,

African Americans make up 13% of the total U.S. population, but 49% of new HIV infection cases are among African Americans.

The CDC has reported the race and ethnicity of persons with HIV/AIDS diagnosed during 2005 as follows:

Because no cures or vaccines for HIV are currently available, prevention is the only means of protection regardless of race or gender.

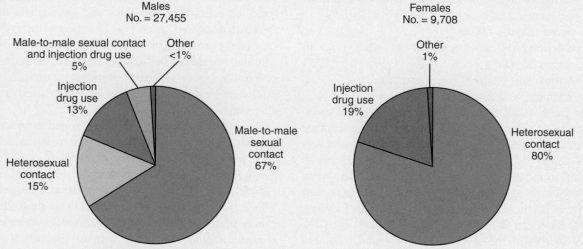

Transmission categories of adults and adolescents with HIV/AIDS diagnosed during 2005. Based on data from 33 states with long-term, confidential, name-based reporting.†

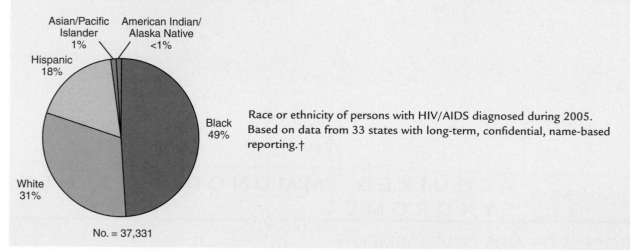

Race or ethnicity of persons with HIV/AIDS diagnosed during 2005. Based on data from 33 states with long-term, confidential, name-based reporting.†

*Centers for Disease Control and Prevention: *HIV/AIDS surveillance report, 2005*, vol. 17, rev ed. Atlanta, 2007, U.S. Department of Health and Human Services.
†Reprinted from Centers for Disease Control and Prevention: *A glance at the HIV/AIDS epidemic, www.cdc.gov/hiv/resources/factsheets/PDF/At-A-Glance.pdf,* accessed October 2007.

Evolution of Human Immunodeficiency Virus

Early Pandemic Spread

The earliest known case of AIDS was identified in a blood sample collected in 1959 from a Bantu man living in what is currently called the Democratic Republic of Congo, an area from which the current world epidemic is believed to have originated.[27] Early in the 1960s in the African country of Uganda, strange deaths began to occur from simple common infections such as pneumonia that did not respond to the usual antibiotic drugs. By the late 1970s and early 1980s the same strange deaths were occurring in Europe and America. Similar reports of unexplained immune system failure increased rapidly in various parts of the world, and the pandemic spread. These early cases came from people with diverse social and medical backgrounds, including heterosexual and homosexual men, IV drug users, and recipients of transfused blood and blood products (e.g., patients with hemophilia and medical and surgical patients). After feverish research, the underlying infectious agent was finally discovered in May 1983. The French scientist Luc Montagnier, a leading pioneer of AIDS research, reported that he and his team at the Pasteur Institute in Paris had isolated the viral cause, now known as the *human immunodeficiency virus (HIV)*.

Evolution and Spread of the Virus

Where did this deadly virus come from, and how did it gain such strength so rapidly? From studies thus far, scientists are beginning to find some answers. Apparently HIV is not a new virus but an old one that only recently grew deadly in human beings while gaining strength during the social upheavals of the 1960s and 1970s. The uprooting effect of rapid social change, urbanization, and world travel allowed the virus to spread rapidly through world populations and reproduce aggressively in its human host.

Parasitic Nature of the Virus

No virus can have a life of its own. By their structure and reproductive nature, viruses are the ultimate parasites. They are mere shreds of genetic material, a small packet of genetic information encased in a protein coat. Viruses only contain a small chromosome of nucleic acids (RNA or DNA), usually with fewer than five genes. They can live only through a host, whom they invade and infect, hijacking the host's cell machinery to make a multitude of copies of itself. Scientists agree that HIV, which is genetically similar to viruses found in African primates (e.g., simian immunodeficiency virus), was probably transmitted to human beings in an earlier age as ancient hunters accidentally cut themselves while butchering their kills for food. The deadly strength of HIV results from its aggressive growth within an increasing number of hosts. Worldwide, 33.2 million people are living with HIV/AIDS, of which 1.3 million are in North American.[28]

Stages of Disease Progression

The individual clinical course of HIV infection varies substantially, but the following three distinct stages mark the progression of the disease:

- Primary HIV infection and extended well period of viral incubation
- HIV-related diseases
- AIDS

Stage 1: Clinical Category A

HIV is transmitted from an infected person to another person through sexual contact (oral, anal, or vaginal), the sharing of needles or syringes, or blood transfusions. Blood donations are now very closely screened for HIV antibodies in most countries, thus reducing this form of transmission. Pregnant women with HIV also may infect their babies during delivery.

Approximately 2 to 4 weeks after initial exposure and infection, a mild flulike episode lasting about 1 week may occur. This brief, mild response reflects the initial development of antibodies to the viral infection. Any subsequent HIV testing is positive. For a number of years the person typically feels well. This long well period is deceptive, however, because it is a critical stage of viral incubation. The virus is hiding in lymphoid tissues (e.g., lymph nodes, spleen, adenoid glands, and tonsils), where it rapidly multiplies in its parasite life cycle within the host, taking over more and more of its special T-helper white

---

pandemic a widespread epidemic, distributed through a region, a continent, or the world.

virus a minute microscopic infectious organism characterized by lack of independent metabolism and the ability to reproduce with genetic continuity only within a living host. Each particle (virion) consists of nucleic acids and a protein shell that protects and contains the genetic material and any enzymes present.

parasite an organism that lives in or on an organism of another species, known as the host, from whom all nourishment is obtained.

BOX 23-2

COMMON TYPES OF OPPORTUNISTIC INFECTIONS IN HIV-INFECTED INDIVIDUALS

Common conditions in clinical category B include the following:
- Bacillary angiomatosis
- Candidiasis, oropharyngeal (thrush)
- Candidiasis, vulvovaginal; persistent, frequent, or poorly responsive to therapy
- Cervical dysplasia (moderate or severe), cervical carcinoma in situ
- Constitutional symptoms, such as fever (38.5° C) or diarrhea lasting longer than 1 month
- Hairy leukoplakia, oral
- Herpes zoster (shingles), involving at least two distinct episodes or more than one dermatome
- Idiopathic thrombocytopenic purpura
- Listeriosis
- Pelvic inflammatory disease, particularly if complicated by tubo-ovarian abscess
- Peripheral neuropathy

Common conditions in clinical category C include the following:
- Candidiasis of bronchi, trachea, or lungs
- Candidiasis, esophageal
- Cervical cancer, invasive
- Coccidioidomycosis, disseminated or extrapulmonary
- Cryptococcosis, extrapulmonary
- Cryptosporidiosis, chronic intestinal (longer than 1 month)
- Cytomegalovirus disease (other than liver, spleen, or nodes)
- Cytomegalovirus retinitis (with loss of vision)
- Encephalopathy, HIV related
- Herpes simplex: chronic ulcer(s) (longer than 1 month in duration); bronchitis, pneumonitis, esophagitis
- Histoplasmosis, disseminated or extrapulmonary
- Isosporiasis, chronic intestinal (longer than 1 month in duration)
- Kaposi's sarcoma
- Lymphoma, Burkitt's (or equivalent term)
- Lymphoma, immunoblastic (or equivalent term)
- Lymphoma, primary, of brain
- *Mycobacterium avium* complex or *M. kansasii,* disseminated or extrapulmonary
- *M. tuberculosis,* any site (pulmonary or extrapulmonary)
- *Mycobacterium,* other species or unidentified species, disseminated or extrapulmonary
- *Pneumocystis carinii* pneumonia
- Pneumonia, recurrent
- Progressive multifocal leukoencephalopathy
- Salmonella septicemia, recurrent
- Toxoplasmosis of brain
- Wasting syndrome from HIV

Reprinted from Centers for Disease Control and Prevention: 1993 revised classification system for HIV infection and expanded surveillance case definition for AIDS among adolescents and adults, *MMWR* 41:17, 1992.

blood cells (CD4 cells) and gaining strength. Researchers emphasize the crucial nature of this incubation period and the importance of earlier medical treatment intervention after a positive HIV test result to slow this viral strengthening time while drugs and vaccines are developed to combat its steady progression.

Stage 2: Clinical Category B

After the extended "well" HIV-positive stage, associated infectious illnesses begin to invade the body. This period of opportunistic illnesses is so named because at this point the HIV infection has killed enough host-protective white blood cells (e.g., T-lymphocytes) to damage the immune system severely and lower the body's normal disease resistance so that even the most common everyday infections have an opportunity to take root and grow (Box 23-2). T-lymphocyte counts are between 200 and 499 cells/mcL during this stage. Common symptoms during this period include persistent fatigue, mouth sores from thrush (oral *Candida albicans*), night sweats, diarrhea, fever greater than 100° F, unintentional weight loss, remarkable headaches, shingles, cervical dysplasia or carcinoma, new or unusual cough, unusual bruises or skin discoloration, and shortness of breath.

Stage 3: Clinical Category C

The terminal stage of HIV infection, designated as AIDS, is marked by rapidly declining T-lymphocyte counts from the normal, healthy level of approximately 800 cells/mcL to less than 200 cells/mcL. At counts this low, various diseases (e.g., tuberculosis, Kaposi's sarcoma) generally occur. Kaposi's sarcoma is the most common AIDS-associated cancer, characterized by malignant, rapidly growing tumors of the skin and mucous linings of the GI and respiratory tracts, where they may cause severe internal bleeding. Low-dose radiation therapy or anticancer drugs may be used to slow the spread of tumors. During severe immunodeficiency, *protozoan parasites* (i.e., primitive single-cell organisms) appear and infect a number of body organs. At counts less than $50/mm^3$, *cytomegalovirus*, a herpes virus causing lesions on mucous linings of body organs, or *lymphoma* (any cancer of the lymphoid tissue), can flourish. This series of HIV effects on the body brings marked changes in body weight in both men and women (wasting syndrome), with women losing disproportionately more body fat. Other common conditions include infection with *Mycobacterium tuberculosis, Pneumocystis carinii* pneumonia, AIDS dementia complex, and progressive multifocal leukoencephalopathy. When the AIDS virus kills enough white cells to overwhelm the immune system's weakened resistance to the disease complications, death follows.

NUTRITION MANAGEMENT IN THE PATIENT WITH HIV/AIDS

Support for Medical Management

Basic Current Goals

Medical management of HIV infection is constantly evolving with intensive medical research. Basic current goals are to achieve the following:

- Delay progression of the infection and boost the immune system
- Prevent opportunistic illnesses
- Recognize the infection early and provide rapid treatment for complications, including infections and cancer

Initial Evaluation: AIDS Team

The initial medical evaluation of a person newly diagnosed with HIV is critical to provide guidelines for ongoing comprehensive care by the AIDS team. This professional team includes medical, nutrition, nursing, and psychosocial health care specialists. Box 23-3 outlines an initial evaluation guide that emphasizes special coordinated medical care and the importance of nutrition, nursing, and psychosocial support.

Drug Therapy

Developing effective drugs is difficult because of the highly evolved nature of the virus. One of the earliest findings in the drug research for HIV has been a group of compounds called *nucleoside/nucleotide reverse transcriptase inhibitors* (NRTIs) that inhibit the virus's necessary enzyme for copying itself, thus effectively preventing viral increase. Multiple toxic side effects have been reported, however, some of which (e.g., nausea) may be helped by dietary modifications (Table 23-3). Other types of antiretroviral drugs approved by the FDA and currently in use in the United States are *non-NRTIs* (NNRTIs), *protease inhibitors* (PIs) and, most recently, *fusion inhibitors.*[29] NNRTIs prevent reproduction of the viral cells by inhibiting reverse transcriptase. PIs help stop HIV by inhibiting the basic enzyme, protease, which is essential to its development. Unfortunately, the virus is capable of mutation in response to some drugs, specifically protease inhibitors, and thus become resistant to treatment.[30] Fusion inhibitors prevent the infection of healthy cells by binding to HIV. In addition to these antiretroviral drugs, many other drugs have been approved by the FDA to prevent or treat AIDS-related illnesses. A list of current drugs can be found at *www.fda.gov/oashi/aids/virals.html.*

BOX 23-3

INITIAL EVALUATION OF NEWLY DIAGNOSED HIV-INFECTED PATIENTS

- History and physical examination
- History of present illness
- Medical history
- Medications and allergies
- Social, sexual, and family histories
- Review of systems (including questions about common HIV infection–related symptoms)
- Baseline evaluation: diagnostic and screening
  - Serologic testing for HIV
  - CD4 cell counts
  - Plasma HIV RNA load
  - HIV resistance testing
  - Complete blood cell count and chemistry panel
  - Glucose-6-phosphate dehydrogenase
  - Tuberculosis screening
  - Serologic testing for *Toxoplasma gondii*
  - Viral hepatitis screening
  - Screening for infections with Cytomegalovirus and other herpes viruses
  - Sexually transmitted disease screening
  - Serologic testing for syphilis
  - Human papillomavirus screening
  - Fasting lipid profiles
  - Testosterone levels
  - Chest radiography
  - Other laboratory tests as indicated
- Special considerations for women
  - Pregnancy testing
  - Gynecologic evaluation for cervical cancer screening and prevention
  - Mammography

Data from Aberg JA and others: Primary care guidelines for the management of persons infected with human immunodeficiency virus: recommendations of the HIV Medicine Association of the Infectious Diseases Society of America, *Clin Infect Dis* 39:609, 2004.

Vaccine Development

A successful HIV vaccine would train the body's immune system to identify and destroy the virus. The development and testing of vaccines takes several years. Once a potential vaccine is identified, it must go through the following three phases of testing and be determined effective before the FDA can approve it for public use:

- *Phase I:* The vaccine is tested in small groups of healthy, low-risk participants. This phase lasts 12 to 18 months.

TABLE 23-3

INITIAL ANTIRETROVIRAL THERAPY AND MAJOR TOXIC EFFECTS AND CAUTIONS

DRUG	MAJOR TOXIC EFFECTS AND CAUTIONS
NRTIs	
Tenofovir/emtric-itabine (or lamivu-dine)	Baseline renal function should be evaluated before initiating tenofovir
	Use with caution or avoid in patients with renal dysfunction
Zidovudine/lamivudine (or emtricitabine)	Headache, nausea
	Anemia
	Lipoatrophy
Abacavir/lamivudine (or emtricitabine)	Hypersensitivity syndrome in 5% to 8% of patients
NNRTIs	
Efavirenz	Central nervous system toxic effects may be limiting
	Teratogenic in first trimester of pregnancy
Nevirapine	Rash
	Hepatotoxicity
	Hypersensitivity syndrome
	Avoid in women with >250 CD4 cells/μL and men with >400 CD4 cells/μL
Ritonavir-Boosted PIs	
Ritonavir-boosted lopinavir	Gastrointestinal adverse effects
	Hyperlipidemia
	Lipodystrophy
	Insulin resistance
Ritonavir-boosted atazanavir	Hyperbilirubinemia
	Avoid concomitant antacid use
	Do no use concomitant proton pump inhibitors
Ritonavir-boosted fosamprenavir	Rash
Ritonavir-boosted saquinavir	Gastrointestinal toxic effects with soft-gel formulation; incidence diminished with hard-gel formulation

Modified from Hammer SM and others: Treatment for adult HIV infection: 2006 recommendations of the International AIDS Society, USA Panel, *JAMA* 296(7):827, 2006.

- *Phase II:* The vaccine is tested in hundreds of high- and low-risk participants. This phase can last up to 2 years.
- *Phase III:* Thousands of high-risk participants are tested for both safety and effectiveness of the vaccine. This phase usually lasts an additional 3 to 4 years.

In February 1999, Thailand became the first country to begin a phase III HIV vaccine trial. The CDC and the NIH are involved in coordinating vaccine research in the United States and are working in conjunction with other agencies worldwide to expedite the development of an effective vaccine. More information about preventative and therapeutic vaccines can be found at *http://aidsinfo.nih.gov/*.

Wasting Effects of HIV Infection on Nutritional Status

Severe Malnutrition and Weight Loss

Patients with HIV typically have decreased appetite and insufficient energy intake coupled with elevated resting energy expenditure. Major weight loss follows and eventually leads to extreme cachexia, similar to that seen in patients with cancer. Malnutrition suppresses cellular immune function, thus perpetuating the onset of opportunistic infections, the primary cause of death in patients with AIDS. The chronic, relentless body wasting of AIDS is so striking that in Africa it is called "slim disease." This wasting process plays a major role in patients' decreased quality of life, debilitating weakness, and fatigue.

Causes of Body Wasting

The characteristic body wasting of HIV infection may result from any of the following processes, alone or in combination:

- *Inadequate food intake:* An important factor in the profound weight loss is severe *anorexia*, or loss of appetite. This state is probably related to the patient's life-changing situation as well as the body's physiologic changes from the disease.
- *Malabsorption of nutrients:* Diarrhea and malabsorption are common in AIDS. These symptoms are related to drug-diet interactions and the progressive effects of HIV infection. The viral infection causes blunting of the intestinal villi and secretion of abnormal intestinal enzymes. In later stages of AIDS, the damaged intestinal tissues are open to opportunistic organisms, resulting in severe diarrhea and malabsorption.
- *Disordered metabolism:* In the final stage of weight loss in patients with AIDS, changes in metabolism (e.g., hypermetabolism and altered energy metabolism) occur. Progressive depletion of lean body mass and increased resting energy expenditure also result.

Lipodystrophy

Encouraging results initially came with the drug megestrol (Megace) in treating cachexia and wasting syndrome in patients with AIDS or cancer. This drug is a synthetic hormone similar to the natural hormone progesterone, which improves appetite and food intake, leading to weight gain. However, the majority of the weight gained is fat mass as opposed to lean tissue. Disproportionate gaining of fat mass, lipodystrophy, and continued wasting of lean tissue contribute to the abnormal body composition changes seen in patients with AIDS. Human growth hormone and resistance training appear to be more effective in preventing lean tissue losses.[31]

Nutrition Assessment

A comprehensive nutrition assessment provides the baseline information necessary for starting and continuing nutrition care. The clinical dietitian on the AIDS team conducts this assessment and calculates daily energy and protein needs, assessing and monitoring weight changes and evaluating laboratory test results. These tests and evaluations are especially necessary for certain patients on enteral or parenteral nutrition support. Further person-centered nutrition care necessary for all HIV-infected patients is evident in the ABCDEFs of nutrition assessment (see the Clinical Applications box, "The ABCDEFs of Nutrition Assessment for Patients with AIDS").

Suggestions for nutrition-related symptom management are outlined in Table 23-2.

Nutrition Counseling, Education, and Supportive Care

Counseling Principles

The basic goal of nutrition counseling is to make the least amount of changes necessary in a person's lifestyle and food patterns to promote optimal nutritional status while providing maximal comfort and quality of life.

In this person-centered care process, the following counseling principles are particularly important:

- *Motivation:* Changes in behavior in any area require the motivation, desire, and ability to achieve one's goals. AIDS is no exception. Until a patient perceives food patterns and behaviors as appropriate goals, wait for a better time and simply start with establishing a general supportive climate in which to continue working together. Any specific obstacle raised by the patient (e.g., time, physical limitations, money, increased anxiety) can be met with related suggestions to consider.
- *Rationale:* Any diet or food behavior change, with possible benefits or risks, must be clearly explained to the patient. Patients with AIDS are more vulnerable to the lure of unproven therapies.
- *Provider-patient agreement:* When the patient is ready, any change must be an agreement and must fit daily routines and include caregivers as needed. Throughout the process, the nutrition counselor should provide necessary information and encouragement.
- *Manageable steps:* All information and actions should proceed in manageable steps, as small as necessary and in order of complexity and difficulty. Do simple, easy things first. Information overload can discourage anyone. Clinicians also should keep in mind any brain or CNS decline in the patient. Such decline may contribute to memory loss and inability to follow nutrition advice. Include support persons in consultations.

Personal Food Management Skills

The patient's living situation and general practical skills in planning, purchasing, and preparing food must be considered. Need for information and guidance in developing these skills or locating sources of help should be addressed.

CLINICAL APPLICATIONS

THE ABCDEFs OF NUTRITION ASSESSMENT FOR PATIENTS WITH AIDS

The initial nutrition assessment visit with a patient infected with HIV is important because it sets the pattern and direction for all the continuing nutrition care that follows.

This vital encounter serves both informational and relational functions. It provides the necessary baseline information for planning practical, individual nutrition support. More importantly, however, the initial visit establishes the essential provider/patient relationship, which is the human context in which continuing nutrition care and support are provided. The basic ABCDs of nutrition assessment (*A*nthropometry, *B*iochemical tests, *C*linical observations, and *D*ietary evaluations) provide a practical guide (see Chapter

17), with two more points added for HIV-infected patients.

*E*nvironmental, behavioral, and psychological assessment
- Living situation, personal support
- Food environment, types of meals, eating assistance needed

*F*inancial Assessment
- Medical insurance
- Income, financial support through caregivers
- Ability to afford food, enteral supplements, additional vitamins or minerals

Community Programs

Information about available community food programs (e.g., Meals on Wheels for delivery of prepared meals when the patient is too ill to shop for food or prepare it) may be needed. Information about food assistance programs (e.g., food stamps or food commodities [see Chapter 13]), for which lower income persons may qualify, may be warranted.

Psychosocial Support

In the final analysis every aspect of care provided should be given in a form and manner that provide genuine psychosocial support. All health care providers working with HIV-infected patients must be particularly sensitive to the psychological and social issues that confront them. Major stress areas include issues relating to autonomy and dependency, a sense of uncertainty and fear of the unknown, grief, change and loss, fear of symptoms and abandonment, and spiritual questions that arise when confronting a life-threatening disease. Common emotions are hostility, denial, withdrawal, depression, anxiety, guilt, and confusion. Health care providers always must be aware of how the patient and caregivers relate to the disease, using the assistance of social workers and clinical psychologists as needed. Stress-reduction groups and activities, including exercise training, are helpful, as in other life-threatening conditions (e.g., cancer and coronary heart disease).

Health care workers also must examine their own stresses, values, and fears about sexual orientation and behavior, IV drug use, and fear of AIDS transmission. Preconceived judgments are easily sensed by patients and threaten the provider-patient relationship. Before they can be effective with patients, all health care workers must first deal with their own fears and prejudices and learn to let go of judgmental behavior.

SUMMARY

The general term *cancer* is given to various abnormal, malignant tumors in different tissue sites. The cancer cell is derived from a normal cell that loses control over its growth and reproduction. Cancer cell development occurs by mutation of regulatory genes and is influenced by environmental chemical carcinogens, radiation, and viruses. Other lifestyle factors associated with an increased risk for cancer include poor diet, excessive alcohol use, and smoking as well as physical and psychological stress. Cell integrity is mediated by the body's immune system, primarily through its two types of white blood cells: T-cells that kill invading agents that cause disease and B-cells that make specific antibodies to attack these agents.

Cancer therapy primarily consists of surgery, radiation, and chemotherapy. Supportive nutrition care must be highly individualized according to body responses to the disease and its treatment. This care is based on nutrition assessment and provided by the following routes: oral, tube feeding, or TPN. In any case, nutrition management must meet the physical and psychological needs of individual patients.

Likewise, nutrition care of patients with AIDS must be built on knowledge and compassion, with a sensitivity and concern for individual patient needs. The current worldwide spread of HIV and its fatal consequences have reached epidemic proportions and are still growing. The overall disease progression follows the three distinct stages: (1) category A, HIV infection; (2) category B, symptomatic disease with opportunistic infection and illnesses; and (3) category C, symptomatic AIDS with complicating diseases leading to death.

Medical management of HIV infection, which is still without a cure or vaccine, involves supportive treatment of associated illnesses and diseases. In the terminal AIDS stage, the virus eventually gains enough strength to destroy the host's immune system, and death follows. New drugs are useful in slowing the disease process while intensive ongoing research seeks a vaccine and cure.

Nutrition management centers on providing individual nutrition support to counteract the severe body wasting and malnutrition characteristic of the disease. The process of nutrition care involves comprehensive nutrition assessment and evaluation of personal needs, planning care with patient and caregivers, and meeting food needs.

CRITICAL THINKING QUESTIONS

1. What is cancer? Describe several major causes of cancer cell formation. Why is cancer an increasing health problem?
2. In what two main ways does nutrition relate to cancer? Give examples of each.
3. Describe the types of defense cells that are the major components of the body's immune system. How does nutrition relate to immunity?
4. Describe nutrition problems associated with each of the three medical treatments of cancer. Outline the general procedure for nutrition management of a patient with cancer.
5. List and describe the reasoning behind each of the American Cancer Society's dietary guidelines for reducing the risk for cancer.
6. Describe the evolutionary history of HIV and its current worldwide epidemic spread. How is it transmitted, and why has the virus spread so rapidly? Identify major population groups at risk.
7. Outline basic parts of a comprehensive initial nutrition assessment of a patient with HIV infection and describe the reasons for each piece of information and its evaluation.
8. Describe the general process of planning nutrition care on the basis of the patient assessment information and the main types of nutrition problems in patients with HIV. Devise a related plan of action for each type of problem. Give an example of how you might follow up to see what did or did not work and make adjustments.

CHAPTER CHALLENGE QUESTIONS

True-False

Write the correct statement for each statement that is false.

1. *True or False:* A cancer cell is unrelated to a normal cell.
2. *True or False:* Genes consist of cell nucleus material that controls protein synthesis and transmits hereditary information.
3. *True or False:* Chemical carcinogens are substances that can cause cancer to develop.
4. *True or False:* The incidence of cancer is not related to age.
5. *True or False:* Cancer-causing mutant genes may be inherited, making a person more susceptible to the influence of some carcinogenic environmental agent.
6. *True or False:* Antigens are specialized protein components of the immune system that protect against disease.
7. *True or False:* Cachexia is a muscle wasting syndrome occurring only in patients with AIDS.
8. *True or False:* Unlike patients with cancer, individuals with AIDS do not require nutrition support.
9. *True or False:* Lipodystrophy is the abnormal fat redistribution syndrome characteristic in some patients with AIDS who have protein wasting and body fat gain, often in abnormal places.
10. *True or False:* Individuals with AIDS have severely weakened immune systems, such that parasites and bacteria that are not normally lethal could result in death.

Multiple Choice

1. Special blood cells that are major components of the immune system are
   a. erythrocytes.
   b. lymphocytes.
   c. neurotransmitters.
   d. platelets.
2. A serious primary problem resulting from prolonged vomiting from cancer chemotherapy relates to
   a. nitrogen balance.
   b. calcium balance.
   c. fluid and electrolyte balance.
   d. vitamin E balance.
3. Side effects of cancer chemotherapy that reflect the toxic effect of the drugs on rapidly reproducing cells include
   a. severe headaches.
   b. GI symptoms.
   c. increased urination.
   d. increased appetite.
4. An adequate amount of high-quality protein is essential in the diet of a patient with cancer to
   a. prevent catabolism.
   b. meet increased energy demands.
   c. prevent anabolism.
   d. stimulate hypermetabolism.

5. Small amounts of which of the following types of food would most likely help treat the nausea caused by cancer chemotherapy?

a. Hot liquids
b. Dry, spicy foods
c. Warm, fat-seasoned foods
d. Soft, cold foods

6. Which of the following is not a method by which HIV can be transmitted?

a. Sexual contact
b. Social kissing
c. Sharing needles
d. Blood transfusions

7. An individual with HIV infection is said to have AIDS when

a. he or she loses 10 pounds.
b. he or she has a rapid increase in T-helper lymphocytes.
c. he or she starts taking medications such as protease inhibitors.
d. he or she has a rapid decrease in T-helper lymphocytes.

8. Body wasting in the patient with AIDS usually is a result of which of the following?

a. Inadequate food intake
b. Malabsorption of nutrients
c. Disordered metabolism
d. All the above

---

evolve Please refer to the Students' Resource section of this text's Evolve Web site for additional study resources.

REFERENCES

1. Pleis JR, Lethbridge-Çejku M: Summary health statistics for U.S. adults: national health interview survey, 2005, National Center for Health Statistics, *Vital Health Stat* 10(232), 2006.
2. Miller DP and others: Association between self-reported environmental tobacco smoke exposure and lung cancer: modification by GSTP1 polymorphism, *Int J Cancer* 104(6):758, 2003.
3. Settimi L and others: Prostate cancer and exposure to pesticides in agricultural settings, *Int J Cancer* 104:458, 2003.
4. McGlynn KA and others: Serum concentrations of 1,1,1-trichloro-2,2-bis(p-chlorophenyl)ethane (DDT) and 1,1-dichloro-2,2-bis(p-chlorophenyl)ethylene (DDE) and risk of primary liver cancer, *J Natl Cancer Inst* 98(14):1005, 2006.
5. Ries LAG and others, editors: *SEER cancer statistics review, 1975-2004,* http://seer.cancer.gov/csr/1975_2004, accessed March 2008.
6. Jain RV and others: Cancer incidence in the south Asian population of California, 1988–2000, *J Carcinog* 4:21, 2005.
7. Lillberg K and others: Stressful life events and risk of breast cancer in 10,808 women: a cohort study, *Am J Epidemiol* 157(5):415, 2003.
8. Valko M and others: Free radicals and antioxidants in normal physiological functions and human disease, *Int J Biochem Cell Biol* 39(1):44, 2007.
9. Ames BN, Wakimoto P: Are vitamin and mineral deficiencies a major cancer risk? *Natl Rev Cancer* 2:694, 2002.
10. Norat T and others: Meat, fish, and colorectal cancer risk: the European Prospective Investigation into cancer and nutrition, *J Natl Cancer Inst* 97(12):906, 2005.
11. Berzofsky JA and others: Progress on new vaccine strategies for the immunotherapy and prevention of cancer, *J Clin Invest* 113(11):1515, 2004.
12. Waldmann, TA: Immunotherapy: past, present and future, *Nat Med* 9:269, 2003.
13. Xu J and others: Preoperative enteral immunonutrition improves postoperative outcome in patients with gastrointestinal cancer, *World J Surg* 30(7):1284, 2006.
14. Laviano A and others: Therapy insight: cancer anorexia-cachexia syndrome—when all you can eat is yourself, *Nat Clin Pract Oncol* 2(3):158, 2005.
15. Palesty JA, Dudrick SJ: What we have learned about cachexia in gastrointestinal cancer, *Dig Dis* 21(3):198, 2003.
16. Doyle C and others: Nutrition and physical activity during and after cancer treatment: an American Cancer Society guide for informed choices, *CA Cancer J Clin* 56(6):323, 2006.
17. Center for Food Safety and Applied Nutrition, U.S. Food and Drug Administration: *Qualified health claims,* www.cfsan.fda.gov/~dms/lab-qhc.html, accessed April 2007.
18. Kushi LH and others: American Cancer Society Guidelines on Nutrition and Physical Activity for cancer prevention: reducing the risk of cancer with healthy food choices and physical activity, *CA Cancer J Clin* 56(5):254, 2006.
19. U.S. Department of Health and Human Services: *Dietary guidelines for Americans,* 2005, Washington, DC, 2005, U.S. Government Printing Office.
20. U.S. Department of Health and Human Services: *Healthy people 2010. understanding and improving health,* Washington, DC, 2000, U.S. Government Printing Office.
21. Fernandez E and others: Nutrition and cancer risk: an overview, *J Br Menopause Soc* 12(4):139, 2006.
22. Gallus S and others: Mediterranean diet and cancer risk, *Eur J Cancer Prev* 13(5):447, 2004.
23. Davies AA and others: Nutritional interventions and outcomes in patients with cancer or preinvasive lesions: systematic review, *J Natl Cancer Inst* 98(14):961, 2006.
24. Mansky PJ, Wallerstedt DB: Complementary medicine in palliative care and cancer symptom management, *Cancer J* 12(5):425, 2006.
25. Centers for Disease Control and Prevention, National Center for Chronic Disease Prevention and Health Promotion: *Chronic disease prevention-preventing and controlling cancer: the nation's second leading cause of death,* www.cdc.gov/nccdphp/publications/aag/dcpc.htm, accessed April 2007.
26. National Center for Health Statistics: *Health, United States, 2006 with chartbook on trends in the health of Americans,* Hyattsville, MD, 2006, U.S. Government Printing Office.

27. Tuofu Z and others: An African HIV-1 sequence from 1959 and implications for the origin of the epidemic, *Nature* 391(6667):594, 1998.

28. Joint United Nations Programme on HIV/AIDS and World Health Organization: *AIDS epidemic update*, Geneva, Switzerland, 2007, *http://data.unaids.org/pub/EPISlides/2007/2007_epiupdate_en.pdf*, accessed March 2008.

29. U.S. Food and Drug Administration: *Drugs used in the treatment of HIV infection*, *www.fda.gov/oashi/aids/virals.html*, accessed April 2007.

30. Wu TD and others: Mutation patterns and structural correlates in human immunodeficiency virus type 1 protease following different protease inhibitor treatment, *J Virol* 77(8):4836, 2003.

31. Engelson ES: HIV lipodystrophy diagnosis and management. Body composition and metabolic alterations: diagnosis and management, *AIDS Read* 13(4 suppl):10, 2003.

FURTHER READING AND RESOURCES

National Cancer Institute: *www.cancer.gov*

American Cancer Society: *www.cancer.org*

CDC: *www.cdc.gov*

AIDS.gov, *Basic Health and Nutrition Tips*: *www.aids.gov/treatment/nutrition/index.html*

AIDS, the official journal of the International AIDS Society: *www.aidsonline.com*

AIDS Treatment News, part of AIDS.org: *www.aids.org/index.html*

Johns Hopkins AIDS service: *www.hopkins-aids.edu*

National Center for HIV/AIDS, Viral Hepatitis, STD, and TB Prevention: *www.cdc.gov/nchstp/od/nchstp.html*

CDC: *Cases of HIV infection and AIDS in the United States and Dependent Areas, 2005: www.cdc.gov/hiv/topics/surveillance/resources/reports/2005report/default.htm*

The National Institute of Allergy and Infectious Diseases, *HIV/AIDS Vaccines: www.niaid.nih.gov/daids/vaccine/news.htm*
> *These organizations and societies provide current information and updates on research, education, treatment, incidence, and mechanism of prevention for cancer or AIDS.*

Kushi LH and others: American Cancer Society Guidelines on Nutrition and Physical Activity for cancer prevention: reducing the risk of cancer with healthy food choices and physical activity, *CA Cancer J Clin* 56(5):254, 2006.

Doyle C and others: Nutrition and physical activity during and after cancer treatment: an American Cancer Society guide for informed choices, *CA Cancer J Clin* 56(6):323, 2006.
> *These articles explore the role of nutrition and physical activity in the prevention of cancer and during and after cancer treatment. The authors provide recommendations and guidelines for each.*

Nerad J and others: General nutrition management in patients infected with Human Immunodeficiency Virus, *CID* 36(2 suppl):52, 2003.
> *The authors give an overview of the nutrition management, levels of care, and appropriate screening tools involved in the care of HIV-infected patients. This article also includes a table of HIV medications and common food interactions.*

Cholesterol Content of Select Foods

ITEM	SERVING SIZE	CHOLESTEROL (mg/SERVING)	ITEM	SERVING SIZE	CHOLESTEROL (mg/SERVING)
Beef			Ice cream		
Ground, medium fat, pan fried	3 oz	75	Premium	½ cup	70
			Low fat	½ cup	20
Steak	3 oz	75	Lamb, leg, meat only	3 oz	76
Thinly sliced	5 slices (21 g)	9	Liver		
Butter	1 pat (5 g)	11	Chicken, simmered	3 oz	38
Cheese			Beef, pan fried	3 oz	409
Cheddar	½ cup (66 g)	69	Lobster	1 cup	104
Cottage, 2% fat	½ cup (113 g)	10	Margarine	1 Tbsp	0
Cream	1 Tbsp	16	Milk, liquid		
Hard (asiago, parmesan)	1 oz	20	Buttermilk	1 cup	9
Chicken			Condensed	½ cup	52
Breast, no skin	3 oz	47	Low fat, 2%	1 cup	18
Breast, with skin	3 oz	50	Skim	1 cup	4
Dark meat, no skin	3 oz	87	Whole	1 cup	33
Dark meat, with skin	3 oz	90	Oysters, raw	3 oz	21
Clam	3 oz	57	Pork		
Crab meat	3 oz	62	Bacon	3 slices (19 g)	16
Cream, whipping, heavy	½ cup	82	Chopped	3 oz	14
			Ham slices	1 oz	16
Egg			Tenderloin	3 oz	69
Whole	1 large	213	Sausage	1 oz	20
White only	¼ cup	0	Shrimp	3 oz	165
Fish			Sour cream	½ cup	51
Halibut	3 oz	65	Turkey		
Salmon	3 oz	88	Breast, with skin	3 oz	83
Tuna, yellowfin	3 oz	50	Dark meat, roasted	3 oz	77
Yellowtail	3 oz	102	Light meat, roasted	3 oz	81
Frozen yogurt	½ cup	5	Veal	3 oz	100

Dietary Fiber in Selected Plant Foods

FOOD	AMOUNT	WEIGHT (g)	TOTAL DIETARY FIBER (g)	NONCELLULOSE POLYSACCHARIDES (g)	CELLULOSE (g)	LIGNIN
Apple, flesh	1 medium	138	1.96	1.29	0.66	0.01
Apple, skin	1 medium	100	3.71	2.21	1.01	0.49
Banana	1 small	119	2.08	1.33	0.44	0.31
Beans, baked	1 cup	225	18.53	14.45	3.59	0.48
Beans, green, cooked	1 cup	125	4.19	2.31	1.61	0.26
Bread, white	1 slice	25	0.68	0.50	0.18	Trace
Bread, whole meal	1 slice	25	2.13	1.49	0.33	0.31
Broccoli, cooked	1 cup	155	6.36	4.53	1.78	0.05
Brussels sprouts, cooked	1 cup	155	4.43	3.08	1.24	0.11
Cabbage, cooked	1 cup	145	4.10	2.55	1.00	0.55
Carrots, cooked	1 cup	155	5.74	3.44	2.29	Trace
Cauliflower, cooked	1 cup	125	2.25	0.84	1.41	Trace
Cereal, All-Bran	1 oz	30	8.01	5.35	1.80	0.86
Cereal, Corn Flakes	1 cup	25	2.75	1.82	0.61	0.33
Cereal, Grapenuts	¼ cup	30	2.10	1.54	0.38	0.17
Cereal, Puffed Wheat	1 cup	15	2.31	1.55	0.39	0.37
Cereal, Rice Krispies	1 cup	30	1.34	1.04	0.23	0.07
Cereal, Shredded Wheat	1 biscuit	25	3.07	2.20	0.66	0.21
Cereal, Special K	1 cup	30	1.64	1.10	0.22	0.32
Cherries	10 cherries	68	0.84	0.63	0.17	0.05
Cookies, oatmeal	4 cookies	52	2.08	1.64	0.21	0.22
Corn, fresh or frozen	1 cup	165	7.82	7.11	0.51	0.20
Corn, canned	1 cup	165	9.39	8.20	1.06	0.13
Flour, bran	1 cup	100	44.00	32.70	8.05	3.23
Flour, white	1 cup	115	3.62	2.90	0.69	0.03
Flour, whole meal	1 cup	120	11.41	7.50	2.95	0.96
Grapefruit	½ cup	100	0.44	0.34	0.04	0.06
Lettuce	⅛ head	100	1.53	0.47	1.06	Trace
Onions, raw, sliced	1 cup	100	2.10	1.55	0.55	Trace
Orange	1 cup	200	0.58	0.44	0.08	0.06
Parsnips, raw, diced	1 cup	100	4.90	3.77	1.13	Trace
Peach, flesh and skin	1 medium	100	2.28	1.46	0.20	0.62
Peanuts	1 oz	30	2.79	1.92	0.51	0.36
Peanut butter	1 Tbsp	16	1.21	0.90	0.31	Trace
Pear, flesh	1 medium	164	4.00	2.16	1.10	0.74
Pear, skin	1 medium	100	8.59	3.72	2.18	2.67
Peas, canned	1 cup	170	13.35	8.85	3.91	0.60
Peas, raw or frozen	1 cup	100	7.75	5.48	2.09	0.18
Plums	1 plum	66	1.00	0.65	0.15	0.20
Raisins	1 oz	30	1.32	0.72	0.25	0.35
Strawberries	1 cup	149	2.65	1.39	1.04	0.22
Tomato, raw	1 medium	135	1.89	0.88	0.61	0.41
Tomato, canned, drained	1 cup	240	2.04	1.08	0.89	0.07

Data from Southgate DAT and others: A guide to calculating intakes of dietary fiber, *J Hum Nutr* 30:303, 1976.

APPENDIX C

Sodium and Potassium Content of Foods, 100 g, Edible Portion

FOOD AND DESCRIPTION	SODIUM (mg)	POTASSIUM (mg)
Almonds		
Dried	4	773
Roasted and salted	198	773
Apple brown betty	153	100
Apple butter	2	252
Apple juice, canned or bottled	1	101
Apples		
Raw, pared	1	110
Frozen, sliced, sweetened	14	68
Applesauce, canned, sweetened	2	65
Apricot nectar, canned (approx. 40% fruit)	Trace	151
Apricots		
Raw	1	281
Canned, syrup pack, light	1	239
Dried, sulfured, cooked, fruit, and liquid	8	318
Asparagus		
Cooked spears, boiled, drained	1	183
Canned spears, green		
Regular pack, solids and liquid	236[a]	166
Special dietary pack (low sodium), solids and liquid	3	166
Frozen		
Cuts and tips, cooked, boiled, drained	1	220
Spears, cooked, boiled, drained	1	238
Avocados, raw, all commercial varieties	4	604
Bacon, cured, cooked, broiled or fried, drained	1021	236
Bacon, Canadian, cooked, broiled or fried, drained	2555	432
Baking powder (home use)		
Straight phosphate	8220	170
Special low-sodium preparations	6	10,948
Banana, raw, common	1	370
Barbecue sauce	815	174
Bass, black sea, raw	68	256
Beans, common, mature seeds, dry		
White, cooked	7	416
White, canned, solids and liquid, with pork and tomato sauce	463	210
Red, cooked	3	340
Beans, lima		
Immature seeds		
Cooked, boiled, drained	1	442
Canned		
Regular pack, solids and liquid	236[a]	222
Special dietary pack (low sodium), solids and liquid	4	222
Frozen, thin-seeded types, commonly called baby limas		
Cooked, boiled, drained	129	394
Mature seeds, dry, cooked	2	612

480

FOOD AND DESCRIPTION	SODIUM (mg)	POTASSIUM (mg)
Beans, mung, sprouted seeds, cooked, boiled, drained	4	156
Beans, snap		
Green		
Cooked, boiled, drained	4	151
Canned		
Regular pack, solids and liquid	236[a]	95
Special dietary pack (low sodium), solids and liquid	2	95
Frozen, cut, cooked, boiled, drained	1	152
Yellow or wax		
Cooked, boiled, drained	3	151
Canned		
Regular pack, solids and liquid	236[a]	95
Special dietary pack (low sodium), solids and liquid	2	95
Frozen, cut, cooked, boiled, drained	1	164
Beans and frankfurters, canned	539	262
Beef		
Retail cuts, trimmed to retail level		
Round	60	370
Rump	60	370
Hamburger, regular ground, cooked	47	450
Heart, lean, cooked, braised	104	232
Liver, cooked, fried	184	380
Tongue, medium fat, cooked, braised	61	164
Beef and vegetable stew, canned	411	174
Beef, corned, boneless		
Cooked, medium fat	1740	150
Canned corned beef hash (with potato)	540	200
Beef, dried, cooked, creamed	716	153
Beef potpie, commercial, frozen, unheated	366	93
Beet greens, common, canned, cooked, boiled, drained		
Regular pack, solids and liquid	236[a]	167
Special dietary pack (low sodium), solids and liquid	46	167
Biscuit dough, commercial, frozen	910	86
Biscuit mix, with enriched flour, and biscuits baked from mix		
Dry form	1300	80
Made with milk	973	116
Biscuits, baking powder, made with enriched flour	626	117
Blackberries, including dewberries, boysenberries, and youngberries, raw	1	170
Blackberries, canned, solids and liquid		
Water pack, with or without artificial sweetener	1	115
Syrup pack, heavy	1	109
Blueberries		
Raw	1	81
Frozen, not thawed, sweetened	1	66
Bluefish, cooked		
Baked or broiled	104	—
Fried	146	—
Bouillon cubes or powder	24,000	100
Boysenberries, frozen, not thawed, sweetened	1	105
Bran, added sugar and malt extract	1060	1070
Bran flakes (40% bran), added thiamin	925	—
Bran flakes with raisins, added thiamin	800	—
Brazil nuts	1	715
Bread crumbs, dry, grated	736	152
Bread stuffing mix and stuffing prepared from mix, dry form	1331	172

Continued

FOOD AND DESCRIPTION	SODIUM (mg)	POTASSIUM (mg)
Breads		
Boston brown bread	251	292
Cracked wheat	529	134
French or Vienna, enriched	580	90
Italian, enriched	585	74
Raisin	365	233
Rye, American (⅓ rye, ⅔ clear flour)	557	145
White enriched, made with 3%-4% nonfat dry milk	507	105
Whole wheat, made with 2% nonfat dry milk	527	273
Broccoli		
Cooked spears, boiled, drained	10	267
Frozen, spears, cooked, boiled, drained	12	220
Brussels sprouts, frozen, cooked, boiled, drained	14	295
Buffalo fish, raw	52	293
Bulgur (parboiled wheat), canned, made from hard red winter wheat		
Unseasoned[b]	599	87
Seasoned[c]	460	112
Butter[d]	987	23
Buttermilk, liquid, cultured (made from skim milk)	130	140
Cabbage		
Common varieties (Danish, domestic, and pointed types)		
Raw	20	233
Cooked, boiled until tender, drained, shredded, cooked in small amount of water	14	163
Red, raw	26	268
Cabbage, Chinese (also called *celery cabbage* or *petsai*)	23	253
Cakes		
Homemade		
Angel food	283	88
Fruit cake, made with enriched flour, dark	158	496
Gingerbread, made with enriched flour	237	454
Plain cake or cupcake, without icing	300	79
Pound, modified	178	78
Frozen, commercial, devil's food, with chocolate icing	420	119
Candy		
Caramels, plain or chocolate	226	192
Chocolate, sweet	33	269
Chocolate coated, chocolate fudge	228	193
Gum drops, starch jelly pieces	35	5
Hard	32	4
Marshmallows	39	6
Peanut bars	10	448
Carp, raw	50	286
Carrots		
Raw	47	341
Canned		
Regular pack, solids and liquid	236[a]	120
Special dietary pack (low sodium), solids and liquid	39	120
Cashews	15[e]	464
Catfish, freshwater, raw	60	330
Cauliflower		
Cooked, boiled, drained	9	206
Frozen, cooked, boiled, drained	10	207
Caviar, sturgeon, granular	2200	180
Celery, all, including green and yellow varieties		
Raw	126	341
Cooked, boiled, drained	88	239
Chard, Swiss, cooked, boiled, drained	86	321
Cheese straws	721	63

FOOD AND DESCRIPTION	SODIUM (mg)	POTASSIUM (mg)
Cheeses		
Natural cheeses		
Cheddar (domestic type)	700	82
Cottage (large or small curd)		
Creamed	229	85
Uncreamed	290	72
Cream	250	74
Parmesan	734	149
Swiss (domestic)	710	104
Pasteurized processed cheese, American	1136[f]	80
Pasteurized processed cheese spread, American	1625[f]	240
Cherries		
Raw, sweet	2	191
Canned		
Sour, red, solids and liquid, water pack	2	130
Sweet, solids and liquid, syrup pack, light	1	128
Frozen, not thawed, sweetened	2	130
Chicken, all classes		
Light meat without skin, cooked, roasted	64	411
Dark meat without skin, cooked, roasted	86	321
Gizzard, chicken, all classes, cooked, simmered	57	211
Chicken potpie, commercial, frozen, unheated	411	153
Chicory, Witloof (also called *French* or *Belgian endive*), bleached head (forced), raw	7	182
Chili con carne, canned, with beans	531	233
Chocolate, bitter or baking	4	830
Chocolate syrup, fudge type	89	284
Chop suey, with meat, canned	551	138
Chow mein, chicken (without noodles), canned	290	167
Citron, candied	290	120
Clams, raw		
Soft meat only	36	235
Hard or round meat only	205	311
Clams, canned, including hard, soft, razor, and unspecified solids and liquid	—	140
Cocoa and chocolate-flavored beverage powders		
Cocoa powder with nonfat dry milk	525	800
Mix for hot chocolate	382	605
Cocoa, dry powder, high fat or breakfast		
Plain	6	1522
Processed with alkali	717	651
Coconut cream (liquid expressed from grated coconut meat)	4	324
Coconut meat, fresh	23	256
Cod		
Cooked, broiled	110	407
Dehydrated, lightly salted	8100	160
Coffee, instant, water-soluble solids		
Dry powder	72	3256
Beverage	1	36
Collards, cooked, boiled, drained, leaves (including stems) cooked in small amount of water	25	234
Cookie dough, plain, chilled in roll, baked	548	48
Cookies		
Assorted, packaged, commercial	365	67
Butter, thin, rich	418	60
Gingersnaps	571	462
Molasses	386	138
Oatmeal with raisins	162	370
Sandwich type	483	38
Vanilla wafer	252	72

Continued

FOOD AND DESCRIPTION	SODIUM (mg)	POTASSIUM (mg)
Corn, sweet		
Cooked, boiled, drained, white and yellow, kernels, cut off cob before cooking	Trace	165
Canned		
Regular pack, cream style, white and yellow, solids and liquid	236[a]	(97)
Special dietary pack (low sodium), cream style, white and yellow, solids and liquid	2	(97)
Frozen, kernels cut off cob, cooked, boiled, drained	1	184
Corn fritters	477	133
Corn grits, degermed, enriched, dry form	1	80
Corn products used mainly as ready-to-eat breakfast cereals		
Corn flakes, added nutrients	1005	120
Corn, puffed, added nutrients	1060	—
Corn, rice and wheat flakes, mixed, added nutrients	950	—
Cornbread mix and cornbread baked from mix, cornbread, made with egg, milk	744	127
Cornmeal, white or yellow, degermed, enriched, dry form	1	120
Cornstarch	Trace	Trace
Cowpeas, including black-eyed peas		
Immature seeds, canned, solids and liquid	236[a]	352
Young pods, with seeds, cooked, boiled, drained	3	196
Crab, canned	1000	110
Crackers		
Butter	1092	113
Graham, plain	670	384
Saltines	1072	154
Sandwich type, peanut butter or cheese	992	226
Cranberries, raw	2	82
Cranberry juice cocktail, bottled (approx. 33% cranberry juice)	1	10
Cranberry sauce, sweetened, canned, strained	1	30
Cream, liquid, light, coffee or table, 20% fat	43	122
Cream substitutes, dried, containing cream, skim milk (calcium reduced), and lactose	575	—
Cream puffs with custard filling	83	121
Cress, garden, raw	14	606
Croaker, Atlantic, cooked, baked	120	323
Cucumbers, raw, pared	6	160
Custard, baked	79	146
Dates, domestic, natural and dry	1	648
Doughnuts, cake type	501	90
Duck, domesticated, raw, flesh only	74	285
Eggplant, cooked, boiled, drained	1	150
Eggs, chicken		
Raw		
Whole, fresh and frozen	122	129
Whites, fresh and frozen	146	139
Yolks, fresh	52	98
Endive (curly endive and escarole), raw	14	294
Farina		
Enriched		
Regular	2	83
Dry form	144	9
Cooked		
Quick cooking, cooked	165	10
Instant cooking, cooked	188	13
Nonenriched, regular, dry form	2	83
Figs, canned, solids and liquid, syrup pack, light	2	152
Flat fish (flounder, sole, sand dabs), raw	78	342
Fruit, cocktail, canned, solids and liquid, water pack, with or without artificial sweetener	5	168
Garlic, cloves, raw	19	529
Ginger root, fresh	6	264
Goose, domesticated, flesh only, cooked, roasted	124	605

FOOD AND DESCRIPTION	SODIUM (mg)	POTASSIUM (mg)
Gooseberries, canned, solids and liquid, syrup pack, heavy	1	98
Grapefruit		
Raw, pulp, pink, red, white, all varieties	1	135
Canned, juice, sweetened	1	162
Grapefruit juice and orange juice, blended, canned, sweetened	1	184
Grapes, raw, American type (slip skin), such as Concord, Delaware, Niagara, Catawba, and Scuppernong	3	158
Grape juice, canned or bottled	2	116
Guava, whole, raw, common	4	289
Haddock, cooked, fried	177	348
Hake, including Pacific hake, squirrel hake, and silver hake or whiting, raw	74	363
Halibut, Atlantic, and Pacific, cooked, broiled	134	525
Ham croquette	342	83
Herring		
Raw, Pacific	74	420
Smoked, hard	6231	157
Honey, strained or extracted	5	51
Horseradish, prepared	96	290
Ice cream and frozen custard, regular (approx. 17% fat)	63[g]	181
Ice cream cones	232	244
Ice milk	68[g]	195
Jams and preserves	12	88
Kale, cooked, boiled, drained, leaves including stems	43	221
Lake herring (cisco), raw	83	250
Lamb, retail cuts	70	290
Lemon juice, canned or bottled, unsweetened	1	141
Lettuce, raw crisphead varieties such as iceberg, New York, and Great Lakes	9	175
Lime juice, canned or bottled, unsweetened	1	104
Lobster, northern, canned or cooked	210	180
Loganberries, canned, solids and liquid, syrup pack, light	1	111
Macadamia nuts	—	164
Macaroni, unenriched, dry form	2	197
Macaroni and cheese	802	423
Margarine[h]	987	23
Mayonnaise	597	34
Milk, cow		
Liquid (pasteurized and raw)		
Whole, 3.7% fat	50	144
Skim	52	145
Canned, evaporated (unsweetened)	118	303
Dry, skim (nonfat solids), regular	532	1745
Malted		
Dry powder	440	720
Beverage	91	200
Chocolate drink, liquid, commercial		
Made with skim milk	46	142
Made with whole (3.5% fat) milk	47	146
Molasses, cane		
First extraction or light	15	917
Third extraction or blackstrap	96	2927
Muffin mixes, corn, and muffins baked from mixes		
Made with egg, milk	479	110
Made with egg, water	346	104
Mushrooms		
Raw	15	414
Canned, solids and liquid	400	197
Muskmelon, raw, cantaloupe, other netted varieties	12	251
Mussels, Atlantic and Pacific, raw, meat only	289	315
Mustard greens, cooked, boiled, drained	18	220

Continued

FOOD AND DESCRIPTION	SODIUM (mg)	POTASSIUM (mg)
Mustard, prepared		
Brown	1307	130
Yellow	1252	130
Nectarines, raw	6	294
Noodles, egg, enriched, cooked	2	44
Oat products used mainly as hot breakfast cereals, oatmeal, or rolled oats		
Dry form	2	352
Cooked	218	61
Oat products used mainly as ready-to-eat breakfast cereals, with or without corn, puffed, added nutrients	1267	—
Ocean perch, Atlantic (redfish)		
Raw	79	269
Cooked, fried	153	284
Ocean perch, Pacific, raw	63	390
Oils, salad or cooking	0	0
Okra		
Raw	3	249
Cooked, boiled, drained	2	174
Olives, pickled, canned or bottled		
Green	2400	55
Ripe, Ascolano (extra large, mammoth, giant jumbo)	813	34
Ripe, salt cured, oil coated, Greek style	3288	—
Onions, mature (dry), raw	10	157
Onions, young green (bunching varieties), raw, bulb and entire top	5	231
Orange, raw, peeled, all commercial varieties	1	200
Orange juice		
Raw, all commercial varieties	1	200
Canned, unsweetened	1	199
Frozen concentrate, unsweetened, diluted with three parts water, by volume	1	186
Oysters		
Raw, meat only, Eastern	73	121
Cooked, fried	206	203
Frozen, solids and liquid	380	210
Oyster stew, commercial frozen, prepared with equal volume of milk	366	176
Pancake and waffle mixes and pancakes baked from mixes, plain and buttermilk, made with egg, milk	564	154
Parsnips, cooked, boiled, drained	8	379
Peaches		
Raw	1	202
Canned, solids and liquid, water pack, with or without artificial sweetener	2	137
Frozen, sliced, sweetened, not thawed	2	124
Peanut butters made with small amounts of added fat, salt	607	670
Peanuts		
Roasted with skins	5	701
Roasted and salted	418	674
Pears		
Raw, including skin	2	130
Canned, solids and liquid, syrup pack, light	1	85
Peas, green, immature		
Cooked, boiled, drained, canned, Alaska (early or June peas)		
Regular pack, solids and liquid	236[a]	96
Special dietary pack (low sodium), solids and liquid	3	96
Frozen, cooked, boiled, drained	115	135
Peas, mature seeds, dry, whole, raw	35	1005
Peas and carrots, frozen, cooked, boiled, drained	84	157
Pecans	Trace	603
Peppers, hot, chili, mature, red, raw, pods excluding seeds	25	564
Peppers, sweet, garden varieties, immature, green, raw	13	213
Perch, yellow, raw	68	230
Pickles, cucumber, dill	1428	200

FOOD AND DESCRIPTION	SODIUM (mg)	POTASSIUM (mg)
Pie crust or plain pastry, made with enriched flour, baked	611	50
Pies, baked, pie crust made with unenriched flour		
Apple	301	80
Cherry	304	105
Mincemeat	448	178
Pumpkin	214	160
Pike, walleye, raw	51	319
Pineapple		
Raw	1	146
Frozen chunks, sweetened, not thawed	2	100
Pizza, with cheese, homemade, baked		
With cheese topping	702	130
With sausage topping	729	168
Plate dinners, frozen, commercial, unheated		
Beef pot roast, whole oven-browned potatoes, peas, corn	259	244
Chicken, fried; mashed potatoes; mixed vegetables (carrots, peas, corn, beans)	344	112
Meat loaf with tomato sauce, mashed potatoes, peas	393	115
Turkey, sliced; mashed potatoes, peas	400	176
Plums		
Raw, Damson	2	299
Canned, solids and liquid, purple (Italian prunes), syrup pack, light	1	145
Popcorn, popped		
Plain	(3)	—
Oil and salt added	1940	—
Pork, fresh, retail cuts, trimmed to retail level, loin	65	390
Pork, lightly cured, commercial, ham, medium-fat class, separable, lean, cooked, roasted	930	326
Pork, cured, canned ham, contents of can	(1100)	(340)
Potatoes		
Cooked, boiled in skin	3^i	407
Dehydrated mashed, flakes without milk		
Dry form	89	1600
Prepared, water, milk, table fat added	231	286
Pretzels	1680^j	130
Prunes, dried, softened, cooked (fruit and liquid), with added sugar	3	262
Pudding mixes and puddings made from mixes, with starch base		
With milk, cooked	129	136
With milk, without cooking	124	129
Pumpkin, canned	2	240
Radishes, raw, common	18	322
Raisins, natural (unbleached), cooked, fruit and liquid, added sugar	13	355
Raspberries		
Canned, solids and liquid, water pack, with or without artificial sweetener, red	1	114
Frozen, red, sweetened, not thawed	1	100
Rennin products		
Tablet (salts, starch, rennin enzyme)	22,300	—
Dessert mixes and desserts prepared from mixes		
Chocolate, dessert made with milk	52	125
Other flavors (vanilla, caramel, fruit flavorings)		
Mix, dry form	6	—
Dessert, made with milk	46	128
Rhubarb, cooked, added sugar	2	203
Rice		
Brown		
Raw	9	214
Cooked	282	70
White (fully milled or polished), enriched, common commercial varieties, all types		
Raw	5	92
Cooked	374	28
Wild, raw	7	220

Continued

FOOD AND DESCRIPTION	SODIUM (mg)	POTASSIUM (mg)
Rice products used mainly as ready-to-eat breakfast cereals		
Rice flakes, added nutrients	987	180
Rice, puffed, added nutrients, without salt	2	100
Rice, puffed or open popped, presweetened, honey and added nutrients	706	—
Rockfish, including black, canary, yellowtail, rasphead, and bocaccio, cooked, oven steamed	68	446
Roe, cooked, baked or broiled, cod and shad[k]	73	132
Rolls and buns, commercial, ready to serve		
Danish pastry	366	112
Hard rolls, enriched	625	97
Plain (pan rolls), enriched	506	95
Sweet rolls	389	124
Rusk	246	161
Rutabagas, cooked, boiled, drained	4	167
Rye, flour, medium	(1)	203
Rye wafers, whole grain	882	600
Salad dressings, commercial[l]		
Blue and Roquefort cheese		
Regular	1094	37
Special dietary (low calorie), low fat (approx. 5 kcal/tsp)	1108	34
French		
Regular	1370	79
Special dietary (low calorie), low fat (approx. 5 kcal/tsp)	787	79
Thousand Island		
Regular	700	113
Special dietary (low calorie, approx. 10 kcal/tsp)	700	113
Salmon, Coho (sliver)		
Raw	48[m]	421
Canned, solids and liquid	351[n]	339
Salt pork, raw	1212	42
Sandwich spread (with chopped pickle)		
Regular	626	92
Special dietary (low calorie, approx. 5 kcal/tsp)	626	92
Sardines, Atlantic, canned in oil, drained solids	823	590
Sardines, Pacific, in tomato sauce, solids and liquid	400	320
Sauerkraut, canned, solids and liquid	747[o]	140
Sausage, cold cuts, and luncheon meats		
Bologna, all samples	1300	230
Frankfurters, raw, all samples	1100	220
Luncheon meat, pork, cured ham or shoulder, chopped, spiced or unspiced, canned	1234	222
Pork sausage, links or bulk, cooked	958	269
Scallops, bay and sea, cooked, steamed	265	476
Soups, commercial, canned		
Beef broth, bouillon, and consommé, prepared with equal volume of water	326	54
Chicken noodle, prepared with equal volume of water	408	23
Tomato		
Prepared with equal volume of water	396	94
Prepared with equal volume of milk	422	167
Vegetable beef, prepared with equal volume of water	427	66
Soy sauce	7325	366
Spaghetti, enriched, cooked, tender stage	1	61
Spaghetti, in tomato sauce with cheese, canned	382	121

FOOD AND DESCRIPTION	SODIUM (mg)	POTASSIUM (mg)
Spinach		
Cooked, boiled, drained	50	324
Canned		
Regular pack, drained solids	236[a]	250
Special dietary pack (low sodium), solids and liquid	34	250
Frozen, chopped, cooked, boiled, drained	52	333
New Zealand spinach, cooked, boiled, drained	92	463
Squash, summer, all varieties, cooked, boiled, drained	1	141
Squash, frozen		
Summer, yellow crookneck, cooked, boiled, drained	3	167
Winter, heated	1	207
Strawberries		
Raw	1	164
Frozen, sweetened, not thawed, sliced	1	112
Sturgeon, cooked, steamed	108	235
Succotash (corn and lima beans), frozen, cooked, boiled, drained	38	246
Sugars, beet or cane, brown	30	344
Sweet potatoes		
Cooked, all, baked in skin	12	300
Canned, liquid pack, solids and liquid, regular packed in syrup	48	(120)
Dehydrated flakes, prepared with water	45	140
Tangerine, raw (Dancy variety)	2	126
Tapioca, dry	3	18
Tapioca desserts, tapioca cream pudding	156	135
Tartar sauce, regular	707	78
Tea, instant (water soluble solids), carbohydrate added		
Dry powder	—	4350
Beverage	—	25
Tomato catsup, bottled	1042[p]	363
Tomato juice, canned or bottled		
Regular pack	200	227
Special dietary pack (low sodium)	3	227
Tomato juice cocktail, canned or bottled	200	221
Tomato puree, canned		
Regular pack	399	426
Special dietary pack (low sodium)	6	426
Tomatoes, ripe		
Raw	3	244
Canned, solids and liquid, regular pack	130	217
Tuna, canned		
In oil, solids and liquid	800	301
In water, solids and liquid	41[q]	279[q]
Turkey, all classes		
Light meat, cooked, roasted	82	411
Dark meat, cooked, roasted	99	398
Turkey potpie, commercial, frozen, unheated	369	114
Turnips, cooked, boiled, drained	34	188
Turnip greens, leaves, including stems		
Canned, solids and liquid	236[a]	243
Frozen, cooked, boiled, drained	17	149
Veal, retail cuts, untrimmed	80	500
Vinegar, cider	1	100
Waffles, frozen, made with enriched flour	644	158
Walnuts		
Black	3	460
Persian or English	2	450
Watercress leaves including stems, raw	52	282
Watermelon, raw	1	100

Continued

FOOD AND DESCRIPTION	SODIUM (mg)	POTASSIUM (mg)
Wheat flours		
Whole (from hard wheat)	3	370
All-purpose, enriched	2	95
Self-rising flour, enriched (anhydrous monocalcium phosphate used as a baking acid)[r]	1079	—[s]
Yeast		
Baker's, compressed	16	610
Brewer's, debittered	121	1894
Yogurt, made from whole milk	47	132
Zwieback	250	150

Numbers in parentheses denote valued input, usually from another form of the food or from a similar food. Dashes denote lack of reliable data for a constituent believed to be present in measurable amount. Values are selected from Watt BK, Merril AL: *Composition of foods—raw, processed, prepared,* Agriculture handbook No. 8, Washington, DC, 1963, U.S. Department of Agriculture.

[a]Estimated average based on addition of salt in the amount of 0.6% of the finished product.
[b]Processed, partially debranned, whole-kernel wheat with salt added.
[c]Processed, partially debranned, whole-kernel wheat with chicken fat, chicken stock base, dehydrated onion flakes, salt, monosodium glutamate, and herbs.
[d]Values apply to unsalted butter. Unsalted butter contains less than 10 mg of either sodium or potassium per 100 g. Value for vitamin A is the year-round average.
[e]Applies to unsalted nuts. For salted nuts, value is approximately 200 mg per 100 g.
[f]Values for phosphorus and sodium are based on use of 1.5% anhydrous disodium phosphate as the emulsifying agent. If emulsifying agent does not contain either phosphorus or sodium, the content of these two nutrients in milligrams per 100 g is as follows:

FOOD	SODIUM	PHOSPHORUS
American processed cheese	650	444
Swiss processed cheese	681	540
American cheese food	—	427
American cheese spread	1139	548

[g]Value for product without added salt.
[h]Values apply to salted margarine. Unsalted margarine contains less than 10 mg/100 g of either sodium or potassium. Vitamin A value based on the minimum required to met federal specifications for margarine with vitamin A added (15,000 IU/lb).
[i]Applies to product without added salt. If salt is added, an estimated average value for sodium is 236 mg/100 g.
[j]Sodium content is variable. For example, very thick pretzel sticks contain approximately twice the amount listed.
[k]Prepared with butter or margarine, lemon juice, or vinegar.
[l]Values apply to products containing salt. For those without salt, sodium content is low, ranging from less than 10 to 50 mg/100 g; the amount usually is indicated on the label.
[m]Sample dipped in brine contained 215 mg sodium/100 g.
[n]For product canned without added salt, value is approximately the same as for raw salmon.
[o]Values for sauerkraut and sauerkraut juice are based on salt content of 1.9% and 2.0%, respectively, in the finished products. The amounts in some samples may vary significantly from the estimate.
[p]Applies to regular pack. For special dietary pack (low sodium), values range from 5 to 35 mg/100 g.
[q]One sample with salt added contained 875 mg of sodium/100 g and 275 mg of potassium.
[r]The acid ingredient most commonly used in self-rising flour. When sodium and pyrophosphate in combination with either anhydrous monocalcium phosphate or calcium carbonate is used, the value for calcium is approximately 120 mg/100 g; for phosphorus, 540 mg; for sodium, 1360 mg.
[s]Value of 90 mg potassium/100 g contributed by flour. Small quantities of additional potassium may be provided by other ingredients.

Suggestions for Salt-Free Seasoning

FISH

Breaded, battered fillets

Dry mustard, onion, oregano, basil, garlic, thyme

Broiled steaks or fillets

Chili or curry powder, tarragon

Fillets in butter sauce

Thyme, chervil, dill, fennel

Fish soup

Italian seasoning, bay leaf, thyme, tarragon

Fish cakes

Tarragon, savory, dry mustard, white pepper, red pepper, oregano

BEEF

Swiss steak

Rosemary, black pepper, bay leaf, thyme, clove

Roast beef

Basil, oregano, bay leaf, nutmeg, tarragon, marjoram

Beef stew

Chili powder, bay leaf, tarragon, caraway, marjoram

Meatballs

Garlic, thyme, basil, oregano, onion, black pepper, dry mustard

Beef stroganoff

Red pepper, onion, garlic, nutmeg, curry powder

POULTRY AND VEAL

Fried chicken

Basil, oregano, garlic, onion, dill, sesame seed, nutmeg

Roast chicken or turkey

Ginger, garlic, onion, thyme, tarragon

Chicken croquettes

Dill, curry, chili, cumin, tarragon, oregano

Veal patties

Italian seasoning, tarragon, dill, onion, sesame seeds

Barbecue chicken

Garlic, dry mustard, clove, allspice, basil, oregano

GRAVIES AND SAUCES

Barbecue

Bay leaf, thyme, red pepper, cinnamon, ginger, allspice, dry mustard, chili powder

Brown

Chervil, onion, bay leaf, thyme, nutmeg, tarragon

Chicken

Dry mustard, ginger, garlic, marjoram, thyme, bay leaf

Cream

White pepper, dry mustard, curry powder, dill, onion, paprika, tarragon, thyme

SOUPS
Chicken

Thyme, savory, ginger, clove, white pepper, allspice

Clam chowder

Basil, oregano, nutmeg, white pepper, thyme, garlic powder

Mushroom

Ginger, oregano, thyme, tarragon, bay leaf, black pepper, chili powder

Onion

Curry, caraway, marjoram, garlic, cloves

Tomato

Bay leaf, thyme, Italian seasoning, oregano, onion, nutmeg

Vegetable

Italian seasoning, paprika, caraway, rosemary, thyme, fennel

SALADS
Chicken

Curry or chili powder, Italian seasoning, thyme, tarragon

Coleslaw

Dill, caraway, poppy seeds, dry mustard, ginger

Fish or seafood

Dill, tarragon, ginger, dry mustard, red pepper, onion, garlic

Macaroni

Dill, basil, thyme, oregano, dry mustard, garlic

Potato

Chili powder, curry, dry mustard, onion

PASTA, BEANS, AND RICE
Baked beans

Dry mustard, chili powder, clove, onion, ginger

Rice and vegetables

Curry, thyme, onion, paprika, rosemary, garlic, ginger

Spanish rice

Cumin, oregano, basil, Italian seasoning

Spaghetti

Italian seasoning, nutmeg, oregano, basil, red pepper, tarragon

Rice pilaf

Dill, thyme, savory, black pepper

VEGETABLES
Asparagus

Ginger, sesame seeds, basil, onion

Broccoli

Italian seasoning, marjoram, basil, nutmeg, onion, sesame seeds

Cabbage

Caraway, onion, nutmeg, allspice, clove

Carrots

Ginger, nutmeg, onion, dill

Cauliflower

Dry mustard, basil, paprika, onion

Tomatoes

Oregano, chili powder, dill, onion

Spinach

Savory, thyme, nutmeg, garlic, onion

Choose Your Foods: Exchange Lists for Diabetes*

HOW THIS EXCHANGE LIST WORKS WITH MEAL PLANNING

This exchange list contains three main groups of food based on the macronutrients: carbohydrates, protein, and fat. Each food list contains foods grouped together by similar nutrient content and serving sizes. Each serving of a food has approximately the same amount of macronutrients and calories as the other foods on the same list.

- Foods on the **Starch** list, **Fruits** list, **Milk** list, and **Sweets, Desserts, and Other Carbohydrates** list are similar because they contain 12 to 15 g carbohydrate per serving.
- Foods on the **Fats** list and **Meat and Meat Substitutes** list usually do not have carbohydrate (except for the plant-based meat substitutes such as beans and lentils).
- Foods on the **Starchy Vegetables** list (part of the **Starch** list and includes foods such as potatoes, corn, and peas) contain 15 g carbohydrate per serving.

- Foods on the **Nonstarchy Vegetables** list (e.g., green beans, tomatoes, and carrots) contain 5 g carbohydrate per serving.
- Some foods have so little carbohydrate and calories that they are considered "free" if eaten in small amounts. You can find these foods on the **Free Foods** list.
- Foods that have different amounts of carbohydrates and calories are listed as **Combination Foods** (such as lasagna) or **Fast Foods.**

---

*Reprinted from American Diabetes Association, American Dietetic Association: *Choose your foods: exchange lists for diabetes,* Chicago/Alexandria, VA, 2007, American Diabetes Association, American Diatetic Association. Reprinted with permission.

FOOD LISTS

The following chart shows the amount of nutrients in one serving from each list.

FOOD LIST	CARBOHYDRATE (g)	PROTEIN (g)	FAT (g)	CALORIES (g)
Carbohydrates				
Starch: breads, cereals and grains; starchy vegetables; crackers and snacks; and beans, peas, and lentils	15	0-3	0-1	80
Fruits	15	—	—	60
Milk				
Fat free, low fat, 1%	12	8	0-3	100
Reduced fat, 2%	12	8	5	130
Whole	12	8	8	150
Sweets, desserts, and other carbohydrates	15	Varies	Varies	Varies
Nonstarchy vegetables	5	2	—	25
Meat and Meat Substitutes				
Lean	—	7	0-3	45
Medium fat	—	7	4-7	75
High fat	—	7	8+	100
Plant-based proteins	Varies	7	Varies	Varies
Fats	—	—	5	45
Alcohol	Varies	—	—	100

STARCH

Cereals, grains, pasta, breads, crackers, and snacks; starchy vegetables; and cooked beans, peas, and lentils are starches. In general, one starch is equivalent to the following:

- ½ cup of cooked cereal, grain, or starchy vegetable
- ½ cup of cooked rice or pasta
- 1 oz of a bread product, such as 1 slice of bread
- ¾ oz to 1 oz of most snack foods (some snack foods also may have extra fat)

Nutrition Tips

- A choice on the **Starch** list has 15 g carbohydrate, 0 to 3 g protein, 0 to 1 g fat, and 80 calories.
- For maximal health benefits, eat three or more servings of whole grains each day. A serving of whole grain is approximately ½ cup of cooked cereal or grain, 1 slice of whole-grain bread, or 1 cup of whole-grain cold breakfast cereal.

Selection Tips

- Choose low-fat starches as often as you can.
- Starchy vegetables, baked goods, and grains prepared with fat count as 1 starch and 1 fat.
- For many starchy foods (bagels, muffins, dinner rolls, buns), a general rule of thumb is 1 oz equals 1 serving. Always check the size you eat. Because of their large size, some foods have a lot more carbohydrate (and calories) than you might think. For example, a large bagel may weigh 4 oz and equal 4 carbohydrate servings.
- For specific information, read the Nutrition Facts panel on the food label.

Bread

FOOD	SERVING SIZE
Bagel, large (approx. 4 oz)	¼ (1 oz)
Biscuit, 2½ inches across ●	1
Bread ●	
Reduced calorie	2 slices (1½ oz)
White, whole grain, pumpernickel, rye, unfrosted raisin	1 slice (1 oz)
Chapatti, small, 6 inches across	1
Cornbread, 1¾-inch cube ●	1 (1½ oz)
English muffin	½
Hot dog bun or hamburger bun	½ (1 oz)
Naan, 8 inches by 2 inches	¼
Pancake, 4 inches across, ¼-inch thick	1
Pita, 6 inches across	½
Roll, plain, small	1 (1oz)

Stuffing, bread ●	⅓ cup
Taco shell, 5 inches across ●	2
Tortilla, corn, 6 inches across	1
Tortilla, flour, 6 inches across	1
Tortilla, flour, 10 inches across	⅓ tortilla
Waffle, 4-inch square or 4 inches across ●	1

● More than 3 g dietary fiber per serving; ● Extra fat or prepared with added fat (add an extra fat choice); ● ≥480 mg or more of sodium per serving. For foods listed as a main dish or meal on the **Combination Foods** and **Fast Foods** lists only, the ● represents more than 600 mg.

Cereals and Grains

FOOD	SERVING SIZE
Barley, cooked	½ cup
Bran, dry	
Oat ●	¼ cup
Wheat ●	½ cup
Bulgur (cooked) ●	½ cup
Cereals	
Bran ●	½ cup
Cooked (oats, oatmeal)	1½ cup
Puffed	½ cup
Shredded Wheat, plain	
Sugar coated	½ cup
Unsweetened, ready to eat	¾ cup
Couscous	⅓ cup
Granola	
Low fat	¼ cup
Regular ●	¼ cup
Grits, cooked	½ cup
Kasha	½ cup
Millet, cooked	⅓ cup
Muesli	¼ cup
Pasta, cooked	⅓ cup
Polenta, cooked	⅓ cup
Quinoa, cooked	⅓ cup
Rice, white or brown, cooked	⅓ cup
Tabbouleh (tabouli), prepared	½ cup
Wheat germ, dry	3 Tbsp
Wild rice, cooked	½ cup

Tip: An open handful is equal to approximately 1 cup or 1 to 2 oz of snack food.

● More than 3 g dietary fiber per serving; ● Extra fat or prepared with added fat (add an extra fat choice); ● ≥480 mg or more of sodium per serving. For foods listed as a main dish or meal on the **Combination Foods** and **Fast Foods** lists only, the ● represents more than 600 mg.

Starchy Vegetables

FOOD	SERVING SIZE
Cassava	⅓ cup
Corn	½ cup
On cob, large	½ cob (5 oz)

Hominy, canned ●	¾ cup
Mixed vegetables with corn, peas, or pasta ●	1 cup
Parsnips ●	½ cup
Peas, green ●	½ cup
Plantain, ripe	⅓ cup
Potato	
Baked with skin	¼ large (3 oz)
Boiled, all kinds	½ cup or ½ medium (3 oz)
Mashed, with milk and fat ●	½ cup
French fried (oven baked)	1 cup (2 oz)
Pumpkin, canned, no sugar added ●	1 cup
Spaghetti or pasta sauce	½ cup
Squash, winter (acorn, butternut) ●	1 cup
Succotash ●	½ cup
Yam, sweet potato, plain	½ cup

● More than 3 g dietary fiber per serving; ● Extra fat or prepared with added fat (add an extra fat choice); ● ≥480 mg or more of sodium per serving. For foods listed as a main dish or meal on the **Combination Foods** and **Fast Foods** lists only, the ● represents more than 600 mg.

Crackers and Snacks

FOOD	SERVING SIZE
Animal crackers	8
Crackers	
Round butter ●	6
Saltine	6
Sandwich, cheese or peanut butter filling ●	3
Whole-wheat regular ●	2-5 (¾ oz)
Whole-wheat lower fat or crispbreads ●	2-5 (¾ oz)
Graham cracker, 2½-inch square	3
Matzoh	¾ oz
Melba toast, approximately 2-inch by 4-inch piece	4 pieces
Oyster crackers	20
Popcorn (microwave popped)	
With butter ● ●	3 cups
No fat added ●	3 cups
Lower fat ●	3 cups
Pretzels	¾ oz
Rice cakes, 4 inches across	2
Snack chips	
Fat free or baked (tortilla, potato), baked pita chips	15-20 (¾ oz)
Regular (tortilla, potato) ●	9-13 (¾ oz)

● More than 3 g dietary fiber per serving; ● Extra fat or prepared with added fat (add an extra fat choice); ● ≥480 mg or more of sodium per serving. For foods listed as a main dish or meal on the **Combination Foods** and **Fast Foods** lists only, the ● represents more than 600 mg.

Beans, Peas, and Lentils

The choices on this list count as 1 starch + 1 lean meat.

FOOD	SERVING SIZE
Baked beans ●	⅓ cup
Beans, cooked (black, garbanzo, kidney, lima, navy, pinto, white) ●	½ cup
Lentils, cooked (brown, green, yellow) ●	½ cup
Peas, cooked (black-eyed, split) ●	½ cup
Refried beans, canned ● ●	½ cup

● More than 3 g dietary fiber per serving; ● Extra fat or prepared with added fat (add an extra fat choice); ● ≥480 mg or more of sodium per serving. For foods listed as a main dish or meal on the **Combination Foods** and **Fast Foods** lists only, the ● represents more than 600 mg.

FRUITS

Fresh, frozen, canned, and dried fruits and fruit juices are on this list. In general, 1 fruit choice is equivalent to the following:

- ½ cup of canned or fresh fruit or unsweetened fruit juice
- 1 small fresh fruit (4 oz)
- 2 Tbsp of dried fruit

Nutrition Tips

- A choice on the **Fruits** list has 15 g carbohydrate, 0 g protein, 0 g fat, and 60 calories.
- Fresh, frozen, and dried fruits are good sources of fiber. Fruit juices contain little fiber. Choose fruits instead of juices whenever possible.
- Citrus fruits, berries, and melons are good sources of vitamin C.

Selection Tips

- Use a food scale to weigh fresh fruits. Practice builds portion skills.
- The weight listed includes skin, core, seeds, and rind.
- Read the Nutrition Facts on the food label. If 1 serving has more than 15 g carbohydrate, you may need to adjust the size of the serving you eat or drink.
- Portion sizes for canned fruits are for the fruit and a small amount of juice (1 to 2 Tbsp).
- Food labels for fruits may contain the words "no sugar added" or "unsweetened." This means that no table sugar (sucrose) has been added.

- Fruit canned in "extra-light syrup" has the same amount of carbohydrate per serving as the "no sugar added" or the "juice pack." All canned fruits on the **Fruits** list are based on one of these three types of packing. Avoid fruit canned in heavy syrup.

Fruit

The weight listed includes skin, core, seeds, and rind.

FOOD	SERVING SIZE
Apple, unpeeled, small	1 (4 oz)
Apples, dried	4 rings
Applesauce, unsweetened	½ cup
Apricots	
Canned	½ cup
Dried	8 halves
Fresh •	4 whole (5½ oz)
Banana, extra small	1 (4 oz)
Blackberries •	¾ cup
Blueberries	¾ cup
Cantaloupe, small	⅓ melon or 1 cup cubed (11 oz)
Cherries	
Sweet, canned	½ cup
Sweet fresh	12 (3 oz)
Dates	3
Dried fruits (blueberries, cherries, cranberries, mixed fruit, raisins)	2 Tbsp
Figs	
Dried	1½
Fresh •	1½ large or 2 medium (3½ oz)
Fruit cocktail	½ cup
Grapefruit	
Large	½ (11 oz)
Sections, canned	¾ cup
Grapes, small	17 (3 oz)
Honeydew melon	1 slice or 1 cup cubed (10 oz)
Kiwi •	1 (3½ oz)
Mandarin oranges, canned	¾ cup
Mango, small	½ fruit (5½ oz) or ½ cup
Nectarine, small	1 (5 oz)
Orange, small •	1 (6½ oz)
Papaya	½ fruit or 1 cup cubed (8 oz)
Peaches	
Canned	½ cup
Fresh, medium	1 (6 oz)
Pears	
Canned	½ cup
Fresh, large	½ (4 oz)
Pineapple	
Canned	½ cup
Fresh	¾ cup

Plums	
Canned	½ cup
Dried (prunes)	3
Small	2 (5 oz)
Raspberries •	1 cup
Strawberries •	1¼ cup whole berries
Tangerines, small •	2 (8 oz)
Watermelon	1 slice or 1¼ cups cubes (13½ oz)

• More than 3 g dietary fiber per serving; ● Extra fat or prepared with added fat (add an extra fat choice); ◗ ≥480 mg or more of sodium per serving. For foods listed as a main dish or meal on the **Combination Foods** and **Fast Foods** lists only, the ◗ represents more than 600 mg.

Fruit Juice

FOOD	SERVING SIZE
Apple juice or cider	½ cup
Fruit juice blends, 100% juice	⅓ cup
Grape juice	⅓ cup
Grapefruit juice	½ cup
Orange juice	½ cup
Pineapple juice	½ cup
Prune juice	⅓ cup

MILK

Different types of milk and milk products are on this list. However, two types of milk products are found in other lists:

- Cheeses are on the **Meat and Meat Substitutes** list because they are rich in protein.
- Cream and other dairy fats are on the **Fats** list.

Milks and yogurts are grouped in three categories (fat free or low fat, reduced fat, or whole) based on the amount of fat they have. The following chart shows what 1 milk choice contains:

	CARBOHY-DRATE (g)	PROTEIN (g)	FAT (g)	CALORIES
Fat free (skim), low fat (1%)	12	8	0-3	100
Reduced fat (2%)	12	8	5	130
Whole	12	8	8	150

Nutrition Tips

- Milk and yogurt are good sources of calcium and protein.

- The higher the fat content of milk and yogurt, the more saturated fat and cholesterol it has.
- Children older than 2 years and adults should choose lower fat varieties such as skim, 1%, or 2% milk or yogurt.

Selection Tips

- 1 cup equals 8 fl oz or ½ pint.
- If you choose 2% or whole-milk foods, be aware of the extra fat.

Milk and Yogurts

FOOD	SERVING SIZE	COUNT AS
Fat free or low fat (1%)		
Milk, buttermilk, acidophilus milk, Lactaid	1 cup	1 fat-free milk
Evaporated milk	½ cup	1 fat-free milk
Yogurt, plain or flavored with an artificial sweetener	⅔ cup (6 oz)	1 fat-free milk
Reduced fat (2%)		
Milk, acidophilus milk, kefir, Lactaid	1 cup	1 reduced-fat milk
Yogurt, plain	⅔ cup (6 oz)	1 reduced-fat milk
Whole		
Milk, buttermilk, goat's milk	1 cup	1 whole milk
Evaporated milk	½ cup	1 whole milk
Yogurt, plain	8 oz	1 whole milk

Dairy-Like Foods

FOOD	SERVING SIZE	COUNT AS
Chocolate milk		
Fat free	1 cup	1 fat-free milk + 1 carbohydrate
Whole	1 cup	1 whole milk + 1 carbohydrate
Eggnog, whole milk	½ cup	1 carbohydrate + 2 fats
Rice drink		
Flavored, low fat	1 cup	2 carbohydrates
Plain, fat free	1 cup	1 carbohydrate
Smoothies, flavored, regular	10 oz	1 fat-free milk + 2½ carbohydrates
Soy milk		
Light	1 cup	1 carbohydrate + ½ fat
Regular, plain	1 cup	1 carbohydrate + 1 fat
Yogurt		
And juice blends	1 cup	1 fat-free milk + 1 carbohydrate
Low carbohydrate (<6 g carbohydrate per choice)	⅔ cup (6 oz)	½ fat-free milk
With fruit, low fat	⅔ cup (6 oz)	1 fat-free milk + 1 carbohydrate

SWEETS, DESSERTS, AND OTHER CARBOHYDRATES

You can substitute food choices from this list for other carbohydrate-containing foods (such as those found on the **Starch, Fruit,** or **Milk** lists) in your meal plan even though these foods have added sugars or fat.

Nutrition Tips

- A carbohydrate choice has 15 g carbohydrate, variable grams of protein, variable grams of fat, and variable calories.

- The foods on this list do not have as many vitamins, minerals, and fiber as the choices on the **Starch, Fruits,** or **Milk** lists. When choosing sweets, desserts, and other carbohydrate foods, you should also eat foods from other food lists to balance out your meals.
- Many of these foods do not equal a single choice. Some also count as one or more fat choices.
- If you are trying to lose weight, choose foods from this list less often.
- The serving sizes for these foods are small because of their fat content.

Selection Tips

- Read the Nutrition Facts on the food label to find the serving size and nutrient information.
- Many sugar-free, fat-free, and reduced-fat products are made with ingredients that contain carbohydrates. These types of foods usually have the same amount of carbohydrates as the regular foods they are to replace. Talk with your RD and find out how to fit these foods into your meal plan.

Common Measurements

Dry:

3 tsp = 1 Tbsp
4 oz = ½ cup
8 oz = 1 cup

Liquid:

4 Tbsp = ¼ cup
8 oz = ½ pint

Beverages, Soda, and Energy or Sports Drinks

FOOD	SERVING SIZE	COUNT AS
Cranberry juice cocktail	½ cup	1 carbohydrate
Energy drink	1 can (8.3 oz)	2 carbohydrates
Fruit drink or lemonade	1 cup (8 oz)	2 carbohydrates
Hot chocolate		
Regular	1 envelope added to 8 oz water	1 carbohydrate + 1 fat
Sugar free or light	1 envelope added to 8 oz water	1 carbohydrate
Soft drink (soda), regular	1 can (12 oz)	2½ carbohydrates
Sports drink	1 cup (8 oz)	1 carbohydrate

Brownies, Cake, Cookies, Gelatin, Pie, and Pudding

FOOD	SERVING SIZE	COUNT AS
Brownie, small, unfrosted	1¼-inch square, ⅞ inch high (approx. 1 oz)	1 carbohydrate + 1 fat
Cake		
Angel food, unfrosted	1⁄12 of cake (approx. 1 oz)	2 carbohydrates
Frosted	2-inch square (approx. 2 oz)	2 carbohydrates + 1 fat
Unfrosted	2-inch square (approx. 2 oz)	1 carbohydrate + 1 fat
Cookies		
Chocolate chip	2 cookies (2¼ inches across)	1 carbohydrate + 2 fats
Gingersnap	3 cookies	1 carbohydrate
Sandwich, with crème filling	2 small (approx. ⅔ oz)	1 carbohydrate + 1 fat
Sugar free	3 small or 1 large (¾-1 oz)	1 carbohydrate + 1-2 fats
Vanilla wafer	5 cookies	1 carbohydrate + 1 fat
Cupcake, frosted	1 small (approx. 1¾ oz)	2 carbohydrates + 1½ fats
Fruit cobbler	½ cup (3½ oz)	3 carbohydrates + 1 fat
Gelatin, regular	½ cup	1 carbohydrate
Pie		
Commercially prepared fruit, two crusts	⅙ of 8-inch pie	3 carbohydrates + 2 fats
Pumpkin or custard	⅛ of 8-inch pie	1½ carbohydrates + 1½ fats
Pudding		
Regular (made with reduced-fat milk)	½ cup	2 carbohydrates
Sugar free or sugar and fat free (made with fat-free milk)	½ cup	1 carbohydrate

Candy, Spreads, Sweets, Sweeteners, Syrups, and Toppings

FOOD	SERVING SIZE	COUNT AS
Candy bar, chocolate/peanut	2 mini bars (1 oz)	1½ carbohydrates + 1½ fats
Candy, hard	3 pieces	1 carbohydrate
Chocolate "kisses"	5 pieces	1 carbohydrate + 1 fat
Coffee creamer		
Dry, flavored	4 tsp	½ carbohydrate + ½ fat
Liquid, flavored	2 Tbsp	1 carbohydrate
Fruit snacks, chewy (pureed fruit concentrate)	1 roll (¾ oz)	1 carbohydrate
Fruit spreads, 100% fruit	1½ Tbsp	1 carbohydrate
Honey	1 Tbsp	1 carbohydrate
Jam or jelly, regular	1 Tbsp	1 carbohydrate
Sugar	1 Tbsp	1 carbohydrate
Syrup		
Chocolate	2 Tbsp	2 carbohydrates
Light (pancake type)	2 Tbsp	1 carbohydrate
Regular (pancake type)	1 Tbsp	1 carbohydrate

Condiments and Sauces

FOOD	SERVING SIZE	COUNT AS
Barbeque sauce	3 Tbsp	1 carbohydrate
Cranberry sauce, jellied	¼ cup	1½ carbohydrate
Gravy, mushroom, canned ●	½ cup	½ carbohydrate + ½ fat
Salad dressing, fat free, low fat, cream based	3 Tbsp	1 carbohydrate
Sweet and sour sauce	3 Tbsp	1 carbohydrate

● More than 3 g dietary fiber per serving; ● Extra fat or prepared with added fat (add an extra fat choice); ● ≥480 mg or more of sodium per serving. For foods listed as a main dish or meal on the **Combination Foods** and **Fast Foods** lists only, the ● represents more than 600 mg.

Doughnuts, Muffins, Pastries, and Sweet Breads

FOOD	SERVING SIZE	COUNT AS
Banana nut bread	1-inch slice (1 oz)	2 carbohydrates + 1 fat
Doughnut		
Cake, plain	1 medium (1½ oz)	1½ carbohydrates + 2 fats
Glazed	3¾-inch diameter (2 oz)	2 carbohydrates + 2 fats
Muffin (4 oz)	¼ muffin (1 oz)	1 carbohydrate + ½ fat
Sweet roll or danish	1 (2½ oz)	2½ carbohydrate + ½ fat

Frozen Bars, Frozen Desserts, Frozen Yogurt, and Ice Cream

FOOD	SERVING SIZE	COUNT AS
Frozen pops	1	½ carbohydrate
Fruit juice bars, frozen, 100% juice	1 bar (3 oz)	1 carbohydrate
Ice cream		
Fat free	½ cup	1½ carbohydrates
Light	½ cup	1 carbohydrate + 1 fat
No sugar added	½ cup	1 carbohydrate + 1 fat
Regular	½ cup	1 carbohydrate + 2 fats
Sherbet, sorbet	½ cup	2 carbohydrates
Yogurt, frozen		
Fat free	⅓ cup	1 carbohydrate
Regular	½ cup	1 carbohydrate + 0–1 fat

Granola Bars, Meal Replacement Bars and Shakes, and Trail Mix

FOOD	SERVING SIZE	COUNT AS
Granola or snack bar, regular or low fat	1 bar (1 oz)	1½ carbohydrates
Meal replacement bar, small	1 bar (1⅓ oz)	1½ carbohydrates + 0–1 fat
Meal replacement bar, large	1 bar (2 oz)	2 carbohydrates + 1 fat
Meal replacement shake, reduced calorie	1 can (10–11 oz)	1½ carbohydrates + 0–1 fat
Trail mix		
Candy or nut based	1 oz	1 carbohydrate + 2 fats
Dried fruit based	1 oz	1 carbohydrate + 1 fat

NONSTARCHY VEGETABLES

Vegetable choices include vegetables in this **Nonstarchy Vegetables** list and the **Starchy Vegetables** list found within the **Starch** list. Vegetables with small amounts of carbohydrate and calories are on the **Nonstarchy Vegetables** list. Vegetables contain important nutrients. Try to eat at least 2 to 3 nonstarchy vegetable choices each day (as well as choices from the **Starchy Vegetables** list). In general, 1 nonstarchy vegetable choice is:

- ½ cup cooked vegetables or vegetable juice
- 1 cup raw vegetables

If you eat 3 cups or more of raw vegetables or 1½ cups of cooked vegetables in a meal, count them as 1 carbohydrate choice.

Nutrition Tips

- A choice on this list (½ cup cooked or 1 cup raw) equals 5 g carbohydrate, 2 g protein, 0 g fat, and 25 calories.
- Fresh and frozen vegetables have less added salt than canned vegetables. Drain and rinse canned vegetables to remove some salt.
- Choose dark green and dark yellow vegetables each day. Spinach, broccoli, romaine, carrots, chilies, squash, and peppers are great choices.
- Brussels sprouts, broccoli, cauliflower, greens, peppers, spinach, and tomatoes are good sources of vitamin C.
- Eat vegetables from the cruciferous family several times each week. Cruciferous vegetables include bok choy, broccoli, Brussels sprouts, cabbage, cauliflower, collards, kale, kohlrabi, radishes, rutabaga, turnip, and watercress.

Selection Tips

- Canned vegetables and juices are also available without added salt.
- A 1-cup portion of broccoli is a portion approximately the size of a regular light bulb.
- Starchy vegetables such as corn, peas, winter squash, and potatoes that have more calories and carbohydrates are on the **Starchy Vegetables** section in the **Starch** list.
- The tomato sauce referred to in this list is different from spaghetti or pasta sauce, which is on the **Starchy Vegetables** list.

Nonstarchy Vegetables

Amaranth or Chinese spinach	Bean sprouts	Cauliflower
Artichoke	Beets	Celery
Artichoke hearts	Borscht •	Chayote •
Asparagus	Broccoli	Coleslaw, packaged, no dressing
Baby corn	Brussels sprouts •	Cucumber
Bamboo shoots	Cabbage (green, bok choy, Chinese)	Eggplant
Beans (green, wax, Italian)	Carrots •	Gourds (bitter, bottle, luffa, bitter, melon)

Green onions or scallions
Greens (collard, kale, mustard, turnip)
Hearts of palm
Jicama
Kohlrabi
Leeks
Mixed vegetables (without corn, peas, or pasta)
Mung bean sprouts
Mushrooms, all kinds, fresh

Okra
Onions
Oriental radish or daikon
Pea pods
Peppers (all varieties) •
Radishes
Rutabaga
Sauerkraut •
Soybean sprouts
Spinach
Squash (summer, crookneck, zucchini)

Sugar pea snaps
Swiss chard •
Tomato
Tomatoes, canned
Tomato sauce •
Tomato or vegetable juice •
Turnips
Water chestnuts
Yard-long beans

● More than 3 g dietary fiber per serving; • Extra fat or prepared with added fat (add an extra fat choice); • ≥480 mg or more of sodium per serving. For foods listed as a main dish or meal on the **Combination Foods** and **Fast Foods** lists only, the • represents more than 600 mg.

MEAT AND MEAT SUBSTITUTES

Meat and meat substitutes are rich in protein. Foods from this list are divided into four groups based on the amount of fat they contain. These groups are lean meat, medium-fat meat, high-fat meat, and plant-based proteins. The following chart shows what one choice includes.

	CARBOHYDRATE (g)	PROTEIN (g)	FAT (g)	CALORIES
Lean meat	—	7	0-3	45
Medium-fat meat	—	7	4-7	75
High-fat meat	—	7	8+	100
Plant-based protein	Varies	7	Varies	Varies

Selection Tips

- Read labels to find foods low in fat and cholesterol. Try for 5 g fat or less per serving.
- Read labels to find unexpected carbohydrate. For example, hot dogs contain a large amount of carbohydrate. Most hot dogs are also high in fat but are often sold in lower fat versions.
- Whenever possible, choose lean meats.
  - Select grades of meat are the leanest.
  - Choice grades have a moderate amount of fat.
  - Prime cuts of meat have the highest amount of fat.
- Fish such as herring, mackerel, salmon, sardines, halibut, trout, and tuna are rich in omega-3 fats, which may help reduce the risk of heart disease. Choose fish (not commercially fried fish fillets) two or more times each week.
- Bake, roast, broil, grill, poach, steam, or boil instead of frying.
- Trim off visible fat or skin.
- Roast, broil, or grill meat on a rack so the fat will drain off during cooking.
- Use a nonstick spray and a nonstick pan to brown or fry foods.
- Some processed meats, seafood, and soy products contain carbohydrate. Read the food label to see if the amount of carbohydrate in the serving size you plan to eat is close to 15 g. If so, count it as 1 carbohydrate choice and 1 or more meat choice.
- Meat or fish that is breaded with cornmeal, flour, or dried bread crumbs contains carbohydrate. Count 3 Tbsp of one of these dry grains as 15 g carbohydrate.

Lean Meats and Meat Substitutes

FOOD	AMOUNT
Beef: Select or choice grades trimmed of fat: ground round, roast (chuck, rib, rump), round, sirloin, steak (cubed, flank, porterhouse, T-bone), tenderloin	1 oz
Beef jerky ●	½ oz
Cheeses with 3 g fat per oz	1 oz
Cottage cheese	¼ cup
Egg substitutes, plain	¼ cup
Egg whites	2
Fish, fresh or frozen, plain: catfish, cod, flounder, haddock, halibut, orange roughy, salmon, tilapia, trout, tuna	1 oz
Fish, smoked: herring or salmon (lox) ●	1 oz
Game: buffalo, ostrich, rabbit, venison	1 oz
Hot dog with ≤3 g fat per oz ● (8 dogs per 14-oz package) (Note: May be high in carbohydrate)	1
Lamb: chop, leg, roast	1 oz
Organ meats: heart, kidney, liver (Note: May be high in cholesterol)	1 oz
Oysters, fresh or frozen	6 medium
Pork, lean	
Canadian bacon ●	1 oz
Rib or loin chop or roast, ham, tenderloin	1 oz
Poultry, without skin: Cornish hen, chicken, domestic duck or goose (well drained of fat), turkey	1 oz
Processed sandwich meats with ≤3 g fat or less per oz: chipped beef, deli thin-sliced meats, turkey ham, turkey kielbasa, turkey pastrami	1 oz
Salmon, canned	1 oz
Sardines, canned	2 small
Sausage with ≤3 g fat per oz ●	1 oz
Shellfish: clams, crab, imitation shellfish, lobster, scallops, shrimp	1 oz
Tuna, canned in water or oil, drained	1 oz
Veal, loin chop, roast	1 oz

● More than 3 g dietary fiber per serving; ● Extra fat or prepared with added fat (add an extra fat choice); ● ≥480 mg or more of sodium per serving. For foods listed as a main dish or meal on the **Combination Foods** and **Fast Foods** lists only, the ● represents more than 600 mg.

Medium-Fat Meat and Meat Substitutes

FOOD	AMOUNT
Beef: corned beef, ground beef, meatloaf, prime grades trimmed of fat (prime rib), short ribs, tongue	1 oz
Cheeses with 4-7 g fat per oz: feta, mozzarella, pasteurized processed cheese spread, reduced-fat cheeses, string	1 oz
Egg (Note: High in cholesterol, limit to 3 per week)	1
Fish, any fried product	1 oz
Lamb: ground, rib roast	1 oz
Pork: cutlet, shoulder roast	1 oz
Poultry: chicken with skin; dove, pheasant, wild duck, or goose; fried chicken; ground turkey	1 oz
Ricotta cheese	2 oz or ¼ cup
Sausage with 4-7 g fat per oz ●	1 oz
Veal, cutlet (no breading)	1 oz

● More than 3 g dietary fiber per serving; ● Extra fat or prepared with added fat (add an extra fat choice); ● ≥480 mg or more of sodium per serving. For foods listed as a main dish or meal on the **Combination Foods** and **Fast Foods** lists only, the ● represents more than 600 mg.

High-Fat Meat and Meat Substitutes

These foods are high in saturated fat, cholesterol, and calories and may raise blood cholesterol levels if eaten on a regular basis. Try to eat three or fewer servings from this group per week.

FOOD	AMOUNT
Bacon	
Pork ●	2 slices (16 slices per lb or 1 oz each, before cooking)
Turkey ●	3 slices (½ oz each before cooking)
Cheese, regular: American, bleu, brie, cheddar, hard goat, Monterey jack, queso, Swiss	1 oz
Hot dog: beef, pork, or combination (10 per 1-lb package) ●	1
Hot dog: turkey or chicken (10 per 1-lb package) ●	1
Pork: ground, sausage, spareribs	1 oz
Processed sandwich meals with ≥8 g fat or more per oz: bologna, pastrami, hard salami	1 oz
Sausage with ≥8 g fat per oz: bratwurst, chorizo, Italian, knockwurst, Polish, smoked, summer ●	1 oz

● More than 3 g dietary fiber per serving;   ● Extra fat or prepared with added fat (add an extra fat choice);   ● ≥480 mg or more of sodium per serving. For foods listed as a main dish or meal on the **Combination Foods** and **Fast Foods** lists only, the ● represents more than 600 mg.

Plant-Based Proteins

Because carbohydrate content varies among plant-based proteins, you should read the food label.

FOOD	AMOUNT	COUNT AS
"Bacon" strips, soy based	3 strips	1 medium-fat meat
Baked beans ●	⅓ cup	1 starch + 1 lean meat
Beans, cooked: black, garbanzo, kidney, lima, navy, pinto, white ●	½ cup	1 starch + 1 lean meat
"Beef" or "sausage" crumbles, soy based ●	2 oz	½ carbohydrate + 1 lean meat
"Chicken" nuggets, soy based	2 nuggets (1½ oz)	½ carbohydrate + 1 medium-fat meat
Edamame ●	½ cup	½ carbohydrate + 1 lean meat
Falafel (spiced chickpea and wheat patties)	3 patties (2-in diameter)	1 carbohydrate + 1 high-fat meat
Hot dog, soy based	1 (1½ cup)	½ carbohydrate + 1 lean meat
Hummus ●	⅓ cup	1 carbohydrate + 1 high-fat meat
Lentils, brown, green, yellow ●	½ cup	1 carbohydrate + 1 lean meat
Vegetarian burger, soy based ●	3 oz	½ carbohydrate + 2 lean meats
Vegetarian burger, 1 patty, vegetable and starch based ●	(approx. 2½ oz)	1 carbohydrate + 2 lean meats
Nut spreads: almond, cashew, peanut, soy nut	1 Tbsp	1 high-fat meat
Peas, cooked: black-eyed and split ●	½ cup	1 carbohydrate + 1 lean meat
Refried beans. canned ●	½ cup	1 starch + 1 lean meat
"Sausage" patties, soy based	1 (1½ oz)	1 medium-fat meat
Soy nuts, unsalted	¾ oz	½ carbohydrate + 1 medium-fat meat
Tempeh	¼ cup	1 medium-fat meat
Tofu	4 oz (½ oz)	1 medium-fat meat
Tofu, light	4 oz (½ oz)	1 lean meat

● More than 3 g dietary fiber per serving;   ● Extra fat or prepared with added fat (add an extra fat choice);   ● ≥480 mg or more of sodium per serving. For foods listed as a main dish or meal on the **Combination Foods** and **Fast Foods** lists only, the ● represents more than 600 mg.

FATS

Fats are divided into three groups based on the main type of fat they contain:

- **Unsaturated fats** (omega-3, monounsaturated, and polyunsaturated) are primarily vegetable and arc liquid at room temperature. These fats have good health benefits.
  - **Omega-3 fats** are a type of polyunsaturated fat and can help lower triglyceride levels and the risk of heart disease.

- **Monounsaturated fats** also help lower cholesterol levels and may help raise HDL (good) cholesterol levels.
- **Polyunsaturated fats** can help lower cholesterol levels.
- **Saturated fats** have been linked with heart disease. They can raise LDL (bad) cholesterol levels and should be eaten in small amounts. Saturated fats are solid at room temperature.
- **Trans fats** are made in a process that changes vegetable oils into semisolid fats. These fats can raise blood cholesterol levels and should be eaten in small amounts. Partially hydrogenated and hydrogenated fats are types of manmade trans fats and should be avoided. Trans fats are also found naturally, occurring in some animal products such as meat, cheese, butter, and dairy products.

Nutrition Tips

- A choice on the **Fats** list contains 5 g fat and 45 calories.
- All fats are high in calories. Limit serving sizes for good nutrition and health.
- Limit the amount of fried foods you eat.
- Nuts and seeds are good sources of unsaturated fats if eaten in moderation. They have small amounts of fiber, protein, and magnesium.
- Good sources of omega-3 fatty acids include:
  - Fish such as albacore tuna, halibut, herring, mackerel, salmon, sardines, and trout
  - Flaxseeds and English walnuts
  - Oils such as canola, soybean, flaxseed, and walnut

Selection Tips

- Read the Nutrition Facts on food labels for serving sizes. One fat choice is based on a serving size that has 5 g fat.
- The food label also lists total fat grams, saturated fat, and trans fat grams per serving. When most of the calories come from saturated fat, the food is part of the Saturated Fats list.
- When selecting fats, consider replacing saturated fats with monounsaturated fats and omega-3 fats. Talk with your RD about the best choices for you.
- When selecting regular margarine, choose those that list liquid vegetable oil as the first ingredient. Soft or tub margarines have less saturated fat than stick margarines and are a healthier choice. Look for *trans* fat–free soft margarines.
- When selecting reduced-fat or lower fat margarines, look for liquid vegetable oil (*trans* fat free). Water usually is the first ingredient.

Fats and oils have mixtures of unsaturated (polyunsaturated and monounsaturated) and saturated fats. Foods on the **Fats** list are grouped together based on the major type of fat they contain. In general, 1 fat choice equals:

- 1 tsp of regular margarine, vegetable oil, or butter
- 1 Tbsp of regular salad dressing

Unsaturated Fats: Monounsaturated Fats

FOOD	SERVING SIZE
Avocado, medium	2 Tbsp (1 oz)
Nut butters (trans fat free): almond, cashew, peanut (smooth or crunchy)	1½ tsp
Nuts	
Almonds	6 nuts
Brazil	2 nuts
Cashews	6 nuts
Filberts (hazelnuts)	5 nuts
Macadamia	3 nuts
Mixed (50% peanut)	6 nuts
Peanuts	10 nuts
Pecans	4 halves
Pistachios	16 nuts
Oil: canola, olive, peanut	1 tsp
Olives	
Black (ripe)	8 large
Green, stuffed	10 large

Unsaturated Fats: Polyunsaturated Fats

FOOD	SERVING SIZE
Margarine: lower fat spread (30%-50% vegetable oil, trans fat free)	1 Tbsp
Margarine: stick, tub (trans fat free), or squeeze (trans fat free)	1 tsp
Mayonnaise	
Reduced fat	1 Tbsp
Regular	1 tsp
Mayonnaise-style salad dressing	
Reduced fat	1 Tbsp
Regular	2 tsp
Nuts	
Walnuts, English	4 halves
Pignoli (pine nuts)	1 Tbsp
Oil: corn, cottonseed, flaxseed, grapeseed, safflower, soybean, sunflower	1 tsp
Oil made from soybean and canola oil (e.g., Enova)	1 tsp
Plant stanol esters	
Light	1 Tbsp
Regular	2 tsp

Salad dressing	
Reduced fat (Note: May be high in carbohydrate) ●	2 Tbsp
Regular ●	1 Tbsp
Seeds	
Flaxseed, whole	1 Tbsp
Pumpkin, sunflower	1 Tbsp
Sesame seeds	1 Tbsp
Tahini or sesame paste	2 tsp

● More than 3 g dietary fiber per serving; ●Extra fat or prepared with added fat (add an extra fat choice); ● ≥480 mg or more of sodium per serving. For foods listed as a main dish or meal on the **Combination Foods** and **Fast Foods** lists only, the ● represents more than 600 mg.

Saturated Fats

FOOD	SERVING SIZE
Bacon, cooked, regular, or turkey	1 slice
Butter	
Reduced fat	1 Tbsp
Stick	1 tsp
Whipped	2 tsp
Butter blends made with oil	
Reduced fat or light	1 Tbsp
Regular	1½ tsp
Chitterlings, boiled	2 Tbsp (½ oz)
Coconut, sweetened, shredded	2 Tbsp
Coconut milk	
Light	⅓ cup
Regular	1½ Tbsp
Cream	
Half and half	2 Tbsp
Heavy	1 Tbsp
Light	1½ Tbsp
Whipped	1 Tbsp
Whipped, pressurized	2 Tbsp
Cream cheese	
Reduced fat	1½ Tbsp (¾ oz)
Regular	1 Tbsp (½ oz)
Lard	1 tsp
Oil: coconut, palm, palm kernel	1 tsp
Salt pork	¼ oz
Shortening, solid	1 tsp
Sour cream	
Reduced fat or light	3 Tbsp
Regular	2 Tbsp

Similar Foods in Other Lists

- Bacon and peanut butter, when used in smaller amounts, are counted as fat choices (see the **Fats** list). When used in larger amounts, they are counted as high-fat meat choices (see the **Meat and Meat Substitutes** list).

- Fat-free salad dressings are on the **Sweets. Desserts, and Other Carbohydrates** list.
- Look for whipped topping and fat-free products, such as margarines, salad dressings, mayonnaise, sour cream, and cream cheese, on the **Free Foods** list.

FREE FOODS

A "free" food is any food or drink choice that has less than 20 calories and 5 g or less of carbohydrate per serving.

Selection Tips

- Most foods on this list should be limited to three servings (as listed here) per day. Spread out the servings throughout the day. Eating all three servings at once could raise your blood glucose level.
- Food and drink choices listed here without a serving size can be eaten whenever you like.

Low-Carbohydrate Foods

FOOD	SERVING SIZE
Cabbage, raw	½ cup
Candy, hard (regular or sugar free)	1 piece
Carrots, cauliflower, or green beans, cooked	¼ cup
Cranberries, sweetened with sugar substitute	½ cup
Cucumber, sliced	½ cup
Gelatin	
Dessert, sugar free	
Unflavored	
Gum	
Jam or jelly, light or no sugar added	2 tsp
Rhubarb, sweetened with sugar substitute	½ cup
Salad greens	
Sugar substitutes (artificial sweeteners)	
Syrup, sugar free	2 Tbsp

Modified Fat Foods with Carbohydrate

FOOD	SERVING SIZE
Cream cheese, fat free	1 Tbsp (½ oz)
Creamers	
Nondairy, liquid	1 Tbsp
Nondairy, powdered	2 tsp
Margarine spread	
Fat free	1 Tbsp
Reduced fat	1 tsp

Mayonnaise-style salad dressing
Fat free	1 Tbsp
Reduced fat	1 tsp

Salad dressing
Fat free or low fat	1 Tbsp
Fat free, Italian	2 Tbsp
Sour cream, fat free or reduced fat	1 Tbsp

Whipped topping
Light or fat free	2 Tbsp
Regular	1 Tbsp

Condiments

FOOD	SERVING SIZE
Barbecue sauce	2 tsp
Catsup (ketchup)	1 Tbsp
Honey mustard	1 Tbsp
Horseradish	
Lemon juice	
Miso	1½ tsp
Mustard	
Parmesan cheese, freshly grated	1 Tbsp
Pickle relish	1 Tbsp
Pickles	
Dill ●	1½ medium
Sweet, bread and butter	2 slices
Sweet, gherkin	¾ oz
Salsa	¼ cup
Soy sauce, light or regular ●	1 Tbsp
Sweet and sour sauce	2 tsp
Sweet chili sauce	2 tsp
Taco sauce	1 Tbsp
Vinegar	
Yogurt, any type	2 Tbsp

● More than 3 g dietary fiber per serving; ● Extra fat or prepared with added fat (add an extra fat choice); ● ≥480 mg or more of sodium per serving. For foods listed as a main dish or meal on the **Combination Foods** and **Fast Foods** lists only, the ● represents more than 600 mg.

Free Snacks

The following foods in these serving sizes are free-food snacks.

- 5 baby carrots and celery sticks
- ¼ cup blueberries
- ½ oz sliced cheese, fat free
- 10 goldfish-style crackers
- 2 saltine-type crackers
- 1 frozen cream pop, sugar free
- ½ oz lean meat

- 1 cup light popcorn
- 2 vanilla wafers

Drinks and Mixes

Any food on this list without a serving size listed can be consumed in any moderate amount.

- Bouillon, broth, consommé ●
- Bouillon or broth, low sodium
- Carbonated or mineral water
- Club soda
- Cocoa powder, unsweetened (1 Tbsp)
- Coffee, unsweetened or with sugar substitute
- Diet soft drinks, sugar free
- Drink mixes, sugar free
- Tea, unsweetened or with sugar substitute
- Tonic water, diet
- Water
- Water, flavored, carbohydrate free

● More than 3 g dietary fiber per serving; ● Extra fat or prepared with added fat (add an extra fat choice); ● ≥480 mg or more of sodium per serving. For foods listed as a main dish or meal on the **Combination Foods** and **Fast Foods** lists only, the ● represents more than 600 mg.

Seasonings

Any food on this list can be consumed in moderate amount.

- Flavoring extracts (for example, vanilla, almond, peppermint)
- Garlic
- Herbs, fresh or dried
- Nonstick cooking spray
- Pimentos
- Spices
- Hot pepper sauce
- Wine, used in cooking
- Worcestershire sauce

COMBINATION FOODS

Many of the foods you eat are mixed together in various combinations, such as casseroles. These combination foods do not fit into any one choice list. This is a list of choices for some typical combination foods. This list will help you fit these foods into your meal plan. Ask your RD for nutrient information about other combination foods you would like to eat, including your own recipes.

Entrees

FOOD	SERVING SIZE	COUNT AS
Casserole type (tuna noodle, lasagna, spaghetti with meatballs, chili with beans, macaroni and cheese) ●	1 cup (8 oz)	2 carbohydrates + 2 medium-fat meats
Stews (beef or other meat and vegetables) ● ●	1 cup (8 oz)	1 carbohydrate + 1 medium-fat meat + 0-3 fats
Tuna salad or chicken salad	½ cup (3½ oz)	½ carbohydrate + 2 lean meats + 1 fat

● More than 3 g dietary fiber per serving; ● Extra fat or prepared with added fat (add an extra fat choice); ● ≥480 mg or more of sodium per serving. For foods listed as a main dish or meal on the **Combination Foods** and **Fast Foods** lists only, the ● represents more than 600 mg.

Other Combination Foods

Your home recipes may be different from similar foods listed here. To figure out your recipe nutrients, follow these steps:

- Find the carbohydrate grams, protein grams, fat grams, and calories for each of the recipe ingredients.
- Total each of the nutrients.
- Divide the totals by the number of servings the recipe yields.
- Compare these numbers with the choices in this booklet.

Frozen Meals and Entrees

FOOD	SERVING SIZE	COUNT AS
Burrito (beef and bean) ● ●	1 (5 oz)	3 carbohydrates + 1 lean meat + 2 fats
Dinner-type meal ●	Generally 14-17 oz	3 carbohydrates + 3 medium-fat meats + 3 fats
Entree or meal with less than 340 calories ●	Approx. 8-11 oz	2-3 carbohydrates + 1-2 lean meats
Pizza		
Cheese or vegetarian, thin crust ●	¼ of a 12-inch pie (4½-5 oz)	2 carbohydrates + 2 medium-fat meats
Meat topping, thin crust ●	¼ of a 12-inch pie (5 oz)	2 carbohydrates + 2 medium-fat meats + 1½ fats
Pocket sandwich ●	1 (4½ oz)	3 carbohydrates + 1 lean meat + 1-2 fats
Pot pie ●	1 (7 oz)	2½ carbohydrates + 1 medium-fat meat + 3 fats

● More than 3 g dietary fiber per serving; ● Extra fat or prepared with added fat (add an extra fat choice); ● ≥480 mg or more of sodium per serving. For foods listed as a main dish or meal on the **Combination Foods** and **Fast Foods** lists only, the ● represents more than 600 mg.

Salads (Deli Style)

FOOD	SERVING SIZE	COUNT AS
Coleslaw	½ cup	1 carbohydrate + 1½ fats
Macaroni or pasta salad	½ cup	2 carbohydrates + 3 fats
Potato salad ●	½ cup	1½-2 carbohydrates + 1-2 fats

● More than 3 g dietary fiber per serving; ● Extra fat or prepared with added fat (add an extra fat choice); ● ≥480 mg or more of sodium per serving. For foods listed as a main dish or meal on the **Combination Foods** and **Fast Foods** lists only, the ● represents more than 600 mg.

Soups

FOOD	SERVING SIZE	COUNT AS
Bean, lentil. split pea •	1cup	1carbohydrate + 1 lean meat
Chowder (made with milk) •	1 cup (8 oz)	1 carbohydrate + 1 lean meat + 1½ fats
Cream (made with water) •	1 cup (8 oz)	1 carbohydrate + 1 fat
Instant •	6 oz prepared	1 carbohydrate
Instant, with beans or lentils •	8 oz prepared	2½ carbohydrates + 1 lean meat
Miso soup •	1 cup	½ carbohydrate + 1 fat
Oriental noodle •	1 cup	2 carbohydrates + 2 fats
Rice (congee)	1 cup	1 carbohydrate
Tomato (made with water) •	1 cup (8 oz)	1 carbohydrate
Vegetable beef, chicken noodle, or other broth type	1 cup (8 oz)	1 carbohydrate

• More than 3 g dietary fiber per serving; • Extra fat or prepared with added fat (add an extra fat choice); • ≥480 mg or more of sodium per serving. For foods listed as a main dish or meal on the **Combination Foods** and **Fast Foods** lists only, the • represents more than 600 mg.

FAST FOODS

The choices in the **Fast Foods** list are not specific fast food meals or items but are estimates based on popular foods. You can get specific nutrition information for almost every fast food or restaurant chain. Ask the restaurant or check its Web site for nutrition information about your favorite fast foods.

Breakfast Sandwiches

FOOD	SERVING SIZE	COUNT AS
Egg, cheese, meat, English muffin •	1 sandwich	2 carbohydrates + 2 medium-fat meats
Sausage biscuit sandwich •	1 sandwich	2 carbohydrates + 2 high-fat meats + 3½ fats

• More than 3 g dietary fiber per serving; • Extra fat or prepared with added fat (add an extra fat choice); • ≥480 mg or more of sodium per serving. For foods listed as a main dish or meal on the **Combination Foods** and **Fast Foods** lists only, the • represents more than 600 mg.

Main Dishes and Entrees

FOOD	SERVING SIZE	COUNT AS
Burrito (beef and beans) • •	1 (approx. 8 oz)	3 carbohydrates + 3 medium-fat meats + 3 fats
Chicken breast, breaded and fried •	1 (approx. 5 oz)	1 carbohydrate + 4 medium-fat meats
Chicken drumstick, breaded and fried •	1 (approx. 2 oz)	2 medium-fat meats
Chicken nuggets •	6 (approx. 3½ oz)	1 carbohydrate + 2 medium-fat meats + 1 fat
Chicken thigh, breaded and fried •	1 (approx. 4 oz)	½ carbohydrate + 3 medium-fat meats + 1½ fats
Chicken wings, hot •	6 (5 oz)	5 medium-fat meats + 1½ fats

• More than 3 g dietary fiber per serving; • Extra fat or prepared with added fat (add an extra fat choice); • ≥480 mg or more of sodium per serving. For foods listed as a main dish or meal on the **Combination Foods** and **Fast Foods** lists only, the • represents more than 600 mg.

Asian

FOOD	SERVING SIZE	COUNT AS
Beef, chicken, or shrimp with vegetables in sauce •	1 cup (approx. 5 oz)	1 carbohydrate + 1 lean meat + 1 fat
Egg roll, meat •	1 (approx. 3 oz)	1 carbohydrate + 1 lean meat + 1 fat
Fried rice, meatless	½ cup	1½ carbohydrates + 1½ fats
Meat and sweet sauce (orange chicken) •	1 cup	3 carbohydrates + 3 medium-fat meats + 2 fats
Noodles and vegetables in sauce (chow mein, lo mein) • •	1 cup	2 carbohydrates + 1 fat

• More than 3 g dietary fiber per serving; • Extra fat or prepared with added fat (add an extra fat choice); • ≥480 mg or more of sodium per serving. For foods listed as a main dish or meal on the **Combination Foods** and **Fast Foods** lists only, the • represents more than 600 mg.

Pizza

FOOD	SERVING SIZE	COUNT AS
Cheese, pepperoni, regular crust ●	⅛ of a 14-inch pie (approx. 4 oz)	2½ carbohydrates + 1 medium-fat meat + 1½ fats
Cheese or vegetarian, thin crust ●	¼ of a 12-inch pie (approx. 6 oz)	2½ carbohydrates + 2 medium-fat meats + 1½ fats

● More than 3 g dietary fiber per serving; ● Extra fat or prepared with added fat (add an extra fat choice); ● ≥480 mg or more of sodium per serving. For foods listed as a main dish or meal on the **Combination Foods** and **Fast Foods** lists only, the ● represents more than 600 mg.

Sandwiches

FOOD	SERVING SIZE	COUNT AS
Chicken sandwich, grilled ●	1	3 carbohydrates + 4 lean meats
Chicken sandwich, crispy ●	1	3½ carbohydrates + 3 medium-fat meats + 1 fat
Fish sandwich with tartar sauce	1	2½ carbohydrates + 2 medium-fat meats + 2 fats
Hamburger		
Large with cheese ●	1	2½ carbohydrates + 4 medium-fat meats + 1 fat
Regular	1	2 carbohydrates + 1 medium-fat meat + 1 fat
Hot dog with bun ●	1	1 carbohydrate + 1 high-fat meat + 1 fat
Submarine sandwich		
Less than 6 grams fat ●	6-inch sub	3 carbohydrates + 2 lean meats
Regular ●	6-inch sub	3½ carbohydrates + 2 medium-fat meats + 1 fat
Taco, hard or soft shell (meat and cheese)	1 small	1 carbohydrate + 1 medium-fat meat + 1½ fats

● More than 3 g dietary fiber per serving; ● Extra fat or prepared with added fat (add an extra fat choice); ● ≥480 mg or more of sodium per serving. For foods listed as a main dish or meal on the **Combination Foods** and **Fast Foods** lists only, the ● represents more than 600 mg.

Salads

FOOD	SERVING SIZE	COUNT AS
Salad, main dish (grilled chicken type, no dressing or croutons) ● ●	Salad	1 carbohydrate + 4 lean meats
Salad, side, no dressing or cheese	Small (approx. 5 oz)	1 vegetable

● More than 3 g dietary fiber per serving; ● Extra fat or prepared with added fat (add an extra fat choice); ● ≥480 mg or more of sodium per serving. For foods listed as a main dish or meal on the **Combination Foods** and **Fast Foods** lists only, the ● represents more than 600 mg.

Sides and Appetizers

FOOD	SERVING SIZE	COUNT AS
French fries, restaurant style		
Small	2.6 oz	3 carbohydrates + 3 fats
Medium	4 oz	4 carbohydrates + 4 fats
Large	6 oz	5 carbohydrates + 6 fats
Nachos with cheese ●	Small (approx. 4½ oz)	2½ carbohydrates + 4 fats
Onion rings ●	1 serving (approx. 3 oz)	2½ carbohydrates + 3 fats

● More than 3 g dietary fiber per serving; ● Extra fat or prepared with added fat (add an extra fat choice); ● ≥480 mg or more of sodium per serving. For foods listed as a main dish or meal on the **Combination Foods** and **Fast Foods** lists only, the ● represents more than 600 mg.

Desserts

FOOD	SERVING SIZE	COUNT AS
Milkshake, any flavor	12 oz	6 carbohydrates + 2 fats
Soft-serve ice cream cone	1 small	2½ carbohydrates + 1 fat

ALCOHOL
Nutrition Tips

- In general, 1 alcohol choice (½ oz absolute alcohol) has approximately 100 calories.

Selection Tips

- If you choose to drink alcohol, you should limit yourself to 1 drink or less per day for women and 2 drinks or less per day for men.
- To reduce your risk of low blood glucose (hypoglycemia), especially if you take insulin or a diabetes drug that increases insulin, always drink alcohol with food.
- Alcohol by itself does not directly affect blood glucose, but be aware of the carbohydrate (e.g., in mixed drinks, beer, and wine) that may raise your blood glucose.
- Check with your RD if you would like to fit alcohol into your meal plan.

ALCOHOLIC BEVERAGE	SERVING SIZE	COUNT AS
Beer		
Light (4.2%)	12 fl oz	1 alcohol equivalent + ½ carbohydrate
Regular (4.9%)	12 fl oz	1 alcohol equivalent + 1carbohydrate
Distilled spirits: vodka, rum, gin, whiskey 80 or 86 proof	1½ fl oz	1 alcohol equivalent
Liqueur, coffee (53 proof)	1 fl oz	½ alcohol equivalent + 1 carbohydrate
Sake	1 fl oz	½ alcohol equivalent
Wine		
Dessert (e.g., sherry)	3½ fl oz	1 alcohol equivalent + 1carbohydrate
Dry, red or white (10%)	5 fl oz	1 alcohol equivalent

YOUR MEAL PLAN

Meal Plan for: _____

RD: _____

Carbohydrate (g) _____

Carbohydrate choices _____

Protein (g) _____

Fat (g) _____

Calories _____

Date: _____

Phone: _____

(% of calories) _____

(servings) _____

(% of calories) _____

(% of calories) _____

	STARCHES	FRUITS	MILK	NONSTARCHY VEGETABLES	MEAT AND MEAT SUBSTITUTES	FATS	MENU IDEAS
Breakfast Time:							
Snack Time:							
Lunch Time:							
Snack Time:							
Dinner Time:							
Snack Time:							

Eating Well with Canada's Food Guide

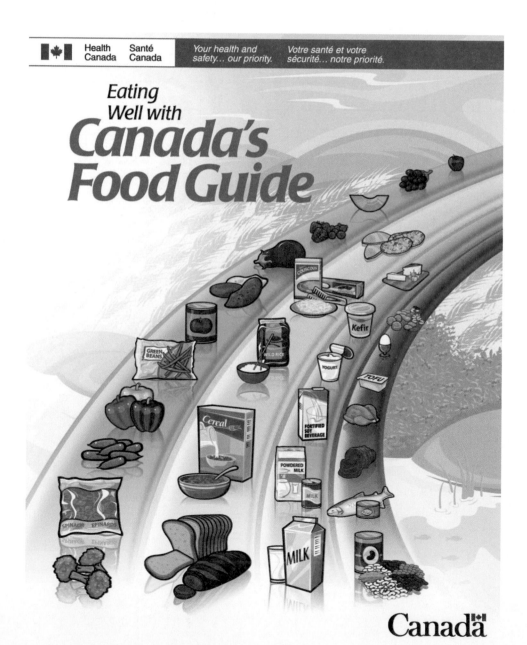

Health Canada Santé Canada

Your health and safety... our priority. *Votre santé et votre sécurité... notre priorité.*

Eating Well with **Canada's Food Guide**

Canada

Recommended Number of Food Guide Servings per Day

Age in Years	Children			Teens		Adults			
	2-3	4-8	9-13	14-18		19-50		51+	
Sex	Girls and Boys			Females	Males	Females	Males	Females	Males
Vegetables and Fruit	4	5	6	7	8	7-8	8-10	7	7
Grain Products	3	4	6	6	7	6-7	8	6	7
Milk and Alternatives	2	2	3-4	3-4	3-4	2	2	3	3
Meat and Alternatives	1	1	1-2	2	3	2	3	2	3

The chart above shows how many Food Guide Servings you need from each of the four food groups every day.

Having the amount and type of food recommended and following the tips in *Canada's Food Guide* will help:
- Meet your needs for vitamins, minerals and other nutrients.
- Reduce your risk of obesity, type 2 diabetes, heart disease, certain types of cancer and osteoporosis.
- Contribute to your overall health and vitality.

What is One Food Guide Serving?
Look at the examples below.

Vegetables and Fruit
Fresh, frozen or canned vegetables 125 mL (½ cup)
Leafy vegetables Cooked: 125 mL (½ cup) Raw: 250 mL (1 cup)
Fresh, frozen or canned fruits 1 fruit or 125 mL (½ cup)
100% Juice 125 mL (½ cup)

Grain Products
Bread 1 slice (35 g)
Bagel ½ bagel (45 g)
Flat breads ½ pita or ½ tortilla (35 g)
Cooked rice, bulgur or quinoa 125 mL (½ cup)
Cereal Cold: 30 g Hot: 175 mL (¾ cup)
Cooked pasta or couscous 125 mL (½ cup)

Milk and Alternatives
Milk or powdered milk (reconstituted) 250 mL (1 cup)
Canned milk (evaporated) 125 mL (½ cup)
Fortified soy beverage 250 mL (1 cup)
Yogurt 175 g (¾ cup)
Kefir 175 g (¾ cup)
Cheese 50 g (1½ oz.)

Meat and Alternatives
Cooked fish, shellfish, poultry, lean meat 75 g (2 ½ oz.)/125 mL (½ cup)
Cooked legumes 175 mL (¾ cup)
Tofu 150 g or 175 mL (¾ cup)
Eggs 2 eggs
Peanut or nut butters 30 mL (2 Tbsp)
Shelled nuts and seeds 60 mL (¼ cup)

Oils and Fats
- Include a small amount – 30 to 45 mL (2 to 3 Tbsp) – of unsaturated fat each day. This includes oil used for cooking, salad dressings, margarine and mayonnaise.
- Use vegetable oils such as canola, olive and soybean.
- Choose soft margarines that are low in saturated and trans fats.
- Limit butter, hard margarine, lard and shortening.

Make each Food Guide Serving count...
wherever you are – at home, at school, at work or when eating out!

▸ **Eat at least one dark green and one orange vegetable each day.**
- Go for dark green vegetables such as broccoli, romaine lettuce and spinach.
- Go for orange vegetables such as carrots, sweet potatoes and winter squash.

▸ **Choose vegetables and fruit prepared with little or no added fat, sugar or salt.**
- Enjoy vegetables steamed, baked or stir-fried instead of deep-fried.

▸ **Have vegetables and fruit more often than juice.**

▸ **Make at least half of your grain products whole grain each day.**
- Eat a variety of whole grains such as barley, brown rice, oats, quinoa and wild rice.
- Enjoy whole grain breads, oatmeal or whole wheat pasta.

▸ **Choose grain products that are lower in fat, sugar or salt.**
- Compare the Nutrition Facts table on labels to make wise choices.
- Enjoy the true taste of grain products. When adding sauces or spreads, use small amounts.

▸ **Drink skim, 1%, or 2% milk each day.**
- Have 500 mL (2 cups) of milk every day for adequate vitamin D.
- Drink fortified soy beverages if you do not drink milk.

▸ **Select lower fat milk alternatives.**
- Compare the Nutrition Facts table on yogurts or cheeses to make wise choices.

▸ **Have meat alternatives such as beans, lentils and tofu often.**

▸ **Eat at least two Food Guide Servings of fish each week.***
- Choose fish such as char, herring, mackerel, salmon, sardines and trout.

▸ **Select lean meat and alternatives prepared with little or no added fat or salt.**
- Trim the visible fat from meats. Remove the skin on poultry.
- Use cooking methods such as roasting, baking or poaching that require little or no added fat.
- If you eat luncheon meats, sausages or prepackaged meats, choose those lower in salt (sodium) and fat.

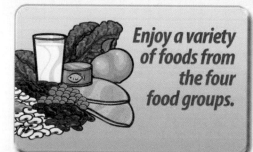

Enjoy a variety of foods from the four food groups.

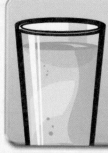

Satisfy your thirst with water!

Drink water regularly. It's a calorie-free way to quench your thirst. Drink more water in hot weather or when you are very active.

* Health Canada provides advice for limiting exposure to mercury from certain types of fish. Refer to www.healthcanada.gc.ca for the latest information.

Eat well and be active today and every day!

The benefits of eating well and being active include:

- Better overall health.
- Lower risk of disease.
- A healthy body weight.
- Feeling and looking better.
- More energy.
- Stronger muscles and bones.

Be active

To be active every day is a step towards better health and a healthy body weight.

Canada's Physical Activity Guide recommends building 30 to 60 minutes of moderate physical activity into daily life for adults and at least 90 minutes a day for children and youth. You don't have to do it all at once. Add it up in periods of at least 10 minutes at a time for adults and five minutes at a time for children and youth.

Start slowly and build up.

Eat well

Another important step towards better health and a healthy body weight is to follow *Canada's Food Guide* by:

- Eating the recommended amount and type of food each day.
- Limiting foods and beverages high in calories, fat, sugar or salt (sodium) such as cakes and pastries, chocolate and candies, cookies and granola bars, doughnuts and muffins, ice cream and frozen desserts, french fries, potato chips, nachos and other salty snacks, alcohol, fruit flavoured drinks, soft drinks, sports and energy drinks, and sweetened hot or cold drinks.

Read the label

- Compare the Nutrition Facts table on food labels to choose products that contain less fat, saturated fat, trans fat, sugar and sodium.
- Keep in mind that the calories and nutrients listed are for the amount of food found at the top of the Nutrition Facts table.

Nutrition Facts		
Per 0 mL (0 g)		
Amount		**% Daily Value**
Calories 0		
Fat 0 g		0 %
Saturates 0 g		0 %
+ Trans 0 g		
Cholesterol 0 mg		
Sodium 0 mg		0 %
Carbohydrate 0 g		0 %
Fibre 0 g		0 %
Sugars 0 g		
Protein 0 g		
Vitamin A 0 %		Vitamin C 0 %
Calcium 0 %		Iron 0 %

Limit trans fat

When a Nutrition Facts table is not available, ask for nutrition information to choose foods lower in trans and saturated fats.

Take a step today...

- ✓ Have breakfast every day. It may help control your hunger later in the day.
- ✓ Walk wherever you can — get off the bus early, use the stairs.
- ✓ Benefit from eating vegetables and fruit at all meals and as snacks.
- ✓ Spend less time being inactive such as watching TV or playing computer games.
- ✓ Request nutrition information about menu items when eating out to help you make healthier choices.
- ✓ Enjoy eating with family and friends!
- ✓ Take time to eat and savour every bite!

For more information, interactive tools, or additional copies visit Canada's Food Guide on-line at:
www.healthcanada.gc.ca/foodguide

or contact:
Publications
Health Canada
Ottawa, Ontario K1A 0K9
E-Mail: publications@hc-sc.gc.ca
Tel.: 1-866-225-0709
Fax: (613) 941-5366
TTY: 1-800-267-1245

Également disponible en français sous le titre :
Bien manger avec le Guide alimentaire canadien

This publication can be made available on request on diskette, large print, audio-cassette and braille.

Advice for different ages and stages...

Children

Following *Canada's Food Guide* helps children grow and thrive.

Young children have small appetites and need calories for growth and development.

- Serve small nutritious meals and snacks each day.
- Do not restrict nutritious foods because of their fat content. Offer a variety of foods from the four food groups.
- Most of all... be a good role model.

Women of childbearing age

All women who could become pregnant and those who are pregnant or breastfeeding need a multivitamin containing **folic acid** every day. Pregnant women need to ensure that their multivitamin also contains **iron**. A health care professional can help you find the multivitamin that's right for you.

Pregnant and breastfeeding women need more calories. Include an extra 2 to 3 Food Guide Servings each day.

Here are two examples:

- Have fruit and yogurt for a snack, or
- Have an extra slice of toast at breakfast and an extra glass of milk at supper.

Men and women over 50

The need for **vitamin D** increases after the age of 50.

In addition to following *Canada's Food Guide*, everyone over the age of 50 should take a daily vitamin D supplement of 10 µg (400 IU).

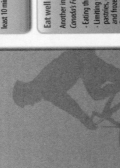

How do I count Food Guide Servings in a meal?

Here is an example:

Vegetable and beef stir-fry with rice, a glass of milk and an apple for dessert	
250 mL (1 cup) mixed broccoli, carrot and sweet red pepper	= 2 **Vegetables and Fruit** Food Guide Servings
75 g (2½ oz.) lean beef	= 1 **Meat and Alternatives** Food Guide Serving
250 mL (1 cup) brown rice	= 2 **Grain Products** Food Guide Servings
5 mL (1 tsp) canola oil	= part of your **Oils and Fats** intake for the day
250 mL (1 cup) 1% milk	= 1 **Milk and Alternatives** Food Guide Serving
1 apple	= 1 **Vegetables and Fruit** Food Guide Serving

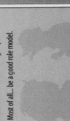

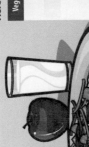

Calculation Aids and Conversion Tables

A group of French scientists created the metric system of weights and measures called the Système International (SI). Here are a few conversion factors to help you make transitions in your necessary calculations.

METRIC SYSTEM OF MEASUREMENT

The metric system is a simple decimal system based on units of 10. It is uniform and used internationally.

Weight Units:

1 kilogram (kg) = 1000 grams (g or gm)
1 g = 1000 milligrams (mg)
1 mg = 1000 micrograms (mcg or μg)

Length Units:

1 meter (m) = 100 centimeters (cm)
1000 meters = 1 kilometer (km)

Volume Units:

1 liter (L or l) = 1000 milliliters (ml or mL)
1 ml = 1 cubic centimeter (cc)

Temperature Units:

The Celsius (C) scale, based on 100 equal units between 0° C (the freezing point of water) and 100° C (the boiling point of water), is used in all scientific work.

Energy Units:

Kilocalorie (kcal) = Amount of energy required to raise 1 kg water 1° C
Kilojoule (kJ) = Amount of energy required to move 1 kg mass 1 m by a force of 1 newton
1 kcal = 4.184 kJ

AMERICAN SYSTEM OF MEASUREMENT

The American system of measurement is not a decimal system, but rather a collection of different units. It has mostly British roots but is now predominately used in the United States only.

Weight Units:

1 pound (lb) = 16 ounces (oz)

Length Units:

1 foot (ft) = 12 inches (in)
1 yard (yd) = 3 feet (ft)

Volume Units:

3 teaspoons (tsp) = 1 tablespoon (Tbsp)
16 Tbsp = 1 cup
1 cup = 8 fluid ounces (fl oz)
4 cups = 1 quart (qt)
5 cups = 1 imperial quart (qt) (used in Canada)

Temperature Units:

The Fahrenheit (F) scale is based on 180 equal units between 32° F (the freezing point of water) and 212° F (the boiling point of water) at standard atmospheric pressure.

CONVERSIONS BETWEEN MEASUREMENT SYSTEMS

Weight:

> 1 oz = 28.35 g
> 2.205 lb = 1 kg

Length:

> 1 in = 2.54 cm
> 1 ft = 30.48 cm
> 39.37 in = 1 m

Volume:

> 1.06 qt = 1 L
> 0.85 imperial qt = 1 L (used in Canada)

Temperature:

Boiling point of water = 100° C = 212° F
Body temperature = 37° C = 98.6° F
Freezing point of water = 0° C = 32° F

Interconversion formulas:

> Fahrenheit temperature (°F) = $\frac{9}{5}$ (°C) + 32
> Celsius temperature (°C) = $\frac{5}{9}$ (°F – 32)

RETINOL EQUIVALENTS

The following internationally accepted definitions and equivalences are provided to calculate retinol-equivalent conversions.

Definitions:

International units (IU) and retinol equivalents (RE) are defined as follows:

> 1 IU = 0.3 mcg retinol (0.0003 mg)
> 1 IU = 0.6 mcg beta-carotene (0.0006 mg)
> 1 RE = 6 mcg retinol
> 1 RE = 6 mcg beta-carotene
> 1 RE = 12 mcg other provitamin A carotenoids
> 1 RE = 3.33 IU retinol
> 1 RE = 10 IU beta-carotene

Conversion Formulas:

On the basis of weight, beta-carotene is half as active as retinol; on the basis of structure, the other provitamin carotenoids are one fourth as active as retinol. In addition, retinol is more completely absorbed in the intestines, whereas the provitamin carotenoids are much less well utilized, with an average absorption of approximately one third. Therefore, in overall activity, beta-carotene is one sixth as active as retinol, and the other carotenoids are one twelfth as active. These differences in utilization provide the basis for the 1:6:12 relation shown in the equivalences given and in the following formulas for calculating retinol equivalents from values of vitamin A, beta-carotene, and other active carotenoids, expressed either as international units or micrograms.

If retinol and beta-carotene are given in micrograms:

> RE = Micrograms of retinol +
> (Micrograms of beta-carotene/6)

If both are given as international units:

> RE = (International units of retinol/3.33) +
> (International units of beta-carotene/10)

If beta-carotene and other carotenoids are given in micrograms:

> RE = (Micrograms of beta-carotene/6) +
> (Micrograms of other carotenoids/12)

APPROXIMATE METRIC CONVERSIONS

WHEN YOU KNOW...	...MULTIPLY BY...	...TO FIND...
Weight		
Ounces	28	Grams
Pounds	0.45	Kilograms
Length		
Inches	2.5	Centimeters
Feet	30	Centimeters
Yards	0.9	Meters
Miles	1.6	Kilometers
Volume		
Teaspoons	5	Milliliters
Tablespoons	15	Milliliters
Fluid ounces	30	Milliliters
Cups	0.24	Liters
Pints	0.47	Liters
Quarts	0.95	Liters
Temperature		
Fahrenheit temperature	$\frac{5}{9}$ (after subtracting 32)	Celsius temperature

Cultural Dietary Patterns and Religious Dietary Practices

Foods specifically associated with these cultural groups are noted. Individuals may consume typical American foods as well; assumptions of dietary patterns cannot be made, but knowledge of these unique foods provides a common understanding of the range of possible food choices.

CULTURAL DIETARY PATTERNS

ETHNIC GROUP	BREAD, CEREAL, RICE, AND PASTA GROUP	VEGETABLE GROUP
Native American Each tribe may have specific foods; listed here are commonly consumed foods.	Blue corn flour (ground dried blue corn kernels) used to make cornbread, mush dumplings; fruit dumplings (walakshi); fry bread (biscuit dough deep fried); ground sweet acorn; tortillas; wheat or rye used to make cornmeal and flours	Cabbage, carrots, cassava, dandelion greens, eggplant, milkweed, onions, pumpkin, squash (all varieties), sweet and white potatoes, turnips, wild tullies (a tuber), yellow corn
African American	Biscuits; cornbread as spoon bread, corn-pone, or hush puppies; grits	Leafy greens including dandelion greens, kale, mustard greens, collard greens, turnips
Japanese	Rice and rice products, rice flour (mo-chiko), noodles (comen, soba), sea-weed around rice with or without fish (sushi)	Bamboo shoots (takenoko), burdock (gobo), cabbage (napa), dried mushrooms (shiitake), eggplant, horseradish (wasabi), Japanese parsley (seri), lotus root (renkon), mustard greens, pickled vegetables, seaweed (laver, nori, wakame, kombu), vegetable soup (mizutaki), white radish (daikon)
Chinese	Rice and related products (flour, cakes, noodles); noodles made from barley, corn, and millet; wheat and related products (breads, noodles, spaghetti, stuffed noodles [wonton], filled buns [bow])	Bamboo shoots; cabbage (napa); Chinese celery; Chinese parsley (corian-der); Chinese turnips (lo bok); dried day lilies; dry fungus (black Judas ear); leafy green vegetables including kale, Chinese cress, Chinese mus-tard greens (gai choy), Chinese chard (bok choy), amaranth greens (yin choy), wolfberry leaves (gou gay), and Chinese broccoli (gai lan); lotus tubers; okra; snow peas; stir-fried vegetables (chow yuk); taro root; white radish (daikon)
Filipino	Noodles, rice, rice flour (mochiko), stuffed noodles (wonton), white bread (pan de sal)	Bamboo shoots, dark green leafy vege-tables (malunggay and salvyot), eggplant, sweet potatoes (camotes), okra, palm, peppers, turnips, root crop (gabi)
Southeastern Asians (Laos, Cambo-dia, Thailand, Vietnam, the Hmong and the Mien)	Rice (long and short grain) and related products such as noodles; Hmong cornbread or cake	Bamboo shoots, broccoli, Chinese parsley (coriander), mustard greens, pickled vegetables, water chestnuts, Thai chili peppers

FRUIT GROUP	MILK, YOGURT, AND CHEESE GROUP	MEAT, POULTRY, FISH, DRY BEANS, EGGS, AND NUTS GROUP	FATS, OILS, AND SWEETS
Dried wild cherries and grapes; wild banana, berries, and yucca	None	Duck, eggs, fish eggs (roe), geese, ground-hog, kidney beans, lentils, nuts (all), pea-nuts, pine nuts, pinto beans, venison, wild rabbit	None
None	Buttermilk	Pork and pork products, scrapple (cornmeal and pork), chitterlings (pork intestines), bacon, pig's feet, pig ears, souse, pork neck bones, fried meats and poultry, or-gan meats (kidney, liver, tongue, tripe), venison, rabbit, catfish, buffalo fish, mackerel, legumes (black-eyed peas, kid-ney beans, navy beans, chickpeas)	Lard
Pear-like apple (nasi), persimmons	None	Fish and shellfish including dried fish with bones, raw fish (sashimi), and fish cake (kamaboko); soybeans as soybean curd (tofu), fermented soybean paste (miso), and sprouts; red beans (adzuki)	Soy and rice oil
Kumquat	None	Fish and seafood (all kinds, dried and fresh), hen, legumes, nuts, organ meats, pigeon eggs, pork and pork products, soybean curd (tofu), steamed stuffed dumplings (dim sum)	Peanut, soy, sesame and rice oil; lard
Avocado, bitter melon (ampalaya), guavas, jackfruit, limes, mango, papaya, pod fruit (tamarind), pomelos, tangelo (na-ranghita)	Custards	Fish in all forms; dried fish (dilis); egg roll (lumpia); fish sauce (alamang and ba-goong); legumes such as mung beans, bean sprouts, chickpeas; organ meats (liver, heart, intestines); pork with chicken in soy sauce (adobo); pork sausage; soy-bean curd (tofu)	None
Apple pear (Asian pear), bitter melon, coconut cream and milk, guava, jackfruit, mango	Sweetened con-densed milk	Beef; chicken; deer; eggs; fish and shellfish (all kinds of freshwater and saltwater); le-gumes including black-eyed peas, pea-nuts, kidney beans, and soybeans; organ meats (liver, stomach); pork; rabbit; soy-bean curd (tofu)	Lard, peanut oil

ETHNIC GROUP	BREAD, CEREAL, RICE, AND PASTA GROUP	VEGETABLE GROUP
Mexican	Corn and related products; taco shells (fried corn tortillas); tortillas (corn and flour); white bread	Cactus (nopales), chili peppers, salsa, tomatoes, yambean root (jicama), yucca root (cassava or manioc)
Caribbean Persons (includes Puerto Rican and Cuban)	Rice; starchy green bananas, usually fried (plantain)	Beets, eggplant, tubers (yucca), white yams (boniato)
Jewish These foods reflect religious and cultural customs of Jewish people. Adherences to religious dietary patterns by followers of the different forms of Judaism (Orthodox, Conservative, Reform, and Reconstructionist) vary. Generally, Orthodox Jews and many Conservative Jews follow kosher dietary rules when eating at home and dining out. Others may only observe these rules when in their own homes. "Keeping kosher" rules are reviewed in the religious dietary pattern section.	Bagel, buckwheat groats (kasha), dumplings made with matzoh meal (matzoh balls or knaidelach), egg bread (challah), noodle or potato pudding (kugel), crepe filled with farmer cheese and/or fruit (blintz), unleavened bread or large cracker made with wheat flour and water (matzoh)	Potato pancakes (latkes); a vegetable stew made with sweet potatoes, carrots, prunes, and sometimes brisket (tzimmes); beet soup (borscht)

Reprinted from Grodner M and others: *Foundations and clinical applications of nutrition,* ed 4, St Louis, 2007, Mosby.

RELIGIOUS DIETARY PRACTICES

	SEVENTH-DAY ADVENTIST	BUDDHIST	EASTERN ORTHODOX
Beef		Avoided by most devout	
Pork	Prohibited or strongly discouraged	Avoided by most devout	
All meat	Avoided by most devout	Avoided by most devout	Permitted but some restrictions apply
Eggs, dairy	Permitted but avoided at some observances	Permitted but avoided at some observances	Permitted but some restrictions apply
Fish	Avoided by most devout	Avoided by most devout	Permitted but some restrictions apply
Shellfish	Prohibited or strongly discouraged	Avoided by most devout	Permitted but avoided at some observances
Meat and dairy at same meal			
Leavened foods			
Ritual slaughter of animals			
Alcohol	Prohibited or strongly discouraged		
Caffeine	Prohibited or strongly discouraged		

Reprinted from Kittler PG, Sucher KP: *Food and culture,* ed 4, Belmont, CA, 2004, Brooks/Cole.

FRUIT GROUP	MILK, YOGURT, AND CHEESE GROUP	MEAT, POULTRY, FISH, DRY BEANS, EGGS, AND NUTS GROUP	FATS, OILS, AND SWEETS
Avocado, guacamole (mashed avocado, onion, cilantro [coriander], chilies), papaya	Cheese, flan, sour cream	Black or pinto beans (rejoles); refried beans (frijoles refritos); flour tortilla stuffed with beef, chicken, eggs, or beans (burrito); corn tortilla stuffed with chicken, cheese, or beef topped with chili sauce (enchilada); Mexican sausage (chorizo)	Bacon fat, lard (manteca), salt pork
Tropical fruits, avocados, plantains, grapefruit, lemons, limes	Flan, hard cheese (queso de mano)	Chicken, fish (all kinds and preparations, including smoked, salted, canned, and fresh), legumes (all kinds, especially black beans), pork (fried), sausage (chorizo)	Olive and peanut oil, lard
None	None	A mixture of fish formed into balls and poached (gefilte fish); smoked salmon (lox)	Chicken fat

HINDU	JEWISH	MORMON	MOSLEM	ROMAN CATHOLIC
Prohibited or strongly discouraged				
Avoided by most devout	Prohibited or strongly discouraged		Prohibited or strongly discouraged	
Avoided by most devout	Permitted but some restrictions apply		Permitted but some restrictions apply	Permitted but some restrictions apply
Permitted but avoided at some observances	Permitted but some restrictions apply			
Permitted but some restrictions apply	Permitted but some restrictions apply			
Permitted but some restrictions apply	Prohibited or strongly discouraged			
	Prohibited or strongly discouraged			
	Permitted but some restrictions apply			
	Practiced		Practiced	
Avoided by most devout		Prohibited or strongly discouraged	Prohibited or strongly discouraged	
		Prohibited or strongly discouraged	Avoided by most devout	

ANSWERS TO CHAPTER CHALLENGE QUESTIONS

CHAPTER 1
True-False
1. F
2. T
3. F
Multiple Choice
1. a
2. d
3. a

CHAPTER 2
True-False
1. F
2. T
3. F
4. T
5. F
6. T
Multiple Choice
1. d
2. b
3. d
4. a
5. c
6. a

CHAPTER 3
True-False
1. F
2. T
3. F
4. F
5. T
Multiple Choice
1. a
2. d
3. b
4. d

CHAPTER 4
True-False
1. F
2. T
3. F
4. F
5. F
6. T
7. T
8. T
9. T
Multiple Choice
1. a
2. d
3. c

CHAPTER 5
True-False
1. F
2. T
3. F
4. T
5. F
6. F
7. T
Multiple Choice
1. d
2. c
3. b
4. d
5. a

CHAPTER 6
True-False
1. F
2. F
3. T
4. F
5. T
6. F
Multiple Choice
1. b
2. c
3. c
4. a
5. d
6. c

CHAPTER 7
True-False
1. F
2. F
3. T
4. F
5. T
6. T
7. F
Multiple Choice
1. c
2. c
3. d
4. b
5. d
6. a
7. d

CHAPTER 8
True-False
1. T
2. T
3. F
4. T
5. F
6. F
7. F

Multiple Choice
1. c
2. a
3. b
4. d
5. a
6. b

CHAPTER 9
Matching
1. k
2. g
3. n
4. a
5. l
6. b
7. f
8. h
9. i
10. p
11. d
12. o
13. j
14. c
15. e
16. m

CHAPTER 10
True-False
1. T
2. F
3. F
4. T
5. F
6. F
7. T
8. T
9. T
10. T
Multiple Choice
1. a
2. d
3. b
4. d
5. c
6. c

CHAPTER 11
True-False
1. F
2. T
3. T
4. F
5. F
Multiple Choice
1. d
2. c
3. b

CHAPTER 12
True-False
1. F
2. F
3. F
4. T
5. F
6. F
Multiple Choice
1. d
2. c
3. b, d
4. a, b, c, d

CHAPTER 13
True-False
1. F
2. F
3. F
4. T
5. F
6. F
7. T
Multiple Choice
1. a, b, c, d
2. c

CHAPTER 14
True-False
1. F
2. T
3. T
4. T
5. F
Multiple Choice
1. d
2. a, c, d
3. a, b
4. b
5. c

CHAPTER 15
True-False
1. F
2. T
3. T
4. T
5. F
6. F
Multiple Choice
1. a, b, c, d
2. a
3. b

CHAPTER 16
True-False
1. F
2. F
3. T
4. F
5. F
6. T
7. T
8. F
9. T

Multiple Choice
1. b
2. d
3. a, b, c
4. a, c
5. c

CHAPTER 17
True-False
1. T
2. F
3. T
4. F
5. F
6. F
7. F
8. F

Multiple Choice
1. a, b, c, d
2. a, b, c, d
3. a, b, c, d
4. a, d

CHAPTER 18
True-False
1. F
2. T
3. T
4. F
5. F
6. T
7. T

Multiple Choice
1. d
2. b
3. b
4. a
5. c

CHAPTER 19
True-False
1. T
2. F
3. F
4. F
5. T
6. T
7. T
8. F
9. F
10. F

Multiple Choice
1. b, c
2. a, c
3. b
4. a

CHAPTER 20
True-False
1. F
2. F
3. F
4. T
5. T
6. T
7. T
8. F
9. F
10. F

Multiple Choice
1. c
2. a, b, c
3. b
4. a, b, c, d

CHAPTER 21
True-False
1. T
2. F
3. F
4. T
5. T
6. F
7. T
8. F
9. T
10. T

Multiple Choice
1. b, d
2. b, c, d
3. a, b, c

CHAPTER 22
True-False
1. T
2. T
3. F
4. T
5. T
6. F
7. F
8. F
9. F
10. T

Multiple Choice
1. a
2. b
3. a
4. a, b, c, d
5. a, b, c, d

CHAPTER 23
True-False
1. F
2. T
3. T
4. F
5. T
6. F
7. F
8. F
9. T
10. T

Multiple Choice
1. b
2. c
3. b
4. a
5. d
6. b
7. d
8. d

GLOSSARY

absorption the process in which nutrients are taken into the cells lining the gastrointestinal tract.

acetone a major ketone compound that results from fat breakdown for energy in uncontrolled diabetes; persons with diabetes periodically take urinary acetone tests to monitor the status of their blood glucose control.

acid and alkaline diets a diet based on the theory that diets high in acidic foods, such as animal protein, caffeine, and simple sugars, disrupt the body's normal pH balance, which is slightly alkaline.

acidosis blood pH less than 7.35. Respiratory acidosis is caused from an accumulation of carbon dioxide (an acid). Metabolic acidosis may be caused by a variety of conditions resulting in excess accumulation of acids in the body or from a significant loss of bicarbonate (base).

adipose fat present in cells of adipose (fatty) tissue.

adipose tissue storage site for fat.

aerobic capacity requiring oxygen to proceed; milliliters of oxygen consumed per kilogram of body weight per minute, as influenced by body composition.

aldosterone a potent hormone of the outside layer of the adrenal glands that acts on the distal nephron tubule to stimulate reabsorption of sodium in an ion exchange with potassium. The aldosterone mechanism is essentially a sodium-conserving mechanism but also indirectly conserves water because water follows sodium.

aldosteronoma excess secretion of aldosterone from the adrenal cortex. Symptoms and complications include sodium retention, potassium wasting (loss in the urine), alkalosis, weakness, paralysis, polyuria, polydipsia, hypertension, and cardiac arrhythmias.

alkalosis blood pH greater than 7.45. Respiratory alkalosis is caused from hyperventilation and excess loss of carbon dioxide. Metabolic alkalosis is seen with extensive vomiting in which significant amounts of bicarbonate are secreted (a base).

allergens food proteins eliciting an immune system response, or allergic reaction. Symptoms may include itching, swelling, hives, diarrhea, difficulty breathing, as well as anaphylaxis in the worst cases.

allergy a state of hypersensitivity to particular substances in the environment; the allergen may be a certain food eaten or a substance (e.g., pollen) inhaled.

amenorrhea absence of a menstrual period in women of reproductive age.

amenorrheic absences or abnormal cessation of menses.

amino acids nitrogen-bearing compounds that form the structural units of protein. After digestion amino acids are available for synthesis of proteins or catabolism for energy production.

aminopeptidase specific protein-splitting enzyme secreted by small glands in the walls of the small intestine that breaks off the nitrogen-containing amino ($-NH_2$) end of the peptide chain, producing smaller chained peptides and free amino acids.

amphophilic molecule containing both hydrophilic and hydrophobic groups.

anabolism the metabolic process of building large substances from smaller parts; the opposite of catabolism.

anaerobic without oxygen.

anaphylaxis severe allergic, sometimes fatal, reaction resulting from exposure to a protein the body perceives as foreign and elicits a systemic response that includes multiple organs.

anemia blood condition characterized by a decreased number of circulating red blood cells, decreased hemoglobin, or both.

anencephaly congenital absence of the brain resulting from the incomplete closure of the upper end of the neural tube.

angina pectoris spasmodic, choking chest pain caused by a lack of oxygen to the heart muscle; symptom of a heart attack; also may be caused by severe effort or excitement.

anorexia nervosa extreme psychophysiologic aversion to food resulting in life-threatening weight loss; a psychiatric eating disorder resulting from a morbid fear of fatness in which a person's distorted body image is reflected as fat when the body is malnourished and extremely thin from self-starvation.

anthropometric measurements physical measurements of the human body used for health assessment, including height, weight, skinfold thickness, and circumference (head, hip, waist, wrist, mid-arm muscle).

antibody protein molecule produced by B cells as a primary immune defense for attaching to specific antigens.

antidiuretic hormone (ADH) a hormone of the pituitary gland that acts on the distal nephron tubule to conserve water by reabsorption; also called vasopressin.

antigen any foreign or non-self substances (e.g., toxins, viruses, bacteria, and foreign proteins) that stimulate the production of antibodies specifically designed to counteract their activity.

anuria an absence of urine production; indicates kidney failure.

appetite-regulating network a hormonally controlled system of appetite stimulus and supression.

arteriole smallest branch of an artery; connects with capillaries.

ascites outflow and accumulation of serous fluid (blood and lymph serum) in the abdominal cavity; also known as abdominal or peritoneal dropsy.

ascorbic acid chemical name for vitamin C, named after its ability to cure scurvy.

atherosclerosis the underlying pathology of coronary heart disease; a common form of arteriosclerosis characterized by the formation of yellow, cheeselike, fatty streaks containing cholesterol that develop into hardened plaques in the inner lining of major blood vessels such as the coronary arteries.

atonic without normal muscle tone.

atrophy tissue wasting.

auscultation listening to the sounds of the gastrointestinal tract with a stethoscope.

azotemia an excess of urea and other nitrogenous substances in the blood.

basal energy expenditure (BEE) the amount of energy (in kcal) needed by the body for maintenance of life when a person is at complete digestive, physical, mental, thermal, and emotional rest (10 to 12 hours after eating, 12 to 18 hours after physical activity, and measured immediately upon waking).

beriberi a disease of the peripheral nerves caused by a deficiency of thiamin (vitamin B_1); characterized by pain (neuritis) and paralysis of legs and arms, cardiovascular changes, and edema. The name is Singhalese for "I can't, I can't."

bile a fluid secreted by the liver and transported to the gallbladder for concentration and storage; it is released into the duodenum with the entry of fat to facilitate enzymatic fat digestion by acting as an emulsifying agent.

binge-eating disorder a psychiatric eating disorder characterized by the occurrence of binge eating episodes at least twice a week for a 6-month period.

blood urea nitrogen (BUN) a basic test of nephron function by measuring its ability to normally filter urea nitrogen, a product of protein metabolism, from the blood.

body mass index (BMI) body weight in kilograms divided by the square of height in meters (kg/m^2). Correlates with body fatness and health risk associated with obesity.

body composition the relative sizes of the four basic body compartments that make up the total lean body mass (muscle mass), fat, water, and bone.

brush border cells located on the microvilli within the lining of the intestinal tract. The microvilli are tiny hairlike projections that protrude from the mucosal cells that help increase surface area for the digestion and absorption of nutrients.

bulimia nervosa a psychiatric eating disorder related to a person's fear of fatness in which cycles of gorging on large quantities of food are followed by compensatory mechanisms to rid the body of excess calories consumed.

cachexia a specific profound syndrome caused by malnutrition and a disturbance in glucose and fat metabolism usually seen in patients with terminal cancer or AIDS; general poor health indicated by an emaciated appearance.

Cajun a group of people with an enduring tradition whose French-Catholic ancestors established permanent communities in the southern Louisiana coastal waterways after being expelled from Acadia (now Nova Scotia, Canada) by the reigning English in the late eighteenth century; developed unique food pattern from the blend of native French influence and mix of Creole cooking found in the new land.

calcitriol the activated hormone form of vitamin D.

callus unorganized meshwork of newly grown, woven bone developed on a pattern of the original clot of fibrin; formed after fracture or surgery and normally replaced in the healing process by hard adult bone.

calorie a measure of heat. The energy necessary to do work is measured as the amount of heat produced by the body's work. The energy value of a food is expressed as the number of kilocalories a specified portion of the food will yield when oxidized in the body.

carboxypeptidase specific protein-splitting enzyme secreted as the inactive proenzyme procarboxypeptidase in the pancreas that is activated by trypsin in the small intestine to break off the acid (carboxyl) end of the peptide chain, producing smaller chained peptides and free amino acids.

carcinogenesis development of cancer.

carotene a group name for three red and yellow pigments (alpha-, beta-, and gamma-carotene) found in dark green and yellow vegetables and fruits. Beta-carotene is most important to human nutrition because the body can convert it to vitamin A.

carotenoids organic pigments found in plants. Known to have functions such as scavenging free radicals, reducing the risk of certain types of cancer, and helping prevent age-related eye diseases. More than 600 carotenoids have been identified, with beta-carotene being the most well known.

catabolism the process by which body tissues are broken down; the opposite of anabolism. Catabolism includes all the processes in which complex substances are progressively broken down into simpler ones, usually with the release of energy. Together, anabolism and catabolism constitute metabolism, which is the coordinated operation of anabolic (building up) and catabolic (breaking down) processes into a dynamic balance of energy and substance.

cellulitis diffuse inflammation of soft or connective tissues from injury, bruises, or pressure sores that lead to infection; poor care may result in ulceration and abscess or gangrene.

cerebrovascular accident (CVA) a stroke, caused by arteriosclerosis within blood vessels of the brain, that cuts off oxygen supply to the affected portion of brain tissue, thus paralyzing body muscle actions controlled by the affected brain area.

chelator a ligand that binds to a metal to form a metal complex.

cholecalciferol the chemical name for vitamin D in its inactive dietary form; often shortened to calciferol.

cholesterol a fat-related compound, a sterol, synthesized only in animal tissues; a normal constituent of bile and a principal constituent of gallstones. In the body, cholesterol is mainly synthesized in the liver. In the diet, it is found primarily in animal food sources.

chronic dieting syndrome the cyclic pattern of weight loss by dieting, then regaining weight by compulsive food binges in response to stress, anxiety, or hunger. This abnormal psychophysiologic food pattern becomes chronic, changing a person's natural body metabolism and relative body composition to the abnormal state of a metabolically obese person of normal weight.

chylomicron lipoprotein formed in the intestinal cell composed of triglycerides, cholesterol, phospholipids, and protein. Allows for absorption of fat into the lymphatic circulatory system before entering the blood circulation.

chyme semifluid food mass in the gastrointestinal tract after gastric digestion.

chymotrypsin a protein-splitting enzyme secreted as the inactive proenzyme chymotrypsinogen by the pancreas that is activated and acts in the small intestine to continue breaking down proteins into shorter chain polypeptides and dipeptides.

clinically severe or significant obesity A body mass index of greater than 40 or a BMI of 35 to 39 with at least one obesity-related disorder.

cobalamin the chemical name for the B-complex vitamin B_{12}; found mainly in animal protein food sources. It is closely related to amino acid metabolism and formation of the heme portion of hemoglobin. Absence of its necessary digestion and absorption agents in the gastric secretions, HCl and intrinsic factor, leads to pernicious anemia and degenerative effects on the nervous system, which require monthly cobalamin injections, bypassing the intestinal absorption defect.

collagen disease a disease attacking collagen tissues, the protein substance of the white fibers (collagenous fibers) of skin, tendon, bone, cartilage, and other connective tissues; any of a group of diseases that cause widespread changes in the connective tissue (e.g., rheumatoid arthritis, lupus erythematosus, scleroderma, and rheumatic fever).

colloidal osmotic pressure (COP) fluid pressure produced by protein molecules in the plasma and cell. Because proteins are large molecules, they do not pass through the separating membranes of the capillary walls. Thus they remain in their respective compartments, exerting a constant osmotic pull that protects vital plasma and cell fluid volumes in these areas.

colostrum a thin, yellow fluid first secreted by the mammary gland a few days after childbirth, preceding the mature breast milk. It contains up to 20% protein including a large amount of lactalbumin, more minerals and immunoglobulins that represent the antibodies found in maternal blood, and less lactose and fat than mature milk.

competitive foods any food or beverage from commercial suppliers served outside federal meal programs regardless of nutritional value.

complex carbohydrates large, complex molecules of carbohydrates composed of many sugar units (polysaccharides). Complex forms of dietary carbohydrates are starch, which is digestible and provides a major energy source, and dietary fiber, which is indigestible (human beings lack the necessary enzymes) and thus provides important bulk in the diet.

conditionally indispensable amino acids six amino acids that normally are considered dispensable amino acids because the body can make them. However, under certain circumstances such as illness, the body cannot make them in high enough quantities and they become indispensable in the diet.

congestive heart failure chronic condition of gradually weakening heart muscle unable to pump normal blood flow through the heart-lung circulation, resulting in congestion of fluids in the lungs.

coronary heart disease term designating the overall medical problem resulting from the underlying disease of atherosclerosis in the coronary arteries.

creatinine nitrogen-carrying product of normal tissue protein breakdown; excreted in the urine.

Cushing's syndrome excess secretion of glucocorticoids from the adrenal cortex. Symptoms and complications include protein loss, obesity, fatigue, osteoporosis, edema, excess hair growth, diabetes, and skin discoloration.

dehiscence a splitting open; the separation of layers of a surgical wound—partial, superficial, or complete—with total disruption and requiring resuturing.

dialysis the process of separating crystalloids (crystal-forming substances) and colloids (gluelike substances) in solution by the difference in their rates of diffusion through a semipermeable membrane; crystalloids (e.g., blood sugar and other simple metabolites) pass through readily, and colloids (e.g., plasma proteins) pass through slowly or not at all.

Dietary Reference Intakes (DRIs) nutrient recommendations for each gender and age group that can be used for assessing and planning diets for healthy populations.

dietetics management of diet and the use of food; the science concerned with the nutrition planning and preparation of foods.

digestion the process in which food is broken down in the gastrointestinal tract, releasing many nutrients in forms the body can use.

dipeptidase specific final enzyme in the protein-splitting system that produces the last two free amino acids.

dispensable amino acids five amino acids that the body can synthesize from other amino acids supplied through the diet and thus do not have to be consumed on a daily basis.

diuresis increased excretion of urine.

diuretic any substance that induces urination and subsequent fluid loss.

diverticulitis inflammation of pockets of tissue (diverticula) in the lining of the mucous membrane of the colon.

dual-energy X-ray absorptiometry (DXA) x-ray machine using two beams (dual) that measures bone density and body composition.

dysphagia difficulty swallowing.

early-onset obesity a genetically associated obesity occurring in early childhood.

edema excess accumulation of fluid in the interstitial spaces (e.g., small structural spaces between tissue parts) of the body.

element a single type of atom. A total of 117 elements have been identified, of which 94 occur naturally on earth. Elements can not be broken down into smaller substances.

elemental formula a nutrition support formula composed of simple elemental nutrient components that require no further digestive breakdown and are thus readily absorbed; formulas with the protein as free amino acids and the carbohydrate as the simple sugar glucose.

emulsifier an agent that breaks down large fat globules into smaller, uniformly distributed particles; the action is chiefly accomplished in the intestine by bile acids, which lower the surface tension of the fat particles, breaking the fat into many smaller droplets and thus greatly increasing the surface area of fat and facilitating contact with the fat-digesting enzymes.

enriched food products that have vitamins and minerals added back after the refining process results in a loss of nutrients. For example, iron may be lost in the refining process of a grain; therefore the product is enriched with additional iron.

enteral a mode of feeding that uses the gastrointestinal tract through oral or tube feeding.

enterokinase an enzyme produced and secreted in the duodenum in response to food entering the small intestine; activates trypsinogen to its active form, trypsin.

enzymes proteins that digest or change nutrients in specific chemical reactions without being changed themselves in the process. Their action is therefore that of a catalyst. Digestive enzymes in GI secretions act on food substances to break them down into simpler compounds. An enzyme usually is named according to the substance (substrate) on which it acts, with common word ending of -ase; for example, sucrase is the specific enzyme for sucrose, which it breaks down into glucose and fructose.

ergogenic the tendency to increase work output; various substances that increase work or exercise capacity and output.

erythropoietin hormone that stimulates the production of red blood cells in the bone marrow.

essential (or primary) hypertension an inherent form of high blood pressure with no specific discoverable cause; considered to be familial.

etiology the cause or origin of a disease.

exogenous originating from outside the body.

exudate various materials such as cells, cellular debris, and fluids, usually resulting from inflammation, that have escaped from the blood vessels and are deposited in or on the surface tissues; protein content is high.

familial hypercholesterolemia genetic disorder resulting in elevated blood cholesterol levels despite lifestyle modifications; caused by absent or nonfunctional low-density lipoprotein receptors and requires drug therapy.

familial hypertriglyceridemia genetic disorder resulting in elevated blood triglyceride levels despite lifestyle modifications; requires drug therapy.

fatty acids the major structural components of fats.

fetal alcohol effects physical and mental birth defects in infants born to mothers who used alcohol during pregnancy. This condition is less severe than fetal alcohol syndrome, occurs three times more often, but is similar in that no cure exists.

fetal alcohol syndrome (FAS) combination of physical and mental birth defects in infants born to mothers who use alcohol during pregnancy.

filé powder substance made from ground sassafras leaves; seasons and thickens the dish being made.

fluorosis excess intake of fluoride causing yellowing of teeth, white spots, and pitting or mottling of tooth enamel.

fortified vitamins and minerals added to foods after processing to improve nutritional value. Such vitamins and minerals may not have been originally present in the food or not in significant quantities. Examples include vitamin

A and D fortified milk, calcium-fortified orange juice, iodine-fortified salt.

galactosemia an autosomal recessive genetic disorder in which the liver does not produce the enzyme needed to metabolize galactose.

gastroscopy examination of the upper intestinal tract by using a flexible tube with a small camera on the end. The tube is approximately 9 mm in diameter and takes color pictures as well as biopsy samples, if necessary.

glomerular filtration rate (GFR) volume of fluid filtered from the renal glomerular capillaries into Bowman's capsule per unit of time; used clinically as a measure of kidney function.

glomerulus the first section of the nephron; a cluster of capillary loops cupped in the nephron head that serves as an initial filter.

glucagon a hormone secreted by the cells of the pancreatic islets of Langerhans in response to hypoglycemia; it has an opposite balancing effect to that of insulin, raising the blood glucose concentration, and thus is used as a quick-acting antidote for a low blood glucose reaction of insulin. It also counteracts the overnight fast during sleep by breaking down liver glycogen to keep blood glucose levels normal and maintain an adequate energy supply for normal nerve and brain function.

gluconeogenesis formation of glucose from noncarbohydrate substances such as amino acids.

glycemic index a system used to rank food according to the increase above fasting blood glucose over 2 hours after ingestion of a constant amount of that food divided by the response to a reference food.

glycerides chemical group name for fats; formed from the glycerol base with one, two, or three fatty acids attached to make monoglycerides, diglycerides, and triglycerides, respectively. Glycerides are the principal constituents of adipose tissue and are found in animal and vegetable fats and oils.

glycogen a polysaccharide, the main storage form of carbohydrate, largely stored in the liver and to a lesser extent in muscle tissue.

glycogenesis formation of stored glycogen from glucose.

glycolipids a lipid with a carbohydrate attached.

goiter an enlarged thyroid gland caused by lack of enough available iodine to produce the thyroid hormone thyroxine.

gynecomastia excessive development of the male mammary gland; frequently the result of increased estrogen levels.

health a state of optimal physical, mental, and social well-being; relative freedom from disease.

health promotion active involvement in behaviors or programs that advance positive well-being.

Heimlich maneuver a first-aid maneuver to relieve a person who is choking from blockage of the airway by a swallowed foreign object or food particle. Standing behind the person, clasp the victim around the waist, placing one fist just under the sternum (breastbone) and grasping the fist with the other hand. Then make a quick, hard, thrusting movement inward and upward to dislodge the object.

hematuria the abnormal presence of blood in the urine.

hemoglobin a conjugated protein in red blood cells composed of a compact, rounded mass of polypeptide chains forming globin, the protein portion, and attached to an iron-containing red pigment called heme. It carries oxygen in the blood to cells.

hepatitis inflammation of liver cells. Symptoms of acute hepatitis (less than 6 months) include flulike symptoms, muscle and joint aches, fever, feeling sick or vomiting, diarrhea and headache, dark urine, yellowing of the eyes and skin. Symptoms of chronic hepatits (longer than 6 months) include jaundice, abdominal swelling and sensitivity, low-grade fever, and fluid retention (ascites).

homeostasis the state of relative dynamic equilibrium within the body's internal environment; a balance achieved through the operation of various interrelated physiologic mechanisms.

hypercholesterolemia condition of elevated blood cholesterol levels.

hyperglycemia condition of elevated blood glucose levels.

hyperhomocysteinemia high levels of homocysteine in the blood; a predictor of cardiovascular disease.

hypertension chronically elevated blood pressure in which systolic blood pressure is consistently 140 mm Hg or greater and/or diastolic blood pressure is consistently 90 mm Hg or greater.

hypoglycemia an abnormally low blood sugar level that may lead to muscle tremors, cold sweat, headache, and confusion. A serious condition in diabetes management that requires immediate sugar intake, followed by a snack of complex carbohydrate food (e.g., bread or crackers) and a protein (e.g., lean meat, peanut butter, or cheese) to maintain normal blood glucose.

hypotension low blood pressure.

idiopathic of unknown cause.

immunocompetence the ability or capacity to develop an immune response (i.e., antibody production or cell-mediated immunity) after exposure to an antigen.

indispensable amino acids nine amino acids that must be obtained from the diet because the body does not make adequate amounts to support body needs.

insulin a hormone produced by the pancreas that attaches to insulin receptors on cell membranes and allows absorption of glucose into the cell.

intrauterine growth restriction (IUGR) a fetus who is less than the 10th percentile of predicted weight for gestational age.

Jambalaya a dish of Creole origin combining rice, chicken, ham, pork, sausage, broth, vegetables, and seasonings.

ketoacidosis excess production of ketones; a form of metabolic acidosis that occurs in uncontrolled diabetes or starvation from burning body fat for energy fuel; a continuing, uncontrolled state that can result in coma and death.

ketones chemical name for a class of organic compounds, including three ketoacid bases that occur as intermediate products of fat metabolism, one of which is acetone.

ketosis the accumulation of ketones, intermediate products of fat metabolism, in the blood.

kilocalorie the general term calorie refers to a unit of heat measure and is used alone to designate the small calorie. The calorie used in nutritional science and the study of metabolism is the large calorie, or kilocalorie, to be more accurate and avoid the use of large numbers in calculations. A kilocalorie, or 1000 calories, is the measure of heat necessary to raise the temperature of 1000 g (1 L) of water 1° C.

kinesiotherapist a health care professional who treats the effects of disease, injury, and congenital disorders through the application of scientifically based exercise principles adapted to enhance the strength, endurance, and mobility of individuals with functional limitations or those requiring extended physical conditioning.

lactated Ringer's solution sterile solution of calcium chloride, potassium chloride, sodium chloride, and sodium lactate in water given to replenish fluid and electrolytes; developed by English physiologist Sidney Ringer (1835-1910).

life expectancy the number of years a person of a given age may expect to live; affected by environment, gender, and race.

linoleic acid (omega-6) essential fatty acid consisting of 18 carbons and two double bonds; found in vegetable oils

linolenic acid (omega-3) essential fatty acid with 18 carbon atoms and three double bonds; found in soybean, canola, and flaxseed oil.

lipectomy surgical removal of subcutaneous fat by suction through a tube inserted into a surface incision or by the removal of larger amounts of subcutaneous fat by major surgical incision.

lipids the chemical group name for organic substances of a fatty nature. The lipids include fats, oils, waxes, and other fat-related compounds such as cholesterol.

lipiduria lipid droplets found in the urine composed mostly of cholesterol esters.

lipogenesis formation of fat.

lipoproteins chemical complex of fat and protein that serve as the major carriers of lipids in the plasma. They vary in density according to the size of the protein load; the lower the density, the lower the protein content. The combination package with water-soluble protein makes possible the transport of non-water-soluble fatty substances in the water-based blood circulation.

macrosomia excessive fetal growth resulting in an abnormally large infant; carries a high risk for perinatal death.

major minerals the group of minerals required by the body in amounts of more than 100 mg/day. The seven major minerals in the body are calcium, phosphorus, sodium, potassium, magnesium, chloride, and sulfur.

masculinization condition marked by the attainment of male characteristics, such as facial hair, either physiologically as a result of male maturation or pathologically by either sex.

medical nutrition therapy (MNT) a specific nutrition service and procedure used to treat an illness, injury, or condition. It involves an in-depth nutrition assessment of the patient or client; nutrition diagnosis; nutrition intervention, which includes diet therapy, counseling, or use of specialized nutrition supplements; and nutrition monitoring and evaluation.

menopause the end of a woman's menstrual activity and capacity to bear children.

metabolic syndrome a combination of disorders that, when occurring together, increase the risk of cardiovascular disease and diabetes. Also known as syndrome X and insulin resistance syndrome.

metabolism the sum of the vast number of chemical changes in the cell, the functional unit of life, which finally produces the essential materials necessary for energy, tissue building, and metabolic controls. Products of the various reactions are called metabolites.

metastasis the spread of cancer to other tissue.

micelles packages of free fatty acids, monoglycerides, and bile salts. The non-water-soluble fat particles are found in the middle of the package, whereas the water-soluble part faces outward and allows for the absorption of fat into the intestinal mucosal cell.

microvilli exceedingly small, hairlike projections covering villi on the surface of the small intestine that greatly increase the total absorbing surface area; visible through an electron microscope.

mucosal folds large visible folds of the mucous lining of the small intestine that increase the absorbing surface area.

mucositis an inflammation of the tissues around the mouth or other orifices of the body.

mutation a permanent transmissible change in a gene.

myocardial infarction (MI) a heart attack; caused by failure of the heart muscle to maintain normal blood circulation because of blockage of the coronary arteries with fatty cholesterol plaques that cut off delivery of oxygen to the affected part of the heart muscle.

MyPyramid a visual pattern of the current basic five food groups (bread/cereal, vegetable, fruit, milk/cheese, meat/dry beans/egg), arranged in a pyramid shape to indicate proportionate amounts of daily food choices.

negative energy balance more total energy is expended than consumed.

neoplasm any new or abnormal cellular growth, specifically one that is uncontrolled and aggressive.

nephron microscopic anatomic and functional unit of the kidney that selectively filters and reabsorbs essential blood factors, secretes hydrogen ions as needed to maintain acid-base balance, reabsorbs water to protect body fluids, and forms and excretes a concentrated urine for elimination of wastes. Each kidney has approximately 1 million nephrons.

nephrosis a nephrotic syndrome caused by degenerative lesions of the renal tubules of the nephrons, especially the thin basement membrane of the glomerulus that helps support the capillary loops; marked by edema, albuminuria, and decreased serum albumin.

nephrotoxic poisonous to the kidney.

niacin chemical name for vitamin B_3; discovered in relation to the deficiency disease pellagra, largely a skin disorder. It is important as a coenzyme factor in many cell reactions related to energy and protein metabolism.

nursing diagnosis a statement about the health of a client based on information gathered during the nursing assessment. The North America Nursing Diagnosis Association defines standard diagnoses.

nursing process a process by which nurses deliver care to patients; includes the steps of assessment, diagnosis, planning, implementation, and evaluation.

nutrition the sum of the processes involved with the intake of nutrients as well as assimilating and using them to maintain body tissue and provide energy; a foundation for life and health.

nutritional integrity defined by the School Nutrition Association as "A level of performance that assures all foods and beverages available in schools are consistent with the Dietary Guidelines for Americans, and, when combined with nutrition education, physical activity, and a healthful school environment, contributes to enhanced learning and development of lifelong, healthful eating habits."

nutritional science the body of science, developed through controlled research, that relates to the processes involved in nutrition—internationally, clinically, and in the community.

oliguria the secretion of small amounts of urine in relation to fluid intake (0.5 ml/kg per hour).

organic farming farming methods that use natural means of pest control and meet the standards set by the USDA National Organic Program. Organic foods are grown or produced without the use of synthetic pesticides or fertilizers, sewage sludge, or ionizing radiation.

osmosis passage of a solvent, such as water, through a membrane that separates solutions of different concentrations, tending to equalize the concentration pressures of the solutions on either side of the membrane.

osmotic pressure pressure produced as a result of osmosis across a semipermeable membrane.

osteoblast cells responsible for mineralization and formation of bone.

osteodystrophy bone disease resulting from defective bone formation. The general term dystrophy applies to any disorder arising from faulty nutrition.

osteopenia used to define individuals with low bone mass and increased risk for fracture.

osteoporosis abnormal thinning of the bone, producing a porous, fragile, latticelike bone tissue of enlarged spaces prone to fracture or deformity; defined as a bone mineral density value more than 2.5 standard deviations below the average 20-year-old sex-matched healthy person.

pancreatic amylase major starch-splitting enzyme secreted by the pancreas that acts in the small intestine.

pancreatic lipase a major fat-splitting enzyme produced by the pancreas and secreted into the small intestine to digest fat.

pandemic a widespread epidemic, distributed through a region, a continent, or the world.

pantothenic acid a B-complex vitamin found widely distributed in nature and occurring throughout the body tissues. Its role, which is major, is as an essential constituent of the body's main activating agent, coenzyme A. This special compound has extensive metabolic responsibility in activating a number of compounds in many tissues; it is a key energy metabolism substance in every cell.

parasite an organism that lives in or on an organism of another species, known as the host, from whom all life cycle nourishment is obtained.

parenteral a mode of feeding that does not use the gastrointestinal tract but provides nutrition support by intravenous delivery of nutrient solutions.

parotid glands the largest of three pairs of salivary glands situated near the ear. The parotid glands lie, one on each side, above the angle of the jaw, below and in front of the ear. They continually secrete saliva, which passes along the duct of the gland and into the mouth through an opening in the inner cheek, level with the second upper molar tooth. Normal saliva flow facilitates the chewing and swallowing of food and prevents dry mouth problems.

pellagra deficiency disease caused by a lack of dietary niacin and an inadequate amount of protein containing the amino acid tryptophan, a precursor of niacin. Pellagra is characterized by skin lesions aggravated by sunlight and by gastrointestinal, mucosal, neurologic, and mental symptoms. The four Ds often associated with pellagra are dermatitis, diarrhea, dementia, and death.

pepsin the main gastric enzyme specific for proteins. Pepsin begins breaking large protein molecules into shorter chain polypeptides; gastric hydrochloric acid is necessary for activation.

peritoneal cavity a serous membrane lining the abdominal and pelvic walls and undersurface of the diaphragm, forming a sac enclosing the body's vital visceral organs within the peritoneal cavity. Peritoneal dialysis is a form of dialysis through the peritoneum into and out of the peritoneal cavity.

pharynx the muscular membranous passage between the mouth and the posterior nasal passages and the larynx and esophagus.

pheochromocytoma tumor of the adrenal medulla or the sympathetic nervous system in which the affected cells secrete increased amounts of epinephrine or norepinephrine and cause headache, hypertension, and nausea.

photosynthesis process by which plants containing chlorophyll are able to manufacture carbohydrate by combining CO_2 and water. Sunlight is used as energy; chlorophyll is a catalyst.

phylloquinone a fat-soluble vitamin of the K group found in green plants or synthetically derived.

plasma protein any of a number of protein substances carried in the circulating blood. Albumin is a major plasma protein which maintains the fluid volume of the blood through its colloidal osmotic pressure.

polarity interaction between the positively charged end of one molecule to the negative end of another or the same molecule.

polydipsia excessive thirst and drinking.

polypharmacy use of multiple medications by a patient.

polyuria excess water loss through urination.

portal an entrance or gateway; for example, the portal blood circulation designates the entry of blood vessels from the intestines into the liver, carrying nutrients for liver metabolism, then draining into the body's main systemic circulation to deliver metabolic products to body cells.

probiotic foods that contain live microbials thought to benefit the consumer by improving intestinal microbial balance (e.g., lactobacilli in yogurt).

proenzyme an inactive precursor (forerunner substance from which another substance is made) converted to the active enzyme by the action of an acid, another enzyme, or other means.

prohormone a precursor substance that the body converts to a hormone. For example, a cholesterol compound in the skin is first irradiated by sunlight and then converted through successive enzyme actions in the liver and kidney into the vitamin D hormone, which then regulates calcium absorption and bone development.

proteinuria an abnormal excess of serum proteins (e.g., albumin) in the urine.

pulmonary edema accumulation of fluid in lungs.

purines nitrogen-containing compounds that yield uric acid as a metabolic end product eliminated in the urine.

pyridoxine the chemical name of vitamin B_6. In its activated phosphate form, B_2PO_4, pyridoxine functions as an important coenzyme factor in many reactions in cell metabolism related to amino acids, glucose, and fatty acids. Clinically pyridoxine deficiency produces a specific anemia and disturbances of the central nervous system.

Ramadan the ninth month of the Muslim year; a period of daily fasting from sunrise to sunset.

Recommended Dietary Allowances (RDAs) recommended dietary allowances of nutrients and energy intake for healthy population groups according to age and sex, with defined weight and height.

refeeding syndrome a potentially lethal syndrome occurring when severely malnourished individuals are fed high-carbohydrate diets too aggressively. A sudden shift in electrolytes and fluid retention coupled with a drastic drop in serum phosphorus levels cause a series of complications involving several organs.

registered dietitian (RD) a professional dietitian, accredited with an academic degree of undergraduate or graduate study program, who has passed the required registration examinations administered by the Commission on Dietetic Registration.

rennin milk-curdling enzyme of the gastric juice of human infants and young animals such as calves. Should not be confused with renin, which is an enzyme produced by the kidney that plays a role in producing angiotensin, a potent vasoconstrictor and stimulant for release of the hormone aldosterone from the adjacent adrenal glands.

resorption the destruction, loss, or dissolution of a tissue or part of a tissue by biochemical activity, such as the loss of bone or tooth dentin.

resting energy expenditure (REE) the amount of energy needed by the body for maintenance of life at rest over a 24-hour period; slightly higher than basal energy expenditure.

retinol the chemical name of vitamin A; derived from its vision function relating to the retina of the eye, which is the back inner lining of the eyeball that catches the lens light refractions to form images interpreted by the optic nerve and brain and makes the necessary light-dark adaptations.

riboflavin chemical name for vitamin B_2; discovered in relation to an early vitamin deficiency syndrome called ariboflavinosis that is mainly evidenced in breakdown of skin tissues and resulting infections. It has a role as a coenzyme factor in many cell reactions related to energy and protein metabolism.

rickets a disease of childhood characterized by softening of the long bones from an inadequate intake and/or synthesis of vitamin D; also associated with impaired calcium and phosphorus metabolism.

saccharide chemical name for sugar molecules. May occur as single molecules in monosaccharides (glucose, fructose, galactose), two molecules in disaccharides (sucrose, lactose, maltose), or multiple molecules in polysaccharides (starch, dietary fiber, glycogen).

salivary amylase a starch-splitting enzyme in the mouth, commonly called ptyalin (from the Greek word *ptyalon,* meaning spittle), that is secreted by the salivary glands.

saturated state of being filled; state of fatty acid components of fats being filled in all their available carbon bonds with hydrogen, making the fat harder and more solid. Such solid food fats are generally from animal sources.

school breakfast and lunch programs federally assisted meal programs operating in public and nonprofit private schools and residential child care institutions. It provides nutritionally balanced, low-cost or free meals to children each school day.

scurvy a hemorrhagic disease caused by a lack of vitamin C. Scurvy is characterized by diffuse tissue bleeding, painful limbs and joints, thickened bones, and skin discoloration from bleeding; bones fracture easily, wounds do not heal, gums are swollen and bleed, and teeth loosen.

secondary hypertension elevated blood pressure for which the cause can be identified and is a symptom or side effect of another primary condition.

secretagogue a substance, such as a hormone or medication, that causes another substance to be secreted. For example, sulfonylureas are medications used to increase the secretion of insulin from beta cells in the pancreas.

senescence the process or condition of growing old.

simple carbohydrates sugars with a simple structure of one or two single-sugar (saccharide) units. A monosaccharide is composed of one sugar unit; a disaccharide is composed of two sugar units.

sorbitol a sugar alcohol digested very slowly by humans. Named for its initial discovery in nature, it is found in ripe berries of the tree *Sorbus acuparia* and also occurs in small quantities in various other berries, cherries, plums, and pears.

speech-language pathologist a specialist in the assessment, diagnosis, treatment, and prevention of speech, language, cognitive communication, voice, swallowing, fluency, and other related disorders.

spina bifida congenital defects in the embryonic fetal closing of the neural tube to form a portion of the lower spine, leaving the spine unclosed and the spinal cord open in various degrees of exposure and damage.

steatorrhea fatty diarrhea; excessive amounts of fat in the feces often caused by malabsorption diseases.

Step I and Step II diets diets previously prescribed to individuals with elevated blood cholesterol to reduce intake of total fat, saturated fat, and cholesterol. These diets have been replaced with the Therapeutic Lifestyle Changes approach.

steroids the group name for lipid-based sterols, including hormones, bile acids, and cholesterol.

stoma the opening established in the abdominal wall, connecting with the ileum or colon, for elimination of intestinal wastes after surgical removal of diseased portions of the intestines.

sugar alcohols nutritive sweeteners that provide 2 to 3 kcal/g; examples include sorbitol, mannitol, and xylitol. Produced in food industry laboratories for use as sweeteners in candies, chewing gum, beverages, and other foods; excess consumption may result in diarrhea.

teratogen drug or substance causing a birth defect.

thermic effect of food an increase in energy expenditure caused by the activities of digestion, absorption, and storage of ingested food. A meal consisting of a usual mixture of carbohydrates, protein, and fat increases the energy expenditure equivalent to approximately 10% of the food's energy content. For example, a 300-kcal piece of pizza would elicit an increase in energy expenditure of 30 kcal.

thiamin chemical name of a major B-complex vitamin; also called vitamin B_1. It was discovered in relation to the classic deficiency disease beriberi and is important in body metabolism as a coenzyme factor in many cell reactions related to energy metabolism.

thyroid-stimulating hormone (TSH) an anterior pituitary hormone that regulates the activity of the thyroid gland; also known as thyrotropin.

thyrotropin-releasing hormone (TSH) a hormone secreted by the hypothalamus that stimulates release of thyroid-stimulating hormone (thyrotropin) by the pituitary.

thyroxine an iodine-dependent thyroid gland hormone that regulates the metabolic rate of the body.

tocopherol the chemical name for vitamin E, which was so named by early investigators because their initial work with rats indicated a reproductive function that is not true with human beings. In human beings, vitamin E functions as a strong antioxidant that preserves structural membranes such as cell membranes.

trace minerals the group of elements required by the body in small amounts of less than 100 mg/day.

transport the movement of nutrients through the circulatory system from one area of the body to another.

triglycerides chemical name for fats in the body or in food; compound of three fatty acids attached to a glycerol base.

trypsin a protein-splitting enzyme secreted as the inactive proenzyme trypsinogen in the pancreas that is activated by enterokinase and acts in the small intestine to break proteins into shorter chain polypeptides and dipeptides.

ultrasonography ultrasound-based diagnostic imaging technique used to visualize muscles and internal organs; also referred to as sonography.

urea chief nitrogen-carrying product of dietary protein metabolism; appears in blood, lymph, and urine.

vagotomy cutting of the vagus nerve, which supplies a major stimulus for gastric secretions.

varices dilated blood vessels within the wall of the esophagus due to cirrhosis of the liver. These vessels can continue to expand to the point of rupturing and can lead to death.

vasculitis inflammation of the walls of blood vessels.

villi small protrusions from the surface of a membrane; fingerlike projections covering mucosal surfaces of the small intestine that further increases the absorbing surface area; visible through a regular microscope.

virus a minute microscopic infectious organism characterized by lack of independent metabolism and the ability to reproduce with genetic continuity only within a living host. Each particle (virion) consists of nucleic acids and a protein shell that protects and contains the genetic material and any enzymes present.

VO_2max Maximal uptake volume of oxygen during exercise; used to measure the intensity and duration of exercise a person can perform.

waist circumference measurement of the waist at its narrowest point width-wise, just above the navel. Waist circumference is a rough measurement of abdominal fat and is a predictor of risk factors for cardiovascular disease. This risk increases with a waist measurement of more than 40 inches in men and more than 35 inches in women.

weaning to accustom a young child gradually to food other than the mother's milk or a bottle-fed substitute formula as the child's natural need to suckle wanes.

Wilson's disease an autosomal recessive genetic disorder in which copper accumulates in tissue and causes damage to organs.

xerostomia condition of dry mouth from a lack of saliva. Saliva production can be hindered by certain diseases, such as diabetes or Parkinson's disease, or by some prescription or over-the-counter medications.

zymogen an inactive enzyme precursor.

INDEX

A

ABCDEFs of nutrition assessment, 473
Absorption
  of fats, 40, 40f
  of iron, 139
  of minerals, 125
  of nutrients, 68-74
    in large intestine, 70-72, 73t
    in small intestine, 69, 72f
    sodium role in, 132
  postoperative considerations in, 440
  of vitamin B_{12}, 112, 113f
  vitamin D role in calcium and phosphorus control, 97
Acarbose, 407t
Acculturation to American diet, 261
Accutane; *See* Isotretinoin
Acetohexamide, 407t
Acetone, 393
Acetyl coenzyme A, 113
Acetylcholine, 115
Achalasia, 341
Acid(s), 163, 164b
  chemical digestion and, 66
  as food additive, 240t
  peptic ulcer disease and, 346
Acid-base balance, 129, 163-164, 164b
Acid-base buffer system, 163-164
Acidic diet, 430
Acidosis, 22, 164
Acquired immunodeficiency syndrome, 467-474
  cultural considerations in, 468
  food intake and, 463, 472
  nutrition assessment in, 473
  nutrition counseling in, 473-474
  nutrition management in, 471b, 471-472, 472t
  opportunistic infections in, 470, 470b
  stages of, 469-470, 470b
  vaccine development for, 471-472
  wasting effects of, 472-473
Active transport, 69, 159
Activities of daily living, 301
Actos; *See* Pioglitazone
Acute cardiovascular disease, 371-372, 373b, 373t
Acute glomerulonephritis, 415-417, 417t
Acute kidney failure, 418, 419t
Acute nephritic syndrome, 417t
Acute pancreatitis, 360-361
Additives to food, 240t, 240-241
Adenosine triphosphate, 74-75
Adequate Intake, 7
  of biotin, 114
  of calcium, 126-127
  of chloride, 135
  of choline, 115
  of chromium, 145
  of cobalamin, 112
  of folate, 111
  of magnesium, 135
  of niacin, 108, 109
  of pantothenic acid, 113
  of phosphorus, 129
  of potassium, 133
  of riboflavin, 107
  of sodium, 132
  of thiamin, 106
  of vitamin B6, 110
  of vitamin D, 97
  of vitamin E, 100
  of vitamin K, 102
  of zinc, 142
Adipose tissue, 36, 75, 77, 81
Adolescence, 189

Adolescent, 205
  daily fluid needs of, 192t
  estimated energy requirements for, 192t
  failure to thrive, 201, 203
  food fads and, 288
  growth patterns of, 206
  mineral needs of, 147
  obesity and, 203-205, 204b
  pregnancy and, 176, 177
  vitamin needs of, 118
  water requirements of, 153t
Adult, 209-229
  aging process and, 214-217, 216f, 217b
  alternative living arrangements and, 226-227
  blood pressure classification for, 375f
  chronic diseases of aging and, 220-221
  government programs for, 221-225
  Healthy People series and, 209, 210b
  impact on health care, 210
  life expectancy and quality of life of, 210
  mineral needs of, 147-148
  nutritional needs of, 214
  nutritional status of, 218, 219f
  physical growth of, 211
  population and age distribution of, 209-210, 211f, 211t
  professional organizations and resources for, 225-226
  psychosocial development of, 212-213, 213f
  racial and ethnic composition of U.S. population, 212
  recommendations for dietary energy intake, 88, 88t
  reduction of risk for chronic disease, 217
  socioeconomic status of, 213-214, 214f
  volumes of body fluid compartments in, 156t
  water requirements of, 153t
  weight management and, 218-220, 220b, 220f
Adulthood, 189
Advanced care planning, 331
Advanced directive, 331
Aerobic capacity, 304, 305
Aerobic exercise, 283, 301-302, 302f, 302t
Afferent arteriole, 412f
Aflatoxin, 248
African American dietary patterns, 259-261, 520-521
Age
  atherosclerosis and, 367
  energy and protein needs from birth to 18 years, 192t
  population and age distribution, 209-210, 211f, 211t
  pregnancy and, 176-177
  target heart rate in aerobic exercise and, 303t
  water requirements and, 152-153, 153t
Aging adult, 209-229
  aging process and, 214-217, 216f, 217b
  alternative living arrangements and, 226-227
  chronic diseases of aging and, 220-221
  government programs for, 221-225
  impact on health care, 210
  life expectancy and quality of life of, 210
  nutritional needs of, 214
  nutritional status of, 218, 219f
  population and age distribution of, 209-210, 211f, 211t
  professional organizations and resources for, 225-226
  reduction of risk for chronic disease, 217
  socioeconomic status of, 213-214, 214f
  vitamin needs of, 118
  weight management and, 218-220, 220b, 220f
Aging process, 214-217
Agricultural pesticides, 237, 237f
AI; *See* Adequate Intake
Air displacement plethysmography, 271, 272f
Alcohol
  cancer risk and, 466
  chronic heart disease and, 374

Alcohol *(Continued)*
  diabetes mellitus and, 397b, 510
  Dietary Guidelines for Americans and, 9f
  digestion and metabolism of, 76
  food-drug interactions and, 333t
  hypertension and, 376t, 378
  peptic ulcer disease and, 346
  tyramine-restricted diet and, 459t
  use during pregnancy, 177-178, 178f
  vitamin needs and, 119
Alcohol-induced thiamin deficiency, 106
Aldosterone, 163, 413
Aldosteronoma, 387
Algal substances, 18, 18t
Alkali as food additive, 240t
Alkaline diet, 430
Alkalosis, 164
Allergens
  food, 353-354
  infant diet and, 199
Allergy
  in celiac disease, 354f, 354-355, 355f, 355t
  food, 353-354
Alpha-glucosidase inhibitors, 407t
Alpha-linolenic acid, 32-33, 33f
  vegetarian diet and, 53
Alpha-tocopherol, 99-101, 101t, 103t
Alternative agriculture, 237f, 237-239, 239f, 240f
Alternative living arrangements, 226-227
Aluminum, 145
Amaryl; *See* Glimepiride
Amenorrhea, 273
American Cancer Society guidelines, 466b, 466-467
American Heart Association
  dietary guidelines of, 369b
  recommendations for lowering cholesterol, 369t
American system of measurement, 516-517
Amino acids, 46-48, 47b, 47f
  dietary protein quality and, 55
  tissue building and, 4-5
  in total parenteral nutrition formula, 444t
Aminopeptidase, 54, 55, 56f
Amphetamines
  athlete and, 312t
  for weight loss, 276
Amphophilic molecule, 34, 35
Amputation, diabetes mellitus-related, 393
Amylase
  pancreatic, 25-26, 27f, 67
  salivary, 23, 65-66
Anabolic steroids, 311, 313t
Anabolism, 48, 74, 75
Anaerobic bacteria, 245
Analgesics, food-drug interactions and, 333t
Anaphylaxis in food allergy, 353-354
Androgenic steroids, 311, 313t
Anemia, 139
  in aging adult, 217, 217b
  in child, 203
  in chronic kidney disease, 419-420
  iron-deficiency, 138, 148
    postoperative, 437
    during pregnancy, 180
  megaloblastic, 111
  pernicious, 112
    during pregnancy, 180
Anencephaly, 172, 173
Angina pectoris, 365
Animal fats, 36-37
Animal starch, 16
Anion, 157, 159t
Anorexia
  in acquired immunodeficiency syndrome, 472
  cancer patient and, 460, 463
  in chronic kidney disease, 420
  dietary modifications for, 464t
  marijuana for, 461
Anorexia nervosa, 205, 291, 292, 292b, 293f